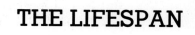

THE LIFESPAN

THE LIFESPAN

GUY R. LEFRANCOIS
University of Alberta

Wadsworth Publishing Company
A Division of Wadsworth, Inc.
Belmont, California

A study guide has been specially designed to help students master the concepts presented in this textbook. Order from your bookstore.

Psychology Editor: **Kenneth King**
Production Editor: **Patricia Brewer**
Designer: **Detta Penna**
Copy Editor: **Patricia Tompkins**
Photo Editors: **Lindsay Kefauver with Jean O'Korn**
Technical Illustrator: **Sirius House**
Cover Photographer: **John William Lund**
Compositor: **Graphic Typesetting Service**

Printed in the United States of America

3 4 5 6 7 8 9 10—88 87 86 85

Library of Congress Cataloging in Publication Data

Lefrançois, Guy R.
  The lifespan.

  Includes bibliographies and index.
  1. Developmental psychology.   I. Title.
BF713.L44   1984   155   83–16760
ISBN 0–534–02969–8

To my grandparents and all the old people without whom we would not be here today.

To my children and all the young people without whom we will not be here tomorrow.

BRIEF CONTENTS

DETAILED CONTENTS

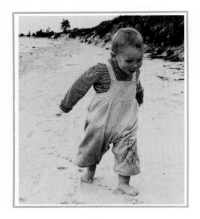

The dwarf sees farther than the giant, when he has the giant's shoulder to stand on.

Samuel Taylor Coleridge
The Friend

> *Nature is often hidden; sometimes overcome; seldom extinguished.*
>
> Francis Bacon
> *Of Nature in Men*

> *Sir Roger told them, with the air of a man who would not give his judgment rashly, that much might be said on both sides.*
>
> Joseph Addison
> *Spectator*, Vol. 1

PART TWO
INFANCY

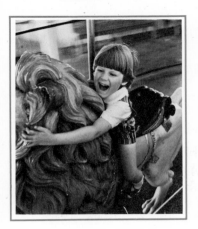

I keep looking back, as far as I can remember, and I can't think what it was like to feel young, really young.

John Osborne
Look Back in Anger

xii

PART THREE
CHILDHOOD

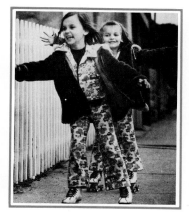

Every time a child says "I don't believe in fairies," there is a little fairy somewhere that falls down dead.

James Matthew Barrie
Peter Pan

More than either, it [England] resembles a family, a rather stuffy Victorian family, with not many black sheep in it but with all its cupboards bursting with skeletons. It has rich relations who have to be kow-towed to and poor relations who are horribly sat upon, and there is a deep conspiracy about the source of the family income. It is a family in which the young are generally thwarted and most of the power is in the hands of irresponsible uncles and bedridden aunts. Still, it is a family.

George Orwell
England, Your England

"I dare say you haven't had much practice," said the Queen. "When I was your age, I always did it for half an hour a day. Why, sometimes I've believed as many as six impossible things before breakfast."

Lewis Carroll
*Through the Looking-Glass
and What Alice Found There*

Go directly—see what she's doing, and tell her she mustn't.

Punch, 1872

10 INTELLIGENCE, CREATIVITY, AND EXCEPTIONALITY 265

See the happy moron,
He doesn't give a damn,
I wish I were a moron,
My God! perhaps I am!

Anonymous
Eugenics Review, 1929

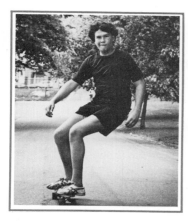
A traveler at Sparta, standing long upon one leg, said to a Lacedaemonian: "I do not believe you can do as much." "True," said he, "but every goose can."

        Plutarch
        Laconic Apothegms

Everybody worships me, it's nauseating.

Noel Coward
Present Laughter

Live as long as you may, the first twenty years are the longest half of your life.

Robert Southey
The Doctor

PART FIVE
ADULTHOOD

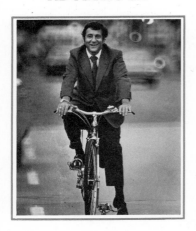

We think so because other people think so,
Or because—or because—after all we do think so,
Or because, we were told so, and think we must think so,
Or because we once thought so, and think we still think so,
Or because having thought so, we think we will think so.

Henry Sidgwick
Lines Composed in His Sleep

Give me chastity and continence, but not yet .

St. Augustine
Confessions

*Happiness in marriage is entirely a
matter of chance.*

> **Jane Austen**
> *Abbey*

*I am convinced digestion is the
great secret of life.*

> **Sydney Smith**
> **In a letter to Arthur Kingslake**

*I silently laugh at my own cenotaph,
And out of the caverns of rain,
Like a child from the womb, like a
ghost from the tomb,
I arise and unbuild it again.*

> **Percy Bysshe Shelley**
> ***The Cloud***

It is always the season for the old to learn.

Aeschylus
Fragments

PART SIX
THE END

So little done, so much to do!

Last words of Cecil John Rhodes

PREFACE

Although prefaces come first, they are usually written last. Perhaps this one should have been written first, because by the time I had finished *The Lifespan,* many of the things that had seemed important at the beginning had been lost in the weeks and months that had gone by. When the time came to write this preface, I found that I had little left to say.

"I have little left to say," I told my editor when he asked me for a preface. And so he sent me copies of dozens of brilliant and stimulating prefaces from which to draw inspiration.

I examined them; I read them; I studied them a little. Frantically, I searched for inspiration. And I discovered something interesting about most college textbooks. Almost every one of them claims to be comprehensive and up-to-date, well organized and clear, lively and interesting, brimming with appeal and relevance, glowing with academic integrity, scholarly and informative, pedagogically sound—and more. Even the dullest of textbooks often boasts a preface that loudly claims an invigorating and lively style; the most pedantic and abstract assures the reader that it is practical and relevant to the daily lives of students; the most selective and biased boasts broad and comprehensive coverage; and each, almost without exception, has the most up-to-date, thorough, and useful ancillary materials available.

Prefaces in textbooks are clearly market oriented. They are designed less to inspire than to sell. They remind me of media advertising—and that is hardly where I would go for truth.

After reading all these prefaces, I now find it difficult to claim that *The Lifespan* is lively and interesting, that it is written with the student in mind, that it conveys some sense of the great mysteries of the human lifespan, that it is a unique work. Indeed, a preface claiming all this (and more) would be not only embarrassing but also largely meaningless, since all books claim all of these things, more or less, in one way or another. Instead, let me just give you some brief facts about this book— no grandiose claims, no superlatives, and no judgments concerning its superiority. Only facts.

■ Coverage and Organization

The Lifespan covers the entire human lifespan from conception to death. The first part gives basic information concerning the scope and methods of research in lifespan development, an account of some of the most important general theories of human development, and a discussion of the two great forces that shape our lives: heredity and environment. The final part reviews the lifespan briefly and presents a philosophical look at living and dying. In between are the four major parts that look in detail at human development from conception to death. The thirteen chapters of these four parts present a comprehensive discussion of the *topics* of development within a chronological superstructure. The emphasis throughout is on practical relevance, thoroughness, and sound scholarship. The bibliography contains more than 1,000 separate entries, many of which were published within the past five years.

■ Special Features

The Lifespan includes a number of special features designed to make it a better teaching-learning tool. Among these are a large number of colored boxes. These boxes are of several types. Research-oriented boxes illustrate methods and problems in psychological research or present examples of outstanding research. Some boxes elaborate on theoretical positions described in the text proper, present new theoretical insights, or apply theory to situations in everyday life. Other boxes present applications of developmental psychology to the family or to education, and a few boxes can't really be classified—for example, definitions and clarifications of difficult concepts. The book also has interviews—transcripts of conversations with individuals whose ages spread over much of the lifespan and who sometimes had interesting things to say.

Another feature of *The Lifespan* is the chapter introductions, which tell the story of a journey I recently undertook with my grandmother and three children. I include the story because much in it is relevant to an understanding of the lifespan, and for whatever motivational qualities it might have. A color rule separates these introductions from the text, for the convenience of those who prefer their psychology "purer" and who wish to omit them.

Other important features of *The Lifespan* are the summaries of key points and the annotated lists of further readings at the end of each chapter, a comprehensive Glossary/Index (items that appear in the glossary are boldface when they first appear in the text), and outlines preceding each chapter. Line drawings and photographs amplify the points and principles of the text.

■ Ancillary Materials

The teaching-learning aids that accompany this text are designed to make life easier for both instructors and students. The student study guide, prepared by George Semb, presents important and useful advice concerning studying, making notes, writing examinations, and learning and using lifespan developmental psychology. The test item manual provides instructors with a carefully prepared and analyzed bank of items for assessing the effectiveness of the teaching-learning process.

■ Writing Style

Reviewers of *The Lifespan* almost invariably commented on its style. *Panache* was the elegant word used by one. A lovely word, panache. Originally, it referred to the long, curled feather worn on the hats of those who, in centuries long before ours, had style. When one bowed, as was the custom in those days, those with style described sweeping curves through the air with their plumes. Nowadays we no longer wear plumes. But those who truly have panache nevertheless do things in such a way that you can almost see a long, curved, graceful plume on their heads. When she looked at this book, my grandmother did not use *panache* to describe its style. But I promised you no superlatives—only facts.

■ Acknowledgments

A bow—graceful, I hope—together with an elegant set of four loops of diminishing size with my panache (my plume is white) to the many people who have contributed in so many positive ways to this project. This text owes a great deal to an outstanding Wadsworth publishing team. My sincere thanks to Ken King, psychology editor; Patricia Brewer, production editor; Patricia Tompkins, copy editor; and Detta Penna, designer. My appreciation, as well, to Sharon Seigel and Judy Cameron for their help with library research. And I especially want to thank the reviewers of the manuscript for their valuable comments: Dan Bellack, University of Kentucky; Michael Bradley, University of North Carolina; Charles F. Halverson, University of Georgia; Seth Kunen, University of New Orleans; Joan N. McNeil, Kansas State University; and Susan Whitbourne, University of Rochester. Finally, I want to thank the many people of all ages who allowed me to interview them while I worked on this manuscript. Unfortunately, space demands and the nature of the book made it impossible for me to use more than a tiny fraction of the resulting wealth of interview material. Please rest assured that even if your words don't appear in the text, you have each had a profound influence on my view of the lifespan. Although you must remain anonymous, you know who you are. And I thank you.

THE LIFESPAN

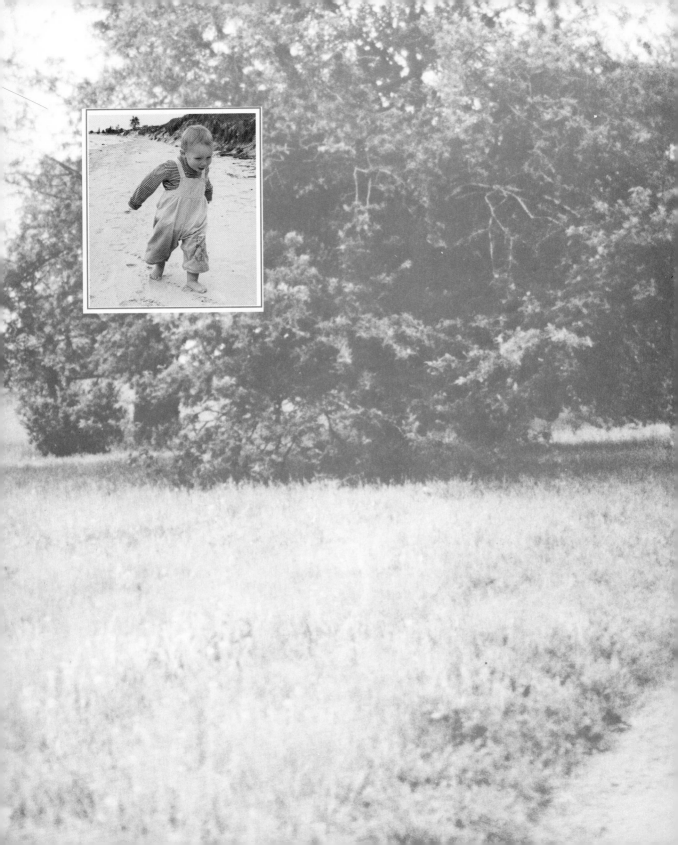

PART ONE   THE BEGINNING

1 SUBJECT AND METHODS

"Begin at the beginning," the King said, gravely, "and go on till you come to the end: then stop."
Lewis Carroll
Alice in Wonderland

T here is more than one door to a pigsty," my grandmother says— a platitude that, at least with respect to the pigsties with which I am most familiar, is plainly wrong. But the meaning is clear and useful—an unobtrusive grain of truth, glowing like a small gem might, even in the mud of a pigsty.

"There is more than one door to a pigsty," she says again, repetition being one of her strong points. I have just pulled the car off the main road—my six-year-old, Marcel, needs to pee. Right now or else. Which is why we have pulled up next to a pigsty.

It's good to stretch our legs. Behind the car, the spring air is heavy with green smells; in front, the green gives way to the browner smell of the pigsty. I stand behind the car with my grandmother and my older son, Paul. He's fifteen. His sister, Denise, is thirteen. She's leaning over the side of the pigpen, trying to entice a pig to where she can pet it while her younger brother pees purposefully between the railings of the pen. Denise is like that. She likes things—dogs, cats, pigs, even people.

We're on a trip, the five of us. I'm taking my grandmother back to where she lived and raised her family and where I too was born and raised. My children have never been there; I haven't gone back for almost two decades. In fact, I haven't been back since I was told I shouldn't. Anne, my wife and mother of my children, told me again this morning that I shouldn't go. She would not come.

The peeing is done now and my people seem restless. I feel a faint sadness at the thought that we get restless so soon even when our heads are full of good green smells and the sky is new-washed blue. We climb back into the car, Paul in front this time and Grandma between Denise and Marcel in the back seat. Grandma knits something small and green. Denise asks her what she meant about doors on pigsties.

"More than one way to dress a cat," she prefaces her explanation. But my mind drifts from the conversation as I pull out again onto the black pavement, easing my way between an oil tanker, "Trimac" emblazoned in fluorescent orange across its back end, and an old pickup. In the rearview mirror, the pickup dances slightly. It seems to be full of Indians. Parts of them stick out of the windows—mostly arms, but at least one foot with an orange sock.

"More than one hole to a fox den. . . ." Small pieces of conversation drift through my consciousness. But my awareness is only partly here, now, in the car. Mostly I am again with you and with this book. I have promised Ken that the first draft will be done by February. And it absolutely must be or, like so many other dreams that I have had, it may never be real. Besides, if Anne is correct, I may not write anymore after we get to where we are now going.

I might as well start, then—now while we drift over the flat miles and I need pay little attention to hills, curves, cliffs, or pickups dancing in my mirror. This book, you see, is a bit like a conversation that we might have, you and I, if you were sitting here in the car with us, and if you were to ask me the right questions. Only a bit like a conversation. Mostly, it's like a textbook; that's what it's meant to be. And that's what it needs to be if it is to find its way into your hands.

"What questions?" you ask. Only one big question, really, could get the whole thing going. There'll be many smaller questions while we travel. And, unfortunately, many questions left over when we finish. But we have to start somewhere. And finish somewhere, too. So you might start by asking me what we, the so-called professionals and experts, know about the span of human life—about the very beginnings of our lives and also about their ends; about the forces that shape our destinies, and about the processes by which we become what we are.

And today, I will begin to answer in the words of my grandmother, since she is here: "There is more than one door to a pigsty, more than one way to dress a cat, more than one hole to a fox den."

And more than one way to approach the search that leads to a book of this kind. Believing, as my grandmother clearly does, that there is some merit in exploring as many doors as possible, I will present you with a text that draws on a multitude of sources ranging across a variety of separate disciplines and representing a great diversity of people. These sources include not only the research and theorizing of people in psychology, sociology, anthropology, medicine, nursing, and other disciplines but include as well episodes and reflections from the lives of the people whose thoughts are found in the Interviews scattered throughout these pages. The people in these Interviews are real (their names have not been included). For this text deals with the lives of people as real as you or me; in fact, it is you and me that it is actually about. The search, in this narrative as in all psychology, is for a greater understanding of human behavior and personality. However, on this trip we will not deal with all psychology, but specifically with the psychology that is important for understanding the span of human life. And in this chapter, while we roll swiftly through the May morning, I will tell you of the subject we will discuss, including something of its history and of its methods.

Lifespan Developmental Psychology

The discipline that concerns itself with the space between conception and death is **lifespan developmental psychology.*** **Psychology** is a general term for the science that studies the behavior of humans (and lower organisms as well); developmental psychology is concerned with changes that occur from childhood through adulthood and with the processes and influences that account for these changes. In other words, *development* refers to changes in behavior over time (Wohlwill, 1973). The task of the developmental psychologist is twofold: to describe changes and to discover their causes. A third, closely related task is to advance theories that organize and interpret observations and are also useful for making predictions.

A *lifespan* view of human development is somewhat different from our traditional views of development. Historically, psychologists have been most concerned with the rapid changes that occur in the early years of life and have often assumed that the end result of these changes is reflected in a developmental peak that occurs in adolescence or early adulthood. According to this view, adulthood is a stable period—a period of little change that might be of concern to a developmental psychologist. Old age, however, brings additional changes, slow at first, but gradually more rapid until they finally approximate the rate of change that is characteristic of infancy. In contrast with this approach, a lifespan view of development not only admits that change occurs at all ages but insists as well that behaviors and changes of adulthood are a product of the individual's history (Baltes, 1973).

Although development refers to changes that occur over time, chronological age is not always the best way of organizing these changes. Relating important developmental changes directly to chronological age would be very convenient, but we cannot always do so. With passing time, chronological age becomes progressively less useful as an indicator of a given individual's most likely characteristics. Our developmental paths seem to diverge more and more as we become older. For example, in terms of their characteristics and capabilities, newborn infants all over the world are highly similar. At the age of one, they might differ from each other a great deal more, but they are still more alike than a group of average forty-year-olds. Thus we can say relatively intelligent and valuable things about the social, emotional, physical, and intellectual development of groups of children sorted according to age (providing we continually bear in mind that although whatever we say might be *generally* true about the average child, it might be quite inaccurate for a given individual). It is more difficult to say intelligent and valuable things about the average middle-aged person or about the average octogenarian. Individuals in these groups vary so much that an average is often totally meaningless. Thus a chronological approach to describing development will be valuable only to the extent that there is a close relationship between age and developmental changes.

How then should we organize our knowledge about development through the lifespan? One useful alternative to a purely chronological approach is based on events in life that have profound effects on us. These *transitions* might include such events as graduation, marriage, becoming a parent, having children leave home, and retiring. To the extent that there is a close relationship between each of these major events and changes in behavior or attitudes, they will be useful to those attempting to understand and explain developmental change.

Another alternative is to organize developmental knowledge by major topics such as intelligence, personality, language, and perception. This alternative generally attempts to provide an in-depth look at each topic and at relevant processes of development throughout the lifespan.

Organization of This Text

In summary, lifespan developmental events are often organized according to chronological age, particularly in the early years of life; later they are often related to major transitions and important topics.

---

*Boldface terms are defined in the Glossary/Index at the end of the book.

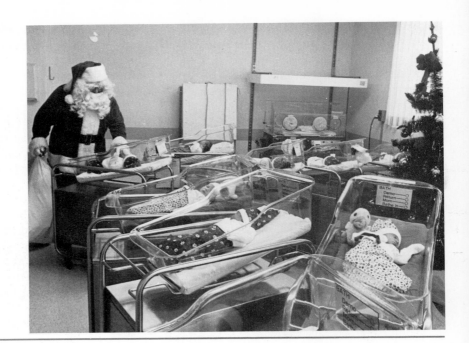

Newborns have similar characteristics and capabilities; it is easier to describe the average infant than the average adult.

Unfortunately, a single book cannot be organized in all possible ways—even a pig whose sty had both back and front doors might eventually develop a preference for one over the other. For convenience and simplicity, the global organization of this text is based on chronological age. Thus we deal sequentially with infancy (birth to two years); childhood (two to twelve years); adolescence (twelve to eighteen years); and adulthood (eighteen years to old age). Adulthood is further divided into three periods: early (eighteen to thirty-five years); middle (thirty-five to sixty-five years); and later (sixty-five years onward) (see Table 1.1). Within each of the major age-periods, we deal with topics and major transitions.

■ Models and Themes in Lifespan Development

Imagine that you have just been presented with this problem: Your psychology instructor has brought into class a smallish thing inside a larger glass thing. You don't know what this smallish thing is. Your task is to decide what the best way would be of discovering all that you can about this thing. Think about the problem for a moment before reading on.

Was there enough information presented so that you could make some reasonably intelligent suggestions? Consider, now, what the nature of your suggestions might have been had I written, "Your instructor has brought into class a smallish animal inside a glass cage." Or if I had written, "Your instructor has brought into class a small piece of machinery inside a glass box." Or, again, "Your instructor has brought into class a strange new fruit in a glass basket." Why is the task of investigating the object so much easier in the last three cases? It is easier simply because you have been presented with information that allows you to classify the object in terms of a something about whose properties and functioning you already know a great deal. You have, in your view of the world, a mental

Table 1.1 Divisions of the lifespan in this text.

Infancy	Birth to 2 years
Childhood	2 to 12 years
Adolescence	12 to 18 years
Adulthood	
Early	18 to 35 years
Middle	35 to 65 years
Late	65 years onward

model of what animals, fruits, and machines are like.

Psychologists investigating human development are, in some ways, in the same position as a student presented with a thing. Initially, it is difficult to know what questions would be the best ones to ask. But if we could look at development in terms of something more familiar, many questions might suggest themselves, not to mention a few answers. And that is, in effect, the starting point of all systematic investigation. We begin with a metaphor—a comparison. We say, this is *like* that, and it might therefore work in the same way as that. The *that* serves as our model.

Models exist at various levels of generality (Reese & Overton, 1970). At a simple, specific level, there are models that describe, for example, how a minute mechanical system might work. At a more complex level, there are models that serve as specific analogies or comparisons (a computer program might be used as a model of human problem-solving processes). And at the most general level, there are models that represent our world views—models of our presuppositions about how things are.

Whereas the term *model* typically refers to broad underlying assumptions or to more specific representations of how things are, **theories** are simply collections of statements that are intended to explain observations and that make it easier for us to make predictions. In this text we deal primarily with theories rather than with models. For example, Chapters 2 and 13 present theories developed by Freud, Piaget, Skinner, Erikson, Levinson, and others. These theories attempt to explain how people function and how they change. And they are inevitably based on a number of basic assumptions that underlie the theorist's model.

Machine-Organism Metaphors

In developmental psychology, two basic models underlie our theories (Reese & Overton, 1970): the **organismic** and the **mechanistic.** The organismic model assumes that people are like active organisms; the mechanistic model assumes that people are like machines. In the first instance, the model is that of a functioning, biological, *active* organism; in the second, the model is that of a *reactive* machine—hence the occasional use of the terms *active* versus *passive* to describe these views.

These underlying models are extremely important in the development of a theory. In effect, they suggest what the theorist will investigate and what the resulting theory will look like. An organismic view (Piaget's, for example) will describe development as a process resulting from self-initiated activities and will look for regularities in behavior in order to understand the wholeness and unity of the organism. In contrast, a mechanistic view (Skinner's, for example) will describe development as a process resulting from reactions to external events and will search for the machine-like predictability that might result, given sufficient knowledge about how the machine reacts to external forces.

You might ask, at this point, which of these two models is correct. The answer is simple: The question is irrelevant. The models are simply metaphors—comparisons. You might as well ask whether "The moon was a ghostly galleon, tossed up on cloudy seas" is more accurate than "That orbed maiden with white fire laden/Whom mortals call the moon." Metaphors are apt and useful or they are clumsy and useless. We might judge our poetic metaphors in terms of the images and feelings they arouse; we can judge our scientific metaphors only in terms of their usefulness.

A number of issues, still largely unresolved, can be identified as major themes in the study of development. These issues, often the subject of considerable controversy, can sometimes be traced to the relatively recent historical roots of the discipline (as they are in a later section of this chapter) and sometimes to the underlying models upon which the theories are based.

One major issue is that raised by the **nature-nurture controversy,** also referred to as the **heredity** versus **environment** question. Extreme points of view on this issue would maintain either that the environment is solely responsible for whatever we become (nurture) or that genetic background (nature) determines the outcome of the developmental process. Although neither of these extreme positions is completely valid, the issue continues to be debated and is discussed in some detail in Chapter 3.

A second issue deals with the question of whether development is a continuous, relatively uninterrupted process or whether it consists of separate stages. Reese and Overton (1970) note that theories based on an organismic model view development as consisting of changes in structure (in knowledge and capabilities) that can be understood in terms of separate stages. In contrast, theories based on a mechanistic view describe development in terms of changes in behavior (changes in reaction), a process best viewed as continuous (one without stages) rather than as discontinuous (with stages).

And a third issue, of considerable importance to our understanding of the later stages of human development, concerns the extent to which our abilities and characteristics deteriorate with the passage of time. Some people believe that decline, both intellectual and physical, is the inevitable consequence of aging; others argue that although physical aging seems impervious to our most determined contrary efforts, intellectual decline can to a large degree be avoided.

As indicated earlier, none of these issues has been clearly resolved; perhaps they cannot be. And perhaps history will show that they were not particularly important in any case. What is important, however, is to keep in mind that what we think and say about children and adults—indeed, the questions we ask and sometimes the answers we are prepared to accept—is strongly influenced by the assumptions we make. It should not be surprising, then, to find that developmental psychology is highly applied in the sense that it is directed toward practical as well as theoretical concerns. The questions that have always seemed most important are those dealing with human welfare. Accordingly, developmental psychologists most concerned with children have looked at questions relating to instruction, discipline and behavior problems, emotional disorders, perceptual problems, language acquisition, social development, morality, and a variety of other topics that are important to teachers, nurses, counselors, physicians, the child welfare profession, religious personnel, and parents. And those concerned with adults and with the processes of aging have tried to understand the changes that occur through adulthood and the adjustments that are required, as well as ways in which the elderly can lead more fulfilling and happier lives and ways in which the pain of dying can be eased—both for those who must die and for those who remain. The study of children and, more recently, the study of the entire span of life grew largely in response to questions that parents, teachers, doctors, and others had about children. Yet these questions have been asked for only a short time, since interest in child development is surprisingly new, and interest in the psychology of adulthood and of aging is even newer.

■ A History of Child Development

Although making children is an ancient art, the scientific study of children is relatively recent. Indeed, for many years animals such as dogs, horses, and sheep were much more likely to be the subjects of detailed observation than were children. And early "teaching" books usually dealt with animal training rather than with child rearing. One probable reason for this lack of information is that dogs and other animals are considered simpler to understand than children. A second reason for the long neglect of child study is rooted in the naive but appealing notion that children and adults are identical—that children are, in effect, miniature adults who differ from normal adults only quantitatively. Perhaps a third reason why the child has just recently become a subject of psychological investigation is the place of children in the affection of adults. Even today, children are not always loved or wanted by their parents; it seems to have been worse yesterday.

In the crowded and diseased slums of eighteenth-century European cities, thousands of parents, ignorant of all but the most difficult birth control methods, bore children whom they promptly abandoned in the streets or on the doorsteps of churches and orphanages. Foundling homes sprang up all over Europe in a futile attempt to care for these children, but the majority died in **infancy**. Kessen (1965, p. 8) reports that of 10,272 infants who were admitted to one foundling home in Dublin in the last quarter of the eighteenth century, only 45 survived. Indeed, until the turn of that century, even if a child were not abandoned, chances of surviving until the age of five were less than one in two. Aries, for example, describes an incident in which a woman who has just given

Society's prevailing attitudes toward children are reflected in the schools, playgrounds, parks, health care, and amusements that are provided for them. These attitudes may also be apparent in practices of emotional or physical abandonment or, as depicted here in an early twentieth-century American factory, in child labor or other forms of exploitation.

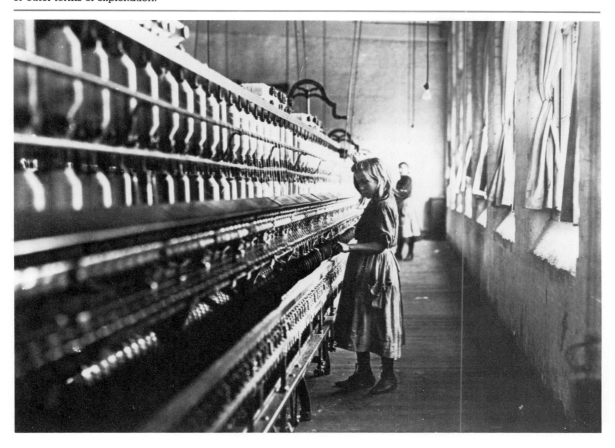

birth to her fifth child (and who is consequently depressed) is consoled by her neighbor: "Before they are old enough to bother you, you will have lost half of them, or perhaps all of them" (Aries, 1962, p. 38). In the face of this tragic mortality rate, it is small wonder that parents were reluctant to become emotionally attached to their children— so reluctant that they could quite callously leave them on an open doorstep, probably to die if they were not rescued before long, probably to die soon in any case. And perhaps nowhere is parental indifference to the fate of their children as obvious as it was in the practice of burying them on thresholds or in the yard much as a dog or cat might be buried (Aries, 1962).

The high mortality rate of abandoned children was not restricted to eighteenth-century Europe, but was characteristic of nineteenth-century America as well. Bakwin (1949) cites evidence indicating that, with few exceptions, children in infant homes (asylums) in the United States prior to 1915 died before the age of two. This well-documented inability of infants to survive in children's homes or in hospitals was labeled **hospitalism** and was identified by symptoms of listlessness, inability to gain weight, unresponsiveness to stimuli, pallor, and eventual death. The cause of death may well have been related to a lack of love between parent and child. It might also, at least in part, have been caused by poor nutrition, lack of stimulation, and poor health care (Bowlby, 1940, 1953).

The nineteenth century brought some improvement in the status of children in Europe; abandonments decreased drastically. Unfortunately this change proved to be due less to increasing love and concern for children and more to their economic value. In nineteenth-century Europe, children became highly prized as workers. In thousands of factories and mines throughout Europe, child labor flourished. The seventh earl of Shaftesbury described in horrid detail the plight of children as young as five or six years, male and female, who worked ten hours a day or more at grueling labor in conditions so hazardous that many became ill and died (Kessen, 1965).

It is difficult to imagine that age from our present perspective, child centered as we are. Yet the shocking pictures of starvation we see on our television sets feature many more children than adults because there are more children than adults starving. Unless humans can satisfy their most basic needs, they are not likely to concern themselves with the more noble sentiments of parental love and **humanitarianism** (Maslow, 1954). But medicine and law have saved the child, not only from death but also from abandonment and excessive abuse, usually. Now, in the wisdom and kindness of a wealthier age, children can be loved and studied, for they are less often an economic burden or an economic necessity.

The widespread social changes that manifested themselves in seventeenth- and eighteenth-century attitudes toward children, together with intellectual movements reflected in the writings of philosophers and early scientists, advances in biology and medicine, and the increasing availability of elementary education, contributed significantly to the development of child psychology. Closely associated with these intellectual movements were John Locke and Jean-Jacques Rousseau. Locke, writing in the late seventeenth century, advanced the notion that the child is essentially a rational creature, born with some limited predispositions, but in the main with a mind comparable to a blank slate (tabula rasa) upon which experience writes messages. The child described by Locke is, in a sense, a passive recipient of knowledge, information, and habits and highly responsive to rewards and punishments. In Locke's words, "If you take away the Rod on one hand, and these little Encouragements which they are taken with, on the other, How then (will you say) shall Children be govern'd? Remove Hope and Fear, and there is an end of all Discipline" (1699).

Rousseau's child, immortalized in the book *Emile*, is, in contrast to the child described by Locke, active and inquiring. Furthermore, this child is not a "blank slate," neither good nor bad until the rewards and punishments of experience exert their influence, but is innately good—a "noble savage." Rousseau (1911) insists that if children were allowed to develop in their own fashion, untainted by the corruption and evil in the world, they would be undeniably good when grown: "God makes all

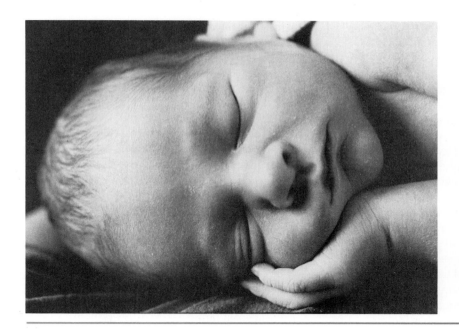

A blank slate, neither good nor bad, as Locke argued? Or, as Rousseau believed, a noble savage, fundamentally good unless corrupted by society?

things good; man meddles with them and they become evil."

Although both Locke and Rousseau are closely associated with the beginning of the study of children, their ideas have led to fundamentally different conceptions of childhood. Locke's description of the child as a passive creature, molded and shaped by the rewards and punishments of experience, has a close parallel in learning-theory descriptions of development, particularly as exemplified in the work of Skinner and Bandura (described in Chapter 2), and clearly represents the *mechanistic* model described earlier. Rousseau's view of an active, exploring child developing through deliberate and purposeful interaction with the environment finds an important place in the work of Jean Piaget (also described in Chapter 2 and elsewhere in this text) and serves as a good illustration of the *organismic* model of child development.

Child psychology as a science did not really begin with these eighteenth-century philosophers. It began, instead, with the first reported systematic observations of children made by such men as Preyer (Dennis, 1949), Darwin (1877), and G. Stanley Hall (1891). Both Darwin and Preyer wrote systematic accounts of the early development of their own children; Hall pioneered the use of the questionnaire as a tool for studying the child, although his questionnaires were presented to parents and teachers rather than to children. Typically they asked adults to try to remember what they had felt and thought when they were children. Thus, although Hall can be credited with pioneering the use of the questionnaire, he made little progress toward an **objective** science of children.

Among other significant figures in the early development of the science of child study was Alfred Binet, who devised the first practical intelligence scale for children (Binet & Simon, 1905), and John B. Watson, who introduced experimental approaches to child study. But more than anyone else, Sigmund Freud is responsible for drawing the attention of both parents and professionals to the importance of the early years of a child's life. Among his major contributions are his emphasis on the effects that the environment has in developing children's personalities.

From Child Development to Lifespan Development

During the hundred or so years since the beginning of scientific psychology, the majority of studies of human development have focused almost exclusively on infancy, childhood, and, to a lesser extent, adolescence. Current interest in adulthood and aging and an increasing tendency to consider development as a lifespan phenomenon are relatively recent. A French mathematician by the name of Quetelet wrote a book about aging as far back as 1835, but almost another hundred years passed before Hall (1922) published a second major book on aging. And although Hall is often associated with the beginnings of the study of aging, there was little activity in the field until recent decades.

There are several reasons why the study of the human lifespan has attained its current importance. Not the least of these is that increased life expectancy together with decreasing birthrates have created a dramatic shift in the proportion of adults relative to younger people. In 1900, for example, life expectancy of a male in North America was only forty-five years, and fewer than one in twenty individuals were over sixty-five. This proportion has now doubled to more than one in ten and could eventually reach one in two or three! (See Figure 1.1.) In addition, the models that are currently used to understand and explain develop-

ment tend to view it as a continuous process that does not culminate with adulthood but rather with death.

Methods of Studying the Lifespan

It is unfortunate that by the time we are able to make sense of the thoughts and emotions of infants, we can no longer remember what it was like to be an infant. It is equally unfortunate that very young children cannot speak. All that we know of the private life of preverbal children is based on inferences that we make. Ideally, these inferences are based not on speculation, inspiration, or the prejudices of grandfathers but on careful, controlled, and replicable observation. Observers of human development may focus on natural events, such as children playing in a park; they may collect information on less naturally occurring events, such as old people being interviewed; or they may collect experimental observations. In addition, lifespan research may often be described as longitudinal (following the same subjects over a long period of time) or cross-sectional (using a *cross section* of different subjects at one point in time). Each of these approaches is described in the following sections. Note that these categories are not mutually exclusive. For example, a lifespan study might be

Figure 1.1
Changes in the United States population over age 65 since 1890. (From U.S. Department of Commerce, 1980.)

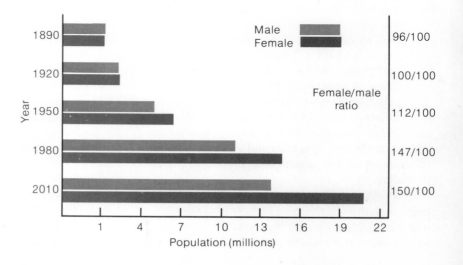

experimental and longitudinal or cross-sectional simultaneously. (See *Some Definitions of Development,* the box on page 14, for further clarification of some terms used in lifespan psychology.)

Observations

Observations are termed *naturalistic* when subjects are observed in natural as opposed to contrived situations. Among the most useful naturalistic methods are diary descriptions, specimen descriptions, time sampling, and event sampling (Wright, 1960).

When investigators record observations daily or at predetermined intervals, frequently in an attempt to arrive at some better understanding of the sequence of development, they are using a **diary description**. Freud, Binet, and Piaget in their early investigations frequently used this approach by keeping diary descriptions of their own children. When investigators observe and record continuous sequences of behavior, they are using a **specimen description.** Such descriptions tend to be highly specific and detailed and are particularly useful for in-depth studies of individuals. Diary descriptions, by contrast, have proven especially useful in developing theories.

Detailed observations made at regular time intervals and for specified periods of time are called **time sampling**. This procedure is useful when the object is to arrive at a general understanding of a person. Its major advantage is that it does not require the investigator to spend a great deal of time with each individual. For example, one person might be observed continuously for five minutes and not be observed again for two hours. In the meantime, the investigator is free to observe another twenty-three people for five minutes each. In this way, a sample of twenty-four could be observed individually and systematically over the entire course of the investigation.

Event sampling takes place when certain types of behavior are observed and recorded and unrelated behaviors are ignored. If the type of behavior in question were aggression, for example, all manifestations of aggression would be recorded. This procedure would be useful if the object of the study were to arrive at an understanding of the various forms that aggressive behavior might take.

Experiments

In an **experiment**, the observer manipulates some aspects of a situation in order to study the effect of an **independent variable** on another variable that is termed **dependent**. A variable always has two or more values and may be a measurement, an outcome, or some way of classifying people or events. For example, an investigator interested in the relationship between teaching methods and verbal ability might simply compare the scores on a test of language skills of children assigned to different teaching methods. In this experiment, the teaching method is an independent variable, and the test score is a dependent variable.

Other experimental procedures involve the use of an **experimental group** and a **control group**. The former is ordinarily composed of subjects treated in some special way. The object of the experiment is, in this case, to discover whether the treatment (independent variable) affects some outcome (dependent variable). To ensure that any changes in the dependent variable are caused by the treatment, it is necessary to use a second group, the control group, which receives no treatment but otherwise is identical to the experimental group in all possible relevant ways (that is, in terms of age, background, personality characteristic, and any other variable that might affect the outcome of the experiment). The effect of the treatment is then assessed by comparing the results of the experimental groups to those of the control group, rather than by comparing scores made by members of the experimental group after treatment to scores made before treatment.*

---

*This is only one of a large variety of experimental designs (arrangements) that are employed in psychological research. For others, see Campbell and Stanley (1963).

SOME DEFINITIONS OF DEVELOPMENT

Development involves growth, maturation, and learning. Although related, each of these terms has its own meaning.

Growth ordinarily refers to physical changes, which are primarily quantitative because they involve addition rather than transformation. Such changes as increasing height and enlargement of the nose are clear examples of growth.

Maturation is a more nebulous term used to describe changes that are relatively independent of the environment. These changes are frequently attributed to heredity. In virtually all aspects of human development, however, there is an interaction between maturation and learning. Learning to walk, for example, requires not only that the child's physical strength and muscular coordination be sufficiently developed but also that there are opportunities to practice the various skills involved.

Learning is defined as change that results from experience rather than from a maturational process. All changes in behavior resulting from experience are examples of learning, provided these changes are not simply the temporary effects of drugs or fatigue (Walker, 1968).

Development, then, is the total process whereby individuals adapt to their environment. And since we adapt by growing, maturing, and learning, these are all aspects of development. The central difference between learning and development is simply that learning is concerned with immediate, short-term adaptation, and development refers to gradual adaptation over a period of years. Learning theorists have traditionally been concerned with discovering the underlying principles of learning, rather than with describing differences between the learning processes of children and adults. Developmental theorists, by contrast, have been largely preoccupied with child-adult differences in learning and behavior and with how a child's learning processes develop chronologically. Developmental psychology, then, has as its subject the human from conception to death. It undertakes two essential tasks: observing humans and their progress in adapting to the world and formulating an explanation of that adaptation.

An Example   A large number of preschool programs have attempted to overcome the cultural and intellectual deficit sometimes found among children from disadvantaged backgrounds. Experimentation has frequently been used to assess the effectiveness of these programs. Weikart and his associates (1968, 1969) report one such experiment, the Ypsilanti project, in which preschoolers previously identified as culturally disadvantaged were given specially designed teaching sessions in their homes. As a major feature of these teaching sessions, mothers were encouraged to become actively involved in both the planning and the execution of the session. The sample, or group of subjects, employed in the study was divided into two groups highly similar with respect to measured intelligence, race, age, and sex—factors that might be related to their performance. The experimental group consisted of those children who had the weekly teaching sessions. The second group served as a control group, and its members received no special treatment.

After approximately ten weeks of treatment, the investigators assessed the effectiveness of the program by administering the Stanford-Binet Intelligence Scale and the Peabody Picture Vocabulary Test to both the experimental group and the control group. Scores obtained by members of each group prior to the experiment (on a pretest) were then compared with those obtained following the experiment (the posttest). The experimental group had gained 8.2 IQ points on the average; the control group had gained 0.9 IQ points. Vocabulary increase as measured by the Peabody Picture Vocabulary Test was 9.9 for the experimental group and 4.0 for the control group. Statistical analyses revealed that the average IQ gain for the experimental group was significantly greater than that for the control group (greater than would be expected by chance alone). Hence the experimenters conclude that their experimental program is effective under these circumstances and with these children in increasing measured intelligence following a ten-week program. They might also generalize, with some confidence, that similar programs with other children might also be effective.

This experiment serves as a good illustration of an experimental method in psychological research. It employed both an experimental group and a control group. Some of the reasons for this are obvious. Measured intelligence and vocabulary scores for both the experimental and the control group could have changed significantly over a ten-week period because of factors entirely unrelated to the experimental program itself. Indeed, a new television program introduced at about the same time could have had similar results. Without a control group, the experimenters might have falsely concluded that their program was effective.

Having highly comparable control and experimental groups is also important. If one of the groups has a greater number of intelligent children, more girls than boys, or more highly educated parents, differences between the two groups might reflect any or all of these factors rather than the experimental treatment. By having comparable groups, we eliminate these factors and thus prevent them from being independent variables that might affect the dependent variables in the experiment: measured intelligence and vocabulary scores. What remains is the most important independent variable: the treatment provided for the experimental group. The investigators predict that their training sessions will affect intelligence and vocabulary. In other words, they predict that the independent variable (home experience) they are manipulating will change the dependent variables (intelligence and vocabulary scores) they are measuring.

Correlational Studies

A great deal of developmental research may be described as follows: Researchers decide to investigate the sources (causes) of specific characteristics in a group of people; people with these characteristics are identified; a comparison group

without these characteristics is also identified. An attempt is now made to obtain historical information about these people (home environment, presence or absence of a father, intelligence, similar characteristics in biological ancestors, and so on). Researchers now compare the two groups with respect to these historical variables. In the end, a relationship (correlation) will be found to exist between specific historical variables and present characteristics, or no relationship will be found.

Largely through studies such as these, research has established relationships between socioeconomic variables such as poverty and delinquency or between the personality characteristics of parents and those of children. Many such studies, sometimes termed *retrospective*, are described in this text. They are called retrospective because they try to establish relationships by looking *backward* at the child's history.

One caution is extremely important in interpreting the results of correlational studies. One of the most common errors in the interpretation of research results stems from the apparently logical but false assumption that if two events are related (correlated), one causes the other. Some studies have demonstrated, for example, that children from disadvantaged homes (low socioeconomic level, low parental education, low academic aspirations, and so on) typically do less well in school than children from more advantaged backgrounds. Given this observation, one might logically assume that home background causes low or high achievement, but the assumption is, in fact, not warranted by the data. At best, correlational studies show relationships or their absence; they do not establish causation. It is possible that home background is related to nutrition, nutrition to intelligence, intelligence to achievement, and hence home background to achievement, with none of these relationships being causal.

These comments should not be interpreted to mean that correlational studies should be avoided and that only experiments should be conducted. Not only are correlational studies often highly informative (when interpreted cautiously) but experiments are also often impossible for practical and ethical reasons. Consider, for example, an experiment designed to investigate the effects of poverty. Such an experiment would require that investigators assign randomly selected (or highly similar) children to precisely defined conditions of wealth or poverty at some critical and presumably early stage in their lives and that these children be examined and compared later. For this, and many other investigations, an experiment is clearly not in order.

Longitudinal and Cross-Sectional Studies

There are two general approaches to the study of human development: the longitudinal and the cross-sectional. A **longitudinal study** is based on observation of the same subjects over a long period of time; a **cross-sectional study** is based on the comparison of different subjects of different developmental levels at the same time. There are two ways, for example, of arriving at some notion about the different rules employed in games played by two-year-old children and six-year-old children. One method is to observe a group of two-year-old children at play and four years later repeat the same procedure with the same children. This is the longitudinal approach, which, for this purpose, is more time-consuming than necessary. The same results could be obtained by observing several groups of two- and six-year-old children at the same time and comparing them directly. Occasionally, however, a longitudinal approach is necessary although it is time-consuming. If investigators wish to discover whether intelligence test scores change with age or remain stable, they could observe the same children at different times. This question could not be answered by employing a cross-sectional approach.

Cross-sectional and longitudinal approaches are both essential for studying human development, and they are often used in combination (see

Table 1.2   A comparison of three approaches in developmental research.

Cross-Sectional Approach	Group	Present Age	Investigation Occurs
Conclusions derive from comparison of three different groups examined at one point in time.	1	10	1984
	2	12	1984
	3	14	1984

Longitudinal Approach	Group	Present Age	Investigation Occurs
Conclusions derive from comparison of same subjects to themselves at different ages.	1	10	1984
			1985
			1986
			1987

Short-Term Longitudinal Approach	Group	Present Age	Investigation Occurs
Conclusions derive from cross-sectional comparison (three groups of different ages each year) and from comparing subjects to themselves at different ages. Study requires four years but spans eight age groups.	1	10	1984 1985 1986 1987 (10) (11) (12) (13)
	2	12	1984 1985 1986 1987 (12) (13) (14) (15)
	3	14	1984 1985 1986 1987 (14) (15) (16) (17)

Table 1.2). Unfortunately, however, each approach has some obvious weaknesses and limitations. As noted earlier, for example, a cross sectional approach cannot give us information concerning changes that occur over time within a single individual, since it looks at each individual only once. Among the problems associated with longitudinal research are its higher cost, the prospect that instruments and methods may become outdated prior to completion, the possibility that some of the research questions will be answered in some other way before the project is finished, and the tremendous amount of time sometimes required.

Often an experiment must be designed to go beyond the lifetime of a single investigator (or team of investigators), particularly if it is intended to examine most or all of the human lifespan. This brings about an additional problem related to subject mortality. The death of subjects not only reduces the size of samples but may also serve to bias the results. If, for example, individuals of a certain personality type die younger than do others, a longitudinal assessment of personality change might reveal some significant changes with old age when such is, in fact, not the case. As a purely hypothetical illustration, if aggressive people die before those who are not aggressive, we might be led to believe that people become less aggressive as they age.

Perhaps the most serious limitation of longitudinal studies is that they must frequently assume that currently valid measures will be equally valid sometime later. This problem is particularly evident in longitudinal studies of vocabulary growth, intelligence, and related variables where rapidly changing cultural conditions may significantly affect the appropriateness of measures employed. Cross-sectional studies sometimes suffer from a similar problem, stemming from their assumption that children at one age level now are comparable to children at that age level at another time. With respect to intelligence, for example, drastic improvements in educational experiences and perhaps in television fare can affect children sufficiently over time that measures of intelligence obtained at one time cannot easily be compared to measures obtained some years earlier from another group of children.

Age, Time, and Cohort in Developmental Research

There are, in effect, three separate sources of variation that cross-sectional and longitudinal studies look at. First, there are changes related to age. Bear in mind, however, that age is neither a cause nor an explanation for human development, although we often treat it that way (Wohlwill, 1970). Second, there are influences related to the time of testing. And third, there is the influence of the **cohort.**

A cohort can be described as a group of individuals who were born within the same range of time. This range is arbitrary but is usually described in terms of a specific time frame. Thus the 1940 cohort includes all individuals who were born during the year 1940, the December 1940 cohort includes all individuals born during December 1940, and the cohort of the fifth decade in the twentieth century includes all individuals born in the ten-year period between January 1940 and December 1949. A cohort is, therefore, of a specific size and composition initially. It does not normally increase in size, but rather decreases as members die, until it has completely disappeared. Its composition also changes gradually in other ways. For example, since men die sooner than women, the male-female ratio of a cohort usually changes over time. Similarly, racial composition might also change as a result of different mortality rates. In the main, then, a cohort is a relatively stable group of individuals born at the same time and therefore of identical (or similar) ages.

What is most important for the lifespan psychologist, however, is not that individuals of a single cohort are of the same age so much as that they may be subject to a variety of experiences very different from those to which members of other cohorts are exposed. For example, cohort groups such as that of my grandmother date to the turn of this century and include people who were born into a world without radios, automobiles, televisions, or computers. These obvious cohort-related influences might be important in attempting to understand why an eighty-year-old person in 1980 might be quite different from an eighty-year-old in 2020 or in 1940. Less obvious cohort-related influ-

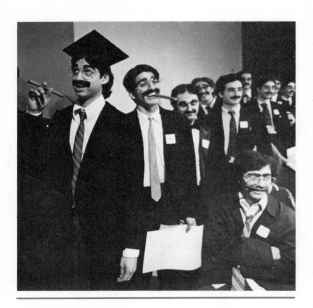

A cohort is a group of individuals born during a single time period and therefore usually subject to similar cultural and historical influences. Research cannot always separate the effects of age from those related to the cohort.

ences would also include changes in medical practices (including the general use of a variety of inoculations, for example), in nutrition, in recreation, in work roles, in morality, and so on. And because of these influences, cohorts that are scarcely separated in time might turn out to be very different in some important ways.

One of the most important problems that has faced developmental research has been the tremendous difficulty experienced in attempting to separate the effects of age, time, and cohort. In both longitudinal and cross-sectional research, two or more of these often cannot be separated. In a cross-sectional design, for example, it is often impossible to determine whether differences between two age groups are age related or whether they are due to generational factors because two different cohorts are being examined. And in a simple longitudinal study, it may be impossible to separate the effects of the time of testing with age. In addition, generalizations derived from a longitudinal study might be applicable only to the specific cohort under investigation.

We can overcome these important research problems in a number of different ways. Most of them relate to Schaie's (1965) *general developmental model*. In complete detail, this model is technical and complex. At a simpler level, however, it may be described as a combination of the longitudinal and the cross-sectional approaches. Sometimes called the **short-term longitudinal approach** or the **longitudinal/cross-sectional approach**, it involves two or more groups of subjects that overlap in age. For example, one group might consist of two-, four-, and six-year-olds; another might consist of six-, eight-, and ten-year-olds. The first group, initially consisting only of two-year-olds, would be tested at the age of two and then again at four and six; the second group would be tested at six, eight, and ten. In this sense, the study is longitudinal and spans a four-year period. But the study is also cross-sectional in that it provides data from two different groups that can be compared directly. Moreover, even though the study spans only four years, it provides longitudinal data over an eight-year period in the subjects' lives.

An Illustration   One example of a problem requiring the longitudinal approach is reported by Hindley, Filliozat, Klackenberg, Nicolet-Meister, and Sand (1966). They compared the ages at which children from different nations first begin to walk unassisted. Although simply interviewing mothers would have provided data for comparison, such data would have reflected the imperfect memories, unintentional exaggerations, and occasional dishonesty of the mothers. The experiment proceeded as follows: Samples of newborn infants in Brussels, London, Paris, Stockholm, and Zurich were selected. An attempt was made to ensure that these children were representative of their respective cities. During extensive interviews with the mothers when the children were nine months, twelve months, eighteen months, and three years of age, the following question was asked: "When did the child first walk alone?" Information gathered in this fashion was assumed to be relatively accurate, though not as accurate as it would have been had the investigators been able to witness the child's

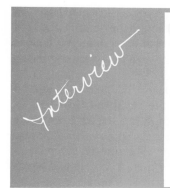

Subject: Male; age seventy-five; retired school teacher.
(on children growing up)

It's going to be a lot different for kids growing up now compared to my day. Just take a few examples like television, which we didn't have. Kids know things now that we didn't even teach when I first started. In some ways, they have to be a lot more intelligent. But in other ways they're sure not. Maybe they don't read as much as we did, because they don't have enough time left over even if they don't have a long list of chores like most of us did. Another thing is their morals are going to be a lot different too. Lots of the things we thought were wrong, nobody even cares about any more. Like not wearing brassieres. It would have shocked us no end. Well, nobody would have done it. It's that simple. Now who cares?

first unassisted steps or had they interviewed the mothers more frequently, particularly during the critical period between eleven and sixteen months when most of the children first began to walk. Nevertheless, this longitudinal study made it possible to establish when children in each of these cities began to walk *on the average* and to compare ages of first walking. It was not possible, however, to establish why there were significant differences in the average age of walking among all five cities, or why children from Stockholm walked at the earliest age (12.44 months) and children from Paris at the latest (13.58).

■ Evaluating Lifespan Research

Truth in psychology, as in most disciplines, is highly relative at best; at worst, it remains an elusive abstraction, seldom attained but occasionally approximated. Hence the validity of conclusions derived from research can seldom be judged in terms of some absolute degree of rightness or wrongness, but must instead be interpreted in terms of usefulness, clarity, logical consistency, and **generalizability**. And of all these criteria, perhaps generalizability is the single most important. Too frequently, results of a specific research project are applicable only to the situation in which they were obtained; they cannot be generalized to other similar situations. The value of such conclusions is limited.

Sampling

One way to ensure that research results will be applicable to a wide variety of situations is to select as representative a sample as possible. Clearly, it would be difficult to obtain valid information concerning the moral beliefs and behaviors of American children by interviewing and observing a sample of subjects from San Francisco or Boston alone. If the results are to be generalized to the entire population, subjects should represent all major geographical areas in the nation. In addition, care must be taken to ensure that all nationalities, major religious groups, socioeconomic levels, occupations, and ages are represented in proportions similar to the entire population. One of the simplest and most effective ways of ensuring that this is the case is to select subjects at random from a group that represents the entire population—in many cases, from the entire population itself.

Memory

Studies of the ages at which girls experience their first menstrual period **(menarche)** have frequently had to rely on the memories of women for whom the event may not be entirely recent; investigations of the ages at which children first walk or talk often base their conclusions on the memories of mothers. Unfortunately, human memory is far from perfect. Not only does it forget but it also distorts—sometimes in predictable ways, sometimes not.

Honesty

Having to rely on the honesty of subjects is a particularly severe problem with questionnaire and interview data, especially when highly personal areas are being researched. Comparisons of contemporary adolescent sexual behavior with behavior characteristic of adolescents several generations ago are typically unreliable primarily for this reason. Given prevailing attitudes toward sexual behavior, it is not unreasonable to suppose that today's adolescent is more likely to be honest about sexual behavior than the adolescent of the 1930s might have been. Hence the finding that there is considerably more premarital sexual activity among contemporary adolescents than there was when their parents were adolescents may be partly confounded by subject honesty.

Experimenter Bias

Rosenthal and Fode (1963) presented some of their psychology students with rats to train. Some students were told that they had been given **maze-bright** rats; others were told they had **maze-dull** rats. Through selective breeding, it has been possible to develop groups of rats that are remarkably different in terms of their ability to learn how to run through a maze or how to solve other typical rat problems. In fact, however, the rats given to these students were all of the same variety. But those students who thought they had bright rats reported considerably more success in training their rats. They also felt that their rats were more gentle, more manageable, and more intelligent than the supposedly dull rats. This experiment illustrates dramatically the power of experimenter bias. Students probably did not lie about their reactions to the rats, but it is highly likely that these largely predetermined reactions affected student observations and perhaps rat behavior as well. The experiment illustrates the potentially prejudicial effects experimenter expectations can have on research outcomes. Although this finding does not call into question experimenter honesty, it does make the honesty of research results somewhat more suspect.

One effective means of guarding against experimenter bias is the **double-blind procedure**. This requires simply that the experimenters and examiners, as well as the subjects, are unaware of the expected outcomes of the research or of which subjects are experimental subjects and which are members of the control group.

Subject Bias

Subject bias may also have an effect on the outcome of an experiment. In a frequently cited experiment, two psychologists (Roethlisberger & Dickson, 1939) compared a number of ways to increase productivity among workers in the Hawthorne plant of the Western Electric Company in Chicago. In successive experiments, the workers were subjected to shorter working periods, longer working periods, better lighting conditions, poorer lighting conditions, long periods of rest, short periods of rest, work incentives such as bonuses, and a variety of other conditions. Under most of these conditions, productivity apparently increased. This observation led to the conclusion that if subjects are aware that they are members of an experimental group, performance may improve simply by virtue of that fact.

Although the "Hawthorne effect," as it is now called, is usually accepted as fact in social science research, its existence has not been well established—in spite of the Hawthorne experiments just described. Following a careful re-examination of the original experiments and interviews with some of the people who were involved at that time, Rice (1982) found little evidence of a Hawthorne effect. He reports that productivity did not increase in many of the experiments, but that later reports of the study usually concentrated on only one experiment in which there was a marked improvement over the five-year course of the study. In this particular experiment, workers (all women) were paid according to the productivity of the entire group (as they were throughout this factory). Since there were only seven or eight women in the group, individual productivity would have a noticeable effect on the pay received by each woman. Accordingly, when several of the experimental group members proved to be slower than the average, the other women became unhappy; as a result, the slower workers were dropped from the group.

Under these circumstances, is it any wonder that the experimental group's performance should improve?

Some Special Problems

Problems involving inadequate sampling, memory distortions, questionable honesty, and experimen-

SUBJECT RIGHTS AND
EXPERIMENTAL ETHICS

In the Western world, it is no longer common to abandon children for fear they will prove too much of an economic burden. And we no longer send them into mines and factories when they are scarcely out of their diapers. Indeed, children have now assumed an importance that is apparent not only in the home but also in the courts, in the schools, and even at the highest level of government. Among the many manifestations of this new importance are the thousands of programs linked directly to the fact that the United Nations designated 1979 as the International Year of the Child (IYC), which increased concern with the social, emotional, and intellectual welfare of children and called attention to a budding concern with their legal rights.

The absolute control that parents and various agencies have long had over the lives and affairs of children has been weakened, although it is far from removed. Nor, of course, should it be, since in a vast majority of cases the control that parents and others exercise over children is to their advantage. Unfortunately, however, this is not always the case. Farleger (1977) reports numerous instances in which children have been "voluntarily" committed to mental institutions by their parents or legal guardians (that is, their parents "volunteered" them). Until recently, these children had virtually no legal recourse, no matter how badly they felt they had been treated, and they would simply remain in the institution until psychiatrists and guardians deemed it appropriate to release them. And if they spent their formative years in a drugged daze, largely ignored by the harried (or calloused) people charged with helping them with whatever real or imagined problems had led to their incarceration, no one was likely to pay a great deal of attention.

Recently, however, a number of major court decisions in the Western world have begun to change this situation. In almost all cases in which institutionalized children have obtained legal aid to establish their right to adequate care or to release, they have been successful. The overriding theme of these court decisions is that laws and their application must protect children rather than the rights of their parents; that societies have a responsibility for the welfare of children that transcends the wishes of parents when these are not in the best interests of the child; that, in short, the rights and privileges that have been guaranteed to adults by the country's Constitution also extend to children.

In spite of these observations, it remains true that children are not always capable of making decisions that are best for their own welfare, and these decisions will continue to be made largely by parents and other "responsible" adults. Increasingly, however, major decisions affecting children will be influenced by their rights.

Evidence of increasing concern with the rights of children is also apparent in the adoption of ethical principles guiding research with children ("Ethical Standards for Research with Children," 1973, published by the Society for Research in Child Development). Establishment of these principles was motivated in part by the observation that research procedures with children can be unethical if they involve coercion, if they subject the child to stress or other potentially damaging conditions, if they involve an invasion of privacy, and so on. The principles specify not only that the consent of parents must be obtained prior to conducting research with children but also that the children themselves must consent. Furthermore, their consent must be "informed" in the sense that they are made aware beforehand of any aspect of the research that might affect their willingness to participate.

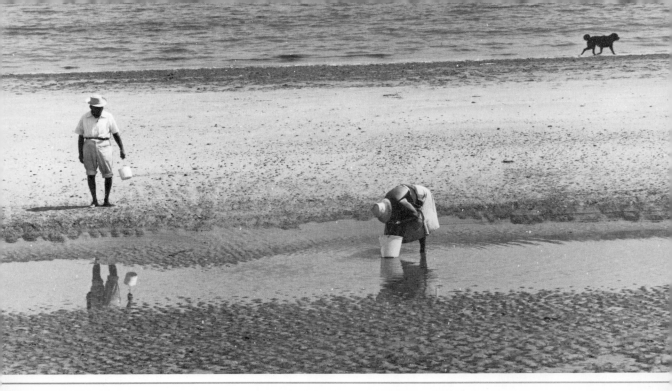

In North American societies, fewer than one in twenty of the very old are in retirement homes or other institutions, which makes it difficult for researchers to obtain
large, representative samples of the elderly.

ter or subject bias may affect research in all areas
of psychology. (See also *Subject Rights and Experimental Ethics*.) In addition, lifespan research is
faced with a handful of unique problems. One such
problem, already mentioned, is that of comparing
different cohorts. Many lifespan questions concern
important changes that occur with advancing age
or follow major transitions. Identifying and investigating these changes frequently require the comparison of different cohorts. Recall that a cohort is
identified in terms of time of birth. Thus people
born in 1950 are one cohort; those born in 1955
may be a different cohort. If, in 1985, we need to
compare thirty-five-year-olds with thirty-year-olds,
we are, in effect, comparing two different cohorts.
And we must now take into consideration the possibility that these two groups will be different in
1985, not because one of them is five years older

than the other but because of certain important
cohort-related historical influences.

A second problem specific to lifespan research
is related to difficulties experienced in obtaining
large, representative samples. Since most children
are in schools for a large part of their lives and are
therefore easily accessible to researchers, this
problem applies much less to them than it does to
older subjects. In fact, approximately only 5 percent of all very old people are in retirement homes
and other institutions for the aged.* Unfortunately,

---

*Although "very old" is uncomfortably vague, our studies and
theories of aging have not yet provided us with terms that are
specific and widely understood to discriminate among older
age groups as the terms *neonate, infant, toddler, child,* and
adolescent distinguish those who are younger. In this context,
the "very old" are above eighty.

this relatively small number of individuals serves as subjects for an overwhelming majority of studies of the aged. Accordingly, investigators must be concerned about whether these subjects are actually representative of others not living in institutions. They must also always keep in mind the point that as people become older and older, they may also become less and less representative. That is, there may be something special that allows ninety-year-olds to live so long. Death does not always select at random.

The use of institutionalized individuals in psychological research poses an additional problem relating to research ethics. First, not all elderly people are capable of informed consent; second, there are sometimes subtle forms of coercion involved in research with those in institutions. Some might feel pressured into participating simply by being members of a group; others might volunteer to please their attendants or to ensure favorable treatment.

■ The Book and Its Subject

A word of caution is appropriate at this point. This book deals in large part with so-called average individuals—with the normal processes of conception, fetal growth, birth, infancy, childhood, adolescence, adulthood, old age, and death. It describes typical behavior and characteristics throughout the lifespan, and it discusses theoretical explanations of normal patterns of development. *But there is no average child, let alone adult!* The concept is a convenient invention, a necessary creation if one is to speak coherently of those aspects of human development that are most important and most general. The reader should bear in mind that each person is a unique individual, that each will differ from the average, and that no one theory will account for all behavior. We are incredibly more complex than any description provided by even the most complex of theories. A theory—and a book—can deal only with the objective details of human behavior, not with its essence.

■ MAIN POINTS

1 The discipline concerned with understanding and explaining changes that occur between conception and death is *lifespan developmental psychology*.

2 Chronological age provides one convenient way of organizing lifespan events. In fact, however, these events are often related more closely to major life transitions (marriage or retirement, for example) than to age.

3 Models are metaphors (comparisons) that exist at different levels of generality. Two general models, the organismic and the mechanistic, underlie much of our developmental theorizing.

4 Organismic theories present a view of active, functioning biological organisms and are exemplified by Piaget's work; mechanistic theories stress the reactive, machinelike predictability of human functioning and are exemplified in Skinner's work.

5 Since models are really metaphors, they cannot be judged in terms of whether or not they are *correct* but in terms of their usefulness.

6 Among the recurring themes in studies of the lifespan are questions relating to the relative influence of heredity and environment, to whether development is continuous or progresses in discrete stages, and to whether development is

primarily linear and characterized initially by increments followed by inevitable decline in the latter stages of life.

7 The study of children is relatively recent in the history of psychology; the study of adult development and aging is even newer.

8 History is replete with evidence of child neglect and abuse, abandonment, exploitation, and shocking mortality rates. Advances in biology and medicine, changing social and economic conditions, the increasing availability of education, and the efforts of early child-study pioneers such as Locke (blank slate), Rousseau (the innocent child corrupted by the environment), Darwin, Binet, Hall, and Freud contributed a great deal to contemporary child psychology.

9 Although Quetelet wrote a book on aging in 1835 and Hall another in 1922, the study of adulthood and the processes of aging has become popular only recently. This new interest stems at least in part from changes in life expectancy and decreasing birthrates, which have resulted in a dramatic increase in the proportion of old to young.

10 Specific observational techniques in the study of human development include diary descriptions, specimen descriptions, time sampling, and event sampling.

11 In an experiment, the investigator assigns subjects to groups and controls relevant variables in an effort to determine whether independent variables affect dependent variables.

12 Correlational studies look at relationships among variables and provide useful information relating to cause-and-effect relationships, *although a correlation is not, by itself, proof of causation.*

13 There are two general approaches to developmental studies: Longitudinal studies examine the same individuals at different periods in their lives; cross-sectional studies compare different individuals at the same time. A combination of these approaches—a short-term longitudinal study—is sometimes employed.

14 Longitudinal and cross-sectional investigations occasionally have difficulty separating effects that are related primarily to age from those related to the time of testing or the cohort.

15 A cohort is a group of individuals born during a single timespan. Not only are these individuals of similar ages but they might also have been exposed to a variety of influences that are unique to their cohort and that might serve to account for important differences between them and members of other cohorts.

16 The validity and reliability of research results are subject to the influences of sample size and representativeness, subject memory and honesty, experimenter and subject biases, and cohort-related experiences. Truth, here as elsewhere, is relative and elusive.

17 The average individual is a conceptually useful invention, but does not exist.

■ FURTHER READINGS

Moving descriptions of changes in the status of children throughout history are provided by:

Aries, P. *Centuries of childhood: A social history of family life* (R. Baldick, Trans.). New York: Alfred A. Knopf, 1962. (Originally published, 1960.)

Kessen, W. *The child*. New York: John Wiley, 1965.

Science, both as a method and as an attitude, need not be nearly so esoteric and difficult as we sometimes imagine. For an entertaining, highly readable, and pertinent discussion of the role of research in the behavioral sciences, see:

McCain, G., & Segal, E. M. *The game of science* (4th ed.). Monterey, Calif.: Brooks/Cole, 1982.

Alternatively, you might consult Asimov's two-volume layperson's approach to understanding science:

Asimov, I. *The intelligent man's guide to science*. New York: Basic Books, 1963.

Not everyone believes that science is the only, or even the best, way of knowing. For a provocative and sometimes challenging view of science and our conception of reality, see:

Pearce, J. C. *The crack in the cosmic egg*. New York: Fawcett, 1971.

Contemporary methods of studying children are described in:

Irwin, D. M., & Bushnell, M. M. *Observational strategies for child study*. New York: Holt, Rinehart & Winston, 1980.

Those interested in a detailed analysis of cross-sectional and longitudinal research and in the development of a research model designed to overcome their limitations are referred to the following article:

Schaie, K. W. A general model for the study of developmental problems. *Psychological Bulletin*, 1965, 64, 92–107.

2 THEORIES OF HUMAN DEVELOPMENT

"Now, what I want is, Facts. Teach these boys and
girls nothing but Facts. Facts alone are wanted
in life. Plant nothing else, and root out everything
else. . . . Stick to Facts, sir!"

Charles Dickens
Hard Times

I do not mind lying, but I hate inaccuracy.

Samuel Butler
Note Books

T|he pickup is no longer behind us. It turned off into Fort Saskatchewan while we continue down the highway between giant petrochemical plants, nickel smelters, and car dealerships. The smell here is far worse than it was by the pigsty; it leaves an unnatural, metallic taste in our mouths, and I find myself driving a little faster, anxious to be where open windows might bring happy surprises of early roses or green alfalfa—or even pigsties.

Grandma is sleeping now. She has finished with doors and holes into pigsties and fox dens, and with dressing cats, and Denise might almost understand what we all know but keep forgetting. There really are many different ways of doing, understanding, and even of being.

I see her in the mirror, my grandmother. Her wire-frame glasses have slipped down her nose, a wisp of silvered hair over one lens. Her face is an elaborate pattern of tiny wrinkles, not even remotely like a dried prune or an aging apple; more like something an artist might do with a single sable hair. She lies there, her left hand on Marcel's head where it rests on her lap—he too, asleep. Her mouth has fallen open and I know that any minute now she will snore abruptly and awaken. And if I tell her that she was sleeping, she will deny it.

While things are quiet in the car, I want to get back quickly to our narrative. In this chapter, we're going to look at theories. An awesome term, *theory*. At worst, it evokes confused impressions of obscure concepts hidden in long, highly technical words; at best it connotes beliefs only slightly removed from outright lies—certainly some distance from fact. My own reactions to the term were initially conditioned by long hours in my grandmother's kitchen, where she would repeatedly and effectively terminate my brave ramblings with the rejoinder, "Yes, but that's just theory. Have you looked at the facts?" And then she would tell me what the facts were; they always contradicted my theory.

I might, to this day, have remained convinced that facts and theory are completely different, and that theory is what one resorts to only when the facts are unknown, had it not been for my grandmother's theory of excrement. (My cousins and I were less polite then; we called it Grandma's ___theory.)

We had been sitting on the porch one soft June night, she knitting and I dreaming, both looking at the garden. A fine garden with potatoes only two hills to a pail and carrots big as my arm. Interrupting my dreams of incredible future glories, I commented on the excellence of my grandmother's garden, taking fine political care to observe that Tremblay's potatoes were never so large or plentiful, and that his carrots were like pathetic shoestrings next to hers.

"It's the horse manure," she said matter of factly, the word being somewhat less offensive in French than in English. *Merde.*

"He uses manure, too," I said, ever ready to contradict the old lady. "Cow manure."

"Cow manure? It's manure, too. Why shouldn't his garden be as good? He uses a lot of it."

"I have a theory about that," said my grandmother. And I jumped right in, a better opportunity never before having presented itself.

"A theory?" Politely, of course. "But the facts, Grandma. We should speak of facts, not theory."

"The facts," she informed me, not unkindly, "are that I have a far better garden than Tremblay, that I use horse manure, and that he uses cow manure."

And the theory, as she explained at great length, simply accounted for the facts: It explained why horse manure favors potatoes and carrots; why chickens' droppings invigorate cabbages; why flattened and dried circles of cow dung excite flowers. It is not a simple theory, nor would it be of much interest to you, sophisticated as you are. But for my grandmother, a proud woman—proud of her favored potatoes and carrots, her invigorated cabbages, her excited flowers—it was of considerable interest.

■ Theory and Science

And for me, it was a lesson in theory—a lesson that I now pass on. Theory need not be a dusty collection of obscure pronouncements, nor does it substitute for fact when fact is absent. In its simplest sense, a theory is no more than an explanation of facts. As Thomas put it, to theorize is to suggest "(1) which facts are most important for understanding ... and (2) what sorts of relationships among facts are most significant for producing this understanding" (1979, p. 3).

Put another way, a theory is a collection of related statements that are intended to organize and explain a set of observations. But the goal of theorizing goes somewhat beyond explanation: In addition, it involves prediction and control. Thus, if my grandmother *understands* why specific man-

ures affect specific crops in given ways, she can not only *predict* these effects but also exercise a high degree of *control* over her garden (barring such acts of God as severe storms, locust infestations, or small boys chasing cats among the turnips).

Theories in human development are also intended to explain (hence lead to understanding); similarly, if they explain adequately, prediction and control should result. For example, if a theory explains why it is that some people are happy and others are not, then it should be possible, given relevant facts, to predict who will be happy. And if the circumstances affecting happiness are under our control, it should also be possible to bring happiness to saddened lives. Thus, theories may have a very practical aspect. At the same time, they are one of science's primary guides for doing research. In large part, it is a theory—sometimes crude, but sometimes elegant and refined—that tells the researcher where to look for a cure for cancer, what the cure will look like when it is found, and how it might be used. In the same way, psychology's theories tell the researcher where and how to look for personality or cognitive change in the lifespan; they also indicate why it might be important to look for this change.

Developing a Theory

Theories are seldom handed to philosophers and scientists carved into rock—or even written on paper. They arise, instead, from observations that are assumed to be factual and that are important enough to require explanation. Since they arise from observations, and since what different individuals choose to observe (that is, what they consider to be important and in need of explanation) may vary a great deal, there are many different theories in most areas of research. And since the underlying assumptions that theorists have about the nature of what they are studying are sometimes very different, so too might these various theories be very different. As we saw in Chapter 1, for example, two fundamental metaphors underlie a great many of our theories of human development: Humans are like machines, reducible to a number of elements whose functions can be precisely predicted, passive reactors to internal and external states (the *mechanistic* model); or humans are like living organisms, complex, exploring, and active (the *organismic* model). These underlying models affect not only what theorists observe but also the explanations they present for these observations.

The types of observations upon which scientific theories are based are seldom of the kind that were of such intimate interest to my grandmother. Science, if nothing else, insists upon a kind of objectivity, precision, and replicability that would have been difficult to obtain, to say the least, in my grandmother's garden. Science is actually less a collection of methods than an attitude. The scientific method that you might have been asked to learn in school (statement of problem, prediction, material, method, observation, conclusion) is simply a means of ensuring that observations are made under sufficiently controlled circumstances that they could be made by anyone else—that, in short, they can be replicated and confirmed. The attitude that characterizes science's search for explanation is precisely one that emphasizes the replicability of observations and demands precision in measuring and observing—hence the importance of the research methods described in the first chapter. If the facts upon which theories are based are themselves suspect, it is clear that the theory is not likely to be useful.

Evaluating Theories

Why, you might ask, must there be a variety of theories if a theory is simply an explanation of facts? Some of the reasons for this state of affairs have already been mentioned. Different theories may be used to explain quite different facts. And even the most general theories of development—those that would attempt to explain all of development—are not all based on the same observations; that is, theorists select observations that need to be explained. Furthermore, given the same set of observations, not all theorists will arrive at the same set of explanations. And, finally, fact (or truth) is no less elusive in developmental psychology than it is elsewhere. Our observations are often relative. They are more or less accurate depending on the precision of our observation (or measurement), and they are often pertinent only in specific circumstances and sometimes for specific individuals. We do not always generalize appropriately. And it is on generalizations that our theories are based.

Given these observations, it becomes apparent that a theory cannot easily be evaluated in terms of its accuracy or truthfulness. But it can be evaluated in other ways, most of which have to do with its usefulness. In other words, theories do not have to be accurate explanations of facts; they can be nothing more than useful attempts to explain important things.

Thomas (1979) suggests a number of criteria that might be employed to judge the "goodness" of a theory. Most important among these criteria are the following: A theory is good if it (1) accurately reflects the facts, (2) is expressed in a clearly understandable way, (3) is useful for predicting events as well as explaining ones that are past, (4) is applicable in a practical sense (that is, has real value for counselors, teachers, pediatricians, and so on), (5) is consistent within itself rather than self-contradictory, and (6) is not based on numerous assumptions (unproven beliefs).

■ Theories of Human Development

The remaining pages of this chapter present some of the most important and most distinctive theoretical approaches to the study of human development. These theories are grouped according to four major orientations: psychoanalytic, cognitive, behavioristic, and humanistic. Although these labels are useful in that they provide distinctions among different concerns and orientations, they can also be misleading if interpreted too narrowly. As will become apparent, most of the theoretical approaches described here have a number of characteristics in common.

Several additional theories of human development are presented in Chapter 13 rather than here because they relate primarily to the adult years of the lifespan. The theories presented here are more useful for understanding childhood and adolescence, as well as for understanding certain basic processes that underlie all of development.

■ Psychoanalytic Approaches

Psychoanalytic approaches are those that attempt to identify deep-seated, usually unconscious forces within individuals. These forces, in interaction with the environment, result in the development of personality.

Sigmund Freud

The name Freud brings to mind visions of a bespectacled and bearded psychiatrist sitting on a chair beside a deeply padded reclining couch upon which lies a patient suffering from some emotional distress. And although the image is appropriate, it is incomplete. Freud's theories do far more than simply provide an approach for understanding and attempting to treat mental disorders. Indeed, they are among the earliest systematic theories of development and are among the most intriguing and the richest in sheer wealth of detail. The picture presented of them here is necessarily highly simplified and somewhat selective.

Basic Ideas   Among the most fundamental Freudian ideas is the notion that human behavior, and consequently the direction that personality development takes, derives from two powerful tendencies: the urge to survive and the urge to procreate (Roazen, 1975). The survival instinct is of secondary importance because it is not usually endangered by our environments. (The Freudian term for environment is *reality*.) The urge to procreate, however, is constantly being discouraged and even prevented by reality; this accounts for the tremendous importance of sexuality in Freud's description of human development.

Sexuality, however, is a very broad term in Freud's writings. It means not only those activities that are clearly associated with sex but other behaviors and feelings, such as affection and love, as well as some behaviors such as eating. Sexual urges are sufficiently important in Freud's system that they are given a special term—**libido**. The libido is the source of energy for sexual urges; accordingly, the urges themselves are referred to as *libidinal urges*.

The General Developmental Process   The newborn infant has a simple, undeveloped personality, consisting solely of primitive, unlearned urges that will be a lifetime source of what Freud called *psychic energy*, the urges and desires that account for behavior. Freud's label for the child's earliest personality is **id**. Very simply, the *id* is made up of all the urges that we inherit. According to Freud, these urges are primarily sexual.

The Freudian infant is all instincts (unlearned tendencies) and reflexes, a bundle of energy seeking, almost desperately, to satisfy urges that are based upon a desire to survive and to procreate. The child has no idea of what is possible or impossible, no sense of reality. An infant has no conscience, no internal moral rules that control behavior. The most powerful urge at this stage is to seek immediate satisfaction of impulses. A child who is hungry does not wait. Now is the time for the nipple and sucking.

Almost from birth, the child's basic urges come into abrupt collision with reality. The hunger urge (linked with survival) cannot always be satisfied immediately. The *reality* of the situation is that the mother is frequently occupied elsewhere and the infant's satisfaction must often be delayed or occasionally denied. Similarly, the child learns that defecation cannot occur at will; parental demands conflict with the child's impulses. This constant conflict between the id and reality develops the second level of personality, the **ego**.

The ego grows out of a realization of what is possible and what is not; it is the rational level of human personality. It comes to include the realization that delaying gratification is often a desirable thing, that long-term goals sometimes require the denial of short-term goals. Although the id wants immediate gratification, the ego channels these desires in the most profitable direction for the individual. Note that the levels of personality represented by the id and the ego are not in opposition. They work together toward the same goal—satisfying the needs and urges of the individual.

The third level of personality—labeled the **superego**—sets itself up in opposition to the first two. The term *superego* refers to the moral aspects of personality. Like the ego, it develops from contact with reality, although it is more concerned with social than physical reality. The development of the superego **(conscience)** does not occur until early childhood. Freud assumed that it resulted

principally from a process of identifying with parents, particularly with the parent of the same sex as the child. To *identify* in a Freudian sense is to attempt to become *like* someone else—to adopt their values and beliefs as well as their behaviors. Thus, by identifying with their parents, children learn the religious and cultural rules that govern their parents' behaviors. These rules then become part of the child's superego. And it is very significant that many religious rules, as well as many social and cultural rules, oppose the urges of the id. Hence, the superego and the id are generally in conflict; Freud assumed that this conflict accounts for much deviant behavior.

In summary, Freud's theory establishes three levels of personality: the id, the ego, and the superego (see Figure 2.1). The first is the source of energy or motivation, deriving from instincts for survival and procreation. The ego is reality oriented and intervenes between the id and the superego to maintain a balance between the id's urges and the superego's rules. It is as though the id were continually saying, "I want to eat; I want to be caressed; I want to possess; I want to kill that sow," while the superego chides (in a grating, confessional voice, to be sure), "Don't you dare; deny your desires; thou shalt not steal or otherwise molest; hands off that sow." And the ego, seated between these warring forces, attempts calmly to make peace: "Have you considered eating only at mealtime and with some moderation? Smoke a cigarette instead. Perhaps you should think of marrying. As for that sow, let the farmer kill it. You can watch. How would that be?"

Psychosexual Stages   Freud's account of the development of the three levels of personality may be interpreted as a description of development. His ideas are also relevant for understanding the motivational changes that occur as an individual develops. Freud divides changes in motivation into a sequence of stages that are distinguishable by the objects or activities necessary for the satisfaction of the individual's urges during that stage (see Table 2.1). The labels for each stage reflect changes

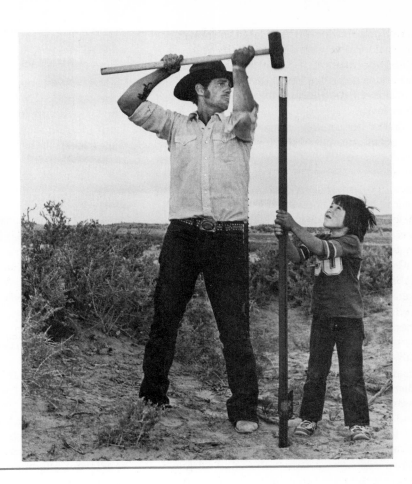

According to Freud, identification is fundamentally involved in the development of conscience (superego). To identify with someone is to do far more than imitate his or her behaviors; it involves attempting to become *like* someone by adopting his or her values and beliefs.

in the areas of sexual satisfaction as the child matures, beginning with the **oral stage** and progressing through the **anal stage**, the **phallic stage**, a **latency stage**, and finally the **genital stage**. Like many other developmental theorists, Freud seemed to believe that human development ends with the onset of adulthood. Accordingly, his developmental theories are more appropriate for understanding the changes of childhood and adolescence than for understanding the changes of adulthood.

Fixation and Regression   In a simplified sense, the development of personality can take three routes. It can follow the normal route described earlier, in which children progress through each stage, developing ego and superego as they mature, so that they become socially well-adjusted individuals. According to Freud, whether or not an individual attains the desired ends depends on the amount of sexual gratification received during each of the phases of development, and if the amount of sexual gratification is too little or too great, one of two possibilities may occur. First, an individual might develop a **fixation**, in which normal development ceases at a certain stage and further development of personality is restricted and incomplete. This is assumed to occur primarily from excessive gratification of sexual impulses at a particular stage. However, when sexual impulses are insufficiently gratified, the individual may *regress* to a previous stage that was happier. **Regression** and fixation are the alternatives to normal, healthy development.

Fixation implies preoccupation with the activities that resulted in sexual gratification while in the fixated stage. Adults partially fixated at the oral stage are described as dependent, demanding, and preoccupied with oral gratification. In this sense, they are very much like infants—unwilling or unable to initiate activities and highly dependent on others. External manifestations of an oral fixation might also include behaviors such as chewing fingernails, smoking, drinking, and otherwise exercising the mouth, lips, and tongue. The anally fixated character is compulsive, stingy, hoarding, and perhaps aggressive. Hoarding compulsions are apparently related to the pleasure an infant derives from withholding feces during the anal phase of development. Similarly, phallic characters are primarily concerned with satisfying sexual urges, without regard for the objects of their sexual gratification. They are the sadists or rapists.

Some Defense Mechanisms   Mention of Freud's theories is incomplete without a consideration of **defense mechanisms**—the common, although sometimes unhealthy, methods many employ to compensate for their inability to satisfy the demands of the id and to overcome the anxiety that accompanies the continual struggle between the id and the superego (Freud, 1946). Defense mechanisms are invented by the ego in its role as a mediator between the id and the superego; they are the ego's attempt to establish peace between the two so that the person can continue to operate in an apparently healthy manner. A number of classical Freudian defense mechanisms are summarized in Table 2.2.

Freud in Review

Freud's theory, despite its tremendous influence in psychology, is open to serious criticism. To begin

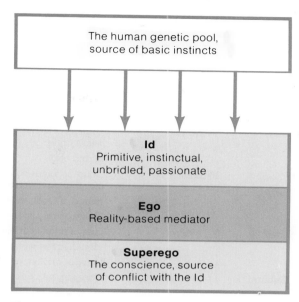

Figure 2.1
The Freudian conception of the three levels of human personality in order of development.

with, it is clearly weak from a scientific standpoint (see Clark, 1980; Fisher & Greenberg, 1977; Rothstein, 1980). The data upon which the theory is based were typically derived from a small number of cases, were obtained in unsystematic fashion, were seldom quantified, and usually depended on the interpretation of a single individual—Freud himself. In addition, the theory is often unclear, uses terms in contradictory fashion, and leads to a variety of competing predictions. Finally, Freud's excessive reliance on sexual and aggressive impulses as the most important forces in shaping personality development proved to be one of the main reasons why a number of his most ardent students and followers eventually departed significantly from his theories. Note, however, that Freud's emphasis on sexual impulses was probably largely a reflection of the Victorian social system—a system characterized by extreme sexual repression (by contemporary standards) and by a firm belief in male superiority.

In spite of its weaknesses, Freud's theory pro-

Table 2.1 Freud's stages of psychosexual development.

Stage	Approximate Age	Characteristics
Oral	0–8 months	Sources of pleasure include sucking, biting, swallowing, playing with lips.
		Preoccupation with immediate gratification of impulses.
		Id is dominant.
Anal	8–18 months	Sources of sexual gratification include expelling feces and urination, as well as retaining feces.
		Id and ego.
Phallic	18 months–6 years	Child becomes concerned with genitals. Source of sexual pleasure involves manipulating genitals.
		Period of Oedipus or Electra complex.
		Id, ego, and superego.
Latency	6–11 years	Loss of interest in sexual gratification.
		Identification with parent of same sex.
		Id, ego, and superego.
Genital	11 onward	Concern with adult modes of sexual pleasure, barring fixations or regressions.

vides an immensely rich basis for understanding personality and has led to the formulation of other major theories, among them that of Erik Erikson, which we look at next.

Erik Erikson

The **developmental theory** advanced by Erik Erikson (1956, 1959, 1961, 1968) draws heavily on the work of Freud but with a number of crucial differences. Recall that one of Freud's primary emphases was on the role of sexuality (libido) as a source of motivation for behavior and the importance of conflicts involving id, ego, and superego in determining personality and mental health. In contrast, Erikson de-emphasizes the importance of sexuality and of psychodynamic conflicts and instead emphasizes the importance of the child's social environment. His theory may be described as a theory of **psychosocial** rather than **psychosexual** development.

A second departure from Freudian theory is Erikson's emphasis on the role of the ego rather than the superego. The theory is essentially more positively oriented, being concerned with the development of a healthy ego (of *identity*, in Erikson's terms) rather than with the resolution of powerful internal conflicts. This—Erikson's concern with the healthy personality—describes a third important difference between his work and that of Freud.

Psychosocial Stages

Erikson describes human development in terms of eight stages, the first five of which span infancy, childhood, and adolescence; the last three describe adulthood. Each of Erikson's stages involves a basic conflict, brought about primarily by a need to adapt to the social environment. Resolution of this conflict results in the development of a sense of competence. Although Erikson's first five stages closely parallel Freud's psychosexual stages in terms of ages, his descriptions and his emphases are quite different. The stages are described briefly here and are summarized in Table 2.3.

Trust Versus Mistrust Erikson (1959) maintains that one of the most basic components of a

Table 2.2 Some Freudian defense mechanisms.

Mechanism	One Possible Manifestation
Displacement A suppressed behavior appears in a more acceptable form.	A potential murderer hunts subhuman primates.
Reaction formation Behavior is the opposite of what the individual would like it to be.	A woman loves an unobtainable man and behaves as though she dislikes him.
Intellectualization Behavior is stripped of its emotional concomitants.	A grown man who loves his mother too dearly treats her with extreme consideration, kindness, and devotion but convinces himself that he is motivated by duty and not by love.
Projection People come to believe that their own undesirable feelings or inclinations are more descriptive of others than of themselves.	A claustrophobic individual who unconsciously avoids closed spaces is amazed at the number of people who suffer from claustrophobia.
Denial Reality is distorted to make it conform to the individual's wishes.	A heavy smoker is unable to give up the habit and decides that there is no substantial evidence linking nicotine with human disease.
Repression Unpleasant experiences are stored deep in the subconscious mind and become inaccessible to waking memory.	A soldier comes very close to death, but remembers no details of the event.

healthy personality is a sense of trust and that this sense of trust toward oneself and toward others develops in the first year of life. The infant is initially faced with a profound conflict between mistrust of a world about which little is known and an inclination to develop a trusting attitude toward that world. Because most initial contact with the environment is through the child's mouth, one of the first developmental tasks is to acquire sufficient trust of the world to explore it willingly with the mouth. With this trust come feelings of security and comfort. These feelings remain in conflict, however, with inclinations not to trust; although the infant will generally have acquired a sense of trust during the first year of life, resolution of this conflict and, indeed, of all others descriptive of the developmental process continues throughout later stages.

Autonomy Versus Shame and Doubt The second of Freud's major stages, the anal stage, corresponds with the second of Erikson's psychosocial stages. During this second stage, children begin to realize that they are authors of their own actions. Initially the child does not deliberately act upon the world, but reacts to it. Sucking, for example, is not engaged in when the child *intends* to suck, but rather when appropriate stimulation is provided. With the recognition that they can carry out some of the behaviors that they intend, children develop a sense of autonomy. This autonomy, however, is threatened by children's inclination to avoid responsibility for their own actions, to go back to the comfort and security that characterized the first stage (Erikson, 1961). But children experience shame and doubt at this inclination; the ultimate resolution of the conflict occurs when they develop a sense of autonomy.

Initiative Versus Guilt By the age of four or five, children have resolved the crises of autonomy; in short, they have discovered that they are somebody. During the next stage, they must discover who it is that they are (Erikson, 1959). True to his Freudian orientation, Erikson assumes that children seek to discover who they are by attempting to be like their parents. It is during this stage that they establish a wider physical environment, made possible by their greater freedom of movement. During this period their understanding of

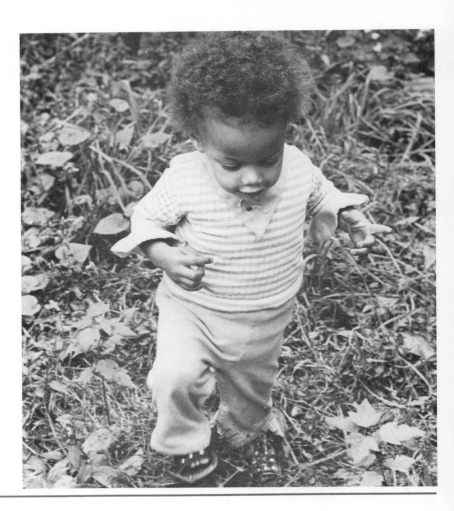

For Erikson, development involves the resolution of important conflicts through acquiring new competencies. For example, as children learn that they can carry out some of the behaviors they intend, they develop a sense of autonomy that surmounts earlier doubts and fears.

language becomes sufficiently advanced for them not only to be able to ask many questions and understand some of the answers but also to permit them to imagine all sorts of possibilities concerning themselves. With their increasing exploration of the environment, children need to develop a sense of initiative with respect to their behaviors. They are autonomous as well as responsible for initiating behavior.

Industry Versus Inferiority   The fourth developmental phase, corresponding to Freud's latency period, is marked by the child's increasing need to interact with and be accepted by peers. It now becomes crucial for children to discover that their selves, their identities, are significant, that they can do things; in short, they find that they are competent. Children now avail themselves of all opportunities to learn those things they think are important to their culture, hoping that by so doing they will become someone. This is the source of their rising feelings of industry. Although this stage corresponds to Freud's latency period, Erikson points out clearly that the only sense in which the child may be considered latent is in the formation

Table 2.3 Erikson's worksheet of developmental phases.

Psychosocial Crises	Radius of Significant Relations	Related Elements of Social Order	Psychosocial Modalities	Psychosexual Stages
1 Trust versus mistrust	Maternal person	Cosmic order	To get To give in return	Oral-respiratory, sensory-kinesthetic (incorporative modes)
2 Autonomy versus shame, doubt	Parental persons	"Law and order"	To hold (on) To let (go)	Anal-urethral, muscular (retentive-eliminative)
3 Initiative versus guilt	Basic family	Ideal prototypes	To make (= going after) To "make like" (= playing)	Infantile-genital, locomotor (intrusive, inclusive)
4 Industry versus inferiority	"Neighborhood," school	Technological elements	To make things (= completing) To make things together	"Latency"
5 Identity and repudiation versus identity diffusion	Peer groups and outgroups; models of leadership	Ideological perspectives	To be oneself (or not to be) To share being oneself	Puberty
6 Intimacy and solidarity versus isolation	Partners in friendship, sex, competition, cooperation	Patterns of cooperation and competition	To lose and find oneself in another	Genitality
7 Generativity versus self-absorption	Divided labor and shared household	Currents of education and tradition	To make be To take care of	
8 Integrity versus despair	"Mankind," "My kind"	Wisdom	To be, through having been To face not being	

Reprinted from Erik H. Erikson, Identity and the life cycle, by permission of W. W. Norton & Company, Inc. Copyright © 1980 by W. W. Norton & Company, Inc. Copyright © 1959 by International Universities Press, Inc.

of heterosexual attachments. In all other ways, children are much more active than latent.

Identity Versus Identity Diffusion   Erikson's fifth developmental stage, corresponding to the beginning of Freud's genital period and dealing directly with the period ordinarily referred to as pre- or early adolescence, involves the development of a sense of identity. Here, Erikson's emphasis on the ego becomes most evident. The development of a strong sense of identity implies the development of a strong ego—hence Erikson's expression, *ego identity*. The crisis implicit in this stage concerns a conflict between a strong sense of **self** and the diffusion of self-concepts.

At a simple level, the formation of an identity appears to involve arriving at a notion not so much of who one is but rather of who one can be. In other words, adolescents are not faced with the task of discovering who they are, but rather of developing one of several potential selves. The source of conflict resides in the various possibilities open to the child—possibilities that are magnified by the variety of models in the environment. Conflict and doubt regarding choice of identity lead to what Erikson terms *identity diffusion*. It is as though adolescents are torn between early acceptance of a clearly defined self and the dissipation of their energies as they experiment with a variety of roles.

Erikson's description of development does not end with adolescence, but continues through the entire lifespan. He describes three additional psychosocial conflicts that occur during adulthood and old age and that require new competencies and adjustments. The first of these, *intimacy and solidarity versus isolation*, relates to the need to develop intimate relationships with others (as oppposed to being isolated) and is particularly crucial for marital and parenting roles. The second, *generativity versus self-absorption*, describes a need to assume social, work, and community responsibilities that will be beneficial to others (that will be generative), rather than remaining absorbed in the self. And the third has to do with facing the inevitability of our own ends and realizing that life has meaning—that we should not despair because its end is imminent. The three Eriksonian stages that span adulthood are discussed in greater detail in Chapter 13.

Erikson in Review

Erikson's theory is referred to as a theory of the life cycle, of ego psychology, of psychosocial development, or as a psychoanalytically oriented theory concerned mainly with the development of a healthy personality. He describes development in terms of a series of crises through which the individual progresses. Each of these involves a conflict between new abilities or attitudes and inclinations that oppose them. The resolution of conflicts results in the development of a sense of competence with respect to a specific capability that is primarily social—hence *psychosocial* development. The resolution of conflicts is never perfected during one developmental phase, but continues through succeeding stages—hence the concept of *life cycle*. Perhaps the most crucial crisis involves the development of a strong sense of identity—hence the concept *ego psychology*.

Note that although Erikson ties ages to each of these psychosocial stages, the ages do little more than indicate a very general sequence. This is particularly true during adulthood, when important social, physical, and emotional events such as retirement, children leaving home, illness, and death occur at widely varying ages and sometimes in a totally unpredictable sequence. Some of the important social and physical changes of childhood are far more predictable; hence ages tied to the psychosocial crises of childhood are more likely to be somewhat accurate.

Erikson's theory, like that of Freud, does not lend itself well to experimental validation. Both are based on untestable assumptions, and neither is particularly useful for making specific predictions about individuals. What Erikson's theory provides is a general framework for describing and interpreting some of the major changes that occur in the lifespan. Its usefulness rests largely in the insights that sometimes result from examining the lives of individuals within the context of the theory.

■ A Cognitive Approach

Whereas psychoanalytic theorists are concerned primarily with personality development, another approach focuses on the cognitive development of children. Chief among cognitive developmental theorists is Jean Piaget, whose work is introduced briefly in the following section and discussed in more detail in sections of subsequent chapters that deal specifically with the intellectual characteristics of children at different ages.

Jean Piaget

The questions people ask when they arrive somewhere unfamiliar to them, or when they begin work in an area previously unknown, are necessarily colored by the information, the prejudices, and the habits that they bring with them. Because Piaget's early training was in biology, it is not surprising that he applied the questions of biology to his study of children. Biologists are concerned with the **adaptation** of species. Accordingly, there are two questions of overriding concern to them: First, they ask what it is that has allowed some organisms to survive while others have passed into oblivion; second, they are concerned with developing classifications of species—with ordering them from the simplest to the most complex, or from the first to the most recent.

Piaget asked two questions about human development that parallel these biological questions. His first question focused on adaptation: What is it in the child's makeup that permits adaptation to this increasingly complex world? Second, he attempted to develop some method for classifying the progressive adaptation of the child: How can human development be organized and classified? In brief, Piaget applied questions of biology to human development. The summary provided in this chapter focuses on his answers to these questions.

Adaptation   Piaget's story of development is a story of adaptation. Children are not born knowing how to cope with the world; indeed, they do not know that the world exists as an external reality until late in the first year of their lives or even in the second. Their simple behaviors are limited to a number of reflexes, some of which are crucial for development. Underlying these simple reflexes are some mental or cognitive representations related to them. That is, there must be some neurological something that underlies sucking, reaching, grasping, and so on. Piaget labels this cognitive (intellectual or mental) representation of a behavior a **scheme** (sometimes used interchangeably with *schema* or *schemata*). Schemes exist at birth but are imperfectly suited for the tasks that face the child. From the first moment, survival demands change. Put another way, survival requires adaptation. And adaptation, according to Piaget, occurs through the interplay of two related processes, **assimilation** and **accommodation**.

Assimilation involves using activities that are already learned. Thus, when infants suck a nipple, they can be said to be assimilating properties of the nipple to the activity of sucking—to the suck-

ing *scheme*, in other words. Frequently, however, the environment requires that behavior change. A lollipop, for example, cannot be sucked in exactly the same manner as a nipple. In this instance, the child must modify behavior to conform to the environment. These changes define accommodation. In short, assimilation is the exercising of an already learned behavior; accommodation involves modification of this behavior. Through the interplay of assimilation and accommodation, the child adapts to a progressively more complex environment throughout the course of development.

Developmental Stages   According to Piaget, development consists of a series of **stages** through which each child passes. Each stage is marked by strikingly different perceptions of the world and adaptations to it; each is the product of learning that occurred during the previous stage and a preparation for the stage that follows. These stages and their major characteristics are discussed briefly here and summarized in Table 2.4.

Sensorimotor Period   During the first two years of life the child is in the **sensorimotor period**, so called because during this period the child understands the world largely through immediate action and sensation. For the infant, the world exists *here and now*. It is real only when it is being acted upon and sensed. When the ball is no longer being chewed, it ceases to be. Although the understanding begins near the end of the first year, it is only toward the end of the second year that children finally realize that objects have a permanence and an identity of their own—that they continue to exist when they are out of sight. Toward the end of the first two years, the child begins to acquire language and progresses slowly from a sensorimotor to a *symbolic* intelligence.

Preoperational Thinking   Following the acquisition of language, the child enters the lengthy period of **preoperational thought** (ages two to seven).

Among the various characteristics of the child's thinking during the preoperational period, one of the more interesting is an excessive reliance on

Table 2.4 Piaget's stages of cognitive development.

Stage	Approximate Age	Some Major Characteristics*
Sensorimotor	0–2 years	Intelligence in action. World of the here and now. No language, no thought in early stages. No notion of objective reality.
Preoperational	2–7 years	Egocentric thought. Reason dominated by perception. Intuitive rather than logical solutions. Inability to conserve.
Concrete operations	7–11 or 12 years	Ability to conserve. Logic of classes and relations. Understanding of number. Thinking bound to concrete. Development of reversibility in thought.
Formal operations	11 or 12 to 14 or 15 years	Complete generality of thought. Propositional thinking. Ability to deal with the hypothetical. Development of strong idealism.

*Each of these characteristics is detailed in appropriate sections of Chapters 5, 7, 9, and 11.

perception rather than on logic. Piaget illustrated this by reference to his famous *conservation* experiments. In one of these experiments, for example, children are presented with two glasses, each of which contains an equal amount of water. The experimenter then pours the contents of one glass into a tall, thin tube—or, alternately, into a low, flat dish. The child is now asked whether each of the containers still has the same amount of water or whether one has more than the other. Preoperational children, relying on the appearance of the two containers, almost invariably say that the tall tube has more because it is higher (or less because it is thinner)—or that the flat dish has more because it is "fatter" (or less because it is shorter). And even when they realize that the water could be poured back into the original container so that both would then be equal, preoperational children continue to rely on perception (on actual appearance) rather than on reasoning.

Concrete Operations   The major acquisition of the next period of development is the ability to think operationally (concrete operations, ages seven or eight to eleven or twelve). An **operation** is a thought—what Piaget called an internalized action. In this sense, **operational thought** is a mental action or, more precisely, an operation performed on ideas according to certain rules of logic. These rules of logic permit the concrete operations child to scoff at the ridiculous simplicity of a conservation problem. Of course, there is the same amount of water in both containers since none has been added or taken away, since one misleading dimension is compensated for by the other (it is taller *but* thinner), and since the act of pouring the water from one container to the other can be reversed to prove that nothing has changed. The concrete operations child is capable of this kind of logic. But this logic is tied to real, concrete objects and events. The child is still unable to reason logically about hypothetical situations or events and cannot go from the real to the merely possible or from the possible to the actual. Thought is bound to the real world, the concrete—hence the label *concrete operations*.

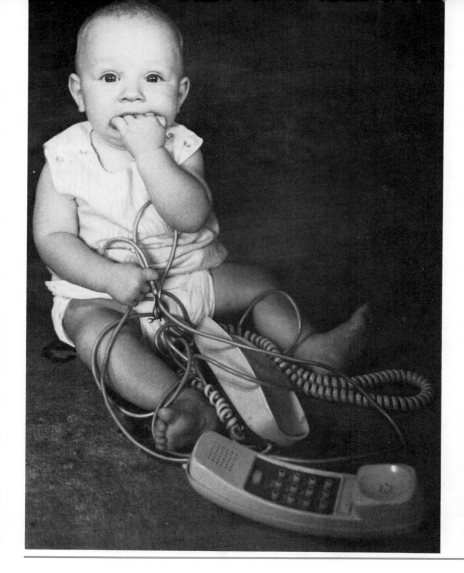

For the sensorimotor infant, the world derives its existence and its meaning from actions that can be performed on it. Thumbs, fingers, entire hands, and even telephones are to chew, suck, smell, taste, and sometimes look at.

Formal Operations   When children finally liberate themselves from the restrictions that have bound them to the concrete world, they enter the last stage of cognitive development—*formal operations*—beginning around the age of eleven or twelve and ending at fourteen or fifteen. During this stage, the child's thought becomes as logical as it will ever be; it is the culmination of a decade of preparation.

Piaget in Review

Development, in Piaget's view, is best described as the emergence of progressively more logical forms of thought—that is, as the development of ways of thinking that become increasingly effective in freeing children from the present and allowing them to use powerful symbols to understand and to manipulate the environment. According to the theory, the major characteristics of thinking in each of the four developmental stages influence all aspects of children's understanding of the world, including their notions of space, time, number, reality, causality, and so on.

A theory such as Piaget's is considerably easier to evaluate objectively than are the psychoanalytic approaches. For example, it makes specific predictions about how average children function intellectually at different age levels. And an enormous number of these predictions have been tested by countless researchers. In general, this research confirms Piaget's initial findings, particularly with respect to the order of stages, although confirmation has not always been obtained concerning the ages at which different children reach specific stages. Note, however, that Piaget has always emphasized that the most important aspects of his stage theory relate to the sequence of intellectual development and not to specific ages.

In summary, Piaget's theory provides a significant contribution to the understanding of intellectual growth. Its major weakness from an applied point of view is that it says relatively little about individual differences among children, about the factors that might account for these differences, or about what can be done to promote intellectual development. In addition, the language and concepts of the theory are sometimes difficult. For example, terms such as *assimilation* and *accom-*

RIEGEL'S DIALECTICAL VIEW OF DEVELOPMENT

Webster's Third New International Dictionary defines *dialectics* as "the process of self-development or unfolding (as of an action, event, idea, ideology, movement, or institution) through the stages of thesis, antithesis, and synthesis...." It then goes on to define *dialectical* as being "marked by a dynamic internal tension, conflict, and interconnectedness of its parts or elements."

And what might dialectics have to do with human development? A great deal according to Klaus Riegel (1970, 1972, 1976), who argues that our conventional views of development as a series of stages or plateaus characterized by a state of balance or equilibrium are incorrect and misleading. According to Riegel, lifespan human development is best viewed in terms of sequences of conflicts, crises, or contradictions and their continued resolution. The concept of *dialectics* is implicit in the view that conflicts or crises arise from contradictory actions and reactions—the classical situation of thesis leading to an antithesis and finally being resolved in a synthesis. But whereas most developmental theories deal primarily with a single facet of development, Riegel's theory applies to development in four dimensions: the inner-biological, individual-psychological, cultural-sociological, and outer-physical.

At a simple level, human development may be seen as progressions in each of these four areas. For example, we grow physically even as hormonal changes lead us to sexual maturity, our intellectual processes alter, and our social positions and interests shift. However, these changes do not always occur in synchrony. For example, sexual maturity might lead a young adolescent toward behaviors that are culturally difficult. From this lack of synchrony conflict arises, and conflict is the root of dialectical processes. Resolution of conflicts may lead to new developments, some of which require major reorganizations in one or more of the four areas of development. And when the reorganization is sufficiently dramatic, we might be tempted to recognize a *stage* or a *plateau*. But a dialectical view does not emphasize the plateau or the equilibrium—as does Piaget's theory, for example. Instead, it views development as a continuous process since the organism and society are never still. Change is constant and complete synchrony is therefore rare and fleeting.

Riegel criticizes Piaget's approach to human development on several grounds. As noted earlier, he feels that the concept of stages characterized by equilibrium is inappropriate in view of the continuous tension, conflict, and change that characterize a *dialectical* progression. In addition, he argues that Piaget considers only limited aspects of human development. With respect to children, for example, Piaget emphasizes the interaction of the child with a variety of objects and events in the environment, but pays too little attention to the most *modation* cannot easily be defined in operational terms; nor is it clear that such concepts provide significant insights into the development and functioning of children. Notwithstanding this, Piagetian theory has been widely and successfully employed in many educational enterprises. (See the box *Riegel's Dialectical View of Development* for additional criticism of Piaget.)

■ Learning-Theory Approaches

The theories presented thus far describe development in terms of progression through a fixed sequence of stages, with approximate ages corresponding to each of these stages. Freud's emphasis is on the development of personality, Erikson's is on social development, and Piaget's emphasis is on intellectual development. In contrast, learning-theory approaches, also called behavioristic approaches, do not describe stages of development; nor are they concerned with the historical causes of behavior. Instead, behavioristic approaches to understanding children attempt to explain how the *environment* influences behavior and development.

According to the behavioristic approaches, there are two broad classes of learning that account for human behavior: classical conditioning and operant conditioning. Conditioning is a general

important of these objects: namely, other children who also interact with the environment, as well as mothers and fathers. Accordingly, while Piaget has succeeded in describing some of the important aspects of the *rational* growth of the child, he has neglected "the fundamental basis of cognitive operations, the social basis of human being" (Riegel, 1976, p. 691).

A final criticism of approaches such as Piaget's is perhaps even more important for a study of the lifespan. Specifically, Riegel argues that in addition to being limited to the "logical" rather than the "artistic and creative," these approaches cannot deal with maturity. They can trace the development of thinking to adolescence, but since the emphasis is always on the the attainment of a stage, they cannot lead us where there are no stages. Since such theories view development as a series of achievements that culminate in adolescence, they have little to say about what might happen following adolescence. When there are no more contradictions to be resolved—no more crises—where does development go?

Riegel's (1973b) answer is simple: There are always more contradictions and more crises. And one of the signs of maturity is the acceptance of contradiction as "a fundamental ingredient of action and thought and not as an insufficiency that has to be denied" (1973b, p. 480). Accordingly, Riegel (1973a) proposes a fifth Piaget-ian stage—a dialectical stage similar to one described by Arlin (1975) as a *problem-finding* stage. In this fifth Piagetian stage, there are no clear plateaus—no levels of cognitive accomplishment clearly evident in the ability to solve a new class of problems. Instead, there is a renewed realization that development occurs on different levels, that it is replete with contradictions, and that different levels of behavior are entirely appropriate. As Riegel notes, a laborer might remain at the level of concrete operations, and a dancer, at a sensorimotor level.

"The developmental and aging processes . . . are founded upon the ability to tolerate contradictions and insufficiencies in action and thought," Riegel informs us; he adds, "this ability has been buried as a consequence of physical restrictions, normative social pressure, and especially, formal education" (1973b, p. 482).

Although it is still too early to evaluate the impact and the usefulness of Riegel's ideas, it is likely that his emphasis on some of the aspects of development that have largely been ignored by other theorists and his insistence that conflict and resolutions continue in dialectical fashion throughout life in all areas of development will eventually be recognized as major contributions to the understanding of our lives.

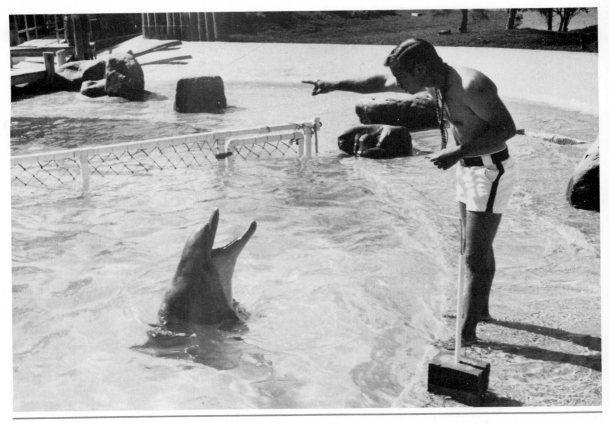

Learning theory approaches to understanding development look at how the environment influences behavior. In *conditioning* procedures such as depicted here, carefully contrived environments that control rewards and punishments are employed to shape highly complex animal behaviors.

term that refers to the various processes by which behaviors (responses) become associated with different circumstances (stimuli). These processes define **classical** and **operant conditioning**—topics that we look at next.

Classical Conditioning

Among early contributors to modern knowledge about human learning was Russian psychologist Ivan Pavlov. In the course of research that he was doing with dogs, Pavlov (1927) observed that the older and more experienced animals in his laboratory began to salivate when they saw their keeper approaching. Because none of the dogs

had ever tasted the keeper, Pavlov reasoned that they were salivating not because they expected to eat him now but probably because they had formed some sort of **association** between the sight of the keeper and the presentation of food. This observation led Pavlov to a series of investigations of a simple form of learning called classical conditioning (see Figure 2.2).

Consider a simple illustration of classical conditioning. I can condition my dog to jump, using a number of different methods. And most of these methods are as gentle and humane as I am. One method, not among the most gentle and humane, would be to approach the beast, say "Jump," and kick him squarely where he sits. That the dog now jumps has nothing to do with the spoken **stimu-**

lus "jump"; rather it has to do with the kick, a far more powerful stimulus for making dogs jump. Now, if I repeat this procedure a number of times, and perhaps over a number of days, the day will surely come when it will no longer be necessary to kick the dog to make it jump. Even a dog as stupid as my George will eventually jump when he hears me say "Jump." In one sense, the stimulus "Jump" can now be substituted for the stimulus kick. Both bring about the same **response.**

The psychology of learning has its own language for the stimuli and responses involved in classical conditioning. The stimulus that is part of the original stimulus-response link (the reflex) is termed the **unconditioned stimulus** (UCS). Food in the mouth of Pavlov's dog, a gentle kick in the other end of mine—both are unconditioned stimuli. They lead to a response without any new learning having taken place. The stimulus that is originally neutral but comes to be effective through repeated pairing with the unconditioned stimulus is called the conditioning or **conditioned stim-**

ulus (CS). The bell or buzzer for Pavlov's dog and the command "Jump" for mine are examples of conditioned stimuli. Eventually these stimuli elicit responses similar to those originally made only for unconditioned stimuli. Corresponding responses are termed the **unconditioned response** (UCR) or the **conditioned response** (CR), depending on whether they occur in response to the unconditioned or the conditioned stimulus. Thus salivating in response to a buzzer is a conditioned response, as is jumping in response to a verbal command. The process involved in classical conditioning is illustrated in Figure 2.2.

A well-known study demonstrating classical conditioning of emotional responses in children is reported by Watson and Rayner (1920). Watson observed that infants react with fear to loud noises, and he deduced that it should therefore be possible to make a child fear any other distinctive stimulus simply by pairing it frequently enough with a loud noise. In this case the noise is an unconditioned stimulus because it elicits a fear

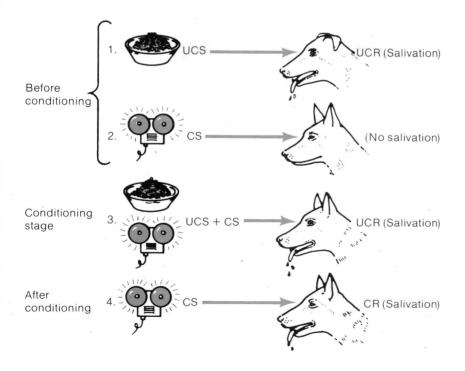

Before conditioning	1. UCS ⟶	UCR (Salivation)
	2. CS ⟶	(No salivation)
Conditioning stage	3. UCS + CS ⟶	UCR (Salivation)
After conditioning	4. CS ⟶	CR (Salivation)

Figure 2.2
Classical conditioning. In 1, an unconditioned stimulus leads to an unconditioned response, whereas in 2 a conditioning stimulus does not lead to the same response. In 3, the unconditioned stimulus is paired with the conditioning stimulus a number of times so that eventually the conditioning stimulus alone elicits the original response, as in 4.

response without any learning having taken place; the responses associated with fear are therefore unconditioned responses. The neutral stimulus that Watson and Rayner chose was a white rat. Contrary to what you might think, a white rat does not usually frighten most young children. The unwitting subject was an eleven-month-old infant named Albert. To demonstrate the effectiveness of classical conditioning in producing emotional reactions, each time Watson and Rayner presented little Albert with the rat, they made a loud noise behind Albert. As was expected, the poor infant reacted with a great deal of fear. After repeating the procedure seven times, Watson and Rayner ceased making the noise, but simply presented the rat to Albert. Now, as soon as the child saw the rat, he was terrified and began to whimper, attempting desperately to crawl away.

Although Watson and Rayner's experiment with Albert is probably more systematic and deliberate than most situations in which we acquire emotional reponses, the results can be generalized to development in general. There is considerable evidence that emotional reactions do transfer from one situation to another. People who react with fear to the sound of a dentist's drill are not trembling because the *sound* of the drill has been responsible for any pain they have felt in the past. But the sound of the drill has previously been associated with pain and has thus acquired the capability of eliciting reactions that are associated with pain. Similarly, children who dislike their teacher and who react negatively to the presence of that teacher may eventually react negatively to the classroom itself, or perhaps to school-related activities, or to adults who resemble the teacher, or to children who resemble other students in the class, or to pencils.

Operant Conditioning

A classical conditioning model is sometimes useful for explaining the learning of simple behaviors that occur in response to specific stimuli. As Skinner (1953, 1957, 1961) has pointed out, however, a great many human behaviors or responses are not **elicited** by any obvious stimuli, but appear instead to be **emitted** by the organism, for whatever reason. Skinner labeled such behavior an **operant**; a response elicited by stimuli, he labeled a **respondent**. Having described these two major classes of behavior, Skinner undertook the work for which he has now become famous: explaining how operant behavior is learned.

The simplest explanation of operant conditioning (also called *instrumental learning*) is that the *consequences* of a response determine whether it is learned or not learned. Put simply, behaviors that are reinforced will tend to be repeated; those that are not reinforced (or that are punished) are less likely to occur again. This is fundamentally different from saying that learning will occur as a function of the pairing of stimuli regardless of consequences. When little Albert reacted with fear to the rat, it was not because his fear responses led to pleasant consequences, but because the rat was paired with some other fear-producing situation.

One of Skinner's first tasks was to define the nature of reinforcement. Because he was determined to be objective and because he did not intend to formulate elaborate theories to explain what he observed, he advanced a simple and objective definition for the term: Whatever increases the probability of a response occurring is reinforcing. A **reinforcer** is the stimulus that reinforces; reinforcement is the *effect* of a reinforcer. Note that reinforcement is defined by its effect; this eliminates a great deal of the confusion concerning the concepts **negative reinforcement** and **punishment.** Negative reinforcement, like positive reinforcement, results in an increase in the probability that a response will reoccur. The difference between the two is that positive reinforcement is effective as a result of a **reward** being added to a situation after the behavior has occurred, whereas negative reinforcement is effective through the removal of an unpleasant stimulus. A simple way of remembering the difference between the two is to remember that positive reinforcement involves a *reward* for behavior; negative reinforcement involves *relief* from something unpleasant. Punishment is distinguished from positive and negative reinforcement by its effects. Whereas reinforcement, whether positive or negative, serves to make a response more likely, punishment does not. (See the box *Expectations and Rewards*.)

There are several different kinds of punishment. The kind that we usually think of first involves a clearly unpleasant consequence. Being beaten with a stick and having one's hair pulled are examples of this kind of punishment. Another kind of punishment involves taking away something that is pleasant. Being prevented from watching television (what psychologists refer to as a *time out* procedure) and having to give up something desirable, such as money or privileges (called *response-cost* punishment), are both examples of this kind of punishment. Distinctions among the various kinds of reinforcement and punishment are illustrated in Figure 2.3. As the illustration makes clear, both may involve pleasant or unpleasant stimuli, but whether these stimuli are added to or removed from the situation determines their effect. It is worth repeating that reinforcement and punishment are defined primarily by their effects.

Shaping According to behaviorists, the majority of human behaviors are operant: They are not elicited as responses to any known stimuli, and they appear to be learned primarily as a function of their consequences. Most of these behaviors are highly complex, however, so that it is difficult to describe learning as simply the emission of an operant followed by reinforcement. In fact, even behaviors that animals can be trained to perform, using operant conditioning, are often sufficiently complex that they are not likely to occur spontaneously. The operant conditioning technique employed in these cases is referred to as **shaping**.

Shaping involves reinforcing any response that brings the behavior of the animal (or person) closer to the desired behavior. For example, a rat that is being conditioned to depress a lever is first trained to become accustomed to eating from the food tray in a special cage (called a *Skinner box*) and to the noise made by the mechanism when it releases food into the tray. Through a process of classical conditioning, the sound of the mechanism comes to be associated with food and may be used as a signal to the rat that food is being provided. Next,

	Nature of stimulus	
	Pleasant	Noxious
Added to the situation	*Positive reinforcement*: Louella is given a jelly bean for being "good"	*Punishment*: Louella has her nose tweaked for being "bad"
Removed from the situation	*Punishment*: Louella has her jelly beans taken away for being "bad"	*Negative reinforcement*: Louella's nose is released because she says "I'm sorry"

Figure 2.3
The four alternatives that define punishment and reinforcement.

it is relatively simple to get the rat to depress the lever, by reinforcing every move that brings it closer to the bar and by not reinforcing any other move. The procedure is also referred to as the *differential reinforcement of successive approximations*.

We can increase our understanding of complex human behaviors by studying Skinnerian shaping techniques. For example, many behaviors require eliminating ineffective responses and modifying effective responses. The reinforcement (for example, applause) that performers receive concerning the quality of their behavior may signal them to modify their behavior to elicit the greatest amount of reinforcement. This reinforcement gradually *shapes* the performer's behavior. Verbal behavior provides yet another example of shaping, since our speech is particularly susceptible to the effects of positive and negative reinforcement. Only the most insensitive people will continue to talk after most of their audience shows signs of falling asleep.

Social Learning

One of the most useful attempts to apply conditioning theory to an understanding of human behavior and development is found in those theories that have attempted to explain *social learn-*

EXPECTATIONS AND REWARDS;
THE OVERJUSTIFICATION HYPOTHESIS

Most of us typically operate under the assumption that the more we are rewarded for doing something, the more we will enjoy whatever it is that is rewarded. And in most cases, this assumption may well be correct. Certainly success (reinforcement) and enjoyment are often closely related—but not always.

Lepper (1981) and his associates (Lepper & Greene, 1978; Lepper, Greene, & Nisbett, 1973) have noted a strange phenomenon that contradicts our belief that reward always leads to enjoyment. In a typical experiment, for example, Lepper and Greene (1975) asked children to solve geometric puzzles. One group was told that they could play with some attractive toys as a reward. A second group was also allowed to play with the same toys but was not told beforehand that there would be a reward for solving the puzzles. Thus one group *expected* a reward, whereas the second did not. Following this initial experimental session, children were later observed unobtrusively to determine whether or not they would continue to play with the geometric puzzles (these were freely available in the classroom). The extent to which they did so would be an indication of their *intrinsic*

interest in the activity. As shown in the figure, significantly more of the children in the *unexpected* reward condition subsequently played with the puzzles. This finding has been replicated in a large number of experiments involving a variety of different activities (Lepper, 1981). How does psychology explain these puzzling findings?

Lepper and his associates suggest that the most reasonable explanation is a *cognitive* one, relating to the fact that we try to make sense of our behavior (and that of others) by understanding its causes. And the causes to which we attribute our behavior are often extrinsic (external rewards), intrinsic (internal satisfaction), or a combination of the two. Thus, when a child engages in an activity in the absence of any expectation of reward for doing so, the most logical cognitive explanation for this behavior is one involving *intrinsic* factors. The expectation of reward, however, introduces an extrinsic motive. Lepper suggests that when the extrinsic reward is striking, the individual tends to attribute the behavior to external rather than to internal causes. In his terms, too great an external reward leads to an *overjustification* of the behavior and a consequent reduction in the importance of intrinsic motivation.

In simple terms, the overjustification argument runs as follows: If I continually engage in a behavior for which there is little external reward, I justify this behavior in terms of the pleasure and enjoyment that I derive from it. But if the activity is subsequently rewarded so that I come to expect a reward for engaging in it, I might, in the end, come to enjoy the activity much less, although I might continue to engage in it. My motives for doing so are now extrinsic rather than intrinsic.

It follows from the overjustification hypothesis that if you pay people a great deal of money to perform some particularly dangerous or distasteful act, you will probably not get them to like the activity any better, although you might well get them to comply with your wishes. It also follows that even dangerous and distasteful activities might be seen as more enjoyable if they are engaged in with no expectation of external reward—providing, of course, that you can get people to do them in the first place.

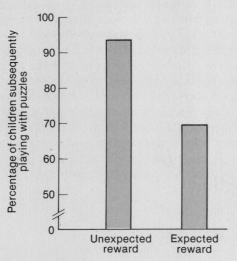

Significantly more of the children who had not expected a reward showed intrinsic interest by subsequently playing with the geometric puzzles. (Data from Lepper and Greene, 1975.)

ing—that is, the learning of behaviors that are appropriate and expected for one's age, sex, social class, occupation, and culture. Among these theories are those advanced by Bandura (1969, 1971, 1977) and Bandura and Walters (1963). Theirs is a theory of **observational learning**. It explains social learning in terms of imitation (hence observation) and explains the effects of imitation in terms of conditioning theory. What the theory says most simply is that children imitate, imitative behavior may be considered an operant, and reinforcement frequently follows imitation. Each of these statements is examined in the following three paragraphs. (See also *Learning Theory Applied to Cultural Differences*.)

First, children do imitate. I once observed my four-year-old son standing in front of the hall mirror, looking at himself and raising his eyebrows to give himself a definitely quizzical expression. He seemed so pleased with himself that I called his mother to see this great display of histrionic ability.

She, not altogether kindly, reminded me that I had indulged in a great deal of eyebrow raising after watching a movie in which the hero had displayed some impressive eyebrow dexterity.

Second, imitative behavior can be considered operant, although a model is ordinarily involved. The model does not usually serve as a direct stimulus for the imitative behavior because it is frequently absent at the time of the imitation. Hence, whatever learning occurs does so in the absence of the model. The model seems to provide a pattern rather than a direct stimulus for the behavior. In most cases, the behavior will not be learned unless some sort of reinforcement follows.

Third, reinforcement does frequently follow imitation. It can take a variety of forms. The behavior itself may often be reinforcing, particularly if it is socially approved. For example, a child who learns to say "milk" from hearing her mother say "milk" may be rewarded with a drink of that precious liquid if she says the proper word at the right time.

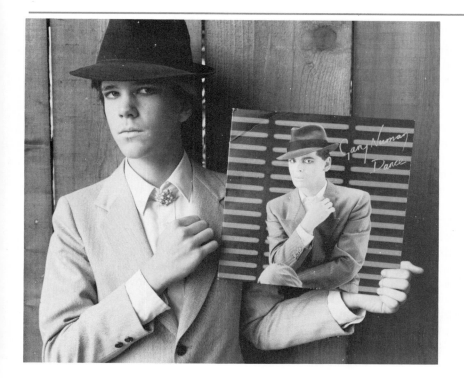

"Look-alikes" illustrate blatant, though often superficial, imitation. In real life, the effects of imitation are often more subtle.

LEARNING THEORY APPLIED TO CULTURAL DIFFERENCES

In one of Margaret Mead's (1937) books, Irving Goldman describes two different cultures: the Kwakiutl Indians of Vancouver Island and the Zuni of New Mexico. The Kwakiutl are aggressive and violent above all else. Their social rank is determined by birth; with high social rank, they inherit not only the prestige that comes with superiority but also a sacred obligation to subjugate and terrorize those of lower rank. In this culture, it is not uncommon for young boys of high social rank to stone, beat, and otherwise abuse those of lower rank. Murder is commonplace and socially accepted. Not only is it accepted, it is also rewarded in that the murderer ordinarily inherits all of the victim's possessions and titles.

In contrast, the Zuni are pacific in the extreme. Social recognition in this culture comes not from possessions or rank; indeed, those who possess too much are considered social misfits. Among the Zuni, the greatest possible honor is to have many friends. Those who can appear at a public festivity dressed entirely in borrowed clothing are the most envied, for their dress says, in effect, "Look at what a lucky person I am to have so many friends that they have dressed me in these beads and feathers."

It is unlikely that the dramatic differences between the Zuni and the Kwakiutl result from different inherited tendencies. It would seem reasonable to suppose, in fact, that if a Zuni infant were exchanged for a Kwakiutl infant shortly after birth, their eventual personalities and behaviors would be highly similar to those that are common in their adoptive cultures—providing, of course, that personality and behavior result at least in part from the experiences that we have. Had you been adopted by a Kwakiutl, do you not think that you too might have proudly paraded in raven feathers and seashells, throwing grand parties (termed *potlatches*) to impress your friends?

Vicarious reinforcement is another source of reinforcement that is important in observational learning. People will frequently imitate the behavior of others and continue to do so, even when they are receiving no reinforcement whatsoever. This type of behavior is apparently related to the imitators' unconscious expectation that if another person is behaving in a specific way and is reinforced for it, then the same manner of behaving will be reinforcing for them, too.

Manifestations of Observation Learning   Imitation frequently involves more than simply copying a model's behavior. Further, a model is not necessarily a person; it can be anything that serves as a pattern for behavior—books, manuals, folk heroes, television heroes, saints, and a host of real and imaginary villains as well. Such models are **symbolic models**; they are probably of greater significance than real-life models in highly technological and relatively impersonal societies.

Bandura and Walters (1963) describe three different effects of imitation on social learning. Acquiring novel behavior, the **modeling effect**, is well illustrated by a child who suddenly begins to say all manner of surprising words in the presence of her grandmother—not because she heard these words at home, of course, but because the neighbor's children do not have such well-behaved parents.

The effects of imitation are also found in the phenomena labeled the **inhibitory effect** (the suppression of deviant behavior) and the **disinhibitory effect** (the appearance of previously suppressed deviant behavior). These effects are usually the result of punishment or reward to the model for engaging in deviant behavior. Consider the hypothetical case of a teenager from an upstanding, conservative, middle-class family whose friends have recently discovered marijuana. The behavior is deviant by the child's own standards, but the amount of reinforcement (in terms of social prestige, acceptance by the group, and so on) that others appear to derive from smoking marijuana may well *disinhibit* this behavior in the child. There is really no new learning involved, as in modeling, but merely the disinhibition of previously suppressed behavior. If this teenager later observes members of her peer group punished by law, parents, or school authorities or experiencing ill effects of the drug, she might suddenly cease engaging in this behavior. Again, there is no new learning involved, although there is a change in behavior resulting from the influence of models; thus, this change illustrates the *inhibitory effect*.

A third effect of imitation is known as the **eliciting effect**: The behavior engaged in by learners as a result of observing a model is not identical to the model's behavior, or deviant, or novel, but is simply related to it. In other words, it is as though the model's behavior suggests some response to the observers and therefore *elicits* that response. For example, if a child "acts up" in school and a number of his classmates also misbehave, it is clear that his behavior has given rise to the related behavior in other children, but it is also clear that they are imitating a *type* of behavior rather than a specific behavior.

Learning Theory in Review

Learning-theory explanations for human development emphasize the role of the environment in shaping our personalities and our behaviors. Unlike psychoanalytic approaches, they are not concerned with psychodynamic conflicts and other hidden causes of behavior, and unlike the more cognitive approaches, they pay relatively little attention to such concepts as *understanding* and *knowing*. Instead, they focus on the role of reinforcement and punishment and on the extent to which behavior can be shaped by its consequences.

One of the principal criticisms of these approaches is that they are poorly suited to explain what are referred to as *higher mental processes*— for example, thinking, feeling, analyzing, problem solving, evaluating, and so on. Their emphasis, and their principal usefulness, relates to actual behav-

ior rather than to thinking and feeling, hence the often-used label, *behavioristic* approaches.

In spite of these shortcomings, learning-oriented approaches are sometimes extremely useful not only for understanding developmental change but also for controlling it. The deliberate application of conditioning principles to change behavior (termed **behavior modification**) has proven extremely useful in a variety of settings, including the classroom, as well as in psychotherapy.

■ Humanistic Approaches

Had I spoken of Piaget or Freud, of learning theories or imitation, in my grandmother's kitchen, the old lady would have listened politely. She is always polite. But in the end she would probably have said, "That's theory. It's all very nice, but what about Frank?" Why Frank? Simply because he was a unique child—as we all were (or are). And although there is little doubt that Freud, Skinner, and Piaget might each have had something very intelligent, and perhaps even useful, to say about Frank's habits of stealing chicken eggs, writing poetry, and dancing little jigs in mudholes, they would have been hard pressed to convince my grandmother that they knew more about Frank than she did. My grandmother is a humanist.

Humanistic psychologists concern themselves with the uniqueness of the individual. A prevalent humanistic notion is that it is impossible to describe the environment in a truly meaningful way, much less a person, since the important features of the environment are particular to each individual. To understand the behavior of others, one must attempt to perceive the world as they see it—from the perspective of their knowledge, experiences, goals, and aspirations. Such an orientation does not imply that it is impossible to understand human nature or human behavior generally, although it renders the task more difficult. It does imply, however, that understanding human behavior in a general sense may be of relatively little value for understanding the behavior of one person. As noted earlier, the individual is one, not an average. There is no average person.

Humanistic concerns with the uniqueness of the individual do not, therefore, lend themselves easily to the formulation of theories that are both highly specific and widely applicable. But they do suggest an attitude toward people, and toward the process of developing, that is of tremendous potential value to those concerned with human welfare. Humanistic orientations tend to personalize (to humanize?) our attitudes toward others; they restore some of the dynamism of the developmental process that our more static and more complex theories might otherwise remove.

Maslow, one of the individuals closely associated with the humanistic movement in psychology, was primarily concerned with the development of the healthy personality. Fundamental to his position is a belief that we are moved by two systems of needs (Maslow, 1970). The **basic needs** are physiological (food, drink) and psychological (security, love, esteem). The **metaneeds** are described as higher-level needs. They manifest themselves in our desire to know, in our appreciation of truth and beauty, and in our tendencies toward growth and fulfillment (termed *self-actualization*) (see Figure 2.4). Alternatively, these two groups of needs are sometimes labeled *growth needs* (metaneeds) and *deficiency needs* (basic needs). The basic needs are termed deficiency needs because, when they are not satisfied, individuals engage in behaviors designed to remedy a lack of satisfaction; for example, hunger represents a deficiency that can be satisfied by eating. The metaneeds are termed growth needs because activities that relate to them do not fulfill a lack, but lead toward growth. These needs are assumed to be hierarchically arranged in the sense that the metaneeds will not be attended to unless the basic needs are reasonably well satisfied. In other words, we pay attention to beauty, truth, and the development of our potential when we are no longer hungry and unloved (at least not terribly so). Put more simply, hunger for food is more compelling than hunger for knowledge.

Chief among Maslow's metaneeds, and most

Figure 2.4
Maslow's hierarchy of needs.

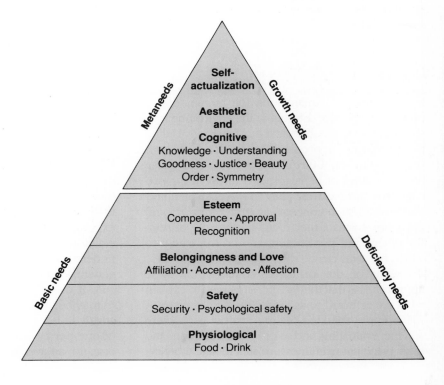

important for understanding human development, is **self-actualization**. By his own admission, the term is difficult to define (Maslow, 1970). He suggests that it is characterized by the absence of "neurosis, psychopathic personality, psychosis, or strong tendencies in these directions" (1970, p. 150). On the more positive side, he claims that self-actualized people "may be loosely described as [making] full use and exploitation of talents, capacities, potentialities, etc." (p. 150). And the reinforcement—the satisfaction associated with true self-actualization—comes from within rather than without. In contrast, satisfaction of lower-level needs, such as those associated with *esteem,* is associated with external sources of reinforcement (approval and recognition). Using this loose definition, Maslow scrutinized 3,000 college students and found only one person he considered to be actualized (although dozens were "potentials").

For our purposes, it is perhaps best to view self-actualization as a process that guides the direction of development rather than as a state that one can attain. The view that we are directed by a need *to become* (to actualize) and that the process of actualization is essentially positive and self-directed presents a subtle but important contrast to the more mechanistic, more passive, and less inner-directed theories that we have considered thus far. And although humanistic theory does not address itself to the specifics of the developmental process, it might in the end serve to explain facts that are not easily explained by other theories.

■ A Final Word About Theories

We began this chapter by insisting that facts and theories are not worlds apart in terms of "truthfulness"—that, actually, theories are intended as explanations of facts. From these explanations, scientists strive for understanding, for prediction, and sometimes for control. But theories do more than explain facts. As Thomas (1979) notes, they suggest which facts are most important for understanding and what relationships among these facts are most likely to lead to understanding. Table 2.5 presents a brief summary of the four approaches to developmental theory discussed in this chapter. History, as is so often its custom, will inform us later about the fruitfulness of these approaches.

Table 2.5   Approaches to development theory.

	Theory	Major Assumption (theoretical belief)	Variables of Greatest Concern
Psychoanalytic	Freud	Individual is motivated by instinctual urges that are primarily sexual and aggressive.	Hypothetical concepts such as id, ego, superego.
	Erikson	Child progresses through developmental stages by resolving conflicts that arise from a need to adapt to sociocultural environment.	Competence, social environment, developmental tasks.
Cognitive	Piaget	Child develops cognitive skills through active interaction with the environment.	Stage, schema, assimilation, accommodation, adaptation.
Behavioristic	Learning theory	Changes in behavior are a function of reinforcement, punishment, and imitation.	Imitation, reinforcement, punishment, stimuli, responses.
Humanist	Humanism	All individuals are unique, but strive toward the fullest development of their potential.	Self, positive growth, metaneeds, self-actualization.

1 A theory is a collection of related statements that are intended to organize and explain observations considered important. Theories are best evaluated in terms of usefulness rather than truthfulness. They should reflect "facts," be understandable, and be useful for predicting events as well as for explaining the past.

2 Freud's theory is useful for understanding the development of personality, especially the abnormal personality.

3 The libido, or source of energy for human behavior and consequently for the formation of personality, derives from powerful instinctual tendencies.

4 The newborn child is all libido—that is, all instinctual urges. The label *id* is applied to the level of personality concerned solely with the gratification of urges—urges that are primarily sexual in Freud's view.

5 Conflict between the id (instinctual urges) and reality develops the ego—the aspect of personality concerned with finding ways for the id to satisfy its basic urges.

6 Later in the course of development, the superego forms as an offshoot of the ego. It represents societal and cultural taboos and restrictions that are imposed on an individual's instinctual urges and is often called conscience.

7 Freud describes development as a progression through five stages, each differentiated from the other primarily by the areas of the child's body that are the principal sources of sexual gratification at that time. The stages in sequence are the oral, the anal, the phallic, a period of latency, and the genital stage.

8 Erikson's *psychosocial* theory of development describes human development in terms of eight stages, each of which involves the resolution of a crisis or conflict that is brought about by a need to adapt to the social environment. Resolution of each crisis results in the development of some new competence.

9 Erikson's stages, in order, are trust versus shame and doubt, initiative versus guilt, industry versus inferiority, identity versus identity diffusion, intimacy versus isolation, generativity versus self-absorption, and integrity versus despair.

10 Piaget's theory describes cognitive development (where *cognition* refers to knowing or understanding). Biologically based, it inquires about the process of adaptation and about how intellectual development can be classified.

11 Piaget believes that adaptation results from interaction with the environment through the processes of using activities already in the child's repertoire (assimilation) and of changing activities to conform to environmental demands (accommodation).

12 Intellectual structure consists of schemes (mental structures corresponding to simple behaviors or reflexes) and later of operations that are progressively more complex. A description of the changes that structure undergoes during development is a description of the sequence of intellectual development (sensorimotor, preoperational, concrete operations, and formal operations).

13 Learning-theory approaches to development focus on immediate behavior and on environmental forces that affect that behavior. The most important concepts for these theories are conditioning and imitation.

14 Classical conditioning describes a simple form of learning, in which a previously neutral stimulus acquires the capability of bringing about a response, following repeated pairing with another stimulus.

15 Operant conditioning results in an increase in the probability of a response following reinforcement. Positive reinforcement (reward) is effective when it follows as a consequence of behavior (wages, for example); negative reinforcement is effective through its removal (relief). Punishment can involve the removal of a pleasant consequence or the presentation of one less pleasant.

16 Shaping is an operant conditioning technique whereby behaviors that are closer and closer approximations to the desired behavior are reinforced. It is useful for teaching animals and humans complex sequences of behavior.

17 Social learning may be explained through observational learning-theories that attempt to explain socialization as a function of imitating models (which can be symbolic as well as actual people). Imitation is often explained in terms of operant conditioning.

18 Three manifestations of observational learning include the learning of new responses (modeling effect), the suppression or reappearance of deviant behaviors (inhibitory-disinhibitory effect), and the emission of behaviors similar but not identical to that of the model (eliciting effect).

19 Humanistic theory is concerned with the uniqueness of the individual child and with the development of human potential. Maslow is an important representative of humanistic concerns.

20 People are incredibly more complicated than this chapter might suggest, but they are easier to understand within the context of the more organized systems provided here than within the context of our more naive intuitions.

■ FURTHER READINGS

Freud and Piaget were voluminous writers. It is often easier and sometimes more valuable to use secondary sources for information about their theories. Nevertheless, the interested student is strongly advised to consult original sources to achieve a better idea of their work. The following are particularly useful starting points:

Baldwin, A. L. *Theories of child development*. New York: John Wiley, 1967

Brill, A. A. (Ed.). *The basic writings of Sigmund Freud*. New York: Random House, 1938.

Inhelder, B., & Piaget, J. *The growth of logical thinking from childhood to adolescence*. New York: Basic Books, 1958.

Piaget, J. *The origins of intelligence in children*. New York: International Universities Press, 1952.

Thomas, R. M. *Comparing theories of child development*. Belmont, Calif.: Wadsworth, 1979.

An imitation-based theory of social learning is presented simply and clearly in:
Bandura, A., & Walters, R. *Social learning and personality development*. New York: Holt, Rinehart & Winston, 1963.

Maslow's humanistic psychology is well explained in:
Maslow, A. H. *Motivation and personality* (2nd ed.). New York: Harper & Row, 1970.

3

HEREDITY AND ENVIRONMENT

His life was gentle, and the elements
So mix'd in him that Nature might stand up,
And say to all the world, "This was a man!"

William Shakespeare
Julius Caesar

I t's mid-morning now. We turn off Highway 55. Bruderheim appears suddenly, directly in front, its three grain elevators maroon sentinels against a pale sky. We cross the railroad tracks, the road becomes street, and I slow down, waking Marcel who wants to know if we're there yet. We have scarcely even left! Again, that faint sadness, this time at the thought that even at the age of six, children might be so anxious to arrive that they will fail to enjoy the journey. How much sadder for us who have far fewer places to go. Rather than answer his question, I look desperately for something interesting that I can point out to him. But Bruderheim distracts me. It floods me with memories of another town, for it was in a town very much like this one that I stole the first chicken. And I wonder now whether I could ever again do what I did in those days. The thought is unbidden, unwelcome, and I urge it back, holding at bay the fear that always follows.

"Let's stop and eat something," Denise suggests, and I quickly put her off.

"There's a service station just down the road." I meet Grandma's eyes in the mirror. She looks away at once, but we both know.

"Service station would be fine," she says, but her needles have stopped clicking. Even she fears my old ghosts. And I drive a little faster, anxious to leave the town behind. Soon we're out on the highway again. The newly planted, rich black fields among green poplar groves relax me, and the ghosts no longer threaten. I want to return to our story quickly now, before we arrive at the service station. We no longer have time for a long and difficult chapter like the last one on theories, but we might almost complete one on the two great forces that seem to hold much of our destinies in their collective hands: our genes and our environments.

■ The Nature-Nurture Question

In a simple sense, nature refers to biology or heredity; nurture refers to upbringing or environment. Thus, the nature-nurture question concerns the ways in which heredity and environment determine the processes and outcomes of development. Development itself may be seen as including the entire evolutionary history of a species—a phenomenon termed *phylogeny* (**phylogenetic development**)—or it may be limited to the development of single individuals within the species—to what is termed *ontogeny*, or **ontogenetic development**. In this text, we are concerned primarily with ontogeny, although ontogeny and phylogeny are clearly related. That is, the development of a single individual is, in some ways, related to the development of the entire species. Many of the behaviors and habits characteristic of an individual are not acquired solely as a function of experience. A moth does not fly into a flame because it has learned to do so; dead moths do not fly. We can therefore assume that the attraction that light has for a moth, like the overpowering urge of a goose to go south or a salmon to swim up a specific river and to a particular place in this river, is the result of inherited or genetic tendencies; in other words, these actions are the result of phylogenetic influences. (See *Wild Children.*)

■ Heredity

Recently, a number of psychologists and other scientists have become intrigued with the possibility of explaining the development of humans at least partly in terms of genetic background. Fishbein (1976), Waddington (1975), and Wilson (1978) (among others) argue that behaviors reinforced through evolution—hence behaviors that are adaptive—become highly probable in succeeding generations. It is as though we are genetically programmed to engage in certain behaviors, to learn certain things and not others. This genetic programming manifests itself not only in those characteristics that are present at birth but also in the unfolding of later abilities and behaviors. This, the unfolding of genetically influenced characteristics, is referred to as **epigenesis**.

The Mechanics of Heredity

The mechanics of heredity are complex and impressive. We know that human life begins with the joining of the mother's **egg cell (ovum)** and the father's **sperm cell**. For life to occur, this union is necessary—and because two people of opposite sexes are involved, it ordinarily* requires a physical union between a male and female as well. The mechanics of this union are not sufficiently academic (or prosaic enough, I might add) to be appropriate for a textbook of this nature. They are therefore left to your imagination.

Enough imagining. A single ovum is produced by a mature and healthy woman usually once every twenty-eight days (sometime between the tenth and the eighteenth day of her menstrual cycle). Some women occasionally produce two or more eggs, or a single fertilized egg sometimes divides, thus making possible multiple births. A mature and healthy man produces several billion sperm cells over the period of a month.

The ovum is the largest cell in the human body. It is approximately 0.15 millimeter in diameter—about half the size of each period (.) on this page. The sperm cell, by contrast, is one of the smallest cells in the body, 0.005 millimeter in diameter. What the sperm cell lacks in size is made up by the length of its tail—fully twelve times longer than the main part of the cell to which it is attached. It is this long tail that enables the sperm to swim toward the ovum.

The egg cell and the sperm cell carry the determiners of heredity. Each initially possesses twenty-three pairs of **chromosomes**, one member of each pair inherited from the father and the other from the mother. These pairs are separated during a series of cell divisions so that the sperm and egg receive only *one* member of each pair. The end result is that each sperm and egg contains twenty-three *single* chromosomes rather than twenty-three *pairs* of chromosomes. These chromosomes are the carriers of heredity.

---

*"Ordinarily" because conception is possible with **artificial insemination**, a procedure that eliminates the need for sexual union. Indeed, recent successful atempts to produce "test tube" babies indicate that conception can occur without the introduction of sperm into the female. Although test tube babies have not yet been developed entirely in test tubes, they originate *in vitro* (in glass). The procedure involves removing an ovum from the mother and sperm from the father, and joining the two outside the mother's body. The fertilized egg is then inserted into the mother and development proceeds as it normally would.

WILD CHILDREN

On a cold, blustery day in the fall of 1797, a group of French peasants caught sight of a naked boy running wildly through the woods. The peasants lay in wait the next day and saw him once more, gathering acorns and roots. The following year, he was seen again by some woodsmen who were able to capture him, although he fought violently. The captured boy was then brought to the nearest village, where he was put on public display. A short time later, he escaped.

A year later, the same boy was again captured. And again, within only a few days, he escaped. But two years later, for some totally unknown reason, the boy walked out of the forest and into a home in a small town next to the forest of Aveyron.

Naked, speechless, and in every way uncivilized, the boy was immediately the subject of great curiosity. At first, he refused all foods except for acorns, chestnuts, walnuts, and potatoes. These he sniffed vigorously before putting them in his mouth. Following extensive examinations, Pinel, one of the leading physicians of the time and an important early advocate of the humane treatment of the insane, pronounced the boy a deaf idiot and predicted that he would never learn anything of any consequence. But one of Pinel's students, Itard, also a physician, was less pessimistic and was accordingly given the task of educating the boy, later named Victor.

In the beginning, Victor continued to refuse meats (raw or cooked), eating only nuts and vegetables. He gave every sign of being deaf; his only verbalizations were sighs, plaintive cries, and a strange series of explosive sounds somewhat like laughter. He had no use for clothing, seemed insensitive to heat or cold, slept as easily on the floor as anywhere else, and carried out his toilet functions as the urge moved him.

And in the end? Did Victor learn what Itard had to teach him? Sadly, no. Life does not always dramatize as fiction might. Victor did not become a statesman or a doctor. Nor was he ever able to sit with Itard and recount stories of his life in the forests. Indeed, although he learned to function in a civilized environment and to recognize familiar objects by name (he was not deaf), he never did learn to speak.

There have been numerous other cases of "wild" children having been dug out of wolf, bear, tiger, or lion dens. When recaptured, many of these children apparently behaved as did their *adoptive* parents; few ever learned to behave as we do. Indeed, of thirty cases of wild children reported by Singh and Zingg (1942), some learned to walk and laugh, a few learned to eat vegetables in addition to meat (or meat in addition to vege-tables), and an even smaller number learned to socialize with other children and with adults, but none learned to speak.

It might appear at first glance that reports of wild children support the belief that a human environment is essential for the development of human characteristics. In other words, it might seem that these children are **retarded**, because they have not had contact with humans during their formative years. Not surprisingly, this view has received wide support in psychological literature (Gesell, 1940; Zingg, 1941). However, the evidence surrounding the reports of feral children is highly circumstantial. In fact, as Dennis (1941b, 1951) points out, there is not a single documented case of a child actually having been raised by a wild animal. The evidence is drawn from reports of children being found with animals or in animal lairs. The identity of these children usually has been unknown, so that the length of time that they spent in isolation can only be guessed, and in no case has anyone actually observed them with their supposed adoptive parents. Dennis suggests that it is likely that the so-called wild children were initially brain damaged or otherwise retarded and that this might explain why they were abandoned by their parents in the first place. He argues strongly that most of the wild children have traits in common with the mentally defective as well as with wild animals and that they were likely mentally defective to begin with and would have continued to be mentally defective, whether with animals or with humans. Thus, accounts of feral children, fascinating as they might be, provide little substantive evidence concerning the heredity-environment question. For answers to this question, science has had to look elsewhere.

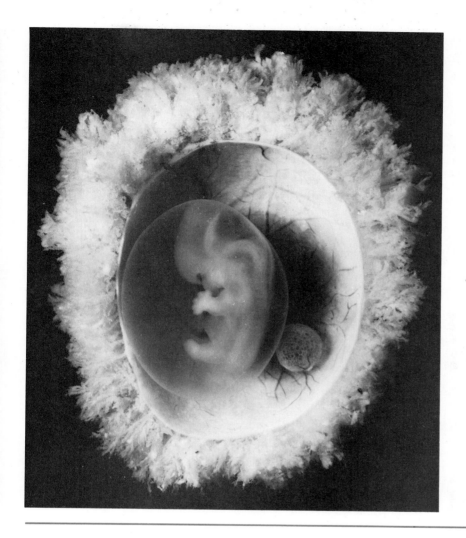

The world in utero, at forty-eight days.

Cells in the human body (except for sex cells) reproduce by means of **mitosis**: the division of a single "parent" cell into two "daughter" cells that are genetically identical to each other and to the parent. Growth of all tissues of an organism is accomplished in this manner, except for the sperm and eggs. Sex cells divide from twenty-three pairs of chromosomes to twenty-three single chromosomes by a process called **meiosis**—a special form of mitosis in which the chromosome number is reduced by one-half. The products of this division, the sperm and eggs, are not genetically identical to the parent cell (see Figure 3.1), thereby accounting for differences between parents and children and between siblings.

Sex Chromosomes   Of the twenty-three chromosomes contained in each sperm and each ovum, one pair is particularly important for determining sex. It is labeled the **sex chromosome** because it determines whether the offspring will be male or female (the other twenty-two are labeled **auto-**

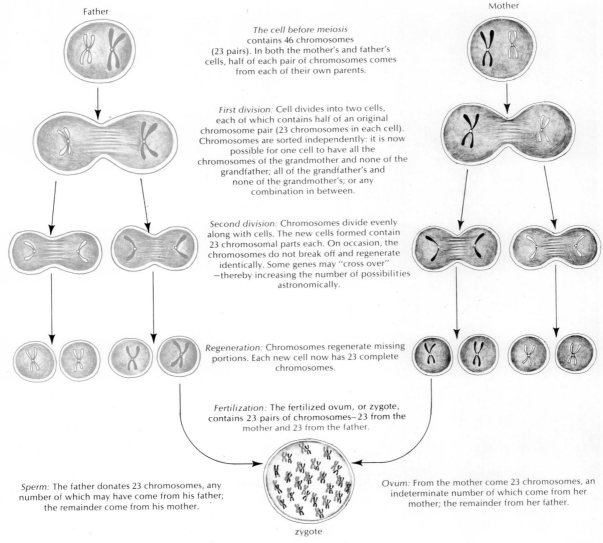

Father

Mother

The cell before meiosis contains 46 chromosomes (23 pairs). In both the mother's and father's cells, half of each pair of chromosomes comes from each of their own parents.

First division: Cell divides into two cells, each of which contains half of an original chromosome pair (23 chromosomes in each cell). Chromosomes are sorted independently: it is now possible for one cell to have all the chromosomes of the grandmother and none of the grandfather; all of the grandfather's and none of the grandmother's; or any combination in between.

Second division: Chromosomes divide evenly along with cells. The new cells formed contain 23 chromosomal parts each. On occasion, the chromosomes do not break off and regenerate identically. Some genes may "cross over" —thereby increasing the number of possibilities astronomically.

Regeneration: Chromosomes regenerate missing portions. Each new cell now has 23 complete chromosomes.

Fertilization: The fertilized ovum, or zygote, contains 23 pairs of chromosomes—23 from the mother and 23 from the father.

Sperm: The father donates 23 chromosomes, any number of which may have come from his father; the remainder come from his mother.

Ovum: From the mother come 23 chromosomes, an indeterminate number of which come from her mother; the remainder from her father.

zygote

Figure 3.1
Meiosis. Cells divide so that the new cells have only half the chromosomes of parent cells. For simplicity, only one of the twenty-three pairs of chromosomes is depicted here. The new cell—the fertilized egg, or zygote—contains the full complement of twenty-three *pairs* of chromosomes.

somes). As shown in Figure 3.2, the father produces two types of sperm, one type with a larger sex chromosome, labeled X, and one type with a smaller sex chromosome, labeled Y. If the sperm that fertilizes the ovum contains an X chromo-

some, the offspring will be a girl; if the sperm cell contains a Y chromosome, the result will be a boy. Because the mother produces only X chromosomes, only the father's sperm determines the sex of the offspring (a fact of which Henry VIII was

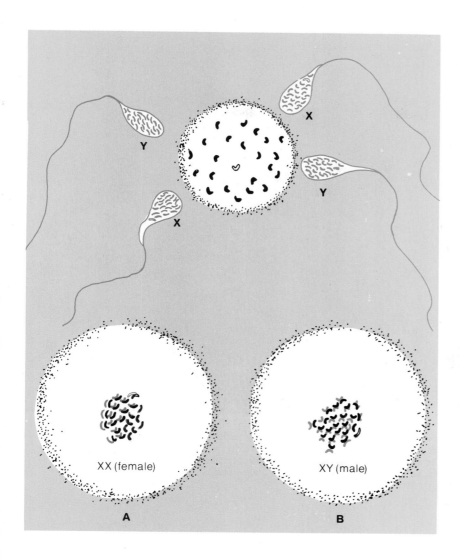

Figure 3.2
Sex determination at fertilization. At the top of the figure are an ovum and four spermatozoa, two with the large X sex chromosome and two with the smaller Y sex chromosome. The ovum always contains only the X sex chromosome. (The sex chromosomes are outlined.) In **A** the zygote (fertilized egg) contains an X spermatozoon and will result in a girl. In **B** the zygote contains a Y spermatozoon and will therefore be a boy.

ignorant as he disposed of his wives for failing to give him sons). The X chromosome contributed by the mother to her son is sometimes the carrier of sex-linked, predominantly male defects and illnesses, such as color blindness, hereditary baldness, and hemophilia.

Genes   The units of heredity carried by the chromosomes are called **genes**. It is estimated that each of the twenty-three chromosomes contains between fifty and one hundred thousand genes, each of which is responsible for determining some characteristic of the offspring (Baskin, 1982).

If the characteristics of an individual were simply determined by the presence or absence of genes, heredity would still be a complex and mysterious process. The concept of heredity is made doubly complex because a child may acquire different forms of the genes from each of his parents and the outcome of this inheritance may be a function of the relative recessiveness or dominance of these genes (or several **recessive** and **dominant**

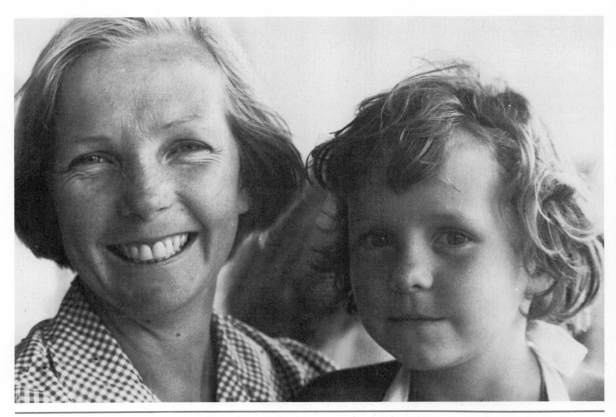

Parents and their children often look very much alike because they have in common certain genes related to physical characteristics. However, the complexity of the processes by which these genes are transmitted, together with the astronomical number of combinations possible, makes it very difficult to predict the nature and extent of family resemblance before the fact.

genes acting in combination, to further complicate the matter). For example, one can greatly oversimplify by stating that there is a gene responsible for the length of an individual's legs: A long gene determines long legs, and a short gene determines short legs (in reality, the "length" of genes is irrelevant). For the sake of simplicity, let us assume further that the gene for long legs is dominant and the one for short legs is recessive. There are clearly three possibilities. Some individuals will have identical corresponding genes for length of leg (either two long or two short genes). Such individuals are described as being **homozygous** with respect to these genes. Those who are **heterozygous** will have different corresponding genes—

in this case, one long and one short. Given two long genes, the individual will have long legs; given two short genes, she will have short legs; but given one of each, she will not have one long leg and one short leg. Because the gene for long legs is dominant, the individual will have long legs. (See Figure 3.3 for a less fictitious illustration.)

So far, our discussion of the genetic basis of human characteristics has been an oversimplification. A more complete (and more complex) discussion of the mechanisms of heredity would discuss the function of various combinations of **deoxyribonucleic acid (DNA)** molecules (Crick, 1962, 1963; Watson, 1963). Among the principal reasons for believing that the DNA molecule is the carrier of hereditary information is the fact that the nucleus of a sex cell is 40 percent DNA molecules, and researchers know that the nucleus of the cell is involved in heredity. DNA is a long, chainlike molecule consisting of different sequences of four chemical subunits. The number of possible combinations of these subunits is literally astronomical.

Genetic Abnormalities

Chromosomal abnormalities are not often related to dominant genes; when they are, they seldom lead to early death or to inability to produce offspring. If they did, the abnormality would quickly be eradicated (because the gene is dominant and all carriers would be affected and die or be infertile). Such is not the case, however, with chromosomal abnormalities related to recessive genes, because many individuals may be carriers of the defective gene without themselves suffering from the disease. (See *Amniocentesis and Genetic Counseling*.)

Down's Syndrome   Mongolism, more recently

called Down's syndrome, is the most common of chromosomal birth defects. It affects approximately 10 percent of all children institutionalized for mental retardation (Thompson, 1975). Children suffering from this defect have an extra piece on one chromosome (chromosome twenty-one, as it is numbered by geneticists). Such individuals will have three of this chromosome rather than a pair—hence the alternative medical label: trisomy 21. Down's syndrome children tend to be short and stocky, have small squarish heads, defective hearts, protruding tongues, and characteristic loose folds of skin over the corners of the eyes, producing an Oriental appearance—hence the label mongolism. Mental retardation is common among these children, although a small number do learn to read. In addition, some are good at imitation, many enjoy music, and they often seem cheerful. Since not all children affected by Down's syndrome manifest all (or most) of these symptoms, they cannot always be easily identified at birth. However, a chromosomal examination provides a sure test.

The probability of producing a child with Down's syndrome has been directly linked with the age of the mother. The incidence ranges from

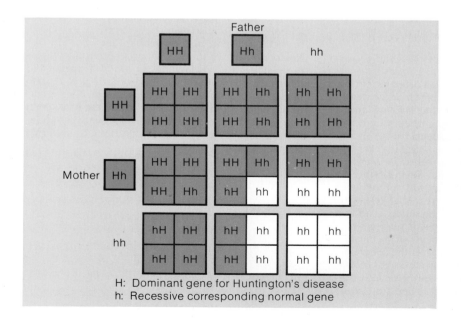

H: Dominant gene for Huntington's disease
h: Recessive corresponding normal gene

Figure 3.3
Huntington's disease (*H*), a disorder involving neurological deterioration and eventual death whose onset usually occurs after the age of twenty, is caused by a dominant gene. Hence, at least one of the parents must suffer from the disorder before the offspring can be affected. The matrix illustrates the possible results of matings between parents who are homozygous with respect to Huntington's disease (*HH*), heterozygous with respect to the disorder (*Hh*—these individuals will also suffer from the disease since the gene is dominant), and homozygous with respect to normality (*hh*).

AMNIOCENTESIS
AND GENETIC COUNSELING

More than forty chromosomal aberrations and other disorders can now be detected in the fetus as a result of advances in medical knowledge and technology (Falek, 1975). In **amniocentesis**, a hollow needle is inserted into the amniotic fluid surrounding the fetus, allowing the physician to obtain fluid containing fetal cells. This procedure is often employed to detect chromosomal defects and disorders. An examination of chromosomes in these cells reveals the absence of chromosomes or the presence of extra chromosomes. In addition, the blood type of the fetus can be detected in this manner, as can the chemical composition of the amniotic fluid; these may provide evidence relating to other diseases that might affect the unborn child. Because the procedure involves a slight risk of infection, it is not routinely performed. It is commonly employed only in those cases in which the mothers are older (over 35) or when there are other factors that might increase the probability of fetal abnormality or other complications.

Although amniocentesis presents a new and powerful tool for detecting possible abnormalities in offspring, other variables such as family background and abnormalities in one or both of the parents as well as in siblings might also provide evidence of risk. And when a probability of some defect is discovered to be higher than usual, potential parents and physicians are faced with decisions that, for some, might entail serious questions of ethics.

Genetic counseling, a branch of medicine or psychology that advises physicians and parents, typically attempts to assess the probability of a defect occurring, its likely seriousness, the extent to which it can be treated and even reversed, and the best action to follow once a decision has been made concerning whether or not to have a child. In many instances, genetic counseling will occur prior to conception and might take into account the age and health of the mother as well as the presence of genetic abnormalities in ancestors or in siblings. In other cases, genetic counseling will occur after conception.

One large-scale genetic counseling service is offered by a University of Michigan free telephone service, which permits physicians and patients throughout Michigan to obtain a wide range of information over the telephone. In appropriate instances, amniocentesis is recommended (for example, when mothers are over age thirty-five or when chromosomal abnormalities are already present in the family). Out of 5,204 calls received between August 1977 and July 1981, some 46 percent were referred for amniocentesis (Rayburn, Wilson, Schreck, Louwsma, & Hamman, 1982). The majority of these involved age (1,232 cases in which mothers were between thirty-five and thirty-nine, 278 cases for mothers between forty and forty-four, and 9 cases for mothers forty-five or older). The second most common reason for calling the center involved genetically linked defects and diseases among family members (for example, Down's syndrome or hemophilia). Other reasons included infants born with some defect, the use of drugs by one or both parents, previous obstetric complications, maternal health problems, and exposure to potential environmental hazards, such as radiation or insecticides.

In spite of the availability of genetic counseling in a number of centers such as the one at the University of Michigan, Weitz (1981) notes that there is still relatively widespread lack of knowledge, both on the part of physicians and on the part of potential clients. In addition, psychological barriers such as fear of genetic diseases, the social stigma attached to them, and values that stress God's will, as well as financial considerations, limit the use of genetic counseling and reduce its effectiveness even when it is available.

Genetic counseling also presents some potential for abuse. In the Ganxiao district of the province of Hubei in northern China, as elsewhere in China, parents take tremendous pride in male children. Accordingly, government regulations limiting parents to a single child have led to the widespread killing of baby girls. In addition, many parents are having the sex of the fetus determined before birth so that female fetuses can be aborted. As a result, there are now five boys for every girl under the age of five in the Ganxiao district ("China Fears Sexual Imbalance," 1983).

one in fifteen hundred for mothers aged fifteen to twenty-four to one in sixty-five for mothers over forty-five (Smith & Wilson, 1973).

Turner's Syndrome   A relatively large, though infrequent, number of chromosomal defects are linked to the sex chromosome. Among them is Turner's syndrome, which affects one out of five thousand female children (Thompson, 1975). These children are born with a missing sex chromosome (designated as XO rather than as XX). Although most such children are aborted spontaneously, those that do survive typically have underdeveloped secondary sexual characteristics, although this is not evident until puberty (Money, 1975). Initial symptoms of the disorder include swelling in the extremities that disappears with age, leaving loose folds of skin (webbing), particularly at the neck, fingers, and toes; dwarfism; occasional mental retardation; low-set ears; and short stubby fingers. Injections of the sex hormone *estrogen* prior to puberty are sometimes helpful in bringing about greater sexual maturation (Timiras, 1972).

Klinefelter's Syndrome   Another chromosomal aberration linked to the sex chromosome involves the presence of an extra X chromosome in a male child (thus XXY) and is called Klinefelter's syndrome. Occurring in one out of four hundred males, it is considerably more common than Turner's syndrome (Thompson, 1975) and is marked by the presence of both male and female secondary sexual characteristics.* Children suffering from this disorder typically have small, undeveloped testicles, more highly developed breasts than is common among boys, high-pitched voices, and little or no facial hair after puberty. Treatment with the male sex hormone, *testosterone,* is often effective in enhancing the development of masculine characteristics and in increasing sex drive

(Johnson, Myhre, Ruvalcaba, Thuline, & Kelley, 1970). Without such treatment, many children suffering from Klinefelter's syndrome remain infertile throughout life.

XYY Syndrome   Males with an extra Y chromosome, sometimes referred to as "super males" because they possess one extra male chromosome, are characteristically tall; frequently, they are also of lower than average intelligence. Some research evidence has linked this syndrome with criminality, following the observation that considerably more of the tall men in prisons are of the XYY type than is true of tall men in the general society (see, for example, Telfer, Baker, Clark, & Richardson, 1968). The theory is that the extra chromosome is linked with greater aggressiveness and hence greater tendencies toward violent crimes. In fact, the syndrome was first discovered among prisoners with violent histories; among them the incidence is between 2 and 12 percent, while only 0.1 percent of the normal population has the syndrome (Jarvik, Klodin, & Matsuyama, 1973). The conclusion that the XYY syndrome is linked with criminality remains extremely tentative (Falek, 1975). Certainly, not all XYY individuals manifest undue aggression. In fact, Witkin et al. (1976) found that imprisoned XYY individuals were more often guilty of nonviolent crimes. Kalat (1981) suggests that one reason why many of these individuals are in jail may be their lower intelligence rather than their greater aggressiveness.

Phenotypes, Genotypes, and Canalization

Your genetic makeup is your *genotype*; it consists of the twenty-three chromosomes you inherited from your mother and the corresponding twenty-three for which your father was responsible. Your *phenotype*, however, is defined by your manifested characteristics. If you have blue eyes, then blue eyes are part of your phenotype. At the same time, the genes that correspond to blue eyes define your genotype. In this simple case, there is a direct correspondence between your genotype and pheno-

---

*Some significantly superior "female" athletes were found to be not females but males with Klinefelter's syndrome—hence the Olympics sex test for female athletes.

type. Because the gene for blue eyes is normally recessive, we can infer your genotype from your phenotype. But if your phenotype were brown eyes, we could not infer your genotype for eye color with certainty. As is shown in Figure 3.4, you might have two dominant genes for brown eyes or only one together with a recessive gene for blue eyes.

Since most human characteristics do not appear to be determined by the presence or absence of a single dominant gene or two recessive genes but by the combined influence of a variety of genes, it is usually difficult to infer genotype from phenotype. To complicate the matter further, phenotype is influenced not only by genotype but also by the environment. Intelligence, for example, is a manifested characteristic (phenotype) that is known to be affected by hereditary forces (genotype) and by environmental factors. One of the most important tasks of psychologists working in this area is to determine the nature and timing of experiences that are most likely to have a beneficial influence on phenotype.

Some manifested characteristics seem to correspond much more closely than others to underlying genetic material. The appearance of these characteristics is, in one sense, predetermined by genotype. This phenomenon is described as **canalization** (Waddington, 1975). Those characteristics that are strongly canalized are less affected by environmental forces. Thus, for a highly canalized characteristic, phenotype corresponds closely to genotype. For characteristics that are not highly

canalized, phenotype may be very different from what might have been predicted on the basis of genetic makeup. Eye color is a highly canalized characteristic; it typically corresponds to genotype and is unaffected by experience. In contrast, many complex intellectual abilities (the ability to learn to speak several languages, for example) do not appear to be highly canalized but result from specific experiences.

Described in evolutionary terms, canalization may be seen as a genetic tendency toward predictable regularity. This predictable regularity ensures that individuals of one species will be much more similar than dissimilar.

■ Environment or Heredity?

Genesis refers to the beginning; it refers, as well, to the development or unfolding of something. In one sense, our genes, aptly named, are our beginnings. Not only do they account for a great many of our obvious physical characteristics, they are also related to the fact that most of us go through similar developmental sequences. This phenomenon, labeled *epigenesis,* is clearly evident in the maturational processes that occur at adolescence. Put in other words, epigenesis is the unfolding of those aspects of human development that appear to be genetically determined.

Although we assume that heredity accounts for most of the physical characteristics of human

Figure 3.4
Phenotype (manifested characteristic) results from genotype (chromosomal makeup), but genotype cannot always be determined from phenotype. A brown-eyed individual might have a recessive gene for blue eyes or two genes for brown eyes.

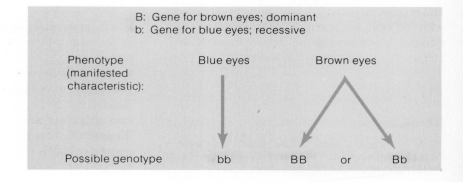

B: Gene for brown eyes; dominant
b: Gene for blue eyes; recessive

Phenotype (manifested characteristic):

Blue eyes   Brown eyes

Possible genotype   bb   BB   or   Bb

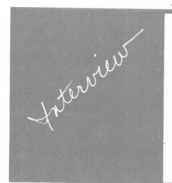

Subject: Female; age sixty-two; married; three children; four grandchildren; not working outside home; husband recently retired.

(referring to a fourteen-year-old grandson who has recently been in a detention center and whose history includes several criminal offenses, some of which are drug related)

Sure, I think he got it from his dad. I *know* he got it from his dad. He was the same way. Always in trouble, but she [her daughter] was in love and there's nothing we could say to stop it. Until it was too late and next thing you knew they had two kids and she had divorced him. Sure he got it from his dad, 'cause his mother sure wasn't like that.

beings, its effect is not necessarily simple and obvious. It is true that such traits as hair or eye color, length of nose, or size of head appear to be clearly hereditary, but not all traits are so obviously genetic. Although weight, height, complexion, and numerous other physical characteristics may be largely determined by genetic endowment, they are also clearly susceptible to the effects of environment, particularly if the environment does not provide sufficient nourishment for the physical development of the individual. This is no less true, but not quite so obvious, in the case of intellectual or personality development. An analysis of the relative contributions of nature (genetic endowment) and nurture (learning and environment) might lead to the conclusion that nature determines the possibilities, whereas nurture makes them either probable or improbable.

In subsequent sections of this chapter, we look at a variety of studies that have attempted to clarify the roles of nature and nurture in our lives. To what extent are our destinies locked into our genes? And to what extent do social realities influence what you and I become?

Family Studies

Literature examining the contributions of heredity and environment to child development is extensive and dates back at least as far as the recognized beginning of psychology as a scientific study. Among

the first well-known names in the controversy that still surrounds the heredity-environment question is Francis Galton, Charles Darwin's cousin (both gifted individuals). Like my grandmother, who believes that the world is populated largely by fools and ignorant people, Galton became concerned that the supply of gifted people in England seemed to be diminishing in relation to the number of less gifted people. He also noted that most of England's outstanding people were either related to each other or came from a very small number of families (Galton, 1896). Galton theorized that genius is hereditary and became convinced that parents should be carefully selected for favorable genetic characteristics, a practice termed **eugenics**.

Among several historical attempts at eugenics was Frederick the Great's effort to produce tall soldiers to serve as honor guards for Prussia's noble families. He tried to accomplish this by mating the tallest and strongest of his soldiers with robust peasant women. Unfortunately (or fortunately), it is not always possible to control the activities of tall soldiers and robust peasant women. Nor was there any scientific documentation of whatever progeny might have resulted from these relatively uncontrolled activities, so that Frederick the Great actually added nothing to our knowledge of human genetics.

A somewhat more successful attempt to employ eugenics was undertaken by John H. Noyes (1937) at Oneida, New York, in a communal religious society. The community flourished for two generations, during which Noyes and other leaders of the group determined which pairs of adults would produce children. The group practiced what they called "multiple marriage." Because this practice appeared to be nothing more than "free love" to outsiders, Noyes's society had to disband when the federal government prosecuted Mormon polygamy in the 1880s. Noyes later claimed that he had succeeded in producing a group of people who were intellectually and physically superior to the normal population. His evidence is totally unverified.

About the time that Noyes and his followers were attempting to produce a race of genetically superior Americans, another group was producing large numbers of apparently intellectually and morally inferior Americans. These notorious families, the Jukes and the Kallikaks, were distinguished by criminal records, immorality, poverty, and a notable lack of intelligence (see Holbrook, 1957). The Jukes, for example, produced more than two thousand people in 130 years, more than half of whom spent time in state institutions for the feebleminded, prisons, and penitentiaries—a fact interpreted by many as further evidence of the inheritability of intelligence, feeblemindedness, and criminality.

Goddard (1914), a prominent and influential individual in the theory and testing of intelligence at that time, gives us a detailed description of the Kallikaks. The Kallikak family had two main branches, each originating from the same father but with strikingly different maternal origins. One branch apparently stemmed from an illicit affair between a soldier and a feebleminded tavern girl. The other began when the young soldier returned from the war and "married into a good family." The progeny from the first branch were not exactly exemplary citizens; indeed, they were reported to have been lazy, criminal, and extremely feebleminded; the descendants from the second branch, however, were normal, reputable people who lived normal, reputable lives. Clear evidence, argued Goddard, that the poor and the stupid should not be allowed to breed.

But is the evidence really clear? Not by a long shot. No clearly reliable instrument had yet been devised to measure intelligence, making it difficult to ascertain whether there was actually as marked a difference between the two branches of the Kallikaks as Goddard believed. In fact, although Goddard had been using his own version of the Binet test to prove that immigrants were feebleminded, he had not bothered to test the Kallikaks. Instead, he sent one of his helpers, a highly "intuitive" woman who, he assures us, could easily recognize feeblemindedness on sight (Gould, 1981). And when she could not see the Kallikaks herself, she relied on accounts provided for her by acquaintances of the Kallikaks and not the family members themselves. Finally, there remains the haunting possibility that Martin Kallikak, the young soldier, was not really the father of the tavern maid's child, whose paternity was established solely on the basis of the mother's testimony. And the mother was supposedly feebleminded.

Animal Studies

It might seem strange to make frequent use of rats in an attempt to understand human behavior. However, there are many things that can be done with social impunity to a rat; the same antics with a human child would be wholly unacceptable. In addition, rats lead relatively uncomplicated lives, reproduce rapidly, and are simple and economical to look after. Children lead complex lives, are quite expensive and difficult to look after, and are usually incapable of reproducing. Hence there are both practical and ethical reasons why the rat is sometimes a preferred subject. Clearly, however, all these studies suffer from the problem of having to generalize from animals to humans.

Among the best-known investigations of the inheritance of learning ability in animals is Tryon's (1940) experiment at the University of California. Tryon attempted to produce a strain of bright rats and one of dull rats through a process of selective breeding. He started with a parent generation of 142 rats, half male and half female. Each rat was run through a seventeen-unit maze for a total of nineteen trials. Tryon counted the total number of errors made by each rat as it learned to run the maze. The count ranged from 14 errors for the brightest rat to 174 for the dullest. Next he mated the bright rats with each other and the dull ones with each other. The progeny from these artificial sexual arrangements were then introduced to the same seventeen-unit maze, and their error scores were tabulated. Now the brightest offspring of the bright rats were mated with each other, while the dullest offspring of the dull rats were mated. The duller rats produced by bright parents (possible even in the best of families) and the brighter rats produced by the dull parents were eliminated. This procedure was continued through a total of eighteen generations, with the brightest of the bright and the dullest of the dull being paired and all others being sacrificed in the interests of science. The experiment was carefully controlled. The offspring from dull parents were occasionally exchanged with those from bright parents, allowing the mother rats to raise offspring that they themselves had not produced. This exchange was designed to eliminate the possibility that early maternal attention was responsible for the apparent difference in brightness, assuming that brighter female rats would be likely to give their offspring the kind of attention particularly beneficial for stimulating their infants' intellectual growth. In addition, errors were scored electronically to eliminate the biases of the experimenter from the final results.

The striking result of this experiment was that the dullest rats among the bright group were brighter than the brightest rats from the dull group; conversely, the brightest rats from the dull group were duller than the dullest ones from the bright group. Indeed, after eighteen generations there was no longer any overlap between the groups (see Figure 3.5).

Searle (1949) later tested the same strains of rats on a variety of other learning tasks and found that the maze-bright rats were not necessarily bright for all tasks. Similarly, the maze-dull rats were not found to be universally dull. Tryon's earlier conclusions regarding maze-learning differences between the two strains were not invalidated, however. Indeed, his conclusions were later reaffirmed by a different experimental procedure. An analysis of the brains of Tryon's two strains of rats performed by Krech, Rosenzweig, Bennett, and Krueckel (1954) revealed marked chemical differences in favor of the maze-bright strain.

Does that mean that the environment has no effect on the intelligence of the rat? No. Krech and his associates (1960, 1962, 1966), assisted by the lowly white Norway rat, provide impressive evidence to the contrary. They too reared groups of rats in either enriched environments or deprived environments. The environment of a laboratory rat is assumed to be enriched when it contains a wide variety of rat toys, such as marbles, exercise wheels, posts to gnaw on, and when the cage is airy and well lighted. A more deprived environment is produced by lining the rat's cage with tin to obscure its view, keeping it dimly lit, preventing the rat from associating with humans or other rats, and keeping all toys out of the cage. It has been demonstrated repeatedly that rats raised in enriched environments are intellectually superior to their less fortunate confreres, at least when intellectual superiority is measured in terms of their ability to learn quickly the pattern of a maze (Hebb, 1949). It has also been discovered that the chemical composition of the brain of a rat that has been raised in an enriched environment is measurably different from that of a rat reared in a deprived environment (Krech, Rosenzweig, & Bennett, 1966).

These objective data argue strongly for varied and plentiful environmental stimulation in the early stages of a rat's life. By extrapolation, the same conclusion may be applied to humans. Fortunately, the evidence supporting this conclusion is not restricted to studies of the behavior of *Rattus norvegicus albinus*; there are studies and naturalistic observations of human children that lead to the same conclusion. However, even in the interests of science, it is not considered proper to decapitate children to examine the chemical structure of their brains. Most of the studies of humans have obviously lacked the experimental controls possible when employing rats; they have also lacked the precision of measurement sometimes possible with the rat. What studies of human children provide that no rat study can offer is the chance to observe and to measure processes considered to

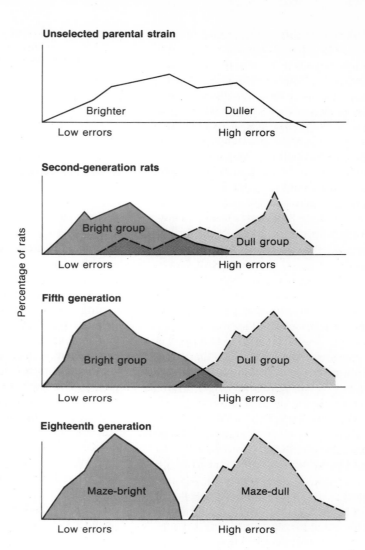

Figure 3.5
An approximate representation of Tryon's successful attempt to produce maze-bright and maze-dull rats through selective breeding. After eighteen generations of selective breeding, the dullest of the bright rats were brighter than the brightest of the dull group, and vice versa. (From *Yearbook of the National Society for the Study of Education.* Copyright 1940 by Guy Montrose Whipple, Secretary of the Society. Used by permission.)

be uniquely human, or at least unavailable to such phylogenetically unfortunate animals as rats.

A number of studies of human children brought up in conditions of varying deprivation, not by experimental design but as a result of the cruel whims of chance, are described in the following section. These studies measure language learning, motor abilities such as walking or creeping, and human intelligence. The rat is ordinarily incapable of communicating by means of lan-

guage, its intelligence is assumed to be quite different from human intelligence, and its ability to walk does not occur at the end of a long period of maturation or learning. Hence these findings are uniquely human.

Children

The Krech studies indicate that enriched environments can be beneficial to rats and that impoverished environments can be detrimental to their development. Although it is probably correct to assume that the same is true for humans, there is a lack of reliable supportive evidence. As noted before, it is usually impossible to restrict the environmental stimulation of young children deliberately to observe the effect on their development. Those studies that address the problem are usually the result of natural rather than contrived circumstances and often lack important experimental controls. For example, children from isolated areas who have not had the same degree or quality of environmental stimulation as children in less isolated regions may also have come from very different genetic backgrounds. It is not altogether unreasonable to assume that frequently those parents who are forced by economic or social conditions to isolate themselves are of inferior intelligence in the first place and that their children might also be of inferior intelligence, regardless of where their parents lived. Thus, it is difficult to determine whether environmental deprivation or heredity was responsible for inferior development. A well-known study that provides controls for this possibility is the study of intelligence test scores of isolated mountain children, known as the Hollow Children, reported by Sherman (1933) and by Sherman and Key (1932).

The Hollow Children were so named because they lived in various isolated hollows, rimmed by the Blue Ridge Mountains, some 100 miles west of Washington, D.C. The hollows were settled by the English and Scotch-Irish immigrants who had been forced to retreat into the mountains when the land on which they lived was granted to German immigrants. There they remained, some more deprived of contact with the external world than others who dwelt closer to civilization. Because the ancestry of each hollow region was the same, we might validly assume that the genetic pool of the area was highly similar.

Four hollows in the Blue Ridge range were selected by Sherman and Key (1932), each characterized by a different degree of isolation. Colvin, the innermost hollow, appeared to be the most isolated. During the previous twelve years (from 1918 to 1930), a school had been in session for a

Table 3.1 Total time school was open in the Hollows from 1918 to 1930.

Hollow	Months of School
Colvin	16
Needles	30
Oakton	66
Rigby	66.5
Briarsville (control group)	108

total of sixteen months. Only three of the adults who lived there were literate, and physical contact with the outside world was virtually impossible and consequently nonexistent. As the researchers proceeded outward toward civilization, passing through Needles Hollow, Oakton Hollow, and finally to Rigby Hollow, schools were in progress for an increasingly longer period of time. In Rigby Hollow, for example, a school had been open for nearly sixty-seven months in the preceding twelve years (see Table 3.1), many of the adults were literate, a road linked the hollow to the outside, a post office provided residents with contact with the world, and many residents subscribed to magazines or newspapers. Briarsville, a small village of the same ancestry as the hollows but situated at the foot of the Blue Ridge Mountains rather than in the isolation beyond the range, was employed as a control group.

The experimenters administered 386 intelligence tests to the Hollow Children and 198 tests in Briarsville. These tests included different measures, ranging from the time-consuming but highly reliable Stanford-Binet to the Goodenough Draw-a-Man Test (which requires only that the subjects draw the "very best" picture they can of a man). Not all tests were given to each child.

Two aspects of this study are particularly important. First, and not surprisingly, as the experimenters moved from the most isolated to the least isolated of the hollows, the performance of the children on the various intelligence tests increased markedly (see Table 3.2). Second, a striking relationship was found between the age of the children at the time of testing and their measured

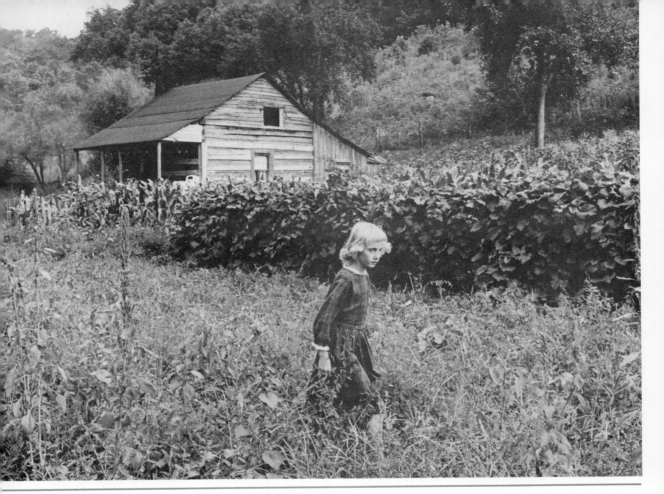

Deprived environments are those that provide too little for the mind. They may occur in the ghettos of our cities or in poetic rural settings such as the one here.

Table 3.2 Comparisons between mountain children and contrast groups on some measures of intelligence.

Measure	Mountain Children	Briarsville Children
National Intelligence Test	61.2	96.1
Pinter-Cunningham	75.9	87.6
Year-Scale Performance Test	83.9	118.6

intelligence (Figure 3.6): the older the children, the lower their IQ scores. Indeed, the very young children were not significantly below the test norms, but the fourteen- and fifteen-year-old children were markedly disadvantaged. Both these observations seem to provide additional evidence that the environment is a potent force in determining the intelligence test scores of individuals. This is somewhat different from saying that their intelligence is itself affected, because it may simply be their ability to take the tests that is affected.

The Sherman and Key study provides evidence that intellectual performance may be negatively affected by the environment. Dennis (1960) conducted a study that demonstrates the effect of impoverished environments on the motor development of children. The subjects for this study were young children who lived in three orphanages in Tehran, the capital of Iran. Two of the orphanages (Institutions I and II) gave their charges similar treatment; the third (Institution III) will be described shortly. The principal difference between Institutions I and II was that the latter accepted children after the age of three, most of whom had spent their first three years in Institution I. Over 90 percent of the children in Institution I were admitted prior to the age of one month and remained until they were between two and three years of age.

Among the most striking features of the children's environment during their first three years in Institution I was the abject poverty. Infants spent almost all their time lying in their cribs, on their backs. They were seldom, if ever, placed on their stomachs—a fact believed to have considerable significance in explaining their retarded motor development. The infants were fed by means of a bottle propped up on a small pillow while lying in their cribs; later, when solid foods were introduced, they were either held for short periods by one of the attendants while being fed or were fed sitting up in their cribs. During these first years, children remained in their cribs continually except when bathed, changed, or, on occasion, fed. When they learned to sit up or to pull themselves to a standing position, they were occasionally removed from the crib and placed on a piece of linoleum on the stone floor. Dennis (1960) reports that two of the rooms had benches along one wall. Children who had learned to sit were often placed on these benches, behind a railing that prevented them from falling. Apart from the cribs and these benches in two of the rooms, none of the rooms had any toys or any other children's furniture. The walls were painted white and were devoid of pictures.

The preceding description makes it clear that

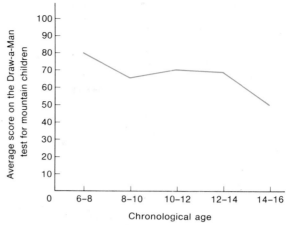

Figure 3.6
One example of increasing retardation with increasing age. (Adapted from Lee, *American Sociological Review* 1951, p. 231. Copyright 1951 by the American Sociological Association. Used by permission of the American Sociological Association and the author.

the amount of human contact for the children in Institution I was minimal. Part of this was due to the extremely high staff-child ratio—one attendant to eight or more children. These attendants were responsible not only for feeding the children but also for bathing and changing them, for changing their beds, and for cleaning the rooms. Conditions in Institution II were similar except that the children were older because they usually came from the first orphanage to the second. Institution III, established mainly to demonstrate better methods of child care, was characterized by a more normal physical and social environment. The ratio of attendants to children was one to three or four; most of the children also came from Institution I, but had been moved to the new orphanage in the early months of their lives. Institution III provided toys and ample opportunity for the children to play. Attendants held the children while feeding them, frequently placed them prone in their cribs, and allowed infants over four months to spend time each day in playpens on the floor.

Dennis's study of these three institutions primarily involved testing motor development and comparing the results among the different insti-

Table 3.3 Percentage of each group passing each test.

Institution	I	I	II	III	III
Number of children	50	40	33	20	31
Age (years)	1.0–1.99	2.0–2.99	3.0–3.99	1.0–1.99	2.0–2.99
Sit alone	42	95	97	90	100
Creep or scoot	14	75	97	75	100
Stand holding	4	45	90	70	100
Walk holding	2	40	63	60	100
Walk alone	0	8	15	15	94

From Wayne Dennis, Causes of retardation among institutional children: Iran. *The Journal of Genetic Psychology*, 1960, pp. 47–59. Used by permission of The Journal Press.

tutions. Table 3.3 summarizes his findings, which clearly demonstrate motor retardation in Institutions I and II. Consider, for example, that in Institution I only 8 percent of the children could walk alone by the age of nearly three years, whereas 94 percent of the children of the same age in Institution III could do so. According to Dennis's data, the pattern is the same for all other aspects of motor development. Interestingly, of those children in Institutions I and II who were capable of locomotion by some means other than walking, only ten did so by creeping; the remaining fifty-seven propelled themselves with their arms and legs while in a sitting position—most of the children moved by **scooting** rather than by creeping. In contrast, in Institution III, all the children who were capable of locomotion but incapable of walking did so by creeping. In explaining the scooting behavior of children in the first two institutions, Dennis maintains that children must have some opportunity to *learn* the abilities involved in creeping—and it is apparent that this learning can be fostered or impeded by the environment. Given Dennis's data, apparently it must be essential for young children to lie prone as well as supine if they are to learn to creep.

The more general conclusion supported by the Dennis experiment is that the motor skills involved in sitting, standing, and walking are not solely the result of genetic processes but may be affected by the environment.

The Effect of Changes in the Environment

Presumably, a good environment will have beneficial effects on a person's development; conversely, a poor environment (as in the Dennis study) may have harmful effects. Can dramatic changes in the environment reverse these effects? Some evidence, such as the classic Lee (1951) study, suggests yes. In this study, several groups of black children were followed through grades one to nine, and intelligence tests were administered to them at various intervals. Some of the subjects had been born in Philadelphia and had remained there; others had been born in the southern United States and had moved to Philadelphia while in grade one or grade four.

To understand the results of the study, it is necessary to accept Lee's assumption that the intellectual stimulation provided for black children in the South during the 1940s was generally inferior to that provided for the same children in Philadelphia schools (this assumption seems reasonable in view of the significant differences in intelligence test scores of comparable groups of black children born in the South and those born in Philadelphia). The data presented in Figure 3.7 show the magnitude of these initial differences and the changes in scores on tests administered after the children had spent some time in Philadelphia. Two aspects of the findings presented in this table are of special note: first, the markedly inferior scores of all groups composed of children who had moved from the South in grade one or later and, second, the increased performance of children who had moved at a younger age. As Bloom (1964, p. 76) notes, "The point of the Lee study is the decreasing effect of an improved environment with increasing age." Bloom contends that the environment will have the greatest effect on a trait during that trait's period of fastest growth.

Dennis (1973) reports a second group of studies with conclusions similar to those of the Lee study. These involved comparisons between two major groups of children: One consisted of orphaned and illegitimate children brought up in extremely unstimulating environments in various *crèches* (French for a cradle or orphanage) in Lebanon; the second also consisted of Lebanese children, but these had been rescued from the crèche through adoption by American parents. The adoptions occurred when the children were between birth and the age of seven. Here, as in the Lee study, various measures of intelligence revealed dramatic differences in favor of children who had been adopted. And the younger the age of adoption, the more dramatic the difference.

The implications of these studies argue strongly for the importance of love and stimulation in infancy and early childhood and demonstrate the harmful effects that the absence of these experiences can have. But they do not deal specifically with the relative contributions of heredity and environment in human development. Studies of twins come closer to this question.

Studies of Twins

"If I had any desire to lead a life of indolent ease," Gould tells us, "I would wish to be an identical twin, separated at birth from my brother and raised in a different social class. We could hire ourselves

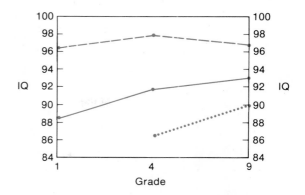

Figure 3.7
Changes in intelligence test scores on measures obtained in first, fourth, and ninth grades for black students born and raised in Philadelphia (dashed line), those born in the South and moving to Philadelphia in the first grade (solid line), and those who did not move to Philadelphia until the fourth grade (dotted line). (Adapted from E. S. Lee, *American Sociological Review*, 1951, p. 231. Copyright 1951 by The American Sociological Association. Used by permission of the American Sociological Association and the author.)

out to a host of social scientists and practically name our fee. For we would be exceedingly rare representatives of the only really adequate natural experiment for separating genetic from environmental effects in humans" (1981, p. 234).

Why is this so? To begin with, identical twins are the only genetically identical individuals that two humans can produce. They are genetically identical because they result from the splitting of a single zygote, a fertilized ovum, that has already obtained its full complement of chromosomes from the sperm and from the ovum. This segmentation results in two fertilized eggs, each with an identical genetic makeup, producing **identical (monozygotic) twins.** The other type of twins, **fraternal** or **dizygotic**, results from the fertilization of two *different* egg cells by two *different* spermatozoa. This is possible only when the mother produces more than one egg and will obviously result in twins who are no more alike genetically than ordinary **siblings**. In comparing the effects of heredity and environment, however, it is customary to assume that fraternal twins have environ-

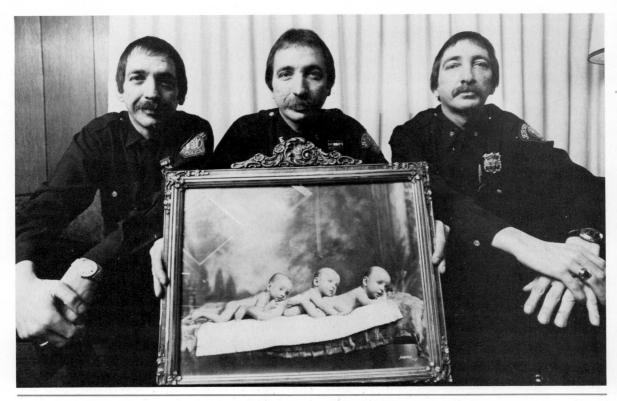

Twins occur rarely in human births and provide researchers with an excellent opportunity to separate the effects of heredity and environment. Triplets, such as the Koralja trio who are Jersey City policemen, are even rarer.

ments that are probably more similar than those of siblings, if only because they share the same womb at the same time and because they are of the same age as they develop. Identical twins are likewise assumed to have highly similar environments.

It follows that any greater similarity between identical twins than between fraternal twins of the same sex (identical twins are always of the same sex) will be due to the influence of heredity. By the same token, if fraternal twins are more alike than ordinary siblings, it would not result from their greater genetic similarity but from their more nearly identical environments, both prenatally and postnatally. Unfortunately for research, the incidence of twins is relatively low—approximately one case in every eighty-six births. Furthermore,

identical twins are much rarer than fraternal twins. The precise causes of twin births are not known, although heredity appears to be a factor, because twins are found relatively frequently in some families and not at all in others. In addition, the age of the parents seems to have some bearing on the probability of giving birth to twins: Krech, Crutchfield, and Livson (1969) report that women between the ages of thirty and thirty-eight are more likely to have twins; similarly, regardless of the age of the mother, older men are more likely to father twins than are younger men.

Numerous studies of twins have been conducted, most of them looking at correlations for intelligence test scores. Recall from Chapter 1 that a correlation is a measure of relationship. It ranges from 0 to plus or minus 1. A high *positive* corre-

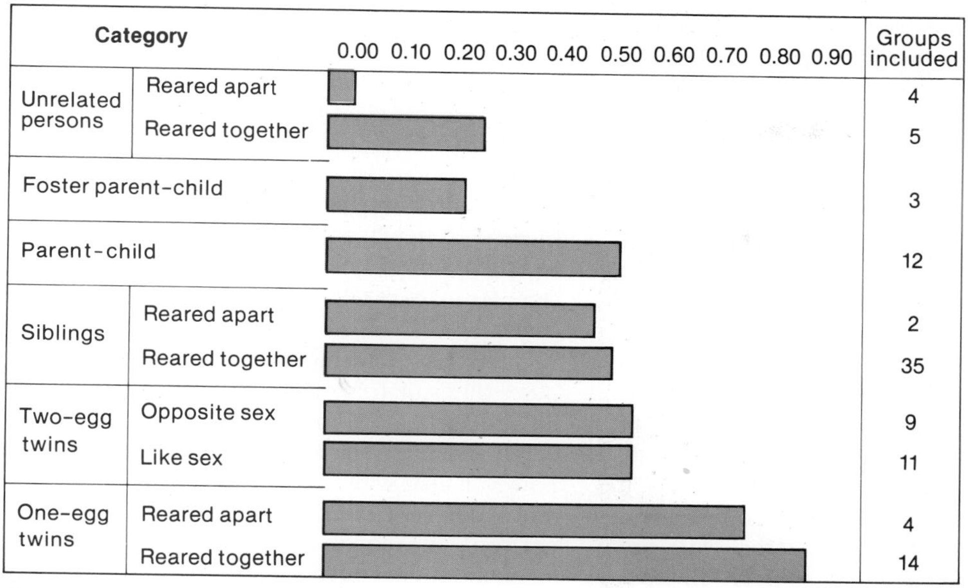

Category		0.00 0.10 0.20 0.30 0.40 0.50 0.60 0.70 0.80 0.90	Groups included
Unrelated persons	Reared apart	▇	4
	Reared together	▇▇▇▇	5
Foster parent–child		▇▇▇▇	3
Parent–child		▇▇▇▇▇▇▇	12
Siblings	Reared apart	▇▇▇▇▇▇	2
	Reared together	▇▇▇▇▇▇▇	35
Two-egg twins	Opposite sex	▇▇▇▇▇▇▇	9
	Like sex	▇▇▇▇▇▇▇	11
One-egg twins	Reared apart	▇▇▇▇▇▇▇▇▇	4
	Reared together	▇▇▇▇▇▇▇▇▇▇	14

Figure 3.8

Correlation coefficients for intelligence test scores from fifty-two studies. The high correlation for identical twins shows the strong genetic basis of measured intelligence. The greater correlation for siblings or twins reared together compared with those reared apart supports the view that environmental forces are also important in determining similarity of intelligence test scores. (From L. Erlenmeyer-Kimling and L. F. Jarvik, Genetics and intelligence: A review. *Science*, 1963, *142*, 1478. Copyright 1963 by the American Association for the Advancement of Science. Used by permission.)

lation—say, +.75 to +1.00—means that if one twin has a high intelligence test score, the corresponding twin is likely to also have a high score (or both are likely to have low or mediocre scores). A high *negative* correlation means that a high score for one would be associated with a low score for the other.

Bouchard and McGue (1981), Hunt (1961), Vernon (1979), and others have summarized some of the correlations of studies of twins. In general, the average correlation for intelligence test scores for identical twins is approximately 0.90, while that for fraternal twins is 0.65. If members of identical and fraternal twin pairs have had similar environments, these correlations may be interpreted as evidence that measured intelligence is at least partly determined by heredity. Related to these studies

is the observation that with decreasing genetic similarity, there is a corresponding decrease in similarity between intelligence scores. Figure 3.8 is a summary of a number of correlations for intelligence test scores. Not surprisingly, the lowest correlation (0.00) is for genetically unrelated children, whereas the highest correspondence (+0.90) is found in the case of identical twins.

These data clearly support a genetic explanation. As the astute reader will note, they can also support an environmental position. For example, it is logical to assume that most sets of identical twins have more similar environments than do cousins or siblings. One may argue, therefore, that the higher correlation between various intelligence measures for identical twins stems at least in part from their more nearly identical environments. The problem is somewhat complicated by the counterargument that many parents of fraternal twins do not realize that their offspring are not identical until their formative years have passed and that many parents would treat fraternal twins just as they would identical twins, particularly if the twins were the same sex. The observed differences between identical twins and fraternal twins, if one assumes that the environments of members of each pair are probably highly similar, must then be due to genetic rather than to environmental factors. Employing the same data, an environmentalist could point to the difference between fraternal twins and siblings as additional evidence that environment influences development. Figure 3.8, for example, reports correlations of 0.65 and 0.50 for intelligence test scores of fraternal twins and siblings, respectively. Because fraternal twins are no more alike genetically than siblings, environmentalists assume that this difference is a result of environmental rather than genetic factors.

Newman, Freeman, and Holzinger (1937) studied twins reared together and twins reared apart. Identical twins reared apart would obviously be unlikely to have similar environments; certainly those reared together would have more nearly identical environments. The data from this study (reported in Table 3.4) provide clear evidence that intelligence, height, and weight are at least partly genetically determined. The power of heredity is evident in the high correlations between members

of twin pairs for each of these measures, whether they were reared together or apart. However, the much lower correlation for intelligence test scores for twins reared apart in comparison to those reared together (0.73 as opposed to 0.92) is evidence that environment is also a powerful factor in determining measured intelligence. The environment's influence on height and weight is apparently much less pronounced, because the correlations are quite close for twins reared together and for those reared apart.

Studies of twins have also compared attributes other than intelligence. For example, Loehlin and Nichols (1976) found that a large number of personality traits are partly inheritable. Note, however, that with increasing age, twins become more different (Henderson, 1982). Clearly, the environment continues to have an influence throughout the course of development.

Perhaps more striking is Gottesman's (1979) finding that various types of mental disorders appear to have a genetic basis. For example, Gottesman and Shields (1982) discovered a significantly higher concordance for schizophrenia between members of identical twin pairs than for members of fraternal twin pairs. The procedure was to identify members of twin pairs from among a population of schizophrenic patients and then to determine how many of these individuals had a twin who was also schizophrenic. Specifically, they found that of twenty-eight pairs of identical twins there was 42 percent concordance—that is, 42 percent of all schizophrenic members of twin pairs had a schizophrenic twin. The concordance between members of fraternal twin pairs was only 9 percent, from a sample of thirty-four pairs.

Further evidence of a genetic factor in schizophrenia is provided by a study conducted by Heston (1966). Children born to mothers who had been diagnosed schizophrenic and institutionalized were taken at birth and placed in adoptive homes. A comparable group of children whose mothers were normal, but who had also been placed for adoption shortly after birth, served as a control group. Of the forty-seven children in the schizophrenic mothers group, five were themselves later diagnosed as schizophrenic, and a large number

Table 3.4 Correlations for intelligence, weight, and height for identical twins reared together and apart.

	Intelligence (group test)	Height	Weight
Identical twins reared together	0.92	0.98	0.97
Identical twins reared apart	0.73	0.97	0.89

Data from H. H. Newman, F. N. Freeman, and K. J. Holzinger, *Twins: A study of heredity and environment*, p. 347. Copyright 1937 by The University of Chicago Press. Used by permission.

of the remaining forty-two were found to suffer from social and emotional problems. Nobody in the comparison group was classified as schizophrenic, and only a few were described as suffering from emotional or social problems. These and similar studies have led to the conclusion that the predisposition to develop schizophrenia may have a significant genetic component (Ehrman & Parsons, 1981; Plomin, DeFries, & McClearn, 1980).

The Jensen Hypothesis

There have been numerous attempts to summarize the data on the inheritance of intelligence. Erlenmeyer-Kimling and Jarvik (1963) looked at more than thirty thousand correlations gleaned from early studies. These studies, with few exceptions, demonstrate an increasing degree of correlation between scores on intelligence tests and the subjects' genetic relatedness. And Vernon (1979), in his review of the literature, concludes that a strong hereditary factor apparently is involved in intellectual *performance* (on intelligence tests). He is careful to point out, however, that heredity is only one of the factors that determines intellectual functioning.

Among the strongest proponents of the theory that heredity accounts for most of the variation in intelligence test scores was Burt (1966), who believed that heredity and environment interact; he went further than most psychologists by stating that the contribution of environment to intelligence is minimal. Jensen's view is similar.

Jensen's (1968) estimates of the heritability of intelligence (heritability coefficients) are based in part on studies of twins (including Sir Cyril Burt's— see the box). The argument is relatively simple. Identical twins, if intelligence were solely determined by heredity, would have IQs that were perfectly correlated (1.00). However, because correlation is less than perfect, the difference between the obtained correlation and a perfect correlation stems from the environment (as well as from errors of measurement). Jensen's interpretation of the relevant research leads him to the conclusion that approximately 80 percent of the variation in intel-

ligence test scores is due to heredity, with only 20 percent being accounted for by the environment. These estimates are now considered to be overestimates. More recent estimates are typically much closer to 50 percent (Henderson, 1982).

Although there is some agreement with Jensen's contention that heredity is more potent than environmental factors in determining variation in measured intelligence, there is considerable disagreement with a second aspect of his work, dealing with genetic differences among races. On measures of intellectual performance, even when care has apparently been taken to ensure that all subjects have at least superficially similar backgrounds, American blacks often score below the average for whites. Given this finding, the apparently high heritability coefficient for intelligence, and the assumption that blacks and whites represent different gene pools, Jensen reasons that racial differences in intelligence test scores may have a genetic component.

The **Jensen hypothesis** has been subjected to severe criticism on a variety of grounds. Kagan (1969) and a number of geneticists point out, for example, that there is so much overlap among racial groups that no single gene exists in one group alone, although it is true that certain genes and clusters of genes are more frequent in some groups than in others. Indeed, there is considerable disagreement among geneticists concerning the concept of race. Although some find it useful and appropriate to divide humanity into varying numbers of races, other contend that the concept of race is no longer tenable or particularly useful. Given the genetic overlap among racial groups, it is presently impossible to prove that IQ differences are genetically determined. Furthermore, IQ differences within a single group are almost invariably five to ten times greater than those between groups. If genetics is so potent, why is there so much variation within groups?

Other critics of Jensen's hypothesis point to his heritability coefficients that cannot really be substantiated (Lerner, 1976), the very small samples in most of the studies from which the heritability coefficients were derived (Crow, 1969), and Jensen's failure to take into account the apparent

SIR CYRIL BURT: FRAUD?

Among the most convincing studies of the inheritability of intelligence were those reported by the late Sir Cyril Burt and used extensively by others to support their genetic arguments (for example, Herrnstein, 1973; Jensen, 1974). These studies ostensibly involved twins, some reared together and some apart—ostensibly because the studies may never have been conducted as reported. Indeed, it now appears that Burt's data may be quite useless (Wade, 1976). Why?

First, Burt's two principal co-workers, authors of numerous articles highly supportive of Burt's argument that intelligence is largely inherited, may never have written any of the articles attributed to them. Margaret Howard and J. Conway could not be found when investigators first began to probe into Burt's research. And when it was later established that they had, in fact, existed, it became apparent that neither could easily have written any of the articles. Furthermore, as Kamin (1974) points out, given the remarkable similarities between the writing styles of these two individuals and Burt, it is difficult to believe that Burt did not write all the material attributed to them (see also Gould, 1981).

Science might, in retrospect, forgive Burt his creation of two fictional characters to assist him in tormenting his detractors and in establishing his point of view. It is less likely to tolerate the errors that have also been found in Burt's work. Among the most obvious of these is the fact that in three separate studies he reports identical correlation coefficients for intelligence test scores of twins raised together and apart. That these scores should be identical, given the highly unreliable nature of the measuring instruments employed, is unlikely at best. In addition, Burt's records frequently fail to provide crucial items of information concerning the tests employed, the age and sex of subjects, and so on.

How devastating is the loss of these data to the hereditarian's argument? Most claim that it is damaging, though not devastating. Jensen points out that most of the important results have already been replicated by others. At worst, estimates of heritability will simply have to be scaled down somewhat. Later reviews of research in this area indicate that most studies still support the view that intelligence is at least partly inherited (DeFries & Plomin, 1978). But few of these studies provide estimates as high as those advanced by Burt (Henderson, 1982; Scarr & Weinberg, 1977).

differences among blacks and whites with respect to such powerful environmental factors as nutrition (Brazziel, 1969). Protein deficiencies that are relatively common in lower socioeconomic groups and in improverished countries have been shown to be related to kwashiorkor (a sometimes fatal deficiency), to significantly below average physical growth, and perhaps to smaller brain size (Lewin, 1975).

Among the most telling criticisms of Jensen's work is that advanced by Crow (1969) concerning Jensen's assumption that the heritability of intelligence is the same in all races. Studies from which heritability coefficients were derived were all conducted on whites; it does not necessarily follow that intelligence is inherited to the same extent in all other racial groups. In addition, as Crow points out, even if 80 percent of the variation in intelligence test scores were determined by heredity, the differences observed between black and white groups still could have resulted from environmental factors. Nutrition is one such factor; perhaps there are others even more subtle. Indeed, as Layzer (1974) convincingly argues, terms such as **heritability coefficient** are largely meaningless in a scientific sense. When applied to the hypothesis of genetic differences among races, they are virtually worthless.

The Stern Hypothesis

A widely accepted point of view in the nature-nurture controversy is implicit in the following "rub-

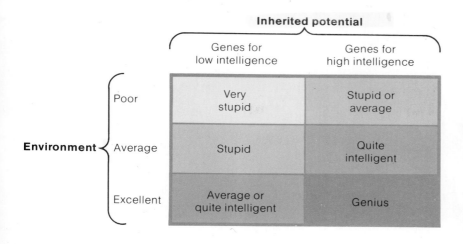

	Genes for low intelligence	Genes for high intelligence
Poor	Very stupid	Stupid or average
Average	Stupid	Quite intelligent
Excellent	Average or quite intelligent	Genius

Environment

Figure 3.9
The Stern hypothesis, an example of gene-environment interaction. Individuals with different inherited potentials for intellectual development can manifest a wide range of measured intelligence as a function of environmental forces.

ber-band" hypothesis from Stern (1956, p. 53; see Figure 3.9):

The genetic endowment in respect to any one trait has been compared to a rubber band and the trait itself to the length which the rubber band assumes when it is stretched by outside forces. Different people initially may have been given different lengths of unstretched endowment, but the natural forces of the environment may have stretched their expression to equal length, or led to differences in attained length sometimes corresponding to their innate differences and at other times in reverse of the relation.

Put somewhat more simply, some of us have short bands (the initial length of the band corresponds to inherited potential for being intelligent); others have longer bands. Some environments (good ones?) stretch bands a great deal; others hardly stretch them. Long bands, of course, stretch to great lengths more easily than short bands. Given the right environment, a short band might in the end be longer than one that was initially quite long—and vice versa.

■ The Issue

A cursory examination of the contents of this chapter might indicate that the central issue is whether environment or heredity is more important in determining the course of human development.

But a more basic issue is implicit in these discussions—the adaptability of humans. Indeed, one might say that the nature-nurture controversy is not really a controversy at all but simply an attempt to answer questions concerning the extent to which human behavior is modifiable. The two hypothetical camps historically aligned on either side of the controversy represent the two extreme responses to the question: that development is entirely genetically ordained and therefore completely unmodifiable (subject to nature) or that development is environmentally determined and therefore completely modifiable (nurture). Both answers are clearly untenable. Neither an exclusive belief in the power of genetics nor the conviction that the environment alone determines human development is acceptable.

■ A Conclusion and a Note on Interaction

The conclusion is clear: Heredity and environment interact to determine human characteristics. What is often unclear, however, is the meaning of this conclusion. Specifically, there are several important points that need to be kept in mind concerning what we mean by *heritability* and by *interaction*.

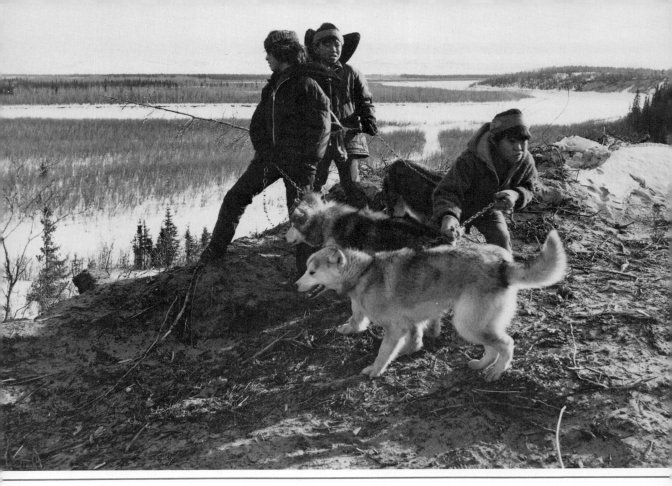

The interaction of heredity and environment is extremely complex. That these Eskimo boys are a product of both might be more clearly evident if we could compare them to who they would have been in different environments. Are dogs less a product of their environments and more of their genes than their masters?

First, heritability describes genetic influences that apply to groups and not to individuals. This means that the influence of heredity for any one individual may be greater or less than for another. Second, numerical estimates of the heritability of something like intelligence are practically worthless, given the unreliability of the tests used to measure it (see Gould, 1981). Third, genes do not *cause* intelligence; they *interact* with the environment and, as a result of this interaction, we behave more or less intelligently.

What, precisely, is interaction? Most of us assume, without really thinking about it, that we

know. Most of us are wrong. We assume, for example, that heredity and environment each account for a percentage of this or that, the sum total being you or me. That is, we assume that if we understood the separate effects of heredity and environment, we would only need to add them to understand their combined effects.

Not so. Interaction is a complex, nonadditive phenomenon. Take something as simple as water and temperature. We know that water and temperature interact to form ice; but can we understand the hardness of ice, its taste, its effect on our skin, solely by understanding temperature and water? And is it not true that steam also results from the interaction of water and temperature? The interaction becomes more complex, but it still appears linear and predictable: More heat equals steam; less heat equals ice. Even here, however, interaction is not quite so simple. With changes in air pressure, the interaction of water and temperature changes. Now an even higher or lower temperature is required for the same effect.

So too with heredity, environment, and human behavior—interaction is not a simple additive affair. Relative contributions of heredity and environment may change with age, might be different in different environments, and might vary from one individual to another. And to the simple questions "What would we be without genetics?" and "What would we be without heredity?" the answer is "Nothing." Clearly, genetics and environment are not additive.

One of the great dangers when considering the effects of heredity and environment is to assume that heredity determines by limiting our possibilities. And while this point of view is at least partly accurate (no amount of nutrition would have been likely to make me 6 feet 9, allowing me to become a basketball star), it is nevertheless true that while we can do little about genetics, we still have considerable control over the environment. It is certainly far more optimistic to adopt a point of view that, with Gould (1981), emphasizes the flexibility and uniqueness made possible by our biological natures. In spite of our tremendous similarities, you and I are really quite different.

■ MAIN POINTS

1 Nature refers to biology or genetics; nurture, to the environment. Hence the nature-nurture question concerns the ways in which heredity and environment interact to determine human development.

2 That genetic information is coded in a DNA molecule is known, but the precise interaction between heredity and environment remains a mystery.

3 The hereditary basis of life resides in the egg cell (ovum) and in the sperm cell (spermatozoon), each of which contains half the number of chromosomes found in ordinary human body cells. In the chromosomes are the carriers of heredity, the genes.

4 Two chromosomes of special importance are the sex chromosomes, X and Y. Only the father can produce a Y chromosome, while both mother and father produce X chromosomes. The presence of a Y chromosome in the fertilized egg determines that the offspring will be male; two X chromosomes determine a female.

5 Among the better-known and most common genetic abnormalities are Down's syndrome, resulting from an extra twenty-first chromosome; Turner's syndrome, affecting females only and linked to an absent sex chromosome (XO rather than XX); the XYY syndrome (super males), affecting males only, and Klinefelter's syndrome, affecting males with an extra X chromosome (XXY). These and other abnormalities may be detected prior to birth through amniocentesis.

6 Galton was one of the first proponents of the theory that intelligence is genetically determined. Highly circumstantial evidence from studies of two families, the Jukes and the Kallikaks, has frequently been employed to support this belief.

7 Tryon's study of rats supports the contention that heredity is of primary importance in the development of intellectual capabilities. Through selective breeding, he succeeded in producing two strains of rats (maze-bright and maze-dull) that were so different that the dullest rats among the bright group were brighter than the brightest rats among the dull group. Krech and his associates and Hebb did the same thing by modifying the rats' environment.

8 Studies of children living in isolated mountain regions (the Hollow Children) provide dramatic evidence of the detrimental effect that deprived and unstimulating environments have on children.

9 The environment's influence on the development of motor skills such as walking is evident in the case of institutionalized children, reared in an unstimulating and undemanding environment, who were markedly retarded in their motor development by the age of two or three years.

10 The damaging effects of early deprivation can sometimes be partially overcome by exposure to a more stimulating environment. In general, a stimulating environment will be more effective during the earlier rather than the later years of childhood.

11 The correlations between various physical and psychological measures for twins frequently indicate that fraternal twins are more closely related than siblings—that is, their scores for various traits tend to be closer than those for siblings. Because fraternal twins are no more alike genetically than siblings and because their environments are in most cases more similar, this greater similarity may be evidence of the environment's influence in determining these traits.

12 Studies of twins also provide evidence that intelligence as well as physical characteristics, some personality traits, and even mental disorders have a genetic basis. The most striking supportive evidence is that the correlation between intelligence test scores for identical twins is approximately 0.90, whereas for fraternal twins it is 0.65.

13 Among proponents of the view that intelligence has a more significant genetic than environmental basis are Burt and Jensen.

14 The Stern hypothesis presents a summary of the evidence relating to the nature-nurture controversy by stating that genetic endowment is like a rubber band that assumes its final length (the actual performance of an individual) as it interacts with the environment. Implicit in this summary is the notion that it is easier to stretch a long band than a short one.

15 Estimates of heritability apply to groups and not to individuals. They are not very useful, given the unreliability and biases of our measures, and they do not establish that genes cause intelligence.

16 The interaction of heredity and environment is complex and nonadditive, so the relative importance of heredity and environment may be very different for different individuals and may change for the same individual under different circumstances.

17 Our genes are more than our limits; they make possible our uniqueness and our flexibility.

■ FURTHER READINGS

The classic account of a number of reported cases of wild children is found in:
Singh, J. A., & Zingg, R. N. *Wolf-children and feral man.* New York: Harper & Row, 1942.

For a fascinating account of the Wild Boy of Aveyron, see:
Lane, H. *The wild boy of Aveyron.* London: Allen & Unwin, 1977.

The Singh and Zingg and the Lane books should be followed by Dennis's rebuttals:
Dennis, W. The significance of feral man. *American Journal of Psychology,* 1941, *54,* 425–432.
Dennis, W. A further analysis of reports of wild children. *Child Development,* 1951, *22,* 153–158.

For a more detailed and complete examination of issues in human genetics than is provided in this chapter, see:
Plomin, R., DeFries, J. C., & McClearn, G. E. *Behavior genetics: A primer.* New York: W. H. Freeman, 1980.

Herrnstein and Kamin present two points of view concerning the classic nature-nurture IQ debate:
Herrnstein, R. J. *IQ in the meritocracy.* Boston: Little, Brown, 1973.
Kamin, L. J. *The science and politics of IQ.* Hillsdale, N.J.: Lawrence Erlbaum, 1974.

The relationship of genetic forces to development and children's learning is elaborated in Fishbein's book. His explanations and illustrations of epigenesis and canalization may be of particular value:
Fishbein, H. D. *Evolution, development, and children's learning.* Pacific Palisades, Calif.: Goodyear, 1976.

Stephen Gould's book presents a fascinating account of the history of mental measurement and a strong indictment of historical and some current beliefs concerning the IQ and its heritability in his aptly titled book:
Gould, S. J. *The mismeasure of man.* New York: W. W. Norton, 1981.

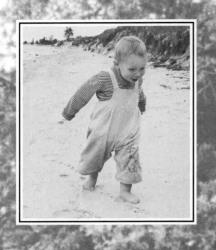

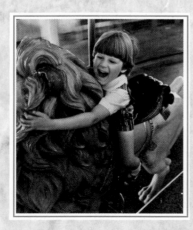

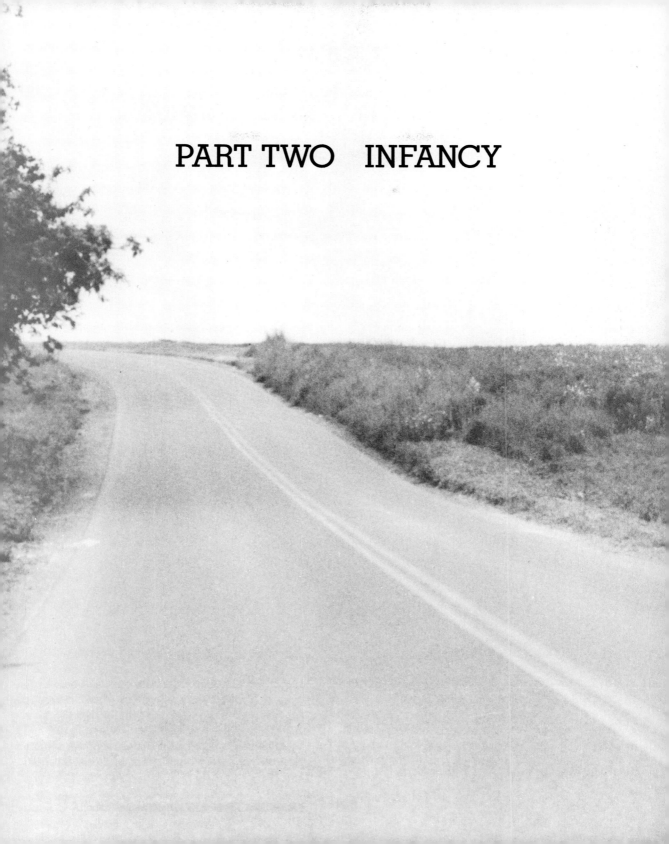

PART TWO   INFANCY

4

PRENATAL DEVELOPMENT AND BIRTH

"Who was your mother?"
"Never had none!" said the child, with another grin.
"Never had any mother? What do you mean? Where were you born?"
"Never was born!" persisted Topsy.
"Do you know who made you?"
"Nobody, as I knows on," said the child, with a short laugh.
"I 'spect I grow'd."

Harriet Beecher Stowe
Uncle Tom's Cabin

The service station is just a short distance off the main road: a pair of Shell gas pumps next to a two-story house sitting boldly a full mile from its closest neighbor. A family lives and works here. They have moved upstairs while a small general store has grown all over the main floor.

Hunger suddenly strikes my brood—as it so often does—and we argue briefly about what they should eat. They vote for potato chips and soft drinks; I argue nutrition and try to tantalize them with the merits of yogurt. There are three of them, and I find that my heart is not in the conflict. Lately the bigger battles consume so much of my energy that I have little left for the smaller skirmishes. And Grandma is not here to take up the slack; she has stayed outside and is talking to the lady planting her garden behind the store.

The store smells of rubber boots and plastic raincoats; I am disappointed. It should smell sweet and somewhat spicy, and only slightly pungent. But I see now that the rubber boots and raincoats are crowded against a southern window where the sun tries to melt them. I give Paul some money and go back outside where the smells are of black loam and new leaves and where the late spring air hums with unseen movements of thousands of little wings. Mostly mosquitoes.

No one seems anxious to leave. Paul and Denise sit on the steps, petting an old black dog; Grandma discusses yellow turnips, and Marcel seems to have disappeared. I ask where he is and someone points to a small shed just beyond the garden.

The shed is very old. It looks as if it was moved here from somewhere else, as if it doesn't really belong. The door has come loose from its top hinge and is now stuck, half open. I walk over and look inside. At first I see nothing, but as my eyes become accustomed to the musty darkness, I find Marcel kneeling by a cardboard box. The writing on the side says "Canadian Club."

"Kittens," he says, pointing. The bottles that might once have been in the box are no longer there; instead, five small kittens, mostly white but with tiny splotches of black and gray here and there. "I wish I could have seen them being born!"

"Why?" I settle back on my heels against the door frame, the sun warm on my left side.

"Denise saw Jimmy's puppies being born and she said it was neat. She said, 'well freak me green.' " Denise says "freak me green" quite a lot lately; the expression is very *au courant* with her crowd.

"Did she tell you how it happens?" I ask him. She didn't, and so as we walk back to the car, I begin to tell him how each tiny pup is born, encased in its little sac, and how the mother cleans it and licks it so that it will start breathing, and how she pushes it along toward her nipples so that it can feed or curl up where it's nice and warm. And soon another little puppy begins to come out. I stop just short of telling him how the mother also eats the afterbirth and umbilical cord.

"How does she know how to do all that?" he asks as we pull back onto the highway. The sun is higher now and gentle heat waves have begun to dance over the black fields; in the mirror, the asphalt shimmers slightly. How, indeed, does a totally uneducated bitch know to do these things?

Here is as good a place as any to get back to your questions about the span of human life. So far we have looked at the history and methods of the study of human development, at theories that have been invented to clarify our understanding, and at heredity and environment, the two great forces that shape our lives. Now, as we hurtle unerringly toward Smoky Lake this Friday morning, we can take a little time to look at human prenatal development and birth.

■ Conception

One might speculate about how a human female would fare if she found herself pregnant and about to give birth to a baby without benefit of the accumulated wisdom of the race in the form of specialized techniques, highly trained personnel, and modern equipment available in today's hospitals. Would she sense an urgency as her time drew near? Would she look for a shed or some other safe and sheltered place in which to give birth to her infant? And when birth finally occurred, would she instinctively stimulate the child's breathing, sever its umbilical cord, and eat the afterbirth (which is rich in nutrients and hormones that would greatly enchance her production of milk)? Or has civilized woman lost all her instinctual tendencies? But before we move too far, let us return again to the beginning.

The beginning of the story of child development was told in Part I, which, surprisingly in this world of unordered things, is entitled "The Beginning." But a smaller and more specific beginning deals not with the human race whose proud members we are, but with the inception of a single individual. This beginning requires the union of a sperm cell with an egg cell, as well as the physical union between the bearers of these cells. But, as I noted earlier, that is a mundane and uninteresting story for people as sophisticated as you are, so we will go directly to **conception**, the union of the two sex cells, rather than the union of the two sexes.

■ Pregnancy

Women find it valuable to be able to detect pregnancy prior to the actual birth of the baby. Although there are few indications of pregnancy that an expectant mother can interpret with certainty prior to the later stages of **prenatal development**, some less certain signs appear relatively soon after conception. They can include cessation of **menses**, morning sickness, changes in the breasts, increased frequency of urination, and **quickening** (movement of the fetus). Most of these symptoms do not occur very early in pregnancy (see the box *Detecting Pregnancy*). Cessation of menses is not usually noticed until at least two weeks of pregnancy have passed, because conception ordinarily occurs approximately two weeks after the last menstrual period. Nor is this a certain sign of pregnancy—many other factors may be its cause. Morning sickness, although it affects approximately two-thirds of all pregnant women, does not ordinarily begin until approximately two weeks after the missed period and can easily be mistaken for some other ailment. Frequent urination is usually relieved by the third month (Reeder et al., 1980). Often during the early stages the breasts enlarge and become slightly sore, and the aureoles darken. Because these symptoms are highly subjective, they are quite unreliable. Quickening, the movement of the **fetus** in the womb, is not noticeable by the mother until the fourth or fifth month, and, by that time, most reasonably intelligent women have realized for some time that they are **pregnant**.

■ Prenatal Development

It is nothing short of phenomenal that an object as physically insignificant as a fertilized egg can become an organism as complex and sophisticated as a child within nine calendar months. The **gestation** period for different species varies considerably. For bovines it is similar to humans; elephants require no fewer than 600 days; dogs come to term in approximately 63 days, rabbits in 31, and chickens in 21.

Fertilization in the woman usually occurs in the **fallopian tubes** that link the **ovaries** to the **uterus** (see Figure 4.1). It results from the invasion of the tubes by sperm cells, one of which successfully penetrates the outer covering of the ovum and unites with it. From that moment a human child begins to form, but it will be approximately 266 days before this individual is freed from the life-giving prison. The gestation period is usually calculated in lunar months, each month consisting of 28 days—hence ten lunar months, or 280 days, for pregnancy when these days are counted from the onset of the last menstrual period, as they usually are. The true gestation period is nevertheless approximately 266 days, because fertilization usually cannot occur until approximately 12 to 14 days prior to the beginning of menses (Pritchard & MacDonald, 1980).

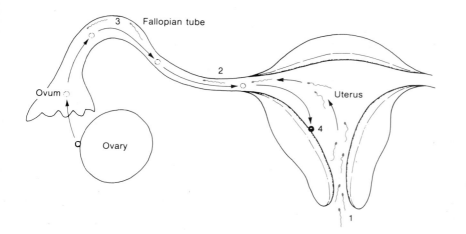

Figure 4.1
Fertilization and implantation. At 1, sperm cells have entered the vagina and are finding their way into the uterus. At 2, some of these spermatozoa are moving up the fallopian tube (there is a similar tube on the other side) toward the ovum. At 3, fertilization occurs. The fertilized ovum drifts down the tube, dividing and forming new cells as it goes, until it implants itself in the wall of the uterus (4) by the seventh or eighth day after fertilization.

DETECTING PREGNANCY:
VIRGIN RABBITS NOW SPARED

In addition to such probable signs of pregnancy as morning sickness and changes in the abdomen or breasts, there are some more *positive* signs. One of these is the ability to hear fetal heartbeats with the aid of a **stethoscope**. Similarly, if fetal movements can be detected by feeling the abdomen, or sometimes simply by observing it, one can be fairly confident that a fetus is present. Other methods for determining the presence of a fetus are to x-ray the mother to detect its outline, to feel it manually through the abdominal wall, or to use *ultrasound*, a high-frequency sonic device that provides a representation of the fetal outline without any of the dangers of X rays. Unfortunately for the woman who must know whether or not she is pregnant immediately after intercourse, none of these positive symptoms develop soon enough, although a fetal heartbeat can be heard four or five weeks into pregnancy.

Several decades ago, the surest early medical test of pregnancy required the aid of a rabbit, a frog, a mouse, or some other unfortunate creature. A small amount of urine from the suspecting mother was injected into an unsuspecting and immature mouse or into a virgin rabbit (if such an animal could be found). If the woman was four weeks (or more) into her pregnancy, the injection caused a rupturing of the follicles on the animal's ovaries. However, even without a **rabbit test**, it was usually possible to detect pregnancy with a fairly high degree of certainty at the end of eight weeks of gestation. Accordingly, many physicians were understandably reluctant to sacrifice the rabbit, mouse, or frog unnecessarily. Fortunately for virgin rabbits and mice, the medical sciences seldom stand still for long. Now certain highly reliable chemical tests are usually employed very early. Virgin rabbits have been spared.

The American College of Obstetrics and Gynecology has standardized the terminology employed in describing prenatal development by identifying three developmental stages with clear time boundaries. The stage of the **fertilized ovum** (also called the germinal stage) begins at fertilization and ends with implantation at approximately the end of the first week. The **embryo** stage follows and terminates at the end of the eighth week (calculated from the onset of the last menses rather than from fertilization), when true bone cells are starting to form. The final stage, the fetus, lasts from the end of the second lunar month until the birth of the baby.

The Fertilized Ovum

After fertilization, the ovum is carried toward the uterus by currents in the fallopian tubes, a procedure requiring between five and nine days. Cell divisions occur during this time, so that the fertilized ovum, which initially consisted of a single egg cell and a single sperm cell, now contains many more cells. It is still no larger at the end of the first week than it was at the time of fertilization, mainly because its multiplying cells are considerably smaller than the unfertilized ovum. This lack of growth is not surprising, because the ovum has received no nourishment from any source other than itself. At the end of the first week, the ovum is no larger than a pinhead but is ready to implant itself in the uterine wall.

The Embryo

The stage of the embryo begins with the implantation of the fertilized ovum in the wall of the uterus. The ovum facilitates this process by secreting certain enzymes and producing minute, tentaclelike growths, called *villi*, that implant themselves in the lining of the uterus to obtain nutrients from blood vessels. This is the beginning of the **placenta**, the organ that, while keeping the blood of the mother and of the fetus separate, allows nutrients to pass to the fetus (or embryo) and allows waste materials to be removed. In time, the placenta and the fetus are connected by the **umbilical cord**, a long, thick cord that is attached, at one end, to the placenta and, at the other, to what will be the child's navel. The umbilical cord consists of two arteries and one large vein and is approximately twenty inches long. It contains no nerve cells, so there is no connection between the mother's nervous system and that of the child **in utero** (a common medical term meaning "in the uterus").

The normal course of physiological development in utero is highly predictable. By the end of the first lunar month (very early in the embryonic stage), the fetus is still only a fraction of an inch long and weighs much less than an ounce. Despite the size, not only has there been cell differentiation into future skin cells, nerves, bones, and other body tissue, but the rudiments of such organs as the eyes, ears, and nose have begun to appear as well. In addition, some of the internal organs are beginning to develop. In fact, by the end of the first month, a primitive, U-shaped heart-to-be is already beating! By the end of the second lunar month (the end of the period of embryonic development), the embryo is between one and one-half and two inches long and weighs close to two-thirds of an ounce. All the organs are now present, the whole mass has assumed the curled shape characteristic of the fetus, and the embryo is clearly recognizable as human. Arm and limb buds have appeared and begun to grow, resembling short, awkward paddles. External **genitalia** have also appeared.

The Fetus

It is now the end of the second lunar month; the woman is six weeks pregnant. She has missed two menstrual periods or is currently missing her second. She is definitely pregnant, although the absolute mass of the organism that she carries inside her is still quite unimpressive. By the end of the third month, it may reach a length of three inches but will still weigh less than an ounce. The head of the fetus is one-third of its entire length and will

have changed to one-fourth by the end of the sixth lunar month and slightly less than that at birth.

During the third month of pregnancy, the fetus is sufficiently developed so that if it is aborted it will make breathing movements and will give evidence of a primitive **sucking reflex** and of the **Babinski reflex** if stimulated appropriately. Such a fetus will, however, have no chance of survival if born at this stage of development.

During the fourth lunar month of pregnancy, the fetus grows to a length of six inches and weighs approximately four ounces. The bones have begun to form, all organs are clearly differentiated, and there may even be evidence of some intrauterine movement. During the fifth month, a downy covering, called **lanugo**, begins to grow over most of the child's body. This covering is usually shed during the seventh month but is occasionally still present at birth. The fetus weighs approximately eleven ounces and may have reached a length of ten inches by the end of the fifth lunar month.

Toward the end of the sixth month, an obstetrician can feel the baby through the mother's abdomen. The heartbeat, faintly discernible in the fifth month, can now be heard clearly with the aid of a stethoscope.

The eyelids have separated so that the fetus can open and close its eyes. It is approximately a foot long and weighs close to twenty ounces. It would have some chance of surviving in a modern hospital if born at this time, although that chance would be minimal given the immaturity of its digestive and respiratory systems.

The fetus's growth in size and weight becomes more dramatic in the last few months of the final stage. Brain development is also particularly crucial during the last three months of pregnancy, as it will continue to be after birth, especially for the first two years of life. The unborn child's sensitivity to malnutrition is assumed to be related to neurological growth during the latter stages of fetal development. This sensitivity is sometimes evident in lower developmental scores during infancy and impaired mental functioning among children born to malnourished mothers (Lewin, 1975).

Most of the physical changes that occur after the seventh month are quantitative, a matter of

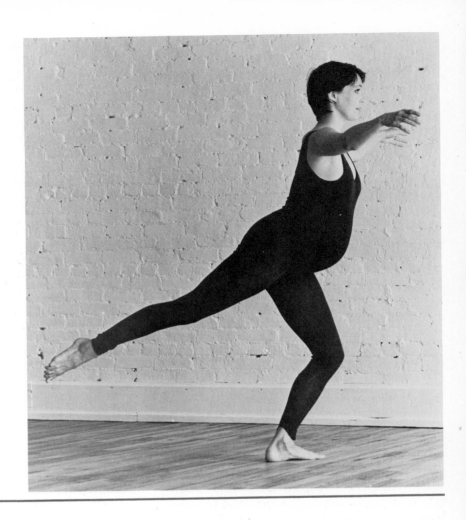

Growth in fetal weight and size becomes more dramatic in the final few months of gestation.

sheer physical growth: from 15 inches in the seventh month (2.6 pounds) to 16 inches in the eighth (4 pounds) and from 17.5 inches in the ninth (4.7 pounds) to 19.6 inches (7 pounds) at the end of the tenth month (see Figures 4.2 and 4.3).

Two terms are sometimes employed to describe the general pattern of fetal development: **proximodistal** and **cephalocaudal**. Literally, these terms mean *from near to far* (proximodistal) and *from the head to the tail* (cephalocaudal). They refer to the fact that among the first aspects of the fetus to develop are the head and internal organs; the last are the limbs and digits.

After 266 days of intrauterine development, the fetus is ready to be born—although some appear to be ready earlier and some later. But before we look at birth, we turn to a discussion of the factors that may be important to the normal or abnormal development of the fetus.

■ Factors Affecting Prenatal Development

It is nearly impossible to provide an exhaustive listing and description of the factors that influence

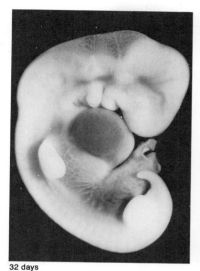
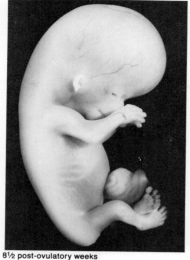
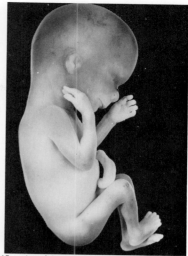

32 days   8½ post-ovulatory weeks   15 post-ovulatory weeks

Figure 4.2
Prenatal development. This figure uses the lunar-month method of calculating duration of pregnancy. The first month begins at the onset of the last menstrual period rather than at estimated time of conception, and each month consists of twenty-eight days.

Age	Weight	Length	Characteristics
1st month	Negligible	Negligible	Cell differentiation into those that will be bones, nerves, or other cells
2nd month	⅔ ounce	1½–2 inches	All organs present; leg buds and external genitalia just appearing
3rd month	⅞ ounce	3 inches	If aborted, will make primitive breathing movements and suck; bones forming, organs differentiated
4th month	4 ounces	6 inches	
5th month	11 ounces	10 inches	Fetal movement (quickening); lanugo appears
6th month	20 ounces	12 inches	Heartbeat clearly discernible; eyelids present
7th month	2.6 pounds	15 inches	
8th month	4 pounds	16 inches	All major changes have now occurred; development is largely a matter of increasing weight and length
9th month	4.7 pounds	17.5 inches	
10th month	7 pounds	19.6 inches	

prenatal development, given the highly circumstantial nature of much of the evidence that has been gathered to support various points of view. In many ways, it is a confused area, not only because it is by nature extremely complex but also because many potentially helpful experiments cannot be performed for ethical or moral reasons. In addition, there is a frequent confounding of causes, as well as some confusion of causes and effects in the experiments performed. Consider, for example, the apparently simple problem of determining whether a particular drug affects the fetus. All that is required, it would appear, is to obtain a group of women to whom the drug has been administered and observe their offspring for any signs of possible effects of the drug. The women, however, have usually been given the drug for a particular reason. The investigator is often unable to determine whether differences between the children produced by women who have taken the drug and a control group are caused by the ailment for which the drug was taken or by the drug itself. For obvious ethical reasons, it is not usually possible to administer the drug simply to observe its effect. Furthermore, the effects of prenatal environments are

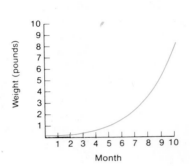

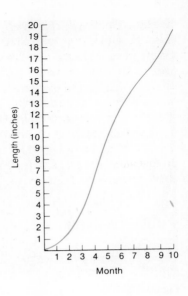

Figure 4.3
Approximate weight and length of the fetus at the end of each lunar month of prenatal development.

sometimes so subtle that they are not easily detected. Despite the difficulties encountered in the field, however, we do have considerable information about the various effects of prenatal conditions on the development of the fetus.

The World in Utero

The world of the embryo and the fetus is difficult for us to imagine, although we have all been through it. It is probably a relatively comfortable place, being so admirably suited to the developing organism that it houses. The temperature is always optimal; adequate nourishment is provided with no effort required of the little parasite, and the environment is absolutely quiet and peaceful—or is it?

Evidence suggests that the fetus is sensitive to vibrations. Bernard and Sontag (1947) found that during the last ten weeks of pregnancy, it is possible to produce marked cardiac acceleration in the fetus with tones of varying intensity. They interpret this as evidence that the fetus is sensitive to sounds. Spelt (1948) provided further corroborating evidence with fetuses conditioned to react to a low-intensity tone during the last two months of pregnancy. Conditioning was accomplished by pairing a loud noise with a door chime that had

been soldered shut. The chime, placed directly on the mother's abdomen, produced a vibration sensation rather than a sound and, prior to conditioning, elicited no discernible response from the fetus. Following fifteen to twenty pairings of the chime with the loud noise, a definite response was obtained with the chime alone. However, because a number of researchers have not always been able to replicate these findings, some doubt remains about the possibility of conditioning the fetus.

The world in utero is not completely noiseless, and noises such as stomach gurgles and loud environmental sounds may affect the captive occupant. But since fetuses have thick wax in their ears, and since all sounds must pass not only through the mother's skin and tissue but also through the amniotic fluid, these sounds are probably muffled and unclear at best.

What other characteristics of that world affect the unborn child? Years ago a common folk-belief was that the mother's emotional states can be communicated directly to the child. If the pregnant woman worried too much, her child would be born with a frown; if she had a particularly traumatic experience, it would mark the infant, perhaps for life; if she was frightened by a rabbit, the result might be a child with a harelip. She must try to be happy and have pleasant experiences so that the child could be born free of negative influences. Most of these tales concerning pregnancy are simply tales. Because there is no direct link between the mother's nervous system and the child's, there is little possibility that the mother's emotional states or disorders will be communicated *directly* to the unborn child. But because of the intimate relationship between the mother and the child, it is logical to suppose that many of the stimuli that affect her will also have some effect on the child, however indirect.

Maternal Emotions

There is some evidence that maternal emotions affect the child. Increases in fetal activity have been observed following emotional tension in the mother (Sontag & Wallace, 1934). In addition, mothers who are anxious during much of their pregnancy frequently have infants who are more irritable, more hyperactive, and have more feeding problems. These infants also cry for longer periods of time during their first three or four days of life (Ottinger & Simmons, 1964). One prevalent theory is that an anxious mother's chemical balances affect the child physiologically and therefore, indirectly, psychologically (Willemsen, 1979).

These findings must be viewed as highly tentative. Not only is it extremely difficult to arrive at valid and useful measures of emotional states in mother and infant, but it is also often impossible to control a variety of other factors that might also be related. For example, some of the factors sometimes associated with high maternal stress (poverty, inadequate diet, medical problems) might also be associated with fetal problems. Hence conclusive statements concerning the influence of maternal emotional states on the unborn are not warranted.

Drugs

Investigating the effects of drugs on the fetus presents many of the ethical and moral problems implied earlier. It is clearly impossible to use human subjects in controlled investigations with drugs whose effects will probably be harmful to the fetus. The information is therefore based on studies of animals or observations of human infants in poorly controlled situations. Generalizing from studies of animals to humans in the case of drugs presents an additional problem, because it has often been demonstrated that certain drugs may have dramatically different results on members of different animal species, as well as on children relative to adults (Bowes, Brackbill, Conway, & Steinschneider, 1970). Also, keep in mind that normal adult doses of a drug might well represent huge doses for a fetus weighing only ounces, particularly if the drug crosses the placental barrier easily.

The frequency of drug use by pregnant women and the variety of drugs they consume is startling. Heinonen, Slone, and Shapiro (1977) gathered data on more than 50,000 pregnant women and found that the average drug intake during pregnancy was 3.8 drugs. Stewart, Cluff, and Philp (1977) looked at the drug histories of 168 pregnant women and found average drug intake to be eleven different drugs! Similar results were also obtained in another recent survey. Among a group of 156 pregnant women in Houston, an average of ten different drugs were taken during pregnancy, not including anesthetics, cigarettes, vitamins, or iron supplements; in Scotland, 747 pregnant women had an average of four different drugs prescribed ("Drugs and the Human Fetus," 1978). Some 92 percent of all pregnant women take at least one drug during pregnancy (Tucker, 1975). And approximately half of all pregnant women smoke cigarettes (Dalby, 1978). The importance of clarifying the effects of these drugs on the fetus is obvious.

Drugs and other substances that cause malformations and physical defects in the fetus are referred to as **teratogens** (from *teras*, the Greek word for *monster*, so called because such substances are thought to be capable of producing monsters). Among the better-known drugs that apparently have marked effects on the unborn child are thalidomide, which causes severe morphological changes in the embryo (Carmichael, 1970; Lenz, 1966); quinine, which is associated with congenital deafness (Baker, 1960); barbiturates and

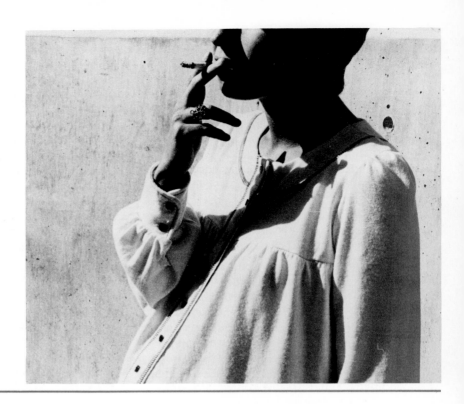

A great number of widely used drugs have harmful effects on the unborn fetus.

other painkillers that reduce the body's oxygen supply, resulting in varying degrees of brain damage; and various anesthetics that appear to cross the placental barrier easily and rapidly and cause depression of fetal respiration and decreased responsiveness in the infant. In one study, infants whose mothers had received a single dose of medication during labor sucked with significantly less pressure and at lower rates and took in less nutrient (Kron, Stein, & Goddard, 1966). Note that the most serious structural changes (physical deformities and abnormalities) that are sometimes associated with drug intake, as well as with other factors such as maternal malnutrition, can occur only during the embryonic stage of development. After this stage, the fetus's basic structure has already been determined and formed and is not highly vulnerable to external influences.

Nicotine is another drug that has long been suspected of having harmful effects on the fetus.

Evidence suggests that smoking increases fetal heart rate and contributes to fetal hyperactivity (Martin, Martin, Lund, & Streissguth, 1977). In addition, it is associated with general retardation of growth in utero. Meredith (1975) also found a significantly higher incidence of premature births among smokers than among nonsmokers. There are indications that the harmful effects of nicotine on the fetus are related to a reduction in the amount of oxygen and other substances that are available to the fetus. Davies, Latto, Jones, Veale, and Wardrop (1979) report that when pregnant smokers stop smoking for forty-eight hours, fetal oxygen levels increase measurably, as does activity of the fetus. However, even among those women who stop smoking while pregnant, there is still a higher probability of problems. Some of these relate to general retardation of fetal growth; others have to do with the observation that implantation of the **zygote** in smoking mothers is apparently more difficult and sometimes occurs too low in the uterus. This can lead to medical problems where the developing placenta eventually covers the opening to the birth canal and can result in serious loss of blood ("Smoking Imperils the Unborn," 1979).

It might be irrelevant to some of you but somewhat disturbing to others to know that alcohol (booze) can sometimes have serious ill effects on the fetus. Evidence suggests that, in sufficient quantities, alcohol consumption by pregnant women may adversely affect the fetus both during fetal development and after birth (Hanson, Streissguth, & Smith, 1978). In serious cases, the newborn may suffer from what is termed **fetal alcohol syndrome (FAS)**. This syndrome is characterized by low birth weight, retarded motor development, and sometimes heart defects and physical abnormalities. (See *Fetal Alcohol Syndrome*.)

Other evidence suggests that intellectual development may also be significantly affected by excessive alcohol consumption. Streissguth, Herman, and Smith (1978) examined a sample of twenty patients, nine months to twenty-one years old, who had all been diagnosed as having a fetal alcohol syndrome at birth. Their average measured IQ was 65 (mildly retarded). In addition, measured IQ was closely related to the severity of their FAS.

A mother suffering from **delirium tremens** is likely to give birth to an infant experiencing a variety of withdrawal symptoms. Such a child will twitch, sweat, be hyperirritable, and probably feverish (Nichols, 1967). The mother may be somewhat uncomfortable as well.

Considerable evidence shows that babies born to narcotics addicts are also addicted. These unfortunate infants suffer a clearly recognizable withdrawal syndrome: hyperactivity, hyperirritability, rapid respiration, vomiting, trembling, perspiring, fevers, and shrill crying. This condition can be fatal (Kron, Kaplan, Phoenix, & Finnegan, 1977). In addition, the use of narcotics has been linked with prematurity and low birth weight as well as with behavior problems such as hyperactivity (Kolata, 1978).

Because of serious research problems, the effects of substances such as LSD and marijuana remain uncertain. For example, pregnant women who smoked marijuana have frequently also smoked tobacco cigarettes, drunk alcohol and coffee, and sometimes taken psychedelic drugs. In many cases, their diets have also been less than optimal. Research with pregnant monkeys that were given LSD has found chromosomal damage in the mothers and a high rate of postnatal death among infants (Kato, 1970).

Although actual documentation of fetal injury related to drug use is not always convincing, it cannot be stated categorically that many drugs are in fact harmless. Bowes et al. (1970) maintain that, at least in the first few weeks of pregnancy, no drug can be considered absolutely safe.

Maternal Health

The mother's health inevitably affects the occupant of her womb; she is responsible for the fetus's comfort and nourishment. A wide range of diseases and infections are also known to affect the fetus. Probably the best known is rubella (German measles); others are syphilis, gonorrhea, poliomyelitis, and diabetes, each of which can cause mental deficiency, microcephaly, blindness, deafness, or a miscarriage. Cretinism (subnormal mental development, undeveloped bones, a protruding abdomen, and rough, coarse skin) may be related to a thyroid malfunction in the mother or to an iodine deficiency in her diet. If the deficiency is not too extreme, it can sometimes be alleviated in the child through continuous medication.

The mother's age also appears to be a factor in the well-being of the fetus. Smith and Wilson (1973) are among the many researchers who have reported a much higher incidence of Down's syndrome among children born to mothers above the age of thirty. Apparently the probability of bearing a mentally defective child increases as the woman nears menopause (Benda, 1956). In addition, older women are more prone to miscarry a child or to have a stillborn infant. Because the reproductive organs and the female skeletal structure do not mature until the early twenties, the best time for a woman to have a child is when she is between twenty-one and twenty-nine years of age.

FETAL ALCOHOL SYNDROME—FAS

Although the medical sciences have known for some time that alcohol consumption by pregnant women may be associated with a variety of defects in their offspring, it is only recently that researchers have recognized a *pattern* of these defects and labeled them *fetal alcohol syndrome* (FAS) (Rosett & Sander, 1979). The major features of this syndrome are problems with the central nervous system sometimes manifested in mental retardation, retarded physical growth, and cranial and facial malformations. These malformations typically include a low forehead, widely spaced eyes, a short nose and long upper lip, and absence of a marked "infranasal" depression (the typical depression above the center of the upper lip, going up toward the nose).

Unfortunately, it is difficult to conduct with humans the types of experiments that would allow researchers to determine precisely what amounts of alcohol, and at what stage of development, will have these effects. Nor is it possible to completely separate the effects of alcohol from those of other drugs that might accompany alcohol use, or from the effects of malnutrition, also a possible corollary of alcohol use. However, research with animals does not pose the same ethical problems. Accordingly, a number of studies have looked at FAS among animals and have found, to no one's great surprise, that injections of ethanol (the type of alcohol that is drunk as opposed to the type that might be rubbed on a horse's sore muscles or that might be burned in an engine) in pregnant mice quite readily produce what appears to be an FAS in their offspring. Not only are these offspring more likely to be born dead, but many of them will also display facial and skull deformations highly reminiscent of those characteristic of FAS children (Rosett & Sander, 1979).

By injecting alcohol directly into mice, by controlling the amount given, and by examining the unborn fetus at different stages of development, it has been possible for researchers to arrive at a clearer picture of FAS than would be possible if observations were limited only to humans. One such study, conducted by Rosett and Sander (1979), presents some surprising and potentially valuable findings. It involved groups of pregnant mice who were injected with two *small* doses of ethanol (0.015 milliliters per gram of body weight of a 25 percent solution of ethanol) on the seventh day of their gestation. Subsequent electron microscope examinations of fetal brains showed significant cellular changes within a single day of the injection—changes that are associated with facial and cranial deformities. It seems clear that alcohol has a striking effect on mouse embryos, even in very small doses, when it is administered at a *critical* period of embryonic development.

Although we cannot generalize directly from these studies to humans, there clearly may be a critical period in human fetal development during which the ingestion of moderate amounts of alcohol might result in a fetus with fetal alcohol syndrome. It is perhaps worth noting that the seventh day of embryonic development in a mouse corresponds to the third week of gestation for humans. At week three, most expectant mothers do not know that they are pregnant.

Maternal Nutrition

Even as the mother's health is of critical importance to fetal development, so is her diet. Although it is extremely difficult to separate the effects of malnutrition from the effects of other variables that often accompany malnutrition (poor medical attention, poor sanitation, drug use, and so on), considerable evidence from animal studies indicates that dietary deficiency can be associated with a wide range of fetal problems. Hepner (1958) reports that serious malnutrition, if it does not lead to fetal death, may result in mental deficiency or such physical abnormalities as rickets, epilepsy, or cerebral palsy. Rosenbaum, Churchill, Shakhashiri, and Moody (1969) investigated the effects in pregnant mothers of proteinuria, a loss of protein that has effects similar to those of low protein intake. Fifty-one mothers with proteinuria were involved in the study. Various assessments of their infants' performances were obtained until the age of four years. Mothers with severe proteinuria gave birth to infants who performed significantly less well neurologically (in terms of motor development, for example) and psychologically (in terms of Bayley mental scores and Stanford-Binet IQs) than average infants from the general population.

Similar studies with pregnant rats that have been systematically malnourished corroborate these findings (Winick, 1968). Offspring of these rats typically have fewer brain cells at birth. Perhaps equally important, even if these brain-deficient rats are themselves well nourished, their offspring will also be inferior in brain development. Thus the effects of malnutrition may continue into the next generation.

Evidence with respect to intellectual development in humans, while still tentative, is highly suggestive. Harrell, Woodyard, and Gates (1955) investigated the effects of diet on the development of two groups of children. Mothers of these children were from deprived environments. The researchers provided an enriched diet to one group; the second group ate as they usually would. Children born to mothers whose diets had been enriched scored appreciably higher on measures of intelligence than their unfortunate counterparts in the control group.

As previously noted, the brain undergoes a developmental spurt during the later stages of fetal development. Lewin (1975) refers to this brain growth spurt as a critical period when inadequate nutrition will have the most serious and the most long-lasting effects. He cites research indicating as well that a significant portion of this growth spurt takes place after birth and that malnutrition in the early years of life can also significantly affect brain development (see, for example, Dobbing, 1974).

However, not all research in this area points to the same conclusion. Stein, Sussen, Saenger, and Marolla (1975) compared groups of eighteen-year-old Dutch men who had been born during the famine of 1944–1945. Since the famine resulted from the German army's blockade of all transportation routes in the country, it affected urban rather than rural food-producing areas. Furthermore, since children were generally provided with adequate nourishment even at the height of the famine, but pregnant mothers were not, the famine affected infants still in utero but not those already born.

Thus war provided a research situation that could not, for obvious ethical reasons, be deliberately duplicated by investigators.

The results? Children born of malnourished mothers had lower birth weights and a higher probability of dying in infancy. Since no systematic effort was made to examine their intellectual performance in infancy, no conclusions can be advanced that might support or refute Lewin's findings (and those of many other researchers) that malnutrition has an adverse effect on intelligence. In any case, by the age of eighteen, those who had been born in areas of famine and those born elsewhere in Holland during this period had no differences in intellectual performance. Note, however, that most of the mothers in this study had been well nourished just prior to pregnancy; in addition, the famine was of relatively short duration (November to May). These observations might well explain why the effects of malnutrition on intellectual development were not apparent eighteen years later.

Certainly, better-controlled research with rat mothers given diets highly restricted in protein from a time *prior* to mating and continuing until after the pups were born resulted in some far-reaching and highly significant outcomes (Zamenhof, van Marthens, & Margolis, 1968). Specifically, infant rats in this study were born with fewer brain cells; in addition, these cells contained less protein than did brain cells of comparable infant rats born to well-nourished mothers.

These and related studies indicate that malnutrition can have detrimental effects on intellectual functioning. Unfortunately, research on malnutrition among humans is seldom experimentally well controlled. That is, investigators have no control over assigning subjects to groups or over the manipulation of treatments. We know that most naturally occurring instances of malnutrition involve many other factors, often including low socioeconomic levels, low educational levels, and low intellectual stimulation. The effects sometimes attributed solely to malnutrition might also, at least in part, be related to these other factors. In addition, malnutrition is seldom limited to the period of prenatal development but usually continues into infancy and even childhood. This was not the case in the Dutch study, where children were given priority for available food. As Stein et al. (1975) note, perhaps the most plausible (though tentative) conclusions are that the effects of malnutrition are a complex interaction of the severity and nature of deprivation, intellectual deficits may result from malnutrition that begins before birth and continues for some time afterward, and some of the short-term effects associated with prenatal malnutrition may be reversible given adequate nourishment after birth.

It is likely that considerably more research will be conducted on the harmful effects of malnutrition within the near future, and perhaps additional steps will be taken to ameliorate present conditions. As Lewin puts it: "An infant deprived of nutrition or stimulation will never develop to full mental capacity. There's no second chance. Today, 70 percent of the world's population seriously risk permanent damage" (1975, p. 29).

Social Class

The greatest single cause of infant death is premature birth. Furthermore, prematurity is among the most direct causes of cerebral palsy and various forms of mental defectiveness. And the factor most closely related to premature births is social rather than medical.

These statements are relatively well-documented facts that are of considerable significance (see Kopp & Parmelee, 1979). Although social class does not, by itself, explain anything, the high correlation between low social class and higher incidence of premature birth suggests that the living conditions and associated emotional and health consequences attributed to poverty are not conducive to the production of healthy full-term babies. Research reviewed in this chapter relating to the effects of maternal malnutrition on the fetus, and subsequently on the infant, is of direct relevance here. There is little doubt that prenatal and postnatal health care of mothers who live in poverty is rarely comparable to that afforded middle-class mothers. General diet, protein intake, and mineral and vitamin intake are often significantly inferior, and the effects of these factors are too often the harsh consequences of an infant being born poor. The social and moral implications are clear.

Rh Incompatibility

There is a particular quality of blood in Rhesus monkeys that is often, though by no means always, present in human blood. Because this factor was first discovered in the Rhesus monkey, it is called the *Rh factor*. Individuals who possess it are termed Rh-positive; those who do not are Rh-negative. Introduction of Rh-positive blood into an individual who is Rh-negative leads to the formation of antibodies to counteract the factor. If these antibodies were then to be introduced into an individual with Rh-positive blood, they would attack that person's blood cells, causing a depletion of oxygen and, in the absence of medical intervention, death.

Unfortunately, this situation can occur in the fetus (termed *fetal erythroblastosis*) in those instances when the fetus has Rh-positive blood and the mother is Rh-negative. The situation will occur only when the father is Rh-positive (and the mother Rh-negative), because the Rh factor is a dominant genetic trait. If blood from the fetus gets into the mother's bloodstream—a common occurrence, usually involving minute ruptures of tiny placental blood vessels—the mother's blood will begin to produce antibodies, but usually not early enough or in sufficient quantities to affect the first child. Subsequent fetuses may be affected, however, when these antibodies cross the placental barrier, enter the fetus's bloodstream, and attack the red blood cells. At one time, this condition was always fatal. Now, doctors are able to monitor antibody levels in the mother's blood, thereby determining when levels are high enough to endanger the fetus. At this point, there are several alternatives. If the fetus is sufficiently advanced, labor might be induced and a complete blood transfusion performed on the infant immediately after birth. In some cases, the blood transfusion may even be performed in utero. Fortunately, this type of medical intervention is not necessary in many cases. Injecting the mother with Rhogam immediately after the first child is born is usually effective in reducing the buildup of antibodies so that other children can then be carried by the mother with little risk of fetal erythroblastosis. Rhogam is Rh-negative blood that already has antibodies, which eventually dissipate but which prevent the formation of additional antibodies.

■ Childbirth

Although the birth of a child in our culture usually occurs within the safe and antiseptic confines of hospital walls, assisted by experts, it has not always been this way. Even today, many children are born in homes or in the fields and forests of the world. I am among those born at home, but unfortunately I remember very little of it. I do remember the births of my younger brothers and sisters, but because I was not permitted to witness the actual deliveries, I cannot draw upon that source of knowledge for this chapter. In those days, my education was limited to dragonflies mating and other quite innocuous events. And when my first child was born, I was not allowed to witness that event, despite my argument that I was teaching a course in child development and had a valid reason for being admitted to the delivery room. The doctor was concerned about the temperament of fathers and had decided that no one but the mother and nursing attendants would be allowed in the delivery room.

The history of **obstetrics** is a long struggle between the traditions and beliefs of generations of midwives and the inevitable progress of science. It begins with Hippocrates' effort to separate labor from religious rites, progresses through the desperate attempts of men like Semmelweis to promote cleanliness in hospitals to combat the dreaded killer of women after childbirth, puerperal fever (dramatized in the novel *The Cry and the Covenant*), and ends with current hospital techniques and procedures. (See Table 4.1 for a sketch of the history of obstetrics.)

Table 4.1 A short history of obstetrics.

400 B.C.	Hippocrates' attempt to separate labor from religious rites.
A.D. 200	Soranus teaches obstetrics to Roman midwives.
1513	Roesslin writes the first printed book on obstetrics.
1560	Pare rediscovers and describes version and breech extraction.
1647	Chamberlen invents obstetric forceps.
1739	Smellie improves the teaching of obstetrics.
1807	The introduction of ergot in obstetrics.
1847	Holmes and Semmelweis fight puerperal fever.
1860	Pasteur discovers streptococci in puerperal fever.
1867	Lister describes asepsis (sterile procedures).
1900	The development of prenatal care and obstetrics in nursing institutions and schools of medicine.
1950	Widespread use of drugs in "assisted" childbirth.
1970	Popularization of "natural" childbirth.

Adapted in part from Bookmiller and Bowen, 1967, pp. 17–18.

A Clinical View

Labor is the process whereby the fetus, the placenta, and other membranes are separated from the woman's body and expelled; it ordinarily occurs approximately 280 days after the beginning of the pregnant woman's last menstrual period, although it can also occur earlier or later than this. The physical status of the child was traditionally classified according to the length of time spent in gestation and by weight. A fetus born before the twentieth week and weighing less than 500 grams (about 1 pound) was termed an **abortion**. A fetus delivered between the twentieth and twenty-eighth week and weighing between 500 and 999 grams (between 1 and 2 pounds) was an **immature birth**. Abortions and immature births are often referred to as miscarriages. An immature birth very rarely survives, although there are several documented cases of fetuses born prior to the twenty-eighth week

Table 4.2 Physical status of child at birth.

Classification by Gestation	Time	Average Weight
Abortion	Before 20th week	Less than 500 grams
Immature birth	20th–28th week	500–999 grams
Premature birth	29th–36th week	1,000–2,499 grams
Mature birth	37th–42nd week	At least 2,500 grams
Postmature birth	After 42 weeks	—

Classification by Weight and Gestation	
SFD (small-for-date)	10 percent less than average infants of same gestational age
AFD (average-for-date)	Within 10 percent of average weight for gestational age
LFD (large-for-date)	10 percent more than average infants of same gestational age

having survived. More often than not, death ensues from respiratory failure.

The birth of a baby between the twenty-ninth and the thirty-sixth week is called a *premature birth,* provided the child weighs between 1,000 and 2,499 grams (between 2 and 5½ pounds). Complications are expected if the child weighs less than 1,500 grams. A **mature birth** occurs between the thirty-seventh and the forty-second week and results in an infant weighing at least 2,500 grams (over 5½ pounds). A late delivery is called a *postmature birth*. Both prematurity and postmaturity are associated with higher risk of postnatal death.

More recent medical terminology classifies newborns as being premature (or preterm) if born before the thirty-seventh week. All newborns, regardless of whether they are premature, are also classified as *small-for-date* (SFD) when they weigh 10 percent less than average newborns of the same gestational age; as *large-for-date* (LFD) when they weigh 10 percent more; or as *average-for-date* (AFD) (see Table 4.2).

The onset of labor is usually gradual and described in three stages. That there are excep-

tions to the normal process is substantiated by numerous fathers who were caught unawares, taxi drivers who drove too slowly, pilots who almost made it, and many others for whom nature would not wait. Although physicians can induce labor, the precise cause of the natural beginning of labor remains unknown. There is no evidence that the procedures doctors employ would normally trigger labor. Labor amazingly begins, more often than not, at the prescribed time. The first stage of labor is the longest, lasting an average of twelve hours for the first baby and varying greatly in length, depending as much on unknown individual factors as on whether the woman has given birth previously. Generally, labor is longest and most difficult for the first delivery.

The first stage of labor consists of contractions of relatively low intensity that are usually spaced far apart at the beginning and eventually occur at shorter intervals. The initial contractions are described as similar to having "butterflies" in one's stomach; they last only a few seconds and are relatively painless. Apparently the "butterflies" become more painful and last considerably longer toward

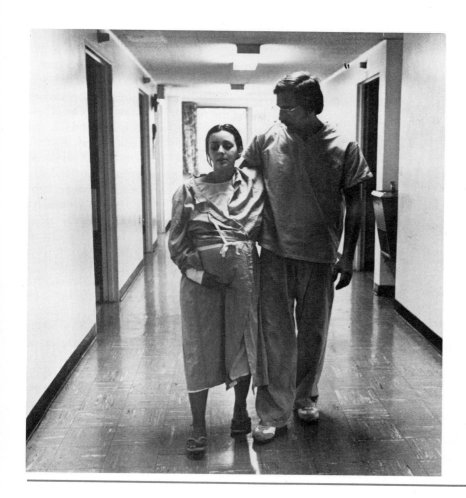

The first stage of labor is usually the longest. It lasts an average of twelve hours for the first infant—less for subsequent births—but varies a great deal for individual women.

the end of the first stage of labor. In this first stage, the **cervix** dilates to allow passage of the baby from the uterus, down through the birth canal, and eventually into the world. Contractions are totally involuntary and exert a downward pressure (equivalent to some 100 pounds of force) on the fetus as well as a distending force on the cervix. If the amniotic sac is still intact, it absorbs much of the pressure in the early stages and transmits some of the force of the contractions to the neck of the cervix. If, however, the sac has ruptured or bursts in the early stages of labor, then the baby's head will rest directly on the pelvic structure and cervix, thus serving as a sort of wedge.

When the cervix is sufficiently dilated, the second stage of labor ensues, beginning with the baby's head (in a normal delivery) at the cervical opening, face to mother's back, and terminating with the birth of the child (see Figure 4.4). The second stage usually lasts no more than an hour and frequently ends in a few minutes. Toward the end of the second stage, the attending physician or nurse severs the neonate's umbilical cord, places silver nitrate or penicillin drops in its eyes to guard against gonococcal infection, and ensures that its breathing, muscle tone, coloration, and reflexive activity are normal and that it is of an appropriate sex. Following this, the physician assists in the third

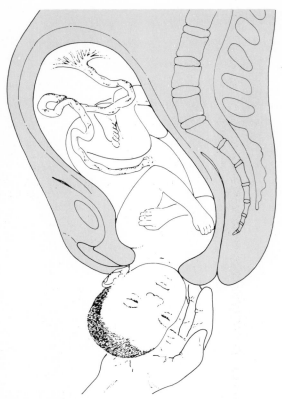

Figure 4.4
This cross section shows the presentation and delivery of a baby.

and final stage of labor and evaluates the condition of the neonate, perhaps by means of the Apgar Scale. (See *Neonatal Scales*.)

In this third stage, the afterbirth—the placenta and other membranes—is expelled. This process usually takes less than five minutes and seldom more than fifteen. The physician examines the afterbirth carefully to ensure that all of it has been expelled. If it is incomplete, surgical procedures may be employed (frequently dilation and curettage, usually referred to as a D & C).

The fetus ordinarily presents itself head first and can usually be born without the intervention of a physician. On occasion, however, complications arise that require some sort of intervention. For example, the head of the fetus is sometimes too large for the opening provided by the mother. In such a case, the physician may make a small incision in the vaginal outlet (an **episiotomy**), which is sutured after the baby is born. If this procedure is not performed, the surrounding tissues may tear and the mother's healing process will be much slower. In fact, in some hospitals it has become routine to perform an episiotomy to guard against this possibility. Complications can also arise from other abnormal presentations of the fetus. Some of these can be corrected prior to birth by turning the fetus manually in the uterus (**version**). Sometimes the fetus is delivered just as it presents itself: **breech** (buttocks first), **transverse** (crosswise), or in a variety of other possible positions, all of which have appropriate medical labels.

At the end of the third stage of labor, the uterus should contract and remain contracted. It may be necessary to massage the abdominal area or administer various drugs to stimulate contraction and to guard against the danger of postpartum (afterbirth) hemorrhage.

In an increasing number of instances, medical intervention bypasses these three stages of birth through a Caesarean delivery. In such cases, birth is accomplished by means of a surgical procedure involving an incision in the mother's abdomen and uterus. Caesarean deliveries may be undertaken when the baby's head is too large for the mother's pelvic opening (or the pelvic opening is abnormally small), when there is some immediate danger to the fetus or mother that requires delivery of the child, or when the normal process of birth cannot be accomplished for some other reason. Although Caesarean deliveries are ordinarily undertaken prior to the onset of labor, they can also be performed later.

A Mother's View: Prepared Childbirth

The preceding discussion of the delivery of a human child is admittedly clinical and perhaps somewhat like the cold, antiseptic hospitals in which most North American babies are born; it fails to uncover and transmit the magic of the process. One can recapture some of the mystery, however, by look-

NEONATAL SCALES

In almost all North American hospitals, it has become routine to evaluate the condition of a newborn by means of the Apgar Scale. The scale, shown below, is almost self-explanatory. Infants receive a score of 0, 1, or 2 for each of five appropriate signs. The maximum score is 10; an average score is usually 7 or better; a score of 4 or less indicates that the neonate must be given special care immediately.

A second important scale for assessing the condition of a newborn infant is the Brazelton Neonatal Behavior Assessment Scale (Brazelton, 1973). Like the Apgar Scale, it may be employed to detect problems immediately after birth. In addition, it provides useful indicators of central nervous system maturity as well as of social behavior. The Brazelton Scale looks at a total of twenty-six specific behaviors, including reaction to light, to cuddling, to voices, and to a pinprick; it also looks at the strength of various reflexes. Indications are that the scale is particularly useful in identifying infants who might be prone to later psychological problems (Als, Tronick, Lester, & Brazelton, 1979). For example, parents of infants who are less responsive to cuddling and to other social stimulation might be alerted to this from the very beginning and might be able to compensate by providing the infant with more loving contact than might otherwise have been the case.

Score	Heart Rate	Respiratory Effort	Muscle Tone	Color	Reflex Irritability
0	Absent	Absent	Flaccid, limp	Blue, pale	No response
1	Slow (less than 100)	Irregular, slow	Weak, inactive	Body pink, extremities blue	Grimace
2	Rapid (over 100)	Good, crying	Strong, active	Entirely pink	Coughing, sneezing, crying

ing at the process from the mother's point of view. In preparation for this discussion, I conferred with several mothers whose experience qualified them to make subjective comments of which I am incapable. One of these experts assured me that childbearing is "as easy as rolling off a log." Another witness, similarly qualified, assured me that "it's a hell of a big log!" Combining these impressions, an absolutely clear picture of the situation emerges. The inexperienced mother sometimes approaches the event with some degree of apprehension; there is often some pain associated with childbirth. However, advocates of natural childbirth (commonly called *prepared* childbirth) claim that through a regimen of prenatal exercises and adequate psychological preparations, many women experience relatively painless childbirths.

Natural childbirth, a phrase coined by a British physician, Grantly Dick Read (1972), refers to the process of having a child without anesthetics. The Read process recommends physical techniques, relaxing exercises, and psychological preparation for the arrival of the child, all directed toward delivery in which painkillers are unnecessary. Natural childbirth is based on the assumption that alleviating the fear of pain, together with training in relaxation, will result in less pain. Read's hypothesis has proved sound. Klusman (1975), for example, found that women who attended childbirth classes experienced less anxiety and easier deliveries.

Two currently popular methods of prepared childbirth are the Lamaze and the Leboyer techniques. The Lamaze method teaches expectant mothers a variety of breathing and relaxation exercises. These are practiced repeatedly, often with the assistance of the father, until they become so habitual that they will be employed almost "naturally" during the actual process of birth. The use of anesthetics during labor is less common among women who are thus prepared. However, the goal of the Lamaze method is not so much to avoid the use of anesthetics as to prepare both father and mother, physically and psychologically, for the birth.

The Leboyer method is concerned more with the delivery of the infant than with advance preparation of the mother. Leboyer's (1975) technique involves delivering the baby in a softly lit room, immersing the infant almost immediately in a lukewarm bath, and then placing the baby directly on the mother's abdomen. These procedures are designed to ease the infant's transition from the womb to the world; thus the need for soft lights, which do not contrast as harshly with the darkness of the womb as does conventional delivery room lighting, and for a lukewarm bath, which might feel something like amniotic fluid. Leboyer claims that his procedures eliminate much of the shock of birth and result in better-adjusted individuals; critics suggest that birth in dimly lit surroundings might contribute to the physician's failing to notice important signs of distress or injury and that the dangers of infection are greater under these circumstances than they are when more conventional hospital practices are employed.

Not only are an increasing number of mothers choosing to have their babies by natural means, but many are also deciding where birth will occur. For some, home is that choice; others choose hospital *birthing rooms*—a homier and more comfortable alternative than a conventional operating or delivery room—or hospital family suites where the father and other siblings can actually stay. There is also some use of midwives in North America, although the practice is far more common in most European countries, where the majority of births are attended by midwives rather than physicians. Although most North American births still occur in hospitals, length of hospitalization is considerably shorter than it once was (often only a matter of hours) and midwifery is now a licensed profession that appears to be growing in at least some states. Pearse (1982) reports that this is the case in upper New England and in the Pacific coast states; however, this does not appear to be a trend in other states. And, in general, relative rates of in-hospital versus out-of-hospital births have remained constant through the late 1970s (see Table 4.3)

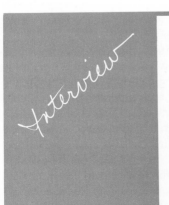

Interview

Subject: Female; age sixty-two; married; three children; four grandchildren; not working outside home; husband recently retired.

(on childbirth)

I wouldn't say I wasn't a bit scared the first time. And every time after that too for that matter. I mean, I looked forward to it, to having the babies because that's what we wanted. Everybody wanted kids in those days. But it wasn't an experience that I could honestly say I looked forward to. It might be different now, I think, with classes and everything. I know, when my daughter had her last one she went to classes, every week I think, and he did too, her husband. And they both said it was such a nice birth. Maybe there's something to it, the classes. We didn't have that when I had my kids. We just saw the doctor maybe once or twice, unless there was problems, and when the time came, we just went ahead and had the baby. But I guess I'd just as soon not have to go through it again.

Table 4.3 Total live births by place of birth and attendant.

Year	MD in-hospital		Not in-hospital			
	Number	Percent	Number	MD (%)	Midwife (%)	Other and not specified (%)
1940	1,316,768	55.8	1,043,631	35.0	8.7	0.6
1950	3,125,975	88.0	428,168	7.1	4.5	0.4
1960	4,114,368	96.6	143,482	1.2	2.0	0.2
1970	3,708,142	99.4	23,244	0.1	0.4	0.1
1973	3,116,901	99.1	27,297	0.4	0.3	0.2
1976	3,138,096	99.0	29,692	0.4	0.3	0.3
1977	3,293,473	99.0	33,159	0.4	0.3	0.3
1978	3,300,659	99.0	32,620	0.4	0.3	0.3
1979	3,460,484	99.0	33,914	0.3	0.3	0.3

From W. H. Pearce, Trends in out-of-hospital births. *Obstetrics and Gynecoloy*, 1970, *60*, 267–270. p. 269. Reprinted with permission from The American College of Obstetricians and Gynecologists.

From one mother's experience, childbirth may be quite painful. For another mother, childbirth may be a slightly painful but intensely rewarding and satisfying experience. (See *A Father's View of Pregnancy and Birth.*) Although the amount of pain can be controlled to some extent with anesthetics, the intensity of the immediate emotional reward will also be dulled by the drugs. In addition, sedatives employed may affect the infant. Children delivered without sedatives are frequently more alert, more responsive to the environment, and better able to cope with immediate environmental demands (Brackbill, 1979). In short, they may have a slight initial advantage, the long-range implications of which are unclear.

A Child's View

How do children, the heroes of the early part of this text, react to the process of birth? Their story begins now, for although life begins at conception, legal existence dates from birth. (In some Oriental countries, the child is considered to be a year old when born, and even there the making of a child does not require more than 266 days.)

Consider the dramatic difference that birth makes. Prior to this moment the child has been living in a completely friendly and supportive environment. The provision of nourishment and oxygen and the elimination of waste products have been accomplished without effort. The uterus has been kept at exactly the right temperature, and the danger of bacterial infection has been relatively insignificant. In addition to the complete biological support provided by the intrauterine environment, there have been no psychological threats. Now, at birth, the child is suddenly exposed to new physiological and, perhaps, psychological dangers. Once mucus is cleared from the mouth and throat, the newborn must breathe for the first time. As soon as the umbilical cord ceases to pulsate, it is unceremoniously clipped an inch or two above the abdomen and tied off with a clamp. The child is now completely alone—singularly dependent and helpless, to be sure, but no longer a parasite (biologically) on the mother.

There are two great dangers of brain damage during the birth of a child. Tremendous pressures are exerted upon the head of the infant during birth, particularly if the first stage of labor has been long and if the amniotic sac has been broken during most of that stage, in which case the head, in a normal presentation, has been repeatedly pressed against the slowly dilating cervix. In addition, the infant suffers passage through an opening so small that it often results in deformation of the head. (For most infants the head usually assumes a more normal appearance within a few days.)

An additional source of pressure on the child's head may be **forceps**, clamplike instruments sometimes employed during delivery. Use of forceps in the first stage of labor (called "high forceps"), once considered an emergency procedure, no longer occurs. Forceps in the final stages of delivery are more common ("low forceps") and not very dangerous. Although it is evident that the fetus can withstand considerable pressure on the head, the real danger of such pressure is that it may rupture blood vessels and cause subsequent

hemorrhaging. In severe cases, death may ensue; otherwise, brain damage is possible, because cranial hemorrhage can restrict the supply of oxygen available for the brain.

The oxygen supply to the brain can be restricted in another way. The fetus is still dependent on the mother for oxygen during the birth process, obtaining this oxygen through the umbilical cord. There is a constant danger that the cord will become lodged between the child's body and the birth canal through which the child must pass. If this happens, the flow of oxygen through the cord may be stopped (referred to as **prolapsed cord**), also causing brain damage. Symptoms of brain damage often include various motor defects loosely defined as cerebral palsy. Even in cases where there are no overt symptoms of brain dam-

A FATHER'S VIEW OF PREGNANCY AND BIRTH

I thought I was pregnant some years ago. And although I took some small consolation from the fact that I knew who the mother was (with reasonable assurance), it was not an easy time.

Contrary to popular expectation, my pregnancy did not last nine months, only four. My wife, who was undeniably pregnant at the time, was in that condition for a full nine months. We attended Lamaze prenatal classes together, which was convenient because she could drive me there. Together we learned to breathe, to relax, to stretch our muscles, and to wipe our faces with damp sponges. It was relaxing, slightly invigorating, and quite exciting. And to begin with, I didn't even know I was pregnant, but simply attended classes as a dutiful father, preparing myself, along with a half-dozen other fathers, for our day in the delivery room. It was not until the final four months of the affair that I began to notice some unusual occurrences: minuscule abdominal movements in the middle of the night, some slight swelling of the ankles, a tendency toward nausea in the morning. Being fully aware of how empathetic I am, I dismissed these mild symptoms with only slightly less amusement than did my friends whom my wife regaled with tales of my

symptoms of pregnancy. But as the symptoms persisted, I became progressively more uneasy. And it was perhaps more with apprehension than with anticipation that I finally entered the delivery room where my wife delivered a lovely male child and I, with considerably more fuss, rid myself of all my symptoms.

I was reassured, some years later, to read that my experience is not entirely unknown in the world. Among certain peoples whom some anthropologists unkindly label "primitive," it was common practice for husbands to experience many of the symptoms of pregnancy, including the contractions and pains of childbirth. This phenomenon was labeled *couvade*, after a French term for the birthing process.

Although the *couvade* is not common among men in modern societies, with the increasing popularity of prepared childbirth, the delivery rooms of most modern hospitals are no longer closed to fathers; indeed, we are encouraged to be present. For most, the experience is incredibly moving. And this is only one small indication of the increasing importance of the father's role in child rearing.

age, there may be minimal damage. Minimal damage may be tentatively linked with such personality predispositions as hyperactivity and impulsivity (Kagan, 1967).

Anoxia, a shortage of oxygen to the brain, has been extensively researched in medicine. Correlation studies have long suggested that anoxia may be related to impaired neurological, psychological, and motor functioning. These findings have most often been explained in terms of brain damage that may have resulted from a temporary shortage of oxygen. Most of these studies have suffered from the difficulty of determining the actual contribution of anoxia to behaviors later observed in infants and children. Because other complications of birth may have caused the anoxia in the first place, it is almost impossible to determine whether the complication itself or the resulting anoxia is the crucial variable.

A study conducted with rats eliminated this problem by systematically depriving subjects of oxygen for varying periods of time (Meier, Bunch, Nolan, & Scheilder, 1960). Subsequently, the rats were examined in terms of their performance in various puzzle boxes, mazes, and discrimination problems. Rats deprived of oxygen performed less well on a number of tasks only if the deprivation had lasted sufficiently long. For example, thirty minutes of oxygen reduction did not significantly affect the rats' performances, but sixty minutes of deprivation did.

Graham, Ernhart, Thurston, and Craft (1962) investigated 355 children at the age of three. At birth, these children had been classified by hos-

Today's fathers are often far more involved in childbirth than their own fathers were.

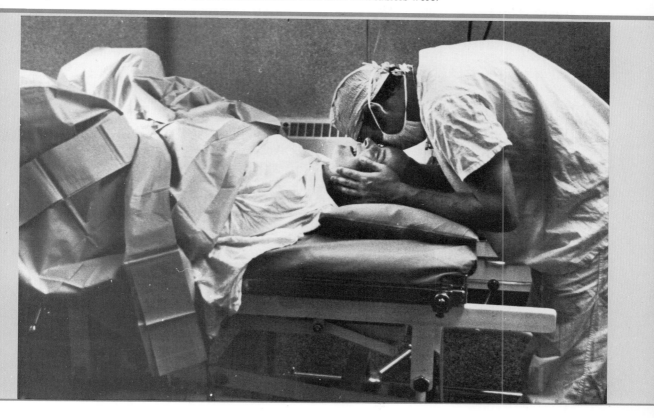

pital staff as either normal full-term newborns, anoxic full-term newborns, or newborns with other complications. Investigators administered a large battery of tests and conducted a variety of observations without knowledge of the individual subject's classification, thus eliminating the possibility that experimenter bias would affect observations. Their single most important finding was that children from the anoxic group did less well on all tests of intellectual functioning (Stanford-Binet, vocabulary tests, concept tests).

In addition to the physiological **trauma** that accompanies birth, there is a remote possibility of psychological trauma. Rank's (1929) theory of the trauma of birth maintains that the sudden change from a comfortable, parasitic existence to the cold and demanding world creates great anxiety for the newborn child who is plagued forever after by a desire to return to the womb. Alleged evidence of this unconscious desire is found in the position assumed by many children and adults while sleeping or in times of stress—the characteristic curl of the fetus. However, no substantial evidence supports the theory of birth trauma (Pratt, 1954). Although the physiological trauma of birth may be significant, there is no evidence to support the notion of enduring psychological trauma.

From the child's point of view, then, birth is an indifferent process: The infant cannot reason about it, cannot compare it with other more or less pleasant states, can do nothing deliberately to alter it, and will not even remember it.

■ Prematurity

Prematurity is defined in terms of a short gestation period (thirty-six weeks or less) and in terms of low birth weight (SFD—less than 90 percent of average weight for term, usually less than 5½ pounds, or 2,500 grams). It is one of the more serious possible complications of birth, affecting approximately 10 percent of all infants born in the United States. Incidence of prematurity is considerably higher in some other countries.

Causes

Although it is impossible to state categorically what the precise causes of premature delivery are, a number of factors are related to its occurrence. Malnutrition, a factor implicated in other infant disadvantages, has been found to be related to prematurity (Birch & Gussow, 1970), as have social class, poverty, and race (Wortis, Heimer, Braine, Redlo, & Rue, 1963). It must be emphasized again, however, that such factors as social class and race have no inherent explanatory value. Certainly, neither *causes* prematurity any more than they *cause* the environmental conditions of poverty, ill health, and lower social and economic opportunity with which they are often associated. But it is likely that such associated factors as a poor diet and poor medical attention are directly related to prematurity. Hence the relationship between prematurity and social class.

Numerous studies have also implicated cigarette smoking with prematurity. In some studies, rate of prematurity among smoking mothers is almost twice as high as would normally be expected, with frequency of premature births increasing with amount smoked. Other related factors include toxemia and various illnesses in the mother while she is pregnant; also related is the mother's age, with increasing age being positively related to incidence of premature births. Youth is also closely associated with prematurity. Teenage mothers are far more likely to give birth to premature and SFD infants and to infants who suffer from various birth defects (Siegel & Morris, 1974). In addition, infants from multiple births are much more frequently premature than are infants from single births, probably because of space limitations within the uterus.

Effects

One of the most obvious possible effects of prematurity is death. Indeed, chances of death for a premature infant weighing between 4½ and 5½ pounds are approximately six times greater than

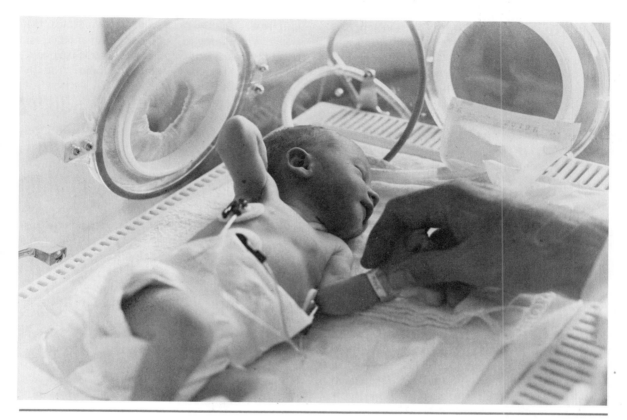

Prematurity is one of the leading causes of infant death. Advances in medical knowledge and technology have greatly increased the premature infant's chances of surviving.

for a child weighing 6 pounds 10 ounces or more. The probability of death increases dramatically with lower birth weights. The most common cause of death, as was mentioned earlier, is respiratory failure. With advances in medical knowledge and technology, however, a premature infant's chances of survival are increasing rapidly.

Among premature infants, measured intelligence is frequently lower than normal (Caputo & Mandell, 1970). Corroboration of this frequently replicated finding has also been obtained in studies of twins: The heavier of two identical twins tends to have the higher measured intelligence (Churchill, 1965). The advantage of these studies of twins is that they naturally control for such

important factors as sex, race, social class, and numerous environmental variables.

Other studies have demonstrated higher incidences of cerebral palsy, autism, physical defects, and hyperkinesis (hyperactivity) among premature infants (Caputo & Mandell, 1970; Wiener, 1970).

In view of these rather alarming findings, and given the highly likely relationship between nutrition and prematurity, probably a great deal can be done for unborn children and their mothers through programs of education, nutrition, and housing. But lest these findings appear too biased, it should also be pointed out that not all premature infants suffer noticeable disadvantages relative to their mature peers. Rawlings, Reynolds, Steward, and Strang (1971) examined sixty-eight infants who had weighed less than four pounds at birth and found that 87 percent of them were apparently normal. A more pessimistic review of these findings would point out that 13 percent of them were not fully normal (in the sense that averages are considered normal) and that this number far exceeds the incidence of abnormality in the general population.

More optimistically, however, prematurity is not necessarily and inevitably linked with physical, psychological, or neurological inferiority. Research has now shown that with adequate care and stimulation, many premature babies fare as well as normal babies. Scarr-Salapatek and Williams (1973) compared two groups of premature infants. The first of these was treated in the conventional manner. That is, the infants were kept in incubators with a minimum of human contact, a practice that is premised on the belief that premature infants are particularly susceptible to infection and highly vulnerable once infected. The second group was also kept in incubators, but these infants were taken from the incubators for feeding and were talked to and fondled by their nurses. In addition, their incubators were decorated with mobiles, and in follow-up visits after they had left the hospital, they were provided with numerous toys at home. It is highly significant that by the age of one these infants were heavier than infants in the control group and scored higher on developmental scales. Evidence is mounting that the usual "hands-off" treatment accorded most premature infants may not be the best of all possible worlds for them.

■ It Is Not That Bad

It is often disturbing for nonmedical people to consult medical journals and textbooks in search of explanations for their various complaints. Inevitably they discover that they have all the symptoms for innumerable vicious infections and exotic diseases. Thus, if you happen to be pregnant at this moment or are contemplating pregnancy, or are otherwise involved in the business, you might find yourself a little apprehensive. I draw this to your attention only to emphasize that it really is not that bad (pregnancy, that is). The intrauterine world of the unborn infant is less threatening and less dangerous than our world. And it is perhaps reassuring that nature often provides for spontaneous abortions when the embryo or the fetus would have been grossly abnormal (Potter, 1957). In most cases the fetus comes to term; when it reaches this stage, the probability that the child will be normal and healthy far outweighs the possibility that it will suffer any of the defects or abnormalities described in this chapter.

■ MAIN POINTS

1 Pregnancy is caused; it does not just happen.

2 Early symptoms of pregnancy are notoriously uncertain, although in combination they provide relatively reliable information. Pregnancy is often ascertained through chemical tests.

3 The gestation period for humans is nine calendar months, which is more commonly computed as 10 lunar months (40 weeks or 280 days), beginning from the onset of the last menses.

4 Prenatal physiological development occurs in three stages: the periods of the ovum (one week), the embryo (two to eight weeks), and the fetus (eight to forty weeks).

5 The fertilized ovum moves from the fallopian tubes to the uterus and imbeds itself in the wall of the uterus approximately seven days after fertilization.

6 From week one to week eight, the embryo develops from an almost microscopic speck to a little organism approximately one and one-half to two inches long and weighing close to two-thirds of an ounce. By the end of the eighth week, all the organs of the infant are present. No further structural changes will take place.

7 Fetal growth involves primarily physical changes in size and weight and neurological development. The fetus's chances of survival are low if born before the seventh lunar month.

8 The average size of a newborn infant is approximately 19.5 inches and nearly 7 pounds.

9 Among the factors that affect prenatal development are maternal nutrition, drugs, alcohol (in excessive amounts), narcotics, general health, and age of the mother. There is evidence that the fetus is sensitive to external sounds.

10 Birth ordinarily occurs 266 days after conception; the mature newborn weighs approximately 2,500 grams. Early deliveries are classified as premature (before the thirty-seventh week). Newborns are also classified as small-for-date (SFD) if they weigh 10 percent less than average newborns of the same gestational age.

11 Labor can be considered in three stages: dilation of the cervix in preparation for birth (lasting an average of nine to twelve hours), the actual birth (usually accomplished within an hour), and expulsion of the placenta and other membranes (soon after birth and lasting several minutes).

12 Some mothers think that having a baby is like rolling off a log; others consider it a rather large log from which the fall is quite painful. Advocates of natural childbirth report relatively painless births.

13 Dramatic demands confront newborns immediately upon delivery, not the least of which is that now they must breathe by themselves and obtain their own food—with the aid of adults.

14 Birth poses two great dangers for the neonate: cerebral hemorrhage, resulting from extreme pressures in the uterus, in the birth canal, or from the forceps wielded by the friendly obstetrician; the second is prolapse of the umbilical cord and anoxia (shortage of oxygen).

15 Prematurity appears to be linked to such social-class variables as diet and poor medical attention, to the age of the mother, and to smoking. Its most apparent effects are the greater possibility of death, physical defects, hyperkinesis, and impaired mental functioning.

■ FURTHER READINGS

Among the best sources for more detailed information on prenatal development and birth are the following obstetrics and nursing textbooks:

Clark, A., et al. *Childbearing: A nursing perspective* (2nd ed.). Philadelphia: F. A. Davis, 1979.

Pritchard, J., & MacDonald, P. *Williams obstetrics* (16th ed.). New York: Appleton-Century-Crofts, 1980.

Reeder, S., et al. *Maternity nursing* (14th ed.). Philadelphia: J. B. Lippincott, 1980.

The following is a collection of five sometimes highly technical, but also highly informative, articles dealing with the relationship between nutrition and the development of the brain, as well as with diet patterns in nonhuman and human primates:

Wurtman, R. J., & Wurtman, J. J. (Eds.). *Nutrition and the brain* (Vol. 1). New York: Raven Press, 1977.

Those interested in alternative approaches to childbirth are referred to the original authors of some of the more popular approaches:

Dick Read, G. *Childbirth without fear: The original approach to natural childbirth* (4th ed.). (H. Wessel & H. F. Ellis, Eds.). New York: Harper & Row, 1972.

Lamaze, F. *Painless childbirth: The Lamaze method.* New York: Pocket Books, 1972.

Leboyer, F. *Birth without violence.* New York: Random House, 1975.

5

PERCEPTUAL AND COGNITIVE DEVELOPMENT

An infant crying for the light:
And with no language but a cry.

> Alfred Lord Tennyson
> *In Memoriam*

The Child is father of the Man.

> William Wordsworth
> "My Heart Leaps Up"

E verybody is awake now. At least twice I have been asked when we're going to stop for lunch. Perhaps it was more than twice, but I wasn't always paying attention. I find it difficult to believe that we should be hungry yet.

"Soon," I answer, although the question is now rather old. "We'll eat at the museum." The enthusiasm is not immediately overwhelming, but since nobody objects very loudly, I know that the plan has been approved.

Fort Victoria Museum. A handful of old buildings, freshly whitewashed, snowy pale against the green hills on the northern bank of the North Saskatchewan River, just four or five minutes off the highway. At one time, a ferry crossed the river at this point, and all important roads in the area ended and started here. Indians, missionaries, traders, settlers, oxen, horses, and all the other stuff of which the West was made had their day in Fort Victoria. Now, there is only this group of tired buildings in which are housed the faintly rusty, mildewed, cracked, and cobwebbed relics of lives whose spans have long since ended.

Sitting on the ground, our backs against the sun-warmed logs of the main house, we eat cucumber sandwiches. Below, the river sweeps by, still going east, probably looking very much as it might if I were a trapper sitting here, against these very logs, at about the time that my grandmother was born. I tell her that, and she chuckles quietly. I wonder again whether she has always found life so gently amusing. And why. For me, it is not always gently amusing.

There are no tourists here now. The lady in the house says there are never very many, even in the middle of summer. Few travelers from distant places come this way. And the lake people, who use the nearby highway to go back and forth between their summer cottages and the cities where they work, have little time to stop at museums.

The children have now finished eating; Paul has taken his brother and sister and a fishing rod down to the river. Grandma's head begins to nod slightly toward her green knitting. She sleeps so easily and so frequently. The sleep of babies, angels, and others whose consciences let them be. I sleep less well.

Inside the house, I hear a baby cry, and remember that the lady who looks after the museum has a small infant in a basket by the treadle sewing machine. Perhaps while the children fish and Grandma sleeps, I can do an interview. I hurry into the museum and approach the basket.

How does one interview a newborn? I find an old chair and drag it next to the basket. Its legs scrape a protest across the worn plank floor. I sit, looking at this four- or five-month-old infant—this preverbal bundle that no longer cries but looks directly at me with large bluish eyes. I sit and look. And look.

There is nothing I can ask, even though I have only a handful of the answers. Still, I am not immediately anxious to be on the highway again. And there may be time now to look at the earliest days and months of the human lifespan. We'll look first at physical characteristics of the newborn, before moving to the mind and senses and their development during the years of infancy. Quickly now before the river becomes tiresome or grandmother awakens. Or this straight-haired infant with drying custard all around her mouth and over one ear should decide that I am no longer fascinating.

■ Description of a Neonate

The **neonate** (newborn infant) is not often overwhelmingly attractive. The creature's features are often wrinkled and may be distorted from passage through the birth canal; it sometimes bears the marks of forceps on various parts of its anatomy; its entire skull may be flattened, lengthened, skewed, or otherwise deformed. It is usually covered with remnants of amniotic fluid, matter sometimes oozes from its mouth and nose, its eyes are wrinkled shut, its breathing rasps and wheezes, and it pierces the air with thin, scratchy wails.

Of what is the neonate capable? Formerly, the newborn was thought to be almost insensitive to external stimulation, with responses limited to the repertoire of reflexive activities provided by the genes. More recent evidence suggests that this belief is a myth. Indeed, it can be demonstrated that almost from the moment of birth the child can see, hear, and feel. The infant is far more than a passive little doll.

Piaget describes the world of the young infant as a world of the *here and now*—a world that has meaning only when the child is actually sensing it or acting toward or with it. For this reason, a discussion of the cognitive or intellectual development of the child must begin with behavior and motor learning, as well as with perceptual abilities and perceptual development. We look at these topics in this chapter.

■ The Orienting Response

As defined in this text (as well as in most others), the period of infancy lasts from the first few weeks of life to approximately two years of age. Table 5.1 shows the physical growth typical in infancy. At the beginning of this period, infants might seem relatively unimpressive; at the end they can walk, talk, recognize their dog, ride a tricycle, and tell their daddy and mama that they love them. How a child develops these capabilities is the concern of the developmental psychologist; it is also the question that concerns us here.

Some of the child's most important behaviors are extremely subtle and almost imperceptible. One such behavior has played a significant role in the development of experimental child psychology. It involves our tendency (and that of other animals) to respond to new stimulation by becoming more alert—that is, by attending or orienting to it, hence the label *orienting response.*

In animals such as dogs and cats, the orienting response is clear and obvious. Upon hearing a new

Table 5.1 Height and weight at the fiftieth percentile for American infants.

Age	Height (inches)		Weight (pounds)	
	Girl	Boy	Girl	Boy
Birth	19¾	20	7½	7½
6 months	25¾	26	15¾	16¾
12 months	29¼	29½	21	22¼
18 months	31¾	32¼	24¼	25¼
24 months	34	34½	27	27¾

Adapted by the Health Department, Milwaukee, Wisconsin; based on data by H. C. Stuart and H. V. Meredith, prepared for use in the Children's Medical Center, Boston. Used by permission of the Milwaukee Health Depatment.

sound, for example, a dog will pause, its ears may perk up and turn slightly toward the sound, and its whole attitude says, in effect, "What was that?" The human infant does not respond in identical fashion; the control that we have over the external parts of our ears is rather limited and unimpressive in most cases. But other distinct and measurable changes will take place, and these in combination define the human orienting response. This reaction includes changes in pupil size, heart rate, conductivity of the skin to electricity (**galvanic skin response,** or **GSR**, also termed *electrodermal response*), and other physiological changes that are observable only by using sensitive instruments.

The value of the orienting response to the child psychologist is that it can be used as an indication of attention, since it occurs only in response to novel stimulation to which the individual is then attending. It can also be used as an indication of learning, since it ceases to occur when the stimulation is no longer novel. In other words, when an infant has learned a stimulus (it has become familiar), the orienting reaction will no longer take place. In the same way, a dog might *orient* visibly when it first hears a cow in the distance, but will cease to do so when the sound has been identified. Such a decrease in the orienting reaction is termed *habituation*.

An interesting illustration of the use of the orienting reaction in infant research is provided by Moffitt (1971). In this study, heart rates of infants aged twenty to twenty-four weeks were monitored while the infants heard taped repetitions of the word *gah*. Not much of a word, really, but adequate for these purposes. When infants first heard the word, their heart rates slowed dramatically— clear indication of an orienting response. But with continued repetition of the same word (same voice, same tone, same volume), infants quickly became accustomed to the stimulus and heart rates rapidly returned to normal. Suddenly, with no break in inflection, tone, or volume, the taped recording changed: It said "bah" instead of "gah." And heart rate decelerated dramatically and immediately, an observation that leads clearly to the conclusion that five- to six-month-old infants are able to tell the difference between sounds as similar as "bah" and "gah." Thus, even though infants cannot tell us whether "mother" sounds the same as "father," whether the color blue looks like red, or whether salt tastes like sugar, we can turn to the orienting response and to other subtle behaviors for our answers. (See *Crib Death* for an unanswered question.)

■ Behavior in the Newborn

Most of the behaviors in which the newborn engages are reflexive—that is, they do not require learning and can easily be elicited in the normal child by presenting the appropriate stimulus. Although neonates may engage in some activity that is not reflexive, they probably do not engage in any deliberate activity. In other words, some of the child's generalized behaviors, such as squirming, waving the arms, and kicking, are sometimes too complex and too spontaneous to be classified as reflexes, but they do not appear to be intentional (White, 1975).

Table 5.2 lists some of the newborn's common reflexes. Probably the best known of these is the sucking reflex, which is easily produced by placing an object in the child's mouth (a nipple is considered an appropriate stimulus). Reflexive behavior related to sucking is the **head turning reflex**, also called the **rooting reflex**, which can be elicited by stroking the baby's cheek or the corner of the mouth. The infant will turn toward the side that is being stimulated. This reflex is readily apparent in breast-fed babies, who need to turn in the direction of stimulation if they are to reach the nipple. It is less important to the child who is presented with a bottle.

Swallowing, hiccoughing, sneezing, and vomiting can all be elicited by the appropriate nourishment-related stimulation. They are therefore referred to as the **vegetative reflexes**.

A number of common motor reflexes in the newborn have no particular survival value at this time, but they might well have been useful in some less "civilized" time. These include the startle reaction—throwing out the arms and feet symmetrically and then pulling them back toward the center of the body. There is speculation that this reflex might be important for infants whose mothers live or sleep in trees. If they suddenly fall but react by throwing out arms and legs, they might luckily catch a branch and save themselves. This particular reflex, labeled the **Moro reflex**, is sometimes useful in diagnosing brain damage, because it ordinarily disappears during infancy in the normal child but is often present later in life in cases of impaired motor centers of the brain. Other reflexes that disappear with time are the *Babinski reflex*—the typical fanning of the toes when tickled in the middle of the soles of the feet; the **palmar reflex** (grasping—also called the *Darwinian reflex*), which is sometimes sufficiently pronounced that the neo-

Table 5.2 Some reflexive behavior of the newborn.

Reflex	Stimulus
Sucking	Object in the mouth
Head turning	Stroking the cheek or the corner of the mouth
Swallowing	Food in the mouth
Sneezing	Irritation in the nasal passages
Moro reflex	Sudden loud noise
Babinski reflex	Tickling the middle of the soles
Toe grasp	Tickling the soles just below the toes
Palmar grasp	Placing object in the infant's hand
Swimming reflex	Infant horizontal, supported by abdomen
Stepping reflex	Infant vertical, feet lightly touching flat surface

Based in part on Dennis, 1934.

nate can be raised completely off a bed when grasping an adult's finger in each hand; and the *swimming* and *stepping reflexes*, which occur when one holds the baby balanced on the stomach, or upright with the feet just touching a surface.

■ Motor Development

The helplessness of neonates results mainly from their inability to exercise control over motor movements. Their behavior is a far cry from that of the young of many subhuman species, including precocial birds and most members of the deer family, who are able to follow their mothers and to make considerable efforts to obtain food almost immediately after birth. But the child does not remain physically helpless throughout infancy. Indeed, one of the major acquisitions during this period is the ability to walk. Much before then the infant will have learned to move by creeping and before that will have developed the ability to sit with a little support.

Although the developmental sequence of motor capacities in children seems to be relatively invariable, it is clear that the ages at which different abilities appear vary considerably from one child to another (Dennis, 1941a; Gesell & Amatruda, 1941). It is useful nevertheless to have developmental **norms**, not only as indications of sequence but also as a standard by which to judge the child's rate of development. Here, as elsewhere, there is no *average* child.

Probably the best-known description of the motor sequence from birth to the age of fifteen months is provided by Shirley (1933). Her study employed a painstaking, longitudinal approach, involving many subjects over a long time. The portion of the study that was concerned with infants was not meant to establish ages at which they acquire new motor skills but was designed to discover whether the acquisition sequence was the same for everybody. Shirley made this explicit, claiming that better norms had already been provided by Gesell's (1937) extensive studies. However, her tentative norms are similar to those of Gesell. (See Figure 5.1 for Shirley's sequence of **motor development**.)

Shirley's results offer rather convincing evidence that most infants go through very similar sequences in acquiring early motor skills. She explained this regularity in terms of maturation (or growth) and claimed, specifically, that learning or experience is not involved in any important way in developing the ability to sit, creep, walk, and so

CRIB DEATH:
SUDDEN INFANT DEATH SYNDROME

A short time ago, one of the local newspapers reported the death of a three-month-old infant who had been found lifeless in his crib in the morning. The infant had apparently been vigorous and healthy prior to his sudden death. Police described the death as "suspicious" and were investigating.

Several days later, the newspaper again reported on this death. Medical authorities had now determined that the infant had died of *sudden infant death syndrome* (sometimes popularly referred to as "crib death"), and all "suspicions" had been abandoned. In fact, however, a diagnosis of *sudden infant death syndrome* (SIDS) is really not a diagnosis at all; it is an admission that the cause of death is unknown.

This mysterious cause of infant death accounts for approximately 2 deaths for every 1,000 live births. This makes SIDS the *leading* cause of death between the ages of one month and one year (Naeye, 1980); it accounts for somewhere between ten and twenty thousand deaths per year in the United States alone.

Although the cause of SIDS is still unknown, some SIDS victims have a number of characteristics in common. Among these, the most common is the presence of a mild upper respiratory infection in slightly more than half of all victims (Kahn & Blum, 1982). In addition, victims are almost never in their first week of life; SIDS occurs most frequently between the ages of one and four months of age. It rarely occurs after the age of six months. SIDS is slightly more common among male than female infants and is somewhat more likely to occur among infants whose siblings have also been victims of the syndrome.

Medically, SIDS has often been associated with *apnea*, a sleep disorder characterized by cessation of breathing. Apnea occurs among a number of adults, seems to involve a temporary paralysis or a collapse of throat muscles, and generally causes the person to awaken at once. In severe cases, tracheotomies may be performed to prevent the victim from dying. Victims of SIDS die before recovering from the apnea.

Frequently, parents of potential SIDS victims become aware that something is amiss and are able to revive the infant before death occurs. Some of these infants, called "near misses for SIDS," have been employed in various studies that have attempted to discover the causes of SIDS or the combination of factors that might be most useful for identifying infants who are at risk for the syndrome. One such study, conducted by Duffty and Bryan (1982), involved ten infants who had been observed to have one or more apnea attacks while in the hospital during their first weeks of life. Another seventy-two infants in the study consisted of "near-miss" infants who had on. She also believed that the high degree of similarity among different babies with respect to motor development results from two innate laws of development. These laws also appear to describe some aspects of fetal development and are mentioned briefly in Chapter 4. The first maintains that development is cephalocaudal—it proceeds from the head toward the feet. Thus infants first acquire control over the head—for example, they can control eye movements and raise the head prior to acquiring control over the extremities. Fetal development proceeds in the same manner: The head, eyes, and internal organs develop in the embryo prior to the appearance of the limbs. Hence, Shirley maintained that cephalocaudal growth is a fundamental biological principle of development.

The second developmental principle is based on the observation that development proceeds in an inward-outward direction, referred to as proximodistal. Development is said to be proximodistal in the sense that internal organs mature and function prior to the development of external limbs and in that children acquire control over parts of the body closest to the center before they can control the extremities. Thus children are capable of gross motor movements before they can control hand or finger movement.

Although Shirley's findings concerning the sequence of motor development have not been seriously questioned by subsequent research, her interpretation of causes has. Experience not only drastically affects the age at which various motor

been revived by parents and referred to the investigation by their pediatricians. Another fifty-two infants were siblings of infants who had previously been victims of SIDS.

The procedure in this experiment involved teaching parents resuscitation techniques and teaching them as well about the use of monitors designed to detect cessation of breathing for a period longer than twenty seconds (in effect, an apnea detector) or a heart-rate monitor that would be activated when the infant's heart rate dropped below eighty beats per minute. Parents were asked to keep track of the number of times the monitors sounded the alarms.

Of the ten infants in the sample who had experienced apnea in the first week of life, none had any further recurrences. This confirms the finding that SIDS rarely, if ever, occurs in the first week of life (Duffty & Bryan, 1982).

Among the seventy-two "near-miss" infants, thirty-one experienced prolonged apnea while being monitored at home. Fourteen of these required "vigorous stimulation" for revival on at least one occasion. And among the fifty-two who had a sibling who was a SIDS victim, sixteen had at least one episode, seven of these requiring vigorous intervention. One died after the mother, a trained nurse, had initially revived the infant.

It is perhaps revealing that in the Duffty and Bryan study, a great many of the potential SIDS victims suffered more than one alarm episode. Indeed, some 45 percent experienced more than ten such episodes. And in many of these infants, episodes occurred in clusters, with perhaps three or four occurring in a period of as many days. Some 63 percent of these infants were also experiencing mild upper respiratory infections at the time of these episodes. A number had also recently been exposed to stress in the form of inoculations, traveling, teething, or overtiredness.

In another study of SIDS, Kahn and Blum (1982) also found a relatively high incidence of respiratory infections among victims. In addition, they reported that many of these victims had been given phenothiazines (in the form of a cough syrup).

Again, note that none of the factors most often associated with SIDS has been shown to *cause* it. Although the presence of these factors might be associated with increased risk, it is still true that a large number of SIDS victims do not have colds, have never taken phenothiazines, have experienced no recent stress, and have no siblings who have been victims of SIDS. Small wonder that physicians and parents are baffled and that law-enforcement personnel are occasionally suspicious.

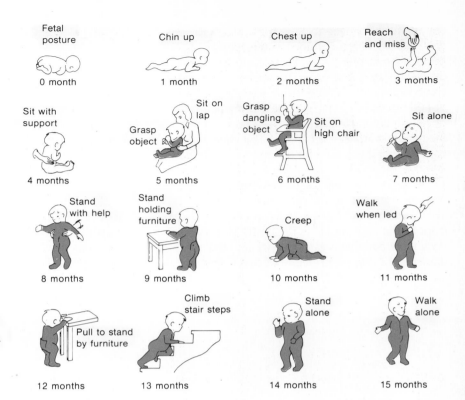

Figure 5.1
Locomotor development in infants (From Mary M. Shirley, *The first two years*. Institute of Child Welfare Monograph No. 7. Used by permission of the Univeristy of Minnesota Press.)

capabilities are attained but can also affect their quality. The Dennis (1960) study of orphaned infants in Iran (see Chapter 3) is a case in point. Recall that this study involved observing the motor development of a group of infants who were raised in pathetically deprived environments in two different institutions. Their motor development was severely retarded, and they preferred scooting to crawling. Infants employed this mode of propulsion not because they preferred it to a more ordinary crawl but because they had not *learned* to crawl, apparently because they had not lain prone in their beds during their infancy. Dennis suggests that the lack of opportunity to exercise the motor activities related to crawling made it unlikely that they would learn to crawl later. Because they had had some experience with sitting, it was not particularly surprising that the mode of propulsion they developed involved sitting and swinging their arms.

Additional evidence that the appearance of infant motor behaviors do follow the same maturational time table in all infants may be found in investigations of infant development in different cultures. For example, Gerber (1958) reports an investigation of 300 Ugandan infants who, a mere two days after birth (all home deliveries without anesthetics), could sit upright, heads held high, with only slight support of the elbows—a feat that most American children cannot accomplish until close to the age of two months (Bayley, 1969). And all 300 of these children were expert crawlers before they were two months of age.

Other research on motor development has attempted to analyze the detailed activities involved in learning various motor activities. Ames (1937), for example, studied films of children creeping and concluded that there are fourteen stages involved in learning to move by creeping. Because of the importance of the ability to move,

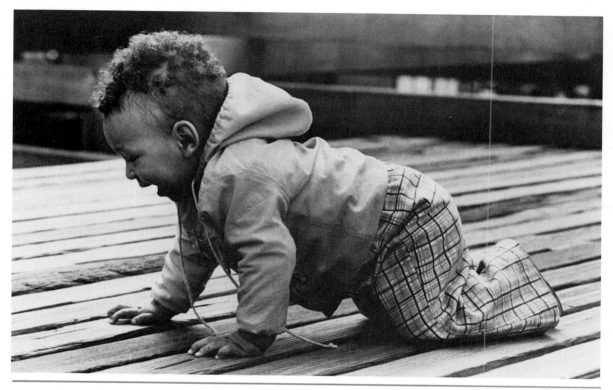

Although maturation of muscular and neural systems is essential for complex motor activities, experience has a great deal to do with learning to creep and crawl, to walk and run, to jump and perhaps to fly.

considerably more research has dealt with locomotion in infants than with other aspects of motor development. Nevertheless, investigations of abilities such as **prehension** also reveal relatively consistent sequences of stages—in this case, ten stages, beginning with the infant incapable of making physical contact with the object and culminating with an adultlike grasp by the age of fifteen months (Halverson, 1931).

■ Perceptual Development

Investigating the sensory capacities and perceptual development of the young infant presents some difficult problems for researchers; most of the difficulties relate to the infant's inability to commu-

nicate directly the effects of sensory experience. Hence investigators have had to rely extensively on nonverbal infant behaviors, including movements of the eyes, time spent looking at stimuli, gross bodily reactions to strong smells or tastes, subtle physiological changes with varying stimulation, and evidence of orienting to sounds.

Vision

For years newborns were assumed to have poorly developed vision, with no ability to discern color patterns, form, or movement. More recent evidence has contradicted many of these early beliefs.

Although no one has yet determined exactly when color vision is first present in the infant, we

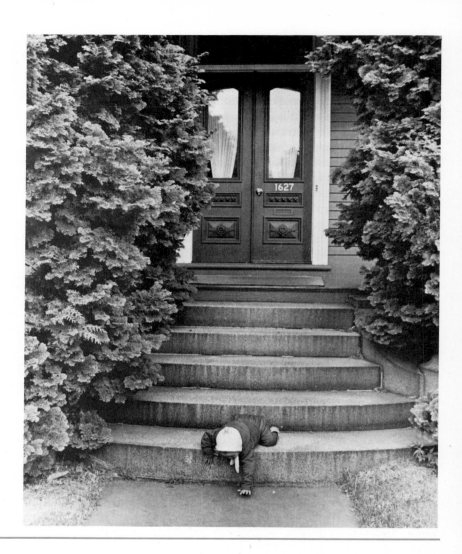

Researchers have subjected the sequence of infants' motor acquisitions to detailed analyses. Most infants go through similar sequences at about the same ages. Some, however, do things their own way.

do know that it is well developed by the age of two to four months (Bornstein, Kessen, & Weiskopf, 1975; Fagan, 1974). By the age of four months, infants even show a *preference* for certain colors; they spend more time looking at pure reds and blues than at other hues (Bornstein & Marks, 1982). **Pupillary reflexes** to changes in the brightness of visual stimulation demonstrate that the neonate is sensitive to light intensity, is capable of visually following a slowly moving object within a few days of birth, and is sensitive to patterns and contours

as early as two days after birth (Fantz, 1961, 1963, 1964, 1965). Cohen (1979) has found that infants under the age of six to eight weeks can perceive contours (or edges) with sufficient contrast but that they cannot yet perceive relationships among different contours or forms.

The extent of the newborn child's awareness of perceptual patterns is difficult to determine. Because infants cannot communicate perceptions and frequently prefer to sleep rather than to participate in psychological investigations, they are

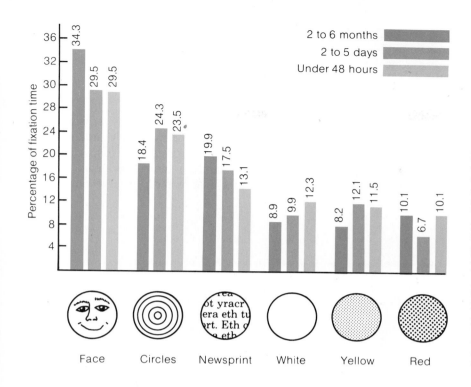

Figure 5.2
Relative duration (percentage of fixation time) of initial gaze of infants in successive and repeated presentations of six circular visual stimuli. The graph depicts infants' preference for the human face and the more complex stimuli. (Based on data in Robert L. Fantz, Pattern vision in newborn infants. *Science*, 1963, *140*, 296–297. Copyright 1963 by the American Association for the Advancement of Science. Used by permission of the American Association for the Advancement of Science and the author.)

rather poor subjects. In one experiment that clearly demonstrates pattern discrimination in the newborn, a criterion for selecting subjects was whether they kept their eyes open long enough to be exposed to the stimulus (Fantz, 1963). Eighteen infants, ranging in age from ten hours to five days, were employed in this experiment. They were shown six circular stimulus patterns of varying complexity, the most complex being a human face. In diminishing order of complexity, the other stimuli included concentric circles, newspaper print, and three unpatterned disks of different colors. Figure 5.2 shows the relative percentage of the total time spent by subjects looking at each of the stimulus figures. The face stimulus was looked at for significantly longer periods of time than the others, indicating not only that infants can discriminate among the various figures but also that they prefer moderate complexity. From their first hours of life, infants' vision seems to be sufficiently developed to allow them to perceive many of the physical

characteristics of their surroundings, when they are awake (Cohen, DeLoache, & Strauss, 1979). (See also *Visual Acuity in the Newborn.*)

In addition to perceiving color, movement, and form and demonstrating preferences among them, young infants apparently can also perceive depth. Gibson and Walk (1960) illustrate this by means of the "visual cliff" studies (see Figure 5.3). The apparatus used in this experiment consists of a heavy sheet of glass over a patterned surface; half of this surface is flush with the glass and half is three feet lower. Thus an adult standing or sitting on the glass can plainly see a drop or cliff where the patterned material falls away from the glass. So can goats that, at the mere age of a day, avoid the deep side, either going around or jumping over it. And so can infants, who, when they are old enough to crawl, typically refuse to cross the deep part, even when their mothers call them from the other side. Thus perception of depth is present at least from the time that the infant can crawl.

For years, a test for depth perception prior to the ability to crawl seemed impossible. With the refinement of physiological measures, however, it became possible to look at changes in heart rate when infants who could not crawl were simply moved from the shallow to the deep side of the visual cliff apparatus. Doing this, Campos, Langer and Krowitz (1970) found heart-rate deceleration in infants who were only a month and a half old. This might not mean that they actually perceive depth (older infants manifest heart-rate *accelera-*

tion in these circumstances) but does indicate that they are perceiving something new or unusual.

Other Senses

The neonate's contact with reality is happily not limited to information derived solely through vision. Unlike the young of many nonhuman species (dogs and cats, for example), there is evidence that the neonate is not deaf at birth. A large number of

VISUAL ACUITY IN THE NEWBORN

One way of describing visual acuity is in terms of what are termed *Snellen* ratings—for example, 20/20, 20/30, or 20/100. We tend to think of 20/20 vision as perfect. Actually, 20/20 indicates something closer to *normal* human vision. A person with 20/20 vision sees at 20 feet what other individuals without visual defects see at 20 feet. A person with 20/100 vision sees approximately as well at 20 feet as people with normal vision see at 100 feet. And there are individuals with better than 20/20 vision (20/15, for example, indicates people who see as clearly at 20 feet as others do at 15).

Among a number of complex and intriguing studies of infant visual perception are those that have attempted to determine the infant's visual acuity. Put more simply, how well can an infant see? Is the world fuzzy and blurred, or is it crisp and clear? Is it 20/20 or better—or worse? How can we possibly find out?

Among the first studies to look at this problem were those that made use of measures of **saccadic motion** (technically, the *optokinetic nystagmus*). Saccadic motion, the extremely rapid side-to-side motion of our eyes when we look at something, is a reflexive response; it changes the pattern of visual stimulation that strikes the retina and is essential for vision. Thus, whenever we are looking at and *seeing* something, our eyeballs are moving. A simple test of visual acuity based on the optokinetic nystagmus presents subjects with a plain background on which are fine vertical lines. As long as these lines are far enough apart, they can be distinguished, and saccadic movements will be observed as the lines move across the infant's field of vision. But if the lines are placed closer and closer together, a point comes when they can

no longer be seen. The field will appear gray, for example, if the background is white and the thin lines are black. Early studies employing this technique found that infants ceased responding to these lines long before an adult with normal vision does. Infant vision apparently is roughly equivalent to somewhere between 20/400 and 20/800 (Kiff & Lepard, 1966).

Subsequent findings revealed, however, that the optokinetic nystagmus might not be a good indicator of visual acuity, since the reflex seems to occur even in animals whose optic nerves have been removed. In addition, the use of corrective lenses with newborn infants does not appear to change their saccadic responses. Other studies have attempted to overcome these problems by looking at the amount of time an infant will gaze at a blank field and comparing it with time spent if the field has a very narrow vertical line through it (for example, Lewis & Maurer, 1977). When the narrow line is below threshold (the infant cannot see it, in other words), the infant should look at the field for about the same amount of time as if it were blank. But when the line is visible, the gazing period is typically longer. Using this technique, Lewis and Maurer report visual acuity figures higher than those found in earlier studies (perhaps 20/150).

In conclusion, the visual acuity of young infants apparently is not nearly as good as that of an adult with normal vision; it does not reach that normal level until somewhere between the ages of six and twelve months (Cohen et al., 1979). Although they are far from blind, the visual world of neonates probably is somewhat fuzzy and blurred.

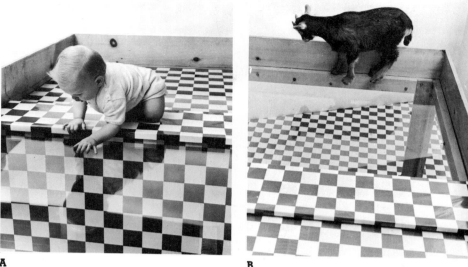

A   **B**

Figure 5.3
Use of the glass-floored visual cliff indicates that depth perception is developed at a very young age in human and other animal babies. In **A,** an infant refuses to cross over the "cliff" to his mother, even when she calls him. In **B,** a baby goat won't step over the cliff—although, unlike the human, it can jump to the other side. Goats show this response at the tender age of one day; humans cannot accurately be tested until they are much older and able to move by themselves.

studies (Eisenberg, Griffin, Coursin, & Hunter, 1964) have shown that the newborn child not only is sensitive to a wide range of sounds but can also detect the location of sound. In addition, sounds of different frequencies have different effects on children, although there are markedly individual responses to auditory stimulation. In general, low-frequency sounds and rhythmic sounds have a calming effect (Brackbill, 1970), whereas higher-frequency signals bring about a more violent reaction (Passman, 1976). Berg and Berg (1979) have found that infants respond more to lower than to higher frequencies. Some researchers have suggested that this might be evidence that the infant's auditory system is pretuned to respond to normal speech frequencies (Eisenberg, 1976).

The newborn is also sensitive to different odors. Infants will attempt to turn away their faces when exposed to a powerful and unpleasant smell such as ammonia (Lipsitt, Engen, & Kaye, 1963). Their sense of taste is less impressive, however

(Pratt, 1954). The distinctive tastes of salt, sugar, citric acid, and water do not bring about different responses, even when placed directly on the tongue, although by the age of two weeks infants will react more greedily to sugar than to salt (Engen, Lipsitt, & Peck, 1974).

Infants are remarkably insensitive to pain (McGraw, 1943). This is probably fortunate (birth might otherwise be quite painful), especially for those male babies whose early experience includes circumcision, usually done in the first week, when the newborn is not expected to feel pain and no anesthetics are used. Newborn girls appear to be more sensitive to pain than are boys (Lipsitt & Levy, 1959).

Neonates are remarkably alert and well suited to their environment. They can hear, see, and smell; they can turn in the direction of food, suck, swallow, digest, and eliminate; they can respond physically to a small range of stimuli; and they can cry and vomit. They are also singularly helpless crea-

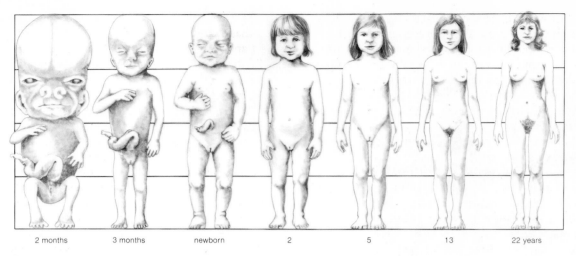

| 2 months | 3 months | newborn | 2 | 5 | 13 | 22 years |

Figure 5.4
Changes in form and proportion of the human body during fetal and postnatal life. (Reproduced with permission from Jensen et al., *Biology*. Belmont, Calif.: Wadsworth, 1979, p. 233.)

tures, who would surely die if the environment did not include an adult intimately concerned with their survival.

A fantastically impressive distance lies between a human adult's responses to the world and the uncoordinated and apparently purposeless movements of a newborn child. The story of the child's progress toward adulthood continues. Figure 5.4 illustrates some of the dramatic physical changes that occur during that progression.

■ The Mind of the Infant

Throughout this text we occasionally pause to insist that the person is really not composed of all the separate layers we have invented to simplify our study. We divide our subject to make it manageable, but we need to constantly remember that we are much more than the sum of these layers.

Thus far in this chapter, we have looked at the simple, unlearned behaviors of newborns and at their motor and perceptual capabilities, as well as the early development of new capabilities. One layer of paramount importance remains; it is inex-

tricably involved with all other aspects of development, but we shall consider it in isolation: the mind of the infant.

Maya Pines (1966) observed that for a long time psychology neglected the infant's mind, as though there was a silent admission that babies did not really have minds or that whatever minds they possessed were relatively unimportant at this stage of development. And Pearce (1977) suggests that we have hardly progressed, that we still think of infants as passive and impotent during the first few months after birth, and that, as a result, we continue to neglect their minds. We, in Pearce's words, have yet to recognize "the magical child."

The first major theorists of child development were more concerned with physical and physiological development, acquisition of language, and emotional and personality development than they were with the mind—with the exception of Jean Piaget. As far back as 1920, Piaget had begun to map the course of the child's cognitive development. Piaget's story of the growth of children's minds deals with their expanding awareness of the world in which they live and their discovery or invention of ways of interacting with this world. It is a complex and fascinating story.

The world of newborn infants begins as a world of the here and now. They have no memories, no hopes, no dreams, no fund of information with which to think. And so they do not think—they behave. Their behavior is of tremendous significance, not only for their motor development but also for the growth of their minds. **Cognition** is rooted in behavior.

The introduction to Piaget's theories (Chapter 2) described the two processes by which children interact with the world: assimilation and accommodation. To assimilate is to incorporate aspects of the environment into existing schemes. Thus, children are born with a primitive ability to suck. As a result, they can *assimilate* suckable objects to their sucking scheme. (*Scheme* is Piaget's term for the infant's simple behaviors.) While they assimilate objects to the sucking scheme, however, infants are forced to make changes in the activity of sucking—hence changes in the sucking scheme. Nipples come in a variety of shapes and sizes and require different positions of the lips and tongue and different sucking motions. In other words, they require *accommodation*. And it is through a continual process of exercising previously learned behaviors (assimilating to previously learned schemes) and changing these behaviors (accommodating) that the infant gradually develops the skills and knowledge that characterize the course of human development. But we are getting ahead of the story.

At the beginning, the world of the infant, while not necessarily William James's "blooming, buzzing mass of confusion," exists only when it is being reacted to and is understood only in terms of those actions. A nipple exists for infants when they look at it, touch it, suck it, or otherwise respond to it; when it is removed from their immediate perception, it ceases to exist. In Piaget's terms, the infant at this stage has not yet achieved the *object concept*—the realization that objects continue to exist even when they are not being sensed.

The process by which objects come to have a permanence and an identity of their own (the *object concept*) is not clearly understood but is of tremendous importance to the child's later cognitive development. To investigate the infant's understanding of objects, Piaget (1954) devised an experiment that involves showing the child an attractive object and then hiding it from view. Piaget argues that if the object exists only when children are perceiving it, they will make no effort to look for it, even when they have seen it being hidden from view. When children begin to look for an object they can no longer see, this is definite evidence that they can imagine it. The object continues to exist for them, even when it is unseen.

Piaget typically classifies his observations by the stages through which children pass. In the earliest stages of the development of the object concept, children do not respond to the object once it is removed. Next, they progress through a number of stages during which they search for the object, but only in the place where they last saw it. Finally, they achieve a complete realization of object permanence and can look for objects in a variety of places. The final stage occurs near the middle of the second year of life.

A number of later investigations of the development of the object concept have attempted to show that the age of acquisition is younger than Piaget suggests. For example, Bower (1971, 1977) used the orienting response of very young infants to determine whether an object ceases to exist when it is removed from sight. In one study, the infant is shown a ball and then a screen is moved between the infant and the ball. A few seconds later, the screen is removed. On some trials, the ball is still there; on others, the ball has been taken away. When infants do not have object permanence, they should not be surprised if the ball is gone. But they would be surprised to see it gone if they expected it to be there—in other words, if they had acquired notions of object permanence. Bower measured surprise by looking at heart rate. Bower's primary finding is that infants as young as three weeks of age appear to have some notion of object permanence, providing the object is hidden from view for only a few seconds. When the object is hidden for longer (15 seconds as opposed to 1½), infants at this age all show surprise when the ball is still present after the screen is removed.

Do studies such as these mean that Piaget was wrong? That infants have a notion of the permanence and independent identity of objects long before the age of eighteen months? No. What the studies indicate is that under the proper circumstances, infants appear to have a rudimentary and short-lived recollection of absent objects. (See *Infants and Spatial Orientation*.) However, this realization is some distance from being able to represent the object *mentally* when it has not just been sensed. It will still be a long time before the infant deliberately searches for an object that has not been present just recently (Haith & Campos, 1977; Ramsay & Campos, 1975). In the next section, we look at some of the events that occur in that long time.

■ Sensorimotor Development

Piaget labels the first two years of the child's life (infancy) the *period of sensorimotor development*. The reason for this is obvious: He believes that children's understanding of the world throughout most of this period is restricted to their perception of it and the activities that they can perform on it—hence, *sensori* and *motor*. Piaget simplifies the infant's development during this period by dividing it into the six substages summarized in Table 5.3 (p. 136). The most important developments during these stages are described on the following pages.

INFANTS AND SPATIAL ORIENTATION

Piaget describes the physical environment of the young infant as a world of the "here and now." Objects do not exist in relation to each other, but only in relation to the child. Thus, when objects are not being sensed directly, they are, in effect, nonexistent.

In recent investigations of the infant's understanding of physical space, Acredolo (1978) provides intriguing corroboration of Piaget's early theorizing. The twenty-four infants in this longitudinal investigation were tested at the ages of six, eleven, and sixteen months. The experimental procedure may be described briefly as follows: Infants were placed in a small enclosure (10 by 10 feet), at the center of which was a table; a baby chair on wheels was attached to the table. The chair could be rotated around the table so that the infant would be facing different walls in the enclosure. Small windows faced each other on two opposing walls. Initially, infants, accompanied by their mothers, were placed in the chair so that one window was on their immediate left, the other on the right. In the training portion of the study, a buzzer sounded and approximately three seconds later the experimenter peeked through one of the windows. The procedure was repeated a number of times, with the experimenter always peeking through the same window (to either the infant's right or left side). When infants had "learned" to expect a face at that window (indicated by looking at the window after the buzzer sounded, but

prior to the appearance of the face), the chair was turned so that the window that had previously been on the left would now be on the right, and vice versa.

In this testing phase of the study, it was possible to determine whether the infants had learned only to turn to the left or right or whether they possessed sufficient knowledge of spatial orientation to interpret the situation objectively (as opposed to *egocentrically*). If, for example, infants had learned only their own response of turning to the left (or right), they would be expected to continue to do so in the testing situation, thus turning toward the wrong window. If, however, they had learned that a face would appear at a particular window, they might be expected to turn in the opposite direction when they had been turned 180 degrees, thus continuing to turn toward the same window.

Acredolo's findings, highly supportive of Piaget's earlier observations, were that the six- and eleven-month-old infants continued to respond egocentrically; they had learned only to turn to their left or right, rather than to turn toward a specific window. By the age of sixteen months, however, responding had become progressively more objective. As long as the infant's interpretation of the world is largely egocentric, spatial orientation and the development of notions of objective reality are likely to be hampered.

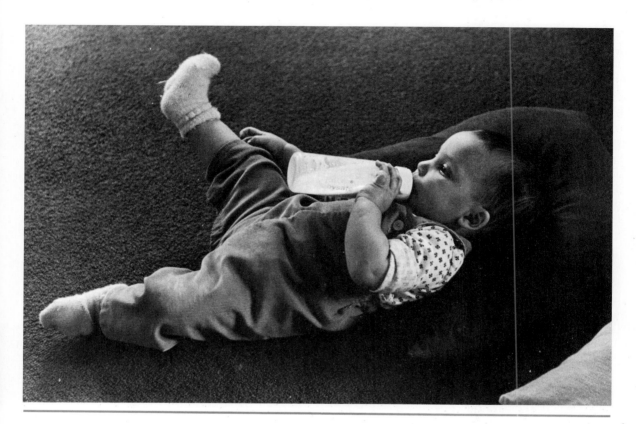

What does an infant think of when he contemplates a foot? Does he even know that this is *his* foot?

Reflexes and Early Learning

The first month of life contains little new learning. Infants spend most of their waking hours exercising the reflexes with which they are born—they suck, look, grasp, and cry. Some children engage in a great deal of the latter activity. The newborn infant also spends much time sleeping. Buhler (1930) reports that newborn infants sleep nearly 80 percent of the time, leaving them with no more than four waking hours per day. Some infants, like mine, have those few waking hours during the night rather than during the day. By the time children are a year of age, however, they spend about as much time awake as asleep.

The child's sucking, reaching, grasping, and looking activities during the first month are not all in vain. Through repeatedly exercising these reflexes, the child eventually gains control over small aspects of the environment (as well as over the activities themselves). By the end of the first month, infants have become relatively proficient at each of these activities, although they still cannot execute more than one action to obtain a single goal. In other words, there is still a lack of coordination between these behaviors. Infants presented with a visually appealing object can look at it but cannot reach toward it. The ability to look at an object and to continue looking at it when it moves (or when the child moves) precedes the ability to direct the hand toward that object (Provine & Westerman, 1979). Deliberately reaching and grasping is therefore a complex activity depending on the purposeful coordination of looking schemes, reach-

Table 5.3 Sensorimotor period: the six substages.

Substage and Approximate Age (months)	Principal Characteristics
1. Exercising reflexes (0–1)	Simple, unlearned behaviors (schemes) such as sucking and looking are practiced and become more deliberate.
2. Primary circular reactions (1–4)	Activities that center on the infant's body and that give rise to pleasant sensations are repeated (thumb sucking, for example).
3. Secondary circular reactions (4–8)	Activities that do not center on the child's body but that lead to *interesting* sights or sounds are repeated (repeatedly moving a mobile, for example).
4. Purposeful coordinations (8–12)	Separate schemes becoming coordinated (ability to look at an object *and* reach for it, for example); recognition of familiar people and objects; primitive beginnings of the understanding of causality implicit in the use of signs to anticipate events.
5. Tertiary circular reactions (12–18)	Experimentation involves repetition with variation (repeating a sound with a number of deliberate changes, for example).
6. Mental representation (18–24)	Transition between *sensorimotor* intelligence and a more *cognitive* intelligence; the internalization of activity so that its consequences can be anticipated prior to its actual performance; increasing importance of language in cognitive development.

ing schemes, and grasping schemes. This coordination is not usually apparent until after the age of three to five months (von Hofsten & Lindhagen, 1979). Until then, infants remain incapable of demonstrating the *intentionality* that Piaget considers essential to intelligent activity.

Early in infancy, children engage in a great deal of repetitive behaviors (thumb sucking, for example) called **primary circular reactions**. They involve reflexive responses that serve as stimuli for their own repetition. For example, the child accidentally gets a hand or a finger into the mouth; this triggers the sucking response, which results in the sensation of the hand in the mouth. That sensation leads to the repetition of the response, which leads to a repetition of the sensation, which

leads to a repetition of the response; this circle of action is in this case a *primary* circular reaction, because it involves the child's own body.

Later circular reactions do not always involve the child's body and are labeled **secondary circular reactions**. Six-month-old infants have numerous secondary circular reactions. They accidentally do something that is interesting, pleasing, or otherwise amusing and proceed to repeat it again and again. By kicking, Piaget's young son caused a row of dolls dangling above his bassinet to dance. The boy stopped to observe the dolls. Eventually he repeated the kicking, not intentionally to make the dolls move, but more likely because they had ceased moving and no longer attracted his attention. The act of kicking had the same effect again,

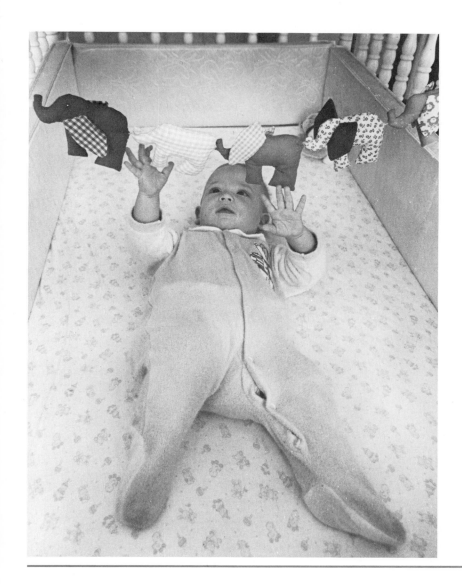

Within days of birth, infants are capable of looking at and following moving objects. Only a few months later the infant is capable of squirming and moving her arms in an apparently deliberate attempt to make these objects move.

and again the boy paused to look at the row of dancing dolls. Soon he was repeating the behavior over and over—hence a circular reaction.

At around the age of one or so, the infant's circular reactions become more experimental; these are **tertiary circular reactions.** The principal difference between these reactions and primary or secondary circular reactions is that the infant now deliberately modifies the response. Instead of saying "aaaagh" 115 times, they now say "aaaagh, aaaaaaaaagh, aaarrgh, aaaarrrrgh, aawooo, awwworrgh." The behavior is still circular, because the response leads to its own repetition, but it is now a repetition that is designed to explore. Children no longer behave simply to behave; they now behave specifically to discover what the effects of

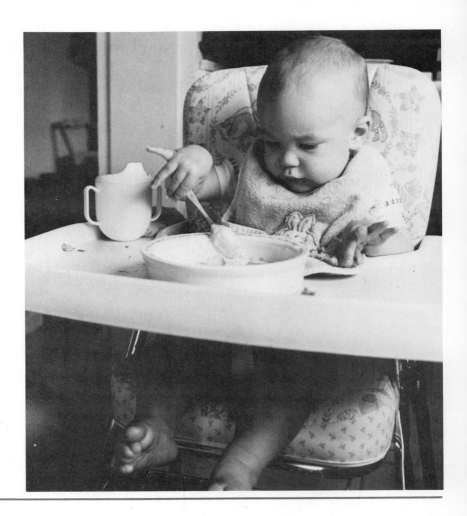

Evidence of intention is clear as the infant eats mostly food rather than fingers and spoon. Is intention still evident when the dish, spoon, and cup are swept off the tray?

their behavior will be. They have actively begun to explore their environment.

As we noted earlier, by the age of eight to twelve months, infants have begun to coordinate previously unrelated behaviors to achieve some desired end. Infants can now look at an object, reach for it, grasp it, and bring it to the mouth specifically to suck it. Throughout this sequence, there is clear evidence of intention. The child has succeeded in distinguishing the means from the end and no longer confuses the object with the activities that are appropriate for it.

Also somewhere between six and twelve months, infants begin to demonstrate their ability to *recognize* familiar objects and people. Phillips (1969) observes that the child is not likely to miss an absent person before being able to recognize that person. And because this ability does not ordinarily develop until the fourth substage (eight to twelve months), the anxiety caused by separation from the mother should not occur prior to this stage. Similarly, fear of strangers (stranger anxiety) should not be common until now. Research reviewed in Chapter 6 indicates that stranger anxiety and the effects of maternal separation are seldom common or serious before six months.

As infants become more familiar with the environment, they begin to use signs to anticipate events: Daddy putting on his jacket is a sign that he is leaving; mother putting on her pajamas is a sign that she is not. Understanding that certain events are *signs* that some other event is likely to occur is closely related to the ability to understand causality. For the young infant, whose logic is not always as perfect as yours or mine, the sign itself is often interpreted as the cause. In other words, a child who realizes that daddy will be leaving when he puts on his jacket *knows* that the cause of leaving is putting on the jacket—just as the *cause* of going to bed is taking a bath, putting on pajamas, getting a good-night kiss, saying prayers, or whatever ritual is common.

Mental Representation

Toward the end of the sensorimotor period, infants begin a transition between the *motoric* intelligence of infancy and the progressively *cognitive* intelligence of childhood. They now begin to represent objects and events mentally and combine these representations to arrive at *mental* solutions for problems. That is, children are now capable of anticipating the consequences of some of their activities prior to actually executing them. Their behavior is consequently no longer restricted to trial and error, as it was previously, but makes use of *mental representation*. In Piaget's terms, the child can now begin to internalize (represent mentally) actions and their consequences, without having to actually carry them out.

An illustration of this growing ability to internalize actions prior to their execution is provided by Piaget's description of the infant's response to a matchbox problem. A partly open matchbox containing a small thimble is given to the child. Because the opening is too small to permit withdrawal of the thimble, the child must open the box first. Earlier, infants would simply grope at the box, attempting in rather clumsy fashion to remove the thimble. Now, however, following initial failure to open the box, infants do not immediately attempt

new solutions, but appear instead to be considering the problem. Some subjects open and close their mouths or hands, very much as though they were providing external manifestations of internal thought processes. The child may subsequently place a thumb or finger directly into the box's partial opening and open it further to remove the thimble.

The ability to conceptualize the environment is also reflected in infants' mushrooming language development, which, according to Piaget, is greatly facilitated by their imitative behavior.

During the early stages of imitation, children are capable of imitating objects, activities, or people that are immediately present. Indeed, some researchers report that at a mere two weeks of age, infants are already able to imitate an adult sticking out the tongue or opening the mouth wide (Meltzoff & Moore, 1977, 1979). However, a number of other researchers do not agree that such young infants are actually imitating when they stick out their tongue in apparent response to a model doing the same thing. Masters (1979) and Jacobson and Kagan (1979) argue that this behavior is largely reflexive, related to feeding, and simply *released* by the nearness of the model rather than being an actual imitation. In any case, infants do not continue to stick out their tongues when the model is no longer present. This may be related to the difficulty they experience in separating the objects they perceive from their perception of them and their consequent failure to realize that objects continue to exist independently of them.

The eventual achievement of object permanence is inferred from what Piaget labels **deferred imitation**—the ability to imitate something or someone no longer present. When a two-year-old child dresses up in her mother's shoes and struts in front of a mirror in the absence of her mother, she is practicing deferred imitation. This behavior is significant, because to imitate a person who is absent, the child must be able to represent that person mentally; similarly, to associate a name with an object not immediately present necessitates representing the object mentally.

Note that when Piaget speaks of the internal representation of an object, he is referring to the

Table 5.4 Average ages for mental development in infants.

Age (months)	Mental Behavior Anticipated
0.2	Regards person momentarily, responding either to speech or to movements.
0.7	Eyes follow moving person.
0.7	Makes definite response to speaking voice.
1.5	Smiles or laughs in response to another person's speaking to and smiling at him or her.
2.0	Visually recognizes mother; expression changes when infant sees mother bending over to talk to him or her.
2.6	Manipulates red ring placed in child's hand or grasped by child.
3.8	Carries red ring to mouth during free play.
3.8	Inspects own hands.
4.1	Reaches for cube, even if not actually touching it.
5.1	Laughs or shows pleasure when held and played with.
5.8	Lifts cup with handle.
6.0	Looks for spoon that has fallen.
9.1	Responds to verbal request *not* accompanied by gesture.
12.0	Turns pages of book, even if effort is clumsy.
14.2	Says two words meaningfully (approximations all right if clear).
20.6	Puts two or more words denoting two concepts into one sentence or phrase.

internalization (or conceptualization) of activities related to the object. Bruner and Kenney (1966) term this **enactive** representation. Children's understanding of objects corresponds to the activities they perform with them. Three-year-olds typically define objects in terms of their function: They are "to do something." A ball is to play with, a bicycle is to ride, and a hole is to dig.

■ A Transition: From Sensation to Representation

The word *infant* derives from the Latin word *infans*. Literally, it means "without speech." And, indeed, throughout much of the period that we arbitrarily label *infancy*, the child is without speech. As noted earlier, the world of infants is initially a world of the here and now, a world populated only by those objects and feelings that are immediately perceived, a world that cannot be represented symbolically but can only be acted upon and felt. But the infant's capacities to act and to feel are far more impressive than we have long believed—perhaps even more impressive than most of us still believe (see Pearce, 1977; Pines, 1982).

Although the term *sensorimotor* describes well the predominant relationship between the infant and the world, it does not describe the most important cognitive achievements of the first two years of life. Some of these achievements are apparent in Table 5.4, which depicts important events in mental development during infancy.

By the time the child is two, the world no longer exists only in the immediate *sensible* present. Objects have achieved a permanence and an identity that no longer depend solely on the child's activities; there is a dawning understanding of cause-and-effect relationships; language is rapidly exercising a profound effect on cognitive development. These achievements, together with children's recognition of their own identities—their selves—represent a dramatic transition from a quasi-animalistic existence to the world of thought and emotions as we know it. But although it is a dramatic transition, at least in its import, it is neither sudden nor startling. Those who follow the lives of individual children closely (and daily) would never see the transition from sensorimotor intelligence to preoperational thought. It happens suddenly and irrevocably on the second birthday only in textbooks. Real life is less well organized.

■ MAIN POINTS

1 The neonate is not a pretty, curly haired, smiling cherub dressed in pink and blue and diminutive bows.

2 The behavioral repertoire of the neonate consists of a large number of reflexes, some of which are important for survival but many of which are not. The sucking reflex, occasionally considered too complex to be a reflex, is elicited by any object put in the infant's mouth.

3 Motor capacities develop in a series of stages. Although there is wide individual variation in the age at which each stage is attained, the sequence of stages appears to be similar among different infants.

4 The perceptual equipment of the neonate is remarkably well developed at birth and matures rapidly with age. Depth perception, response to patterns, and the ability to recognize colors are all present early in life, as is the ability to detect odors and tastes.

5 The infant's world is a world of the *here and now*. The infant does not realize that objects continue to exist even when they are not being sensed. Not until around the age of eighteen months does the child develop a complete understanding of object permanence (the *object concept*).

6 Piaget describes the intellectual development of the sensorimotor child (from birth to two years) in six substages, each of which is identified by the child's characteristic way of reacting to the world and understanding reality.

7 There is little learning in the first month of life, but infants repeatedly practice the simple reflexes with which they were born.

8 Circular reactions are repetitive behaviors in which the response serves as a stimulus for its own repetition. Primary circular reactions center on the infant's body (thumb sucking, for example); secondary circular reactions involve the environment (making a mobile move, for example).

9 Tertiary circular reactions appear in the second year of life and are characterized by the infant's active exploration of the environment, by modifying behaviors to observe their effects on the environment.

10 Somewhere between the ages of eight and twelve months, infants begin to coordinate the various activities they have been practicing. This coordination of schemes allows them to employ activities intentionally to attain goals.

Toward the end of the second year, a transition occurs between the motoric and perceptual intelligence of the preceding stage and the more cognitive intelligence of the succeeding stage. Here the child begins to show evidence, both in language and in behavior, of an ability to conceptualize the environment.

▪ FURTHER READINGS

Two readable and informative references by Bower are directly relevant to this chapter. The first is an article that presents an intriguing account of abilities that are present at one stage in life (sometimes remarkably early), disappear, and sometimes reappear; the second is an introduction to child development, with an emphasis on the power of the infant's mind:

Bower, T. G. R. Repetitive processes in child development. *Scientific American*, 1976, *235*, 38-47.

Bower, T. G. R. *A primer of infant development*. New York: W. H. Freeman, 1977.

A detailed and highly illustrated account of growth and development in the first year of life is provided by:

Caplan, F. (Ed.). *The first twelve months of life: Your baby's growth month by month*. New York: Grosset & Dunlap, 1973.

For a comprehensive collection of research-based articles on various aspects of infant growth and development, see:

Osofsky, J. D. (Ed.). *Handbook of infant development*. New York: John Wiley, 1979.

The following is an extremely simple, nontechnical description of development during the first three years of life; it offers numerous practical suggestions that might be particularly useful for parents interested in understanding and promoting the intellectual development of their infants:

White, B. L. *The first three years of life*. Englewood Cliffs, N.J.: Prentice-Hall, 1975.

Although Piaget's writings are often difficult reading, there are many relatively simple accounts of his principal findings and theoretical beliefs, among them:

Ault, R. L. *Cognitive development: Piaget's theory and the process approach*. New York: Oxford University Press, 1977.

Beard, R. M. *An outline of Piaget's developmental psychology for students and teachers*. New York: Mentor, 1969.

Furth, H. G. *Piaget and knowledge*. Englewood Cliffs, N.J.: Prentice-Hall, 1969.

Ginsberg, H., & Opper, S. *Piaget's theory of intellectual development* (2nd ed.). Englewood Cliffs, N.J.: Prentice-Hall, 1978.

The major premise of this captivating and sometimes disturbing book is that we have grossly underestimated the infant's intellectual capacities and that, worse still, we damage and even destroy much of that capacity:

Pearce, J. C. *Magical child: Rediscovering nature's plan for our children*. New York: Bantam Books, 1977.

6

ATTACHMENT AND SOCIAL-EMOTIONAL DEVELOPMENT

The hand that rocks the cradle
Is the hand that rules the world.

William Ross Wallace
John O'London's Treasure Trove

143

Fort Victoria Museum is only a memory now, rapidly fading as the miles streak blackly beneath us—probably a different memory for each of us. For grandmother, who slept through much of it, another gently pleasant impression to add to her vast collection of indistinct memories. For Marcel, perhaps a fresher, more pointed recollection of a huge and fierce river and great white buildings to add to a smaller store of younger memories. Paul's memories will no doubt be wrapped around the toothy, sharp-spined, wall-eyed pike he caught— as will Denise's, for she helped him clean it. And my memories? Those great blue eyes staring wide, the custard-caked mouth open even wider, and that piercing wail carrying in it faint echoes of another scream that I have been trying to forget, jolting me violently, almost physically. And the scream bringing mother, grandmother, and various children running to see what I had done.

I had done nothing—I think. I had simply been sitting there, absorbed in the telling of the tale of the lifespan.

Ah, the tale of the lifespan! Such a tale it might be if we could tell it whole, the way it really is for each of us. Sadly, we must always divide it into smaller, more manageable pieces—into chapters and topics. And the tale must almost always deal only with the average—seldom with the unique.

There is a quiet space in this early Friday afternoon traffic. Perhaps late lunches or preparations for the weekend keep people off the highway. I know that traffic will become much heavier before nightfall, but by then we should be well beyond the Alberta lake country and into the mixed forests of northern Saskatchewan. For tonight we must be there. I have promised, and I can no longer change my mind in spite of what Anne said this morning before we left.

But there will be time enough to think of these things later. Now, while we pass through the great siesta of the early afternoon, I want to get back to the third chapter in this section on infancy—a chapter in which we look at the social and emotional lives of infants.

■ The Bidirectionality of Influence

Although we have long assumed that parents are actively effectual and children passively affected—in other words, that the direction of parent-child influence is from parent to child—children also affect their parents (Bell, 1968, 1971; Harper, 1971). And to the extent that children are successful in changing the behaviors of their parents, they may also have some influence on the nature and extent to which parents, in turn, affect their children's behavior—hence the expression *bidirectionality of influence.*

Some of the numerous difficulties involved in studying parent-child relationships and social-emotional development are obvious; they include problems of definition, measurement, and identification of causes using studies that do not always have the types of controls necessary for true experiments. Other problems are less obvious but no less serious. Chief among them is the observation that not only are parents different one from the other, sometimes in very subtle ways, but infants too differ greatly one from the other. Perhaps the only valid conclusions we can ever reach in this area will have to take into account very specific characteristics of parents and children. For example, instead of attempting to show that permissiveness or authoritarianism leads to qualities A or B in the child, we might be compelled to qualify by recognizing that permissiveness or authoritarianism in certain parents affects certain children in one way and other children in another.

In spite of these difficulties, there is a great deal of recent and significant research on parent-child interaction and on infants' social-emotional development. Among other things, this research looks at how individual characteristics of infants as well as those of parents influence parent-child interaction; it looks as well at the nature of infants' emotional development, at the development of reciprocal attachment between mother and infant (bonding), and at the role of fathers in the social and emotional development of young children. These complex topics are the subjects of this chapter.

■ Infant States

When discussing the typical characteristics of infants, we tend to assume that all "normal" infants possess the same qualities, that all react in similar, predictable ways, and that individual differences observed in older children are absent or undetectable in the very young infant. In fact, individual differences are detectable very shortly after birth, are consistent, and are related to differences evident later in life. The term *infant state* is employed to describe the general condition of a neonate. And it is in an examination of a specific infant's predominant states that individual differences become most apparent.

Various researchers (for example, Wolff, 1966) have advanced a number of similar classifications of infant states. Thus an infant may be described as being in a state of regular sleep, disturbed sleep, drowsiness, alert activity, or focused activity. Additional states may sometimes be detected by employing physiological measures or more refined observational criteria. For example, Wolff (1959) distinguishes between deep sleep and regular sleep, largely in terms of heart and respiration rate. Similarly, he distinguishes between alert focused activity and inflexibly focused activity in terms of spontaneous changes in the infant's alert responsiveness. Inflexibly focused activity is, in effect, crying.

The most important point to be derived from research on infant states is that individual infants vary consistently in terms of the amount of time spent in each state. Brown (1964) studied states in six babies. Although this group of babies spent approximately one-third of their time in stages of sleep, one infant slept 56 percent of the time. One child was in an alert state only 4 percent of the time; another, 37 percent of the time; one infant cried 39 percent of the time; another, only 17 percent of the time. Additional evidence of striking individual differences among these babies is provided by the observation that one infant responded to 86 percent of all auditory stimuli presented to her or that occurred randomly, regardless of her state. A low-intensity noise would cause her to open her eyes when in a state of apparently deep sleep.

Given these tremendous individual differences, knowledge of the average newborn's daily states is perhaps not especially revealing. Hutt, Lenard, and Prechtl (1969) have found that this hypothetical infant sleeps between 75 and 80 percent of the time and that three-quarters of this time is spent in irregular sleep. The average neonate is drowsy or alert perhaps two or three hours of the day and engages in more intense, focused activity another hour or two. Crying, a common inflexible focused activity, occupies the remainder of the time.

Clearly, environmental conditions play an important role in determining infant states and in bringing about changes from one state to another, although basic differences in predominant states appear to be at least partly genetically based. It is no secret that rocking a child may serve to quiet him, even as feeding may have the same effect (Van den Daele, 1970).

The long-term significance of infant states is still a matter of considerable ongoing research. It appears plausible that predominant infant states have direct effects on parent-child interaction and, consequently, on the type of child (and adult) an infant will eventually become. There remains the practical difficulty of separating causes. In short, it remains impossible to specify the extent to which later individual differences simply reflect initial differences and the extent to which they are influenced by environmental variables such as parenting styles—which are themselves influenced by the infant's initial states.

Consider two hypothetical instances, exaggerated for the sake of illustration. One involves a particularly difficult infant: He cries a great deal, refuses his mother's breast at awkward and unpredictable times, soils his diaper continually, and otherwise makes life miserable for his mother. She, in turn, is an easily annoyed, impatient, highly impulsive, emotional woman, given to temper tantrums and other behaviors that might unkindly be described as childish. A second infant sleeps regularly, seldom cries, loves her mother's breast, and soils her diaper only at regular intervals and in what appears to be an apologetic manner. Her mother is patient, happy, and quite delighted with her child. It might be revealing to speculate on the probable nature of the mother-infant interaction in each of these cases and on the eventual effect of this interaction on both the mother and the child. It might become clearer that infant states are by no means irrelevant to what the child and mother eventually become.

■ Infant Emotions

Any statements about an infant's emotions must be tentative for two reasons: Emotion is a subjective response that cannot easily be interpreted by an observer, particularly when subjects are still incapable of communicating their feelings in language more sophisticated than gurgles, wails, grunts, sighs, sobs, and belches; and situations that adults ordinarily interpret as emotional cannot always be assumed to be emotional for infants. Until children are sufficiently developed that the emotional content of social and physical situations has meaning for them, investigating their emotions is indeed a difficult task.

Nevertheless, beginning with the pioneering work of Watson (1914), a number of psychologists have assumed that the infant is capable of emotional responses from birth; that is, emotional responses are part of the reflexive repertoire. Watson identified three distinct emotional responses of a neonate: fear, rage, and love. He assumed that each of these was a reflex and could therefore be elicited by a specific stimulus. Rage, for example, was thought to result from being confined or from having movements restricted; fear, from a loud noise or from being dropped suddenly; and love resulted from being stroked or fondled. Sherman and Sherman (1929) later suggested that whenever investigators assumed a child was reacting emotionally in response to a particular stimulation, they were subjectively interpreting the infant's behavior in terms of adult and personal predispositions. In other words, adults may attribute motives and emotions to children with no valid basis for doing so. A similar tendency is to anthropomorphize animal behavior—that is, to describe it in human terms. The tendency appears most pronounced when the investigators are most ignorant about their subject.

More recent research on emotional reactions in infants has dealt primarily with expressions of anger, pain, or frustration, with joy and contentment, and with fear.

Crying

Wolff (1969) analyzed tape recordings of infants crying and identified a number of distinct cries that he interprets as expressions of different underlying emotions. Perhaps the most frequent cry is called the rhythmical cry. It not only expresses hunger but is also the type of cry to which most infants eventually revert after initially engaging in another type of crying. The angry cry is characterized by its protracted loudness and results from more air being forced through the vocal cords. A third distinguishable cry is that of pain, characterized by a long wail followed by a period of breath holding.

What this research reveals most clearly is that infants' cries may be distinguished one from the other and appear to fall into identifiable cate-

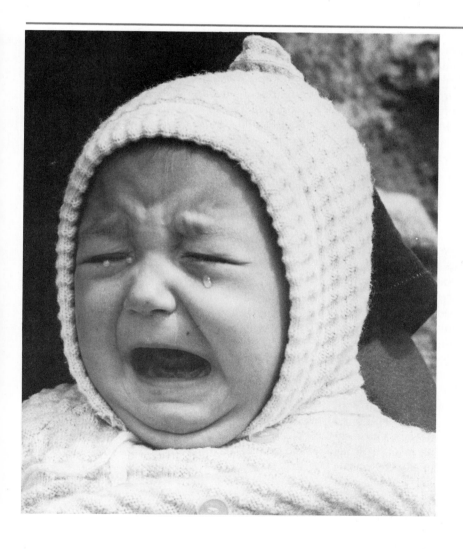

Science tells us there are rhythmic cries, cries of anger, and cries of pain. Literture tells us there are real tears and the tears of crocodiles. Have crocodiles no emotions?

gories. The inference that a long wail followed by breath holding is an expression of pain rather than of anger, for example, can only be based on knowledge of the conditions that led to the cry.

Mothers appear to be remarkably sensitive to the nature of infant cries, although here, too, there are individual differences (Ainsworth & Bell, 1969). Wolff (1969) reports that most mothers respond quickly to hunger cries and even more quickly to cries of anger or pain. Whereas hunger cries often lead to the presentation of food, cries of pain typically elicit comforting behavior or alarm.

The meanings of an infant's cries are apparently not universal. Isabell and McKee (1980) observe that in many primitive cultures where the child is carried about constantly by the mother, mother-infant communication can occur through physical contact. In these cultures, there appears to be little need for the vocal signals of distress that we have come to expect from our infants. For instance, among South American Indian tribes in the northern Andes, infant crying is extremely rare and is invariably interpreted as a sign of illness. Why else would a warm, well-fed, and constantly embraced infant cry?

Fear

Fear reactions in children have been investigated in some detail. Initially, infants appear to react with fear to loud noises and sudden loss of support. Subsequently, some infants come to fear a wide range of stimuli; others remain relatively unperturbed in the face of environmental changes. Fear of heights appears to be almost universal in infants by the age of thirteen to eighteen months and is present in more than 20 percent of all children by the age of seven months (Scarr & Salapatek, 1970). Fear of strangers is not ordinarily manifest until the second half of the child's first year and becomes most common by the age of two years. Other situations that may evoke fear in an infant typically involve some unexpected change. For example, a jack-in-the-box may be frightening—so might an experimenter or parent wearing a mask. (See *A Longitudinal Study of Wariness*.) In addition, sep-

aration from the mother is frightening for some infants, as are sounds presented in irregular fashion (Passman, 1976).

Fears in later life appear to be closely related to parental fears, to socioeconomic level, and to intelligence. Given the close relationship between intelligence and socioeconomic level, however, it is difficult to determine which of these factors is more closely implicated in children's fears. However, Angelino, Dollins, and Mech (1956) have found that lower-class children are more afraid of scolding, starvation, punishment, and divorce; higher-class children are most afraid of being left alone, of being physically hurt, and of being in darkness.

Smiling

Smiling, a universal phenomenon among human cultures, is a fleeting response in the warm, well-fed infant and appears to occur as early as two to twelve hours after delivery (Wolff, 1963). In the weeks and months following birth, infants smile in response to an ever-widening range of sights and sounds. The social smile occurs first in response to a human voice (by the third week). By the age of three and one-half months, infants smile more in response to familiar than unfamiliar faces (Gewirtz, 1965). Accordingly, Gewirtz has identified three stages in the development of smiling behavior. The first phase, spontaneous or reflex smiling, occurs in the absence of readily identifiable stimuli and is often, though perhaps incorrectly, attributed to gas pains. Social smiling, the second phase, occurs initially in response to auditory and visual stimuli that are social in nature— that is, they are related to other humans. Finally, the child manifests the selective social smile, common among children and adults, which occurs in response to social stimuli that the child can presumably identify as familiar. With the appearance of the selective social smile, there is a decline in the frequency with which most children will smile in response to an unfamiliar voice or face and a corresponding increase in withdrawal behavior and other signs of anxiety in the presence of strangers. (More is said about stranger anxiety later.)

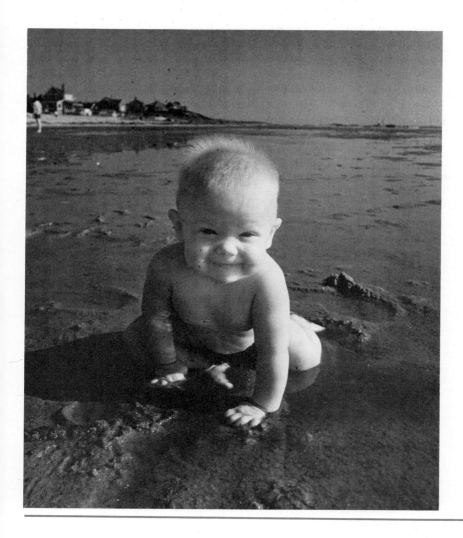
Smiling is a universal human response.

At around the age of four months, infants begin to laugh in addition to smiling. Initially, laughter is most likely to occur in response to physical stimulation such as tickling; later it occurs in response to more social and eventually more cognitive situations (for example, seeing other children laughing) (Sroufe & Wunsch, 1972). Although the function of laughter in infants has never been very clear, perhaps because it has not been investigated much, Sroufe and Waters (1976) suggest that it probably serves to release tension. Fear, by contrast, signifies a continued building up of tension.

Smiling and laughing are undoubtedly of crucial importance in parent-child interaction, particularly since we have come to recognize more clearly that parents and children have a mutual and interdependent effect on each other. In fact, both research evidence and common sense suggest that parents look for smiles and other nonverbal gestures in their infants as evidence that they are themselves worthwhile and loved. There is little reason to suppose that parents are not at least as sensitive as their children are to feelings of rejection.

A LONGITUDINAL STUDY OF WARINESS

Some years ago, I had the misfortune of accepting an invitation to a Halloween costume party. Actually, it was more stupidity than misfortune, but the less said about that, the better.

As part of my "costume," I attempted valiantly to grow a beard. After a number of months, I eventually succeeded in covering parts of my face with dirty-looking tufts of blackish hair. The remainder of my costume required little effort. Or imagination, I might add, although it did demand some courage. Or more of the stupidity about which I prefer not to speak.

Shortly after what I strongly felt to be a miserable excuse of a party, and one at which I remained for only the briefest time, I shaved off all my wild whiskers. And when I walked out of the bathroom clean shaven, my one-year-old daughter took one wide-eyed look at me and turned crying to her mother.

Although I was initially taken aback, my daughter's reaction should not have been unexpected. As is discussed in the text, we know that young infants often react to the unexpected with fear.

One of the classical studies of the roots of fear in infancy is a longitudinal study of wariness conducted by Bronson (1972). In this context, the term *wariness* refers to an uneasiness that is somewhere between mild discomfort or distress and outright fear. The Bronson study involved a relatively small sample of sixteen male and sixteen female infants. Approximately half the sample were Caucasian; the others had at least one parent of Japanese, Chinese, Filipino, Hawaiian, or mixed ancestry. All lived in Honolulu. Infants were observed by one or more investigators at the ages of three, four, six and one-half, and nine months. All observation sessions were videotaped so that they could be analyzed in detail later. In addition, parents were interviewed and questioned at some length. Details of the observation sessions varied, depending on the infants' ages. At the ages of three and four months, infants were observed while they lay on their backs in their cribs. During the observation session, they were presented with a number of novel objects, such as a paper parasol being opened and closed and a mobile over their cribs. In addition, an adult male "stranger" leaned over the crib, smiled slightly at the infant, and asked the infant to smile, using its name repeatedly. This episode lasted for approximately one minute, unless the infant smiled broadly and repeatedly or began to cry.

At the age of six and one-half months, infants were observed as they sat upright in an infant seat on the floor in a familiar room. The infant's mother sat within view a short distance away. The experimenter hid immediately behind a screen in back of the infant's seat and pushed a number of novel objects in front of the infant. Among these objects was a a squarish box covered with red and white crepe paper and equipped with a sound device that transmitted random arrangements of short and long beeps. During the observation period, the experimenter, a male stranger, walked out from behind the screen, squatted in front of the infant, and spoke quietly and in a friendly fashion for one minute unless, again, the child cried or smiled continuously. At the end of the observation session, the stranger picked up the infants, unless his presence had already made them cry.

Observations at the age of nine months took place with the baby on the floor and again involved the beeping object as well as the stranger. As for the infants six and one-half months old, the final episode in the observation involved the stranger placing the infant on his knee for approximately one minute, unless the infant cried or smiled repeatedly earlier.

Examination of videotapes led to the development of a number of categories for classifying infant reactions. These categories present a five-level sequence, ranging from smiling with delight (repeated smile) through smiling (less broad, noncontinuous smile), a neutral reaction (blank expression without vocalization), uneasiness (frowning, vocalizing, squirming, or trying to crawl away), and crying. These five categories present, in effect, a behavioral definition of wariness. At the first level (smiling repeatedly), the infant is totally unwary; at the highest level of wariness, the infant shows definite signs of fear (see table, opposite page).

This study produced a number of important findings. To begin with, it is notable that the most prevalent class of responses for three- and four-month-old infants is one of smiling rather than one of being uneasy or of crying. By the age of six and one-half months, however, there is increasing evidence of wariness. And by nine months, there is evidence of *learned* fears. These findings are in agreement with others (see text) indicating that infants are not likely to display marked stranger anxiety until the second half of the first year of life.

A second intriguing finding relates to the effects of maternal care on the development of wariness in the infant. Observers identified two broad classes of maternal behavior in this study. At one extreme are those mothers who appear particularly adept at recognizing infant moods and needs, who respond sensitively, and who appear to enjoy interacting with their infants. At the other extreme are those who seem quite indifferent to

Coding categories for describing infant reactions: criteria for the affect scale ratings of dominant emotional tone.

Scale Point	Category Description	Criterion Behaviors for Each Age		
		3 and 4 Months	6½ Months	9 Months
1	Smiled with delight	Wiggled or vocalized as smiled	Repeated broad smiles, or smiles with sounds of pleasure	
2	Smiled		Smiled more than once, but not broadly	
3	Neutral		Predominantly blank expression and no vocalization	
4	Uneasy	Severe frown or puckering of chin	Frowned, or sounded unhappy (or, on pickup, turned body away)	Frowned, sounded unhappy, or crawled to mother (or, on pickup, squirmed or turned body away)
5	Cried		Cried or whimpered	

Adapted from G. W. Bronson, "Infants' reactions to unfamiliar persons and novel objects," *Monographs of the Society for Research in Child Development*, 1972, 37, No. 3. © The Society for Research in Child Development, Inc. Used by permission.

infant needs and moods, whose interaction with infants appears more routine and less enjoyable, and who frequently limit this interaction to essential tasks such as feeding, bathing, and changing. For some unknown reason, these two styles of mothering appear to be far more critical for male than for female infants. That is, boys whose mothers were classified in the first group (sensitive, and so on) were less likely to be wary of strangers and of novel objects than boys whose mothers were more indifferent. In this study, as in an earlier Bronson (1971) study, mothering style did not appear to be as important for female infants.

A third important finding is that, at all ages, objects are far less potent than strangers in bringing about reactions of wariness or fear. By the age of nine months, a number of infants had reacted with fear toward strangers and seemed to have learned to associate specific features of a person with fear. Thus some infants consistently react with fear to bearded individuals, to individuals wearing white smocks, or to people with long noses. Similarly, wariness of novel objects was very rare prior to the age of nine months. By that age, mothers reported a number of instances in which many of the infants had responded with fear to something other than a strange person. Situations or objects that make loud noises or move suddenly are most likely to bring about fear reactions in infants (vacuum cleaners, for example).

A fourth finding based on Bronson's investigation relates to the role of temperament and may contribute to an understanding of the development of fear. During their first visits to infants' homes, researchers asked the mothers numerous questions about infants' typical reactivity. Specifically, investigators looked at incidence and persistence of crying, distress reactions during bathing, frequency and intensity of being startled, and the incidence of blinking when presented with novel stimulation. Not surprisingly, infants with the most reactive temperaments, and especially those who startled most easily, were more likely to be wary of strangers later.

Why are infants sometimes wary and sometimes not? The Bronson data suggest that innate temperament in interaction with various experiences is involved. And the relationship of age to the development of fear may, at least in part, indicate that certain experiences are unlikely or at least less frequent at earlier ages, as well as that the *meanings* of some experiences depend on the infant's level of understanding. Clearly, a stranger is not a stranger until a familiar person can be recognized as familiar.

But why should some strangers and some novel objects elicit fear? One plausible explanation is Hebb's (1966) suggestion that infants develop certain expectations about their world and that violation of these expectations *(incongruence* is Hebb's term) may lead to fear.

Which might well be why my infant daughter turned crying to her mother. And then again . . .

A particularly significant but sad finding relating directly to these observations is presented in a study of mothers interacting with their blind children (Fraiberg, 1974, 1975). Blind children do not smile as often as do the sighted, an observation that agrees with the supposition that the true social smile not only occurs in recognition of a familiar face or situation but also appears more readily in response to a smiling face. Perhaps it is not surprising that Fraiberg found that mothers of the ten blind infants in her study felt more distance—less attachment—with their babies.

Blind infants differ from normal infants not only in smiling less but in a number of other ways as well, the most important of which (at least for early mother-child interaction) may be their inability to engage in mutual gazing. In the early stages of infancy, mutual gazing appears to be one of the most frequent and important types of interaction between infant and mother. It becomes less frequent with the infant's increasing ability to coordinate motor activities and to engage in behaviors to which the mother can respond in other ways (Hartup & Lempers, 1973).

The importance for children of visual contact with their mothers is further corroborated in a study where children aged three to four and one-half years were observed in a playroom with their mothers present or with a silent, life-size, color film of their mothers or of some stranger (Passman & Erck, 1978). That children played as long in the presence of their filmed mother as they did in the actual presence of their mother indicates that visual contact alone has an important function in parent-child interactions. It is significant as well that children whose mothers were present, either filmed or in actuality, played longer than did children whose mothers were not present or who were exposed to films of unfamiliar women.

The bidirectionality of mother-child influence is evident in a variety of other situations. Fretting and crying on the part of an infant trigger soothing behavior in the mother: rocking, singing, talking quietly, and so on (Lewis & Lee-Painter, 1974). In turn, the mother's soothing behavior quiets the infant. Perhaps the infant's quiet behavior now leads to a mutual gaze. Has the infant learned to be quiet and loving in response to the mother's soothing behavior? Or has the mother learned to be soothing in response to the infant's crying? Probably both: The influences are bidirectional.

It would be highly misleading, however, to suggest that an infant's being quiet and loving— or not being noisy and irritating—is solely or even primarily a function of interaction between parents and infants. Regardless of their environments, some infants apparently are likely to behave in one way and others in another. Put another way, some important differences among infants appear to be innate rather than learned, and they might have important implications for the infants' development and behavior in later years.

■ Temperament

When psychologists speak of differences in the customary ways of reacting and behaving that differentiate adults from each other, they generally speak of **personality** differences.

When psychologists speak of differences among infants, they rarely use the term *personality*. The term is too global for the characteristics of young infants; it implies a degree of learning that has not yet had time to occur. Instead, psychologists speak of infant **temperament**. The principal difference between *temperament* and *personality* is simply that temperament is assumed to have a primarily genetic basis, whereas personality has developed through interaction with the environment (Plomin, 1982). Thus a child is born with a certain temperament rather than with a certain personality, but the personality that later develops is an outgrowth of innate temperament and environmental influences.

Studying Infant Temperament

The classical studies of infant temperament are those of Thomas, Chess, and Birch (1968, 1970). These investigations, begun in 1956, are known as the New York Longitudinal Study (NYLS). Initial subjects for the NYLS consisted of 85 families with a total of 141 children. Subjects were from highly educated, professional backgrounds. Among the important goals of this study were to develop ways of identifying and classifying infant temperament and to examine the relationship of infant temperament to later adjustment and behavior. The principle data-gathering technique employed in early stages of the study involved regular, structured interviews with parents, as well as direct observations of the infants themselves. Subsequent aspects of the NYLS have involved a variety of testing, interview, and observational approaches.

Types of Temperament

Analysis of the NYLS data has led Thomas, Chess, and Birch to suggest that at least nine different infant characteristics can be observed relatively easily and can be used to differentiate among different infants (see Table 6.1). That is, parents or other observers can rate infants as being *high*, *medium*, or *low* on each of these characteristics, particularly after the infant is two or three months of age.

Further analysis of this data subsequently led to the observation that certain infants seemed to have remarkably similar patterns of characteristics. There are three such patterns, each of which identifies a *type* of infant that parents seemed to recognize readily. For example, infants who might be described as "difficult" were characterized by irregularity (lack of rhythmicity) with respect to such things as eating, sleeping, and toilet functions; withdrawal from unfamiliar situations; slow adaptation to change; and intense as well as negative moods. In contrast, an "easy" temperament is characterized by high rhythmicity (regularity in eating, sleeping, and so on); high interest in new things; high adaptabilty to change; and a preponderance of positive moods, as well as low or moderate intensity of reaction. The third temperament type identified by Thomas, Chess, and Birch is labeled "slow to warm up" and is characterized by low activity level; high initial withdrawal from the unfamiliar; slow adaptation to change; and somewhat negative in mood, but with a moderate or low intensity of reaction.

Table 6.1 Nine temperament characteristics of infants.

1. Level and extent of motor activity
2. Rhythmicity (regularity of functions such as eating, sleeping, and eliminating)
3. Withdrawal or approach in new situations
4. Adaptability to change in the environment
5. Sensitivity to stimuli
6. Intensity (energy level) of responses
7. General mood or disposition (cheerful, cranky, friendly, and so on)
8. Distractibility (how easily infant may be distracted from ongoing activities)
9. Attention span and persistence in ongoing activities

Note: In the Thomas, Chess, and Birch (1970) studies of infant temperament, parents and other observers rated each infant high, medium, or low on each of these characteristics.

Of the original 141 children in the NYLS, 65 percent could be classified as belonging to one of these three temperament types; the remaining 35 percent displayed varying mixtures of the nine temperament characteristics.

The Implications of Infant Temperament

Thomas and his associates (Thomas, Chess, & Birch, 1970; Thomas, Chess, & Korn, 1982) suggest that being able to identify infants on the basis of their predominant temperament characteristics may be highly useful for a number of reasons, including the notion that children of different temperaments may respond in quite different ways to parenting styles. They suggest, for example, that "easy" children, because of their high adaptability, will respond well to a large variety of parenting styles (permissive or authoritarian, for example). In contrast, a more difficult infant may require more careful parenting. Since these children adapt more slowly and respond less well to novelty and change, they require consistent and patient parents. In addition, given their more intense and more negative moods, they are not likely to react well to highly authoritarian or highly punitive parents.

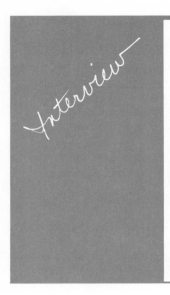

Subject: Female; age forty-eight; widowed; two children, both independent; manager of a cleaning business.

(concerning her children)

They were real different when they were babies, you know. I mean Luke was a holy terror. Just about drove me crazy, always hollering for something or needing a change or falling out of his crib. He did that more than once. Wonder he didn't scramble his brains. And Chris, he was just about the opposite. Never cried or nothing unless he was real sick or hurt. Right through school, too, Chris he never complained. Just done his work, but his brother, he was two years younger. Luke was. Well Luke, he complained, all right, and he got himself into trouble more times! Nothing serious, mind you. Just kid stuff. Never got kicked out of school or anything like that.

. . .

Now? Well, I don't know. They're grown up. They're different all right. I mean Chris is more quiet and all, but Luke settled down a lot when he grew up. Marriage is what did it.

But the importance of identifying infant temperament may not be restricted solely to whatever advice might result with respect to the best child-rearing styles for different children. Thomas et al. (1970) found some important *long-term* implications of temperament. Specifically, infants of difficult temperament are far more likely to manifest problems requiring psychiatric attention. Indeed, of the 42 children (out of a sample of 141) who had such problems, 70 percent had been classified as difficult infants and only 18 percent as easy children.

To the extent that infant characteristics are related to later behaviors, early identification of these characteristics might be of tremendous value for parents, educators, and others concerned with the welfare of children. Thus the NYLS has led to attempts to identify "high-risk" infants, as well as to various suggestions relating to the best way of reacting to this potential risk. However, there are some potential dangers in these attempts. As Rothbart (1982) notes, labeling infants as *difficult*, particularly when parents have not thought of them in that way, may lead parents to expect problems, might change their reactions to their infants, and

might, indirectly, be related to the appearance of problems.

Evaluating Infant Temperament Research

Quite apart from these practical considerations are a number of problems related to definitions of these concepts as well as to the actual research. Kagan (1982) raises two important questions: Are there temperamental traits? How valid are parental reports? A third absolutely critical question concerns the extent to which temperament is a consistent characteristic of human reaction and behavior and the extent to which it is related to later behaviors. In other words, are infants of certain temperament (if there is such a thing as temperament) at greater or lesser risk of emotional and behavior problems later in life?

Answers to these three questions are still somewhat controversial. Bates (1980), for example, insists that temperament does not exist within an individual but is instead a *projection* of the observer. Like a number of personality theorists, he suggests that behavior is as much (or perhaps more) a function of the immediate environment as it is of characteristics within the individual (Mischel, 1979, for example). According to this view, infants are not intrinsically *easy* or *difficult*; parents, psychologists, and other observers simply see them that way. And the remarkably low agreement that often exists between "expert" observer and parent ratings of infant temperament may serve as evidence of this. That is, to the extent that observers *project* characteristics upon individuals, they might be expected to disagree about these characteristics. And to the extent that they simply observe characteristics that actually exist, they would be expected to agree (if they are able to observe these characteristics accurately). That parents tend to agree with each other more than they agree with other observers may simply indicate that they have been likely to discuss characteristics of their infants and to reach some consensus about them (Field & Greenberg, 1982).

Questions relating to the "risk" associated with the difficult temperament cannot easily be answered. Although Thomas et al. (1970) report considerably higher incidence of problems requiring psychiatric help among difficult infants, other analyses of the same data have found that predictions made in infancy are notably unreliable, although predictions made later are somewhat more useful (Rutter, Birch, Thomas, & Chess, 1964). Rothbart (1982) advises that researchers should proceed cautiously, given the dangers of mislabeling infants as "high risk" when they are not, as well as the possibility that such labels might adversely affect parent-infant relations and might also contribute to later problems.

Resolving the Temperament Controversy

Is the concept of infant temperament meaningful? Are parents adequate judges of infant characteristics? Are difficult infants at higher psychological risk?

Unfortunately, much of the data required to answer these questions is not yet gathered. Studies such as the New York Longitudinal Study by Thomas et al. (1970) present a monumental contribution to their answers, however. Indeed, the questions might never have been asked had it not been for the studies.

Kagan (1982), following an examination of these issues, concludes that sufficient evidence exists to accept that children differ in temperament for at least a few years, that reasonably educated parents can detect and accurately report on some of the more obvious of infant characteristics (such as fearfulness or fearlessness), and that knowledge of infant temperament might have important practical implications. In addition, evidence from studies of twins supports the view that temperament has an important genetic basis—that it represents inherited rather than strictly acquired characteristics.

Plomin (1982), another eminent researcher in this area, agrees that the concept of temperament is valid and useful, but *difficult temperament* is a difficult concept.

■ Attachment

Attachment is an emotional bond, not easily defined, impossible for an infant to describe for us, but of tremendous importance for the infant. Measurements of infant attachment are necessarily indirect. Investigators look at behaviors that are directed more often toward the object of attachment than elsewhere (crying, smiling, vocalizing, following, clinging, holding, and so on) (Ainsworth & Bell, 1969); they focus on the infant's reaction to strange situations and on physical contact between parents and infant (for example, Ainsworth, 1972, 1979; Ainsworth, Blehar, Waters, & Wall, 1978); or they look at the infant's reaction to being separated from a parent (Stayton, Ainsworth, & Main, 1973).

One of the problems that affects research in this area is the practical impossibility of conducting the types of controlled experiments that would be most likely to lead to definite answers. Infants cannot be deliberately separated from their mothers at different times in their lives, and for different periods of time, to determine the effects of separation; nor can they be brought up in complete social isolation. Considerations such as these have led to a series of intriguing studies with infant monkeys and their mothers. (See *Surrogate Monkey Mothers.*)

Mother-Infant Bonding

Until recently, most of the research on parent-infant interaction has focused on the effects of this interaction on infants rather than on parents. By the same token, considerations of parent-child attachment have traditionally emphasized the attachment that children form to their parents and the effects of separation and deprivation on children. More recently, a number of researchers have ex-

amined attachment from the parents' point of view—especially the mother's view. **Mother-infant bonding,** the expression coined to label this interest, may be described simply as the emotional or attachment bond that exists between mother and infant. And although *bond* is often used as though it were synonymous with *attachment, mother-infant bonding* refers primarily to the very early, biologically based attachment between mother and infant. *Attachment* is a much more general term that includes not only what is meant by mother-infant bonding but all other positive emotional ties that might exist among parents, children, and other people as well.

Klaus and Kennell (1976), authors of an important book on mother-infant bonding, sug-

SURROGATE MONKEY MOTHERS

Observation of primates in their natural environments leaves little doubt of strong mother-infant attachment. Very young infants spend most, and sometimes all, their time clinging to their mothers. Why does an infant monkey become attached to its mother? Is it, as reinforcement theory would surely predict, because she is always present when he is being fed—just as she is usually present when such comforting things as sleeping and grooming occur?

In a series of experiments, Harlow (1958, 1959; Harlow & Zimmerman, 1959) separated infant monkeys from their mothers shortly after birth and provided them with mother surrogates. The substitute mothers were wire monkey-mother models with interesting wooden heads.

Each infant's cage contained two surrogate mothers: one covered with soft terry cloth, the other left bare. Both models were heated by a light bulb so that their warmth would be approximately equal. In the experiment most relevant here, one surrogate mother had a bottle attached to her chest with the nipple protruding, suggesting to the immature monkey that this was indeed a milk-giving breast. In some cages, the bottle was attached to the wire model; in others, the terry-cloth mother was given the "breast." The seemingly logical prediction is that if the infant monkeys were to develop an attachment to either model, it would be to the milk-giving model.

Harlow measured attachment in two ways: the total time per day that the infant spent embracing one model

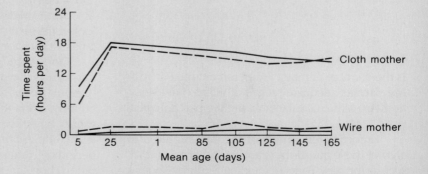

Amount of time spent by infant monkeys on cloth and wire surrogate mothers. The results show a strong preference for the cloth mother, regardless of whether the infant was fed on the wire model (broken line) or on the cloth model (solid line). (From H. F. Harlow, *Scientific American,* 1959, *200,* 68–74. Copyright 1959 by Scientific American, Inc. All rights reserved. Used by permission.)

gest that the mother-infant bond develops as a function of close contact and interaction with the infant from the earliest moments after birth. Thus, although there is a biological predisposition toward the formation of this bond and toward the interaction that is instrumental in its development, the bond does not exist automatically as soon as the child is born. They suggest, as well, that the failure to establish a strong mother-infant bond is detrimental to the future adjustment and emotional health of the child and may be related to such things as child abuse or "growth failure" (a physical-psychological condition characterized by apathy, loss of appetite, illness, and sometimes death).

A number of studies have been conducted to examine the formation and significance of mother-infant bonding. Klaus, Kreger, McAlpine, Steffa, and Kennell (1972) randomly selected a group of twenty-eight low-income mothers and allowed half of them extended contact with their infants immediately after birth (one hour of the first two hours following birth), as well as five additional hours of contact with their infants on each of the first three days following birth. The remaining fourteen mothers served as a control group. Their contact with their infants occurred according to hospital routine, so that they had virtually no contact with the infants for some hours following birth (many hospitals remove the neonate at once). Contact then occurred regularly at feeding time.

One month later, follow-up interviews and filmed observations of mothers and infants at feed-

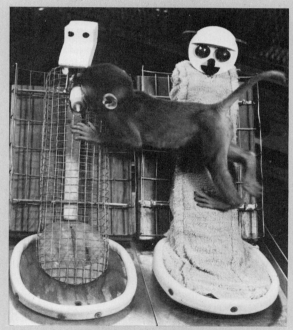

The infant monkey remains on the terry-cloth mother even though he must stretch to the wire model to feed.

or the other, and the infant's response to a fear-producing stimulus such as the plaster cast of a monkey head or a mechanical teddy bear that moved and played a drum. The results? After the age of twenty-five days (presumably some time is required for the attachment to develop), all monkeys spent little time with the naked wire model, but spent over twelve hours a day with the terry-cloth mother. If the models were placed in close proximity, the infant would attempt to feed from the wire model while clinging to the terry-cloth model! Similarly, the infants ran into the arms of the soft mother when shown the frightening stimulus. If she was not present, the infant monkey reacted with much greater fear, frequently cowering in a corner of the cage or the room and adopting a quasi-fetal attitude, occasionally covering its eyes.

The Harlow studies contradict earlier beliefs about the formation of attachments between mother and child and raise some important questions. If her role of food giving does not endear the mother to her child, what does? Does the monkey infant become attached to the terry-cloth mother out of a perverse desire to make things difficult for psychological investigators? Or is Harlow closer to the truth when he suggests that it is the quality of the contact between infant and mother that is most important? Wire models do not make for comfortable contact; terry-cloth ones do.

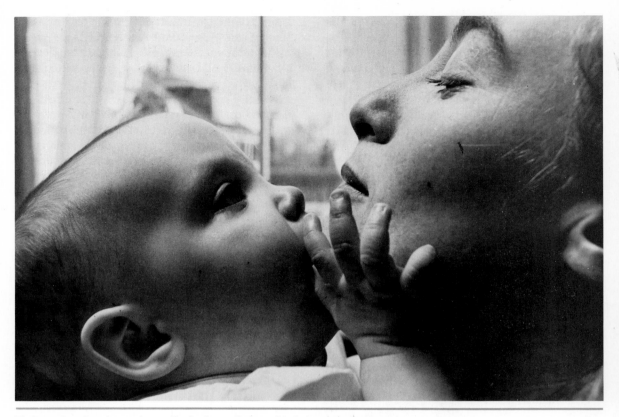

Mother-infant bonding refers to the biologically based link that usually forms between mother and infant beginning shortly after birth. Mutual gazing is thought to be important in the formation of this bond.

ing times indicated that mothers in the extended-contact group were significantly more attached to their infants, showed more concern for them, and expressed considerably more interest in them. These mothers tended to fondle their babies more, to engage in more verbal interaction with them, and to spend more time in mutual gazing.

Follow-up studies of the same infants and mothers, undertaken when the infants were aged one and two, still revealed significant differences between extended-contact and control group mothers, not only in terms of attachment but in terms of verbal interaction as well (Ringler, Kennell, Jarvella, Navojosky, & Klaus, 1975). Other research indicates that extended contact between mother and infant immediately following birth may be manifested in closer mother-infant attachment and in physical development (greater weight gains) as well as in measured intelligence (see, for example, Kennell, Trause, & Klaus, 1975).

In conclusion, early and extended contact between mothers and infants apparently is of fundamental importance for the formation of mother-infant bonds that, in turn, are intimately linked with the healthy development of infants. However, as Wasserman (1980) cautions, the evidence is still not totally convincing that there is a "sensitive period" immediately after birth, and that mother-infant bonding must occur during that time. She argues that the formation of attachments is sufficiently important to human development that it is likely that the infant and mother can take advantage of other opportunities for bonding without harmful consequences. Furthermore, the assumption that limited contact with infants immediately after birth—the usual practice in many hospitals—may lead to bonding failure and subsequent health and adjustment problems has not been supported. In a careful investigation, Egeland and Vaughn (1981) found no greater incidence of abuse, child neglect, illness, or adjustment problems among children who had been separated from their mothers for a period of time immediately after birth. Although early contact between parents and infants is highly desirable, the importance of a crucial few hours immediately after birth has not yet been clearly established.

Other Explanations of Attachment

What other factors may be important in attachment? Bowlby (1958) presents an ethological theory of attachment in which both smiling and crying play major roles. **Ethology** is concerned with the behavior of animals in natural settings and with parallels that exist between nonhuman animal behavior and ours. Bowlby suggests that attachment between mother and infant is the end product of an evolutionary process. Attachment had important survival value at a time when physical survival was threatened by the "hissing serpents and dragons of Eden" (Sagan, 1977). Given the importance of attachment for the infant's survival—and consequently for the survival of the race—one can reasonably suppose that powerful biological forces direct both mother and infant toward mutual attachment. Bowlby goes somewhat further and speculates that attachment is very much like imprinted behaviors such as "following" in young precocial birds—the characteristic way that young chickens or ducks, for example, follow the first moving object they see during a critical period (usually their mother, fortunately). In the same way as imprinting occurs during a critical period, but only in the presence of a suitable stimulus, termed a *releaser*, so attachment between a mother and infant occurs as a function

of the crying and smiling behavior of the infant. Bowlby suggests that these are, in fact, releasers for maternal attachment. When Schaffer and Emerson (1964) studied mother-child interaction during the first eighteen months of the infant's life, they found that the two aspects of the mother's behavior most highly related to her child's attachment to her were the mother's responsiveness to crying and the amount of stimulation that she provided. The nature of the stimulation appeared to be much less important than sheer quantity of stimulation. Thus, it made little difference whether the mother stimulated the child physically (by rocking, for example), whether the stimulation was primarily long range (such as singing), or whether she simply provided objects to play with.

Other theoretical explanations for maternal attachment have also been advanced. Learning-theory explanations maintain that attachment results from the mutual reinforcement that mother and infant provide each other (Bijou & Baer, 1965). From the infant's point of view, the most obvious source of reinforcement is the fact that the mother is the principal (sometimes the only) source of nourishment and comfort. From the mother's point of view, sources of reinforcement are more subtle but might include feelings of accomplishment, power, and worth that result from looking after someone who is virtually helpless. Gewirtz and Boyd (1976) suggest that learning-theory explanations of attachment are not at all incompatible with ethological explanations. Although some genetic tendencies related to mother-infant attachment may exist, they are nevertheless subject to environmental influence.

Fathers and Infant Attachment

And what about the father's relationship with his babies? Our traditional views of the family and of mother-father roles have typically focused on the importance of the mother in the early social development of the infant—and on the father's relative unimportance. Most of our developmental theorists (Freud, for example) argue that the father becomes important some time after the infants reach the age of two or three. Furthermore, many of these theorists have viewed the infant as largely incompetent—as passive and reflexive, as being moved by primitive physiological needs but seldom by a need to discover and to know. Little wonder that the father, and often the mother as well, has not been seen as playing an important role other than as a caregiver.

Several important changes are rapidly altering our conception of the father's role. These include an increasing number of "father-assisted" childbirths, where interaction is possible between father and infant as early as it might occur between mother and infant. In addition, changing work patterns and changing male-female responsibilities in the home among the middle-class majority have done a great deal to change the role of the father with his infant (Pedersen, 1980). As Lamb (1980) notes, mothers continue to be extremely important to the infant, but they are not unique. Fathers and other caretakers are also tremendously important. In fact, considerable research indicates that newborns and young infants may form attachments almost as strong with fathers as with mothers.

Parke and Sawin (1980) observed forty infants (twenty male and twenty female) immediately after birth, three weeks later in their homes, and three months later, also in their homes. Not surprisingly, they found that mothers spent more time than fathers did with infants in routine caretaking roles (feeding, changing, bathing); in contrast, fathers spent more time making faces at their infants and mimicking them. In other words, fathers tended to provide more social stimulation and mothers did more caretaking. Fathers also held their daughters more than their sons, although they provided more visual stimulation for the sons. In contrast, mothers tended to hold their sons more, but provided more stimulation for their daughters.

A study reported by Lamb (1980) had very similar findings. In this investigation, twenty infants were observed between the ages of seven and thirteen months and later between the ages of fifteen and twenty-four months. One of the main purposes of the study was to look at possible differences in the extent to which infants become attached to mothers and fathers, as well as at differences with respect to what are referred to as *affiliative* behaviors. An **affiliation**, or affiliative behavior,

Evidence suggests that given the opportunity, newborns can form attachments with fathers very similar to those they more typically form with mothers.

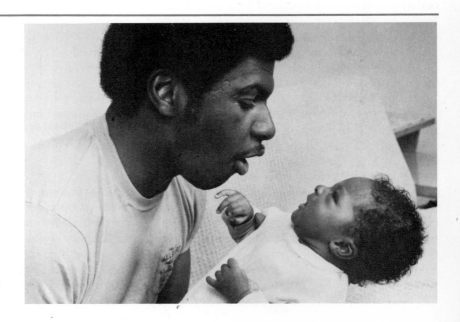

demonstrates a social relationship that stops short of being an attachment. Evidence of affiliation, for example, includes smiling, looking at, laughing, and giving; evidence of attachment might include seeking proximity, approaching, clinging, wanting to be picked up, and putting the head in the lap. Observations of affiliation and attachment were made when both parents were in the room, along with a third person, a visitor.

Contrary to what might have been expected, fathers fared extremely well with respect to the attachment and affiliation that their infants displayed toward them. For younger infants (ages seven to thirteen months), there was no difference in the amount of attachment behavior directed toward mother or father, although both received far more attachment behavior than did the visitor. However, fathers were recipients of more affiliative behaviors (smiling, looking at, vocalizing, laughing, and giving) than were mothers. And for older infants (ages fifteen to twenty-four months), fathers continued to have more affiliative behaviors directed toward them and were now also the objects of more attachment behaviors (seeking proximity, touching, approaching, wanting to be held). The differences between mothers and fathers, with respect to the amount of affiliative and attachment behavior directed toward them by their infants, were minimal, however. In fact, the boys displayed the majority of these behaviors toward their fathers; girls were somewhat less predictable. Lamb suggests that here, at the age of two, is evidence of the beginning of same-sex modeling.

In summary, it appears that infants (especially males) begin to affiliate with their fathers at a very young age, when they are given the opportunity to do so (Parke & O'Leary, 1975). Although fathers seem to interact more (touching and talking) with sons than daughters and with firstborns more than later children, they appear to be as competent as mothers in caregiving roles (feeding, changing, bathing) (Lamb, 1976a, 1976c). And it is significant that in a novel situation, the departure of both the father and the mother is followed by signs of distress, whereas the departure of a stranger leads to an increase in play behavior (Kotelchuck, 1976).

What such studies have established is that the father is far from irrelevant in the early development of the infant. The importance of the father was long neglected by psychological research. It does remain true, nevertheless, that the mother typically has considerably more contact with young infants than does the father (Lamb, 1976b; Rebelsky & Hanks, 1972), although infants and older children frequently prefer to play with the father when they can (Clarke-Stewart, 1980). (See also *A Family Model of Influences*.)

■ Strangers and Separation

Indirect investigations of parent-child attachment have also taken other forms. Perhaps the best known are the numerous studies of maternal deprivation and separation. Clearly, one index of an infant's attachment to parents and of their importance may be derived from the infant's reactions when the parents are gone. Another group of studies has attempted to explore certain dimensions of parent-child attachment by studying the reactions of infants to strangers. If an infant's behavior is identical with respect to all adults, it is unlikely that she has formed a strong, specific attachment to her mother or father. If, however, she reacts with visible fear and anxiety in the presence of strangers, she has at least learned to equate the presence of her parents with comfort and security.

Stranger Anxiety

Fear of strangers occurs in many infants. Although it appears to be most common after the age of nine months, it sometimes occurs before the age of four months and often not at all (Eckerman & Rheingold, 1974; Eckerman & Whatley, 1975). Lack of fear in the first few months of life is assumed to indicate that children do not yet discriminate readily among adults who surround them and that they have not yet formed strong attachments to any particular person. (See *Coping with Anxiety* for another type of attachment.)

A FAMILY MODEL OF INFLUENCES

For many years, a single global model has governed most of the research on parent-infant influence. Specifically, researchers have typically looked at the relationship between parents and infants and have generally focused only on what sociologists refer to as *dyadic* relationships. A dyadic relationship is simply a two-way relationship. Thus researchers initially concentrated almost exclusively on the mother-infant relationship; more recently, however, increasing attention has been devoted to the father-infant dyad.

This model, useful though it continues to be, has one major shortcoming. It fails to take into consideration the *triadic* nature of the majority of the families into which infants are born, as well as the great variety of indirect effects that parents and families can have on infants. Put another way, our prevailing models have been dyadic and psychological, whereas alternative models proposed by individuals such as Parke (1979) and Belsky (1981) are triadic and partly sociological.

This new family-based triadic model differs from the traditional dyadic model in a number of important ways. First, it suggests that far more influences are at work on the infant than just a mother on the one hand and a father on the other. There is, in addition, a family—a social unit made up of husband and wife (as opposed to just father and mother). Second, the model suggests that many complex influences may be at play other than the obvious parent-infant links. Belsky (1981) refers to these as "second-order" effects. Some possible second-order effects include the influence that a father might have on a mother, which might then cause her to interact differently with the infant; the relationship that the mother has with the infant, which might influence the way the father interacts with the infant; the influence that the infant's arrival (or temperament) has on the marriage and the consequent effects this might have on parenting—to name but a few effects.

This type of model suggests new lines of research and new interpretations of older research. It emphasizes the dynamic nature of parenting and points up that parents are more than just mother and father. It reaffirms that, even as parents influence children, so too do infants influence parents. And it further points out that more than two individuals are influenced, by including the full complex of family relationships.

What does research tell us about these relationships? Perhaps not as much as we would like to know, given that many of the results are still unclear or contradictory. To summarize briefly, Belsky (1981) reviews research which indicates that the birth of an infant often changes the relationship between husband and wife (sometimes increasing stress and discord, sometimes having the opposite effect); that discordant and conflict-ridden marriages are sometimes related to the development of antisocial behavior in children; that highly supportive marital relationships are related to caretaking skills with young infants; that the birth of an infant can frequently make a good marriage better, although it is less likely to make a bad one good; and that among the key qualities of parenting reflected in cognitive development and adjustment are *sensitive* mothering (attentiveness, warmth, responsiveness, and stimulation) and *involved* fathering (doing things with infants, including caretaking and playing).

But, as Belsky points out, we still know "very little about the direct influence of the child on marital relations and even less about the reverse process of influence" (1981, p. 17). The adoption of a model that considers the family in addition to the mother and the father may increase our knowledge considerably.

That fear does develop in many infants is perhaps a function of what has been labeled the "incongruity hypothesis" (Hunt, 1964). Essentially, this hypothesis maintains that once children have become familiar with and can recognize their environment, they develop certain expectations. The appearance of unexpected events is incongruous with the infant's expectations and leads to anxiety.

An indirect test of this hypothesis is provided by Schaffer's (1966) investigation of the onset of fear in children. Schaffer examined the relationship between a number of social variables (maternal availability, number of siblings, exposure to strangers) and infant responses when confronted with strangers. Significantly, he found only two variables related to incidence of stranger anxiety:

the number of siblings in the home and exposure to strangers. It appears that infants who are in contact with the largest number of people (strangers and siblings) are less likely to manifest fear, will react with the least amount of fear, and will cease to be afraid of strangers at an earlier age than infants with fewer contacts. This finding is consistent with the incongruity hypothesis, because early exposure to a wide variety of strangers would necessarily eliminate or at least reduce the incongruity associated with the presence of a stranger.

Institutionalized Children

Several naturally occurring situations have provided some indication of the importance of the parents in the life of the child. Spitz (1945, 1954) and Bowlby (1940, 1953) are among many psychologists to describe the harmful effects of naturally occurring parent-child separation. Spitz (1945), reporting the fate of institutionalized children, claimed that they had significantly higher mortality rates, that they were retarded in physical development, and that their emotional development was so severely thwarted by lack of *mothering* that they frequently withdrew, became depressed, and sometimes died as a result. The syndrome, which he explicitly attributed to maternal deprivation, is known as **marasmus** (progressive emaciation) or *anaclitic depression* (a slowing of normal development, weeping, sadness, and an increased susceptibility to disease).

Related studies all conclude that if children are prevented from forming a bond with a primary caretaker for a prolonged time, they will suffer severe emotional disturbances resulting from the lack of maternal love. By implication, then, the studies point to the hypothesis that maternal love or mothering is intimately involved not only in the child's emotional development but also in intellectual development and physical well-being. However, advocates of this hypothesis generally concede that maternal love need not come only from the true mother but may also come from any person who devotes the time, attention, and love to the child that a mother customarily displays.

Note, as well, that the effects of separation are highly dependent upon the age at which the infant is separated from parents. In general, maternal (or parental) separation prior to the age of six months does not have the same consequences as separation that occurs later (Casler, 1961). Children separated from their parents after the age of six months are already likely to have formed a strong attachment to them. Any unhappy effects of institutionalization may be due to rupturing this affectional bond, rather than to the child's being deprived of a mother or father. That is, if children are separated from their mothers before becoming strongly attached to them, one might expect that separation will not be especially traumatic. Additionally, regardless of the children's age when institutionalized, if the institution in which they are housed does not provide sufficient emotional and intellectual stimulation (recall the Tehran institutions described by Dennis), any negative effect on the infants will more likely be due to the nature of the care rather than to the lack of a mother.

Accordingly, Casler concludes that a general lack or impoverishment of stimulation accounts for many of the damaging effects of institutionalization on very young children—not their lack of mothering. Although Casler's conclusion may well be valid, his arguments do not contradict the belief that parental stimulation and love are conducive to an infant's healthy development, a belief supported by experience and by other studies.

Maternal Separation

One study examined seventy adopted children between birth and sixteen months of age (Yarrow & Goodwin, 1973). All these children were in foster homes prior to adoption, and all were assumed to have had normal environments both before and after adoption. This study, then, is one of maternal separation rather than of maternal deprivation. Its aim was to discover the effects on the infant of separation from a parent figure. Because children were adopted at various ages, it was also possible to examine differences in their reactions as a function of age.

COPING WITH ANXIETY:
SECURITY BLANKETS

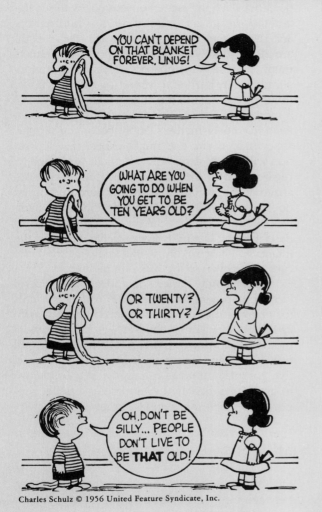

Charles Schulz © 1956 United Feature Syndicate, Inc.

A series of intriguing studies has been looking at the role of the blanket in the life of the American child. No less than half of all middle-class American children exhibit strong attachments to inanimate objects, the most common of which is, not surprisingly, the blanket (Weisberg & Russell, 1971). These children are also attached to their mothers. In one study, Passman and Weisberg (1975) compared the effectiveness of mothers and blankets in reducing a child's anxiety in a strange situation. They found that children who were attached to their blankets displayed no more anxiety than children who were not attached to blankets but whose mothers were present— as long as these children had their blankets close by. In fact, they played and explored more than children who had no mother, favorite toy, or blanket present. Related studies (Passman, 1974, 1977) also found that a blanket was as effective as the mother in a school-like situation for those children who were attached to their blankets. More recent research has shown, however, that in situations of higher stress or arousal, the mother becomes more effective than a blanket or other inanimate attachment object in reducing anxiety (Passman, 1976). When children are playing, pacifiers (Halonen & Passman, 1978), color films of mothers (Passman & Erck, 1978), and monochromatic videotapes of mothers are sometimes as effective as the actual presence of mothers. If you are anxious and cannot bring your mother with you, do bring your blanket . . . or whatever.

Not surprisingly, reactions were least severe for children under three months of age. This finding is consistent with the observation that prior to this age children have not formed any strong attachments. Only nine children were adopted before the age of three months; the remainder were placed at ages ranging from three to sixteen months. Only 15 percent of all the children were completely free of all disturbances; the remainder manifested disturbances of varying severity (see Table 6.2). These disturbances were most obvious in the infant's sleeping schedule and were also evident in feeding behaviors, social reactions (withdrawal, for example), and in emotional behavior (crying). Disruptions in social reactions were manifested in three behaviors: decreased social responsiveness; increased stranger anxiety; and specific disturbances in interactions with the new mother figure, expressed in feeding difficulties, colic, digestive upsets, and, most strikingly, physical rejection of the new mother or excessive clinging to her.

It is also significant that developmental scores, expressed in terms of IQ estimates, were lower in 56 percent of the cases following adoption. Separation from the mother or mother figure apparently has an adverse effect on most significant aspects of the infant's development.

Yarrow and Goodwin (1973) also examined the validity of the critical period hypothesis with respect to maternal separation. As discussed in Chapter 3, this hypothesis maintains that there is a period of time during which exposure to specific situations will lead to predictable behavior, but that exposure to the same situations before and after the critical period is less likely to lead to that behavior. For example, maternal separation prior to the age of three months seems to be not nearly so harmful as separation at the age of nine months. The relationship of age at separation to manifestation of disturbances in the Yarrow and Goodwin study is presented in Table 6.3. Although there does not appear to be a critical period before and after which maternal separation will have no effect, there is a definite relationship between age at separation and disturbances in the infant.

Table 6.2 The immediate impact of mother-child separation.

Impact	Percentage
No disturbances	15
Mild disturbances	36
Moderate disturbances	23
Severe disturbances	20
Extreme disturbances	6

Based on data provided by Yarrow and Goodwin, 1973.

■ Other Related Topics

This chapter has been concerned primarily with the social and emotional development of the young infant, with emphasis on the development of attachment between parents and infant, parent-child interaction, and infant emotions. Other topics that are of increasing relevance to the social and emotional development of the infant include the effect of substitute caregiving in nurseries and day-care centers, of mother or father absence, and of single-parent families. All of these topics are treated in Chapter 8, in a section dealing specifically with the family.

■ The Whole Person

There is something frustrating about categorizing the developing person into such psychologically

Table 6.3 Severity of reaction to maternal separation, according to age.

Severity of Reaction	Under 3 Months	3–4 Months	4–5 Months	6 Months	9 Months
Slight or no reaction	100%	60%	28%	9%	0
Moderately severe to very severe	0	40%	72%	91%	100%

Based on data provided by Yarrow and Goodwin, 1973.

convenient categories as *description of capabilities, physical development, motor development, social-emotional development, intellectual development*, and so on. We lose the individual in the interminable and sometimes confused array of beliefs, findings, tentative conclusions, convincing arguments, and suggestions. The theoretical infant is a hypothetical average. And although a great many infants are very close to the hypothetical average child when they are one month old, fewer are still average at the age of two months, even fewer at the age of six months, and by the age of a year, almost none. By the time the child becomes as old as you or me, the average individual will no longer exist but will appear only in the overly simplified theories of the social scientist or in the files of the market researcher who wants to know what the "average" person is wearing this spring.

Each person is a more or less integrated whole, whose intellect, emotions, and physical being all interact; each part is inextricably linked with and dependent upon every other part of the living organism. However, if we attempt to describe a person in that way, the sheer complexity of the task might drive us mad. And so we continue to speak of the isolated forces that affect human development as though they exist apart from the integrated, whole person. But it bears repeating that our divisions, although necessary, are artificial and somewhat misleading.

■ MAIN POINTS

1 The direction of influence in parent-infant interaction is not solely from parent to child but is mutual—hence the expression "bidirectionality of influence."

2 Infant states reflect basic individual differences very early in life and may be related to differences observed later.

3 Statements about the young child's emotional responses are often subjective. Infants may react to stimulation with a generalized excitement. Research has also differentiated among crying, smiling, and fear responses, some of which occur very early in life.

4 Individual differences among adults are often referred to as *personality* differences; those among infants, as differences in *temperament*. Temperament characteristics are assumed to have a strong genetic basis.

5 The New York Longitudinal Study (NYLS—Thomas, Chess, and Birch, 1970) identified nine characteristics of infant temperament; particular combinations of them are associated with three types of children: difficult, easy, and "slow to warm up."

6 Some evidence suggests that difficult infants (lack of rhythmicity, withdrawal from the unfamiliar, slow adaptation to change, and intense, negative moods) run a higher risk of behavior and emotional problems than do easy children.

7 Attempts to identify high-risk infants on the basis of early assessments of temperament have been criticized on the grounds that the observed relationship between these assessments and later problems is not high, the measures are notably unreliable (there is often little agreement between parents and other observers), individual behavior is often not consistent with apparent temperament or personality characteristics, and there are dangers in labeling certain infants as high risk.

8 Among the earliest forms of social interaction between mother and infant is the mutual gaze.

9 Mother-infant bonding appears to be important to the healthy development and adjustment of the infant. It has not yet been established, however, that there is a critical period during which this bonding must occur or that it can only occur with the mother.

10 An ethological explanation of attachment between mothers and infants maintains that smiling and crying serve as "releasers" for attachment bonds that are genetically influenced.

11 Learning-theory explanations of mother-infant attachment are based on the assumption that the mother's role as caretaker is what endears her to the infant.

12 Infants appear to become equally attached to their mothers and fathers when given the opportunity but display more affiliative behaviors toward their fathers. Boys are especially likely to adopt an attitude of "let's be friends."

13 Fear of strangers occurs in many infants but is less pronounced in those who have been exposed to many people.

14 Infant separation from parents may have harmful effects on the child, particularly after the age of six months but seldom before the age of three months.

15 Although relatively fragmented aspects of the child have been discussed in this chapter, we are concerned with the whole person.

■ FURTHER READINGS

In the following book, Bowlby examines mother-infant interaction with special emphasis on the development of attachment:
Bowlby, J. *Attachment and loss.* New York: Basic Books, 1973.

An extensive and critical review of studies of maternal deprivation is:
Casler, L. Maternal deprivation: A critical review of the literature. *Monograph of the Society for Research in Child Development,* 1961, *26*(2).

Parents and others who are concerned with child rearing might find the following of particular value in applying theory and research:
Stein, S. B. *New parents' guide to early learning.* New York: New American Library, 1976.

An important view of mother-infant bonding is presented in:
Klaus, M., & Kennell, J. *Maternal-infant bonding.* St. Louis: Mosby, 1976.

A collection of major studies of the father's role in the young infant's social development is contained in:
Pedersen, F. A. (Ed.). *The father-infant relationship: Observational studies in the family setting.* New York: Praeger, 1980.

An excellent general coverage of most of the topics discussed in this chapter is provided by:
Maccoby, E. E. *Social development: Psychological growth and the parent-child relationship.* New York: Harcourt Brace Jovanovich, 1980.

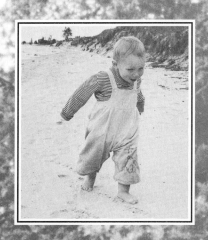

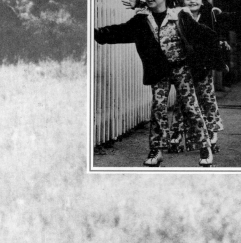

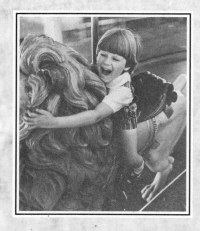

PART THREE   CHILDHOOD

7 COGNITIVE AND LANGUAGE DEVELOPMENT IN EARLY CHILDHOOD

Bliss was it in that dawn to be alive,
But to be young was very heaven.

William Wordsworth
"A Poet's Epitaph"

Sweet childish days, that were as long
As twenty days are now.

William Wordsworth
"To a Butterfly"

The little town of Smoky Lake, sleeping as we angled along her main street between the elevators and the hotel, is now well behind us. We have left Highway 855 and have turned east on 28—east toward my roots, and toward where . . . My hands are suddenly clammy on the steering wheel, and I know that I have not succeeded well in putting it out of my mind. I push the thought back and try to relax again. I have had much practice at trying to relax.

The highway is more serpentine now. It climbs hills among jackpines, whose roots clutch light sands, descends them in rapid curves, and snakes its way among the countless bogs and little lakes scattered in its path. Our windows are open wide; I am fundamentally opposed to air conditioners, although I might change my mind if I drove too often among the petrochemical industry's hulking monsters or among pig farms. Here the air is light with birdsong and bees and it is difficult to remember the smell of factories and farms. The winds of our passing blow wildly through the car, wreaking great havoc with Denise's hair as well as with my grandmother's. Grandma smiles gleefully through her dishevelment, filling her lungs deeply with air that, for her, is redolent with good memories. Denise, less moved by piney scents or by the rich odor of springtime bogs, tries valiantly to hold her hair against the wind. The wind is winning, although she is now sitting in the front, where the turbulence is less extreme and more predictable.

The car always seems to work better on roads like this, as though it is happy to stretch its legs after weeks of running short spurts at erratic speeds among traffic lights and signs and through school zones and construction detours. Now it hums at high speed through this blue spring afternoon, stretching its length low along the uncoiling asphalt.

With only the slightest warning—a hint of the very beginning of a small fishtail—the left rear tire slackens and softens so gently that by the time I have brought the car to a stop, it has just begun to rest on its rim.

"I told you we needed new tires in the back," Paul says. He did. But I had decided to get them after the trip when I had more time. If I had more time.

I pull off the road onto a grassy shoulder. There is no hurry. It isn't winter; there is neither wind nor rain. I have tools and I know how to use them. And I will now teach Paul, and perhaps Marcel and Denise, how one changes a tire. Efficiently, effortlessly, and with a sense of accomplishment.

A jack, first. From the trunk. An ordinary bumper jack, perfectly adequate for jobs of this kind. And a tire wrench to operate the jack and to remove the wheel lugs.

But the tire wrench does not rest where it has customarily rested. In fact, once I have completely emptied the trunk, I realize that it no longer lives in this car. Paul remembers now that he might have used it to fix a bicycle tire. But he thinks he also remembers putting it back in the trunk. I try to repress my anger.

We stand on the road, Paul and I. He, because he feels partly responsible; I, because of some vague feeling that I should somehow teach him how to do this, this standing on highways. Denise and Marcel remain totally unconcerned. They chase each other through the greening ditch, looking for crocuses and wild strawberry blossoms, while grandmother sits regally on the spare tire, knitting her rapidly enlarging green thing.

A truck screeches to a stop; inside, two men, their necks sun reddened, their hands oiled and calloused. Each wears a stained cap set back on the head at a jaunty, almost rakish angle. One says *Massey Ferguson* across its front; the other, *John Deere*.

"How come you ain't got no wrench?" John Deere asks, as I operate the jack with their tire iron.

I begin to explain. At the same time, Paul tries to tell them that it's his fault. I know he fears that I will be angry and is trying to mollify me. The thought makes me slightly angry. I don't like to think that my children manipulate me.

"Ain't nothing worse than having no jack," Massey Ferguson says, apparently forgetting that we do have a jack—that we are lacking only one inconsequential tire iron. "He don't got no jack neither," he continues, nodding his head toward John Deere, and they both laugh hugely at what might be a private joke. Or perhaps "not gotting" a jack is universally hilarious.

"They ain't spoke no English so good," Paul says, as we pull back out onto the highway. I drive gingerly at first, wondering whether I am the only one who doesn't trust spare tires.

"It's because they're dumb," Denise says.

"Maybe it's because their parents didn't speak well," Paul says.

"Maybe they're both university professors who just like to talk that way," Grandma adds, chuckling.

Strangely, nobody asks my opinion in spite of the fact that I am acknowledged, I think, as something of an expert on matters of this nature. The thought nags uncomfortably for a moment, but I set it quickly aside, because as I think of answers that I might have phrased, had someone cared to ask me, I am reminded of where we left off in our narrative. And I am also reminded that we must continue quickly, for there is little time to waste if everything is to be said before we arrive.

Let us turn, then, once more to the lifespan and look at the physical and intellectual development of the young child, as well as at the early development of language. For soon we will be in Vilna, where the tire must be fixed.

■ Physical Growth

A comparison of the six-year-old child with the two-year-old provides some idea of the developmental process during the preschool years. The magnitude of the difference is phenomenal, although the changes that occurred from birth to the end of the child's second year are probably even more striking. The first observation that one can make about the process of development during childhood is that it is generally characterized by a marked slowing of development. For example, the rate of weight gain for the average child is greater during the first year than it is each year between the ages of two and five.

Table 7.1 traces the physical development of boys and girls from the age of two to six. Comparing these data with Table 5.1 reveals a dramatic deceleration in growth rates after the period of infancy, particularly in height. Although the growth rate between the second and fourth year declines, the rate of absolute weight gained increases between the fourth and the sixth year. However, the increase in weight gain is slight and does not significantly change the general pattern of decelerated growth.

Different growth rates for different parts of the body help explain some of the changes that occur between the ages of two and six. The thick layers of baby fat that one-year-old children have begin to disappear slowly during the second year of life and continue to recede gradually. In effect, these tissues grow much more slowly than other tissues, so that by the time children have reached the age of six, their layers of fat are less than half as thick as they were at the age of one. Partly because of this change, they begin to look more like adults.

Other changes as well account for the gradual transition from the appearance of infancy to the

appearance of young boyhood or girlhood. Not only does the relative amount of fatty tissue change during the preschool years but its distribution also changes as a result of the more rapid growth of bone and muscle. The squat appearance of infants is explained by the fact that their waists are at least as large as their hips or chests. Six-year-old children, by contrast, have begun to develop waists that are smaller in girth than their shoulders and hips. This becomes even more evident in early adolescence than at the end of the preschool period.

The girth of infants is also due in part to the relative size of the internal organs, many of which grow much more rapidly than other parts of the body, while all must be accommodated in the space between the child's pelvis and diaphragm. As a

Table 7.1 Height and weight at the fiftieth percentile for American children.

Age	Height (inches)		Weight (pounds)	
	Girl	Boy	Girl	Boy
2 years	34	34½	27	27¾
2½ years	36	36¼	29½	30
3 years	37¾	38	31¾	32¼
3½ years	39¼	39¼	34	34¼
4 years	40½	40¾	36¼	36½
4½ years	42	42	38½	38½
5 years	43	43¼	41	41½
5½ years	44½	45	44	45½
6 years	45½	46¼	46½	48¼

Adapted by the Health Department, Milwaukee, Wisconsin; based on data by H. C. Stuart and H. V. Meredith, prepared for use in Children's Medical Center, Boston. Used by permission of the Milwaukee Health Department.

result, their abdomens protrude. As they grow in height during the preschool years, their abdomens gradually become more like those of healthy adults.

Figure 5.4 portrays other changes in body proportions that account for the different appearance of the six-year-old. That figure shows that the head of a two-month fetus is approximately half the length of the entire body. At birth the head is closer to one-fourth the size of the rest of the body. By the age of six, it is close to one-eighth the size, which is a short step removed from the head-to-body relationship typical of the normal adult with a normal-sized head: one-tenth. From the age of two to six, the head changes from approximately one-fifth to one-eighth of total body size—a noticeable change. Because of this change and because of changes in the distribution of fat and in the space that the child now has for internal organs, the six-year-old looks remarkably like an adult; the two-year-old looks more like a typical baby.

■ Motor Development

Infants' most significant motor achievement is learning to walk. At the same time that they learn to walk, they also learn to coordinate other motor activities that they have been practicing, so that by the age of two they are remarkably adept at picking up objects, stacking blocks, unlacing shoes, and a host of other motor activities that are more or less pleasing for mothers. The close relationship between motor and cognitive development during infancy is explicit in the theories of Jean Piaget. According to Piaget, during the sensorimotor period, the infant has difficulty separating action from thought—hence the close alliance between activity and early intellectual development.

The course of motor development during infancy involves the acquisition of abilities such as those involved in locomotion and in grasping. Children continue to make progress in motor development during the preschool period; their locomotion becomes more certain as they lose the characteristic wide-footed stance of the toddler (from eighteen months to two and one-half years).

As their equilibrium stabilizes and their feet move closer together, their arms and hands also move closer to their bodies. Thus, they lose both the wide stance and the appearance of a tightrope walker; they no longer need to maintain a precarious balance with both arms and feet. As their walking improves, they acquire the ability to climb stairs standing upright and completely unassisted and eventually to hop with two feet and to skip.

Gesell (1925) provides norms for motor behavior between the ages of two and five; these are additional evidence of increased perceptual-motor coordination. He reports that the three-year-old is capable of copying either a circle or a horizontal line, both of which are ordinarily impossible for a two-year-old child. The four-year-old has acquired the ability to copy a cross, which is a much more difficult figure. In addition, four-year-olds can copy a diamond and button their own clothes. The five-year-old is also capable of all these skills and in addition can copy a triangle or a prism and is capable of lacing (or unlacing) shoes.

Additional corroboration of Gesell's findings is provided by Cratty (1970), who employed a sample of 170 middle-class children in an attempt to determine the order of difficulty in copying various geometric designs. His sample did not include subjects younger than four years, so the age comparison must begin from there. Cratty found that children could not copy a triangle until the age of six, but that rectangles, circles, and squares could be copied correctly before six. He also found that the diamond was considerably more difficult than other forms, and that few subjects could copy it correctly prior to the age of seven. Cratty reports a study conducted by Ilg and Ames (1965), which found that the order of difficulty for figures, beginning with the easiest, is the circle, the square, the triangle, the cross, the divided rectangle (a rectangle with diagonals and vertical and horizontal bisecting lines drawn in), and the diamond. Ilg and Ames indicate that three-year-olds can copy a circle, just as Gesell reported. However, whereas Gesell reported that a four-year-old could copy a cross, Ilg and Ames found that a cross could only be drawn correctly by six-and-one-half-year-olds. Like Gesell, though, they report that the diamond and

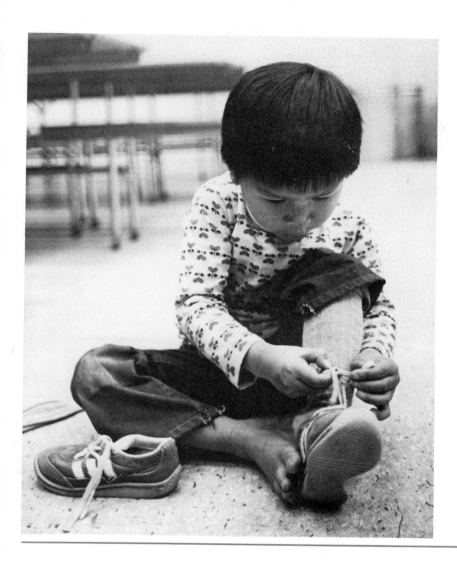

Tying shoelaces is far more complex and difficult than unlacing shoes; it requires great concentration and skill, not to mention a little luck.

the divided rectangle could not be copied correctly before the age of eight or nine. All these figures can be copied in almost recognizable fashion considerably earlier, however, probably accounting for the minor contradictions among the findings of Cratty, Ilg and Ames, and Gesell.

The most striking observation is that the order of difficulty for these geometric designs is virtually the same for every reported study. Because of the close relationship between motor development and general intellectual development, a variety of measures of intelligence use these geometric forms. The revised Stanford-Binet, for example, asks subjects at the ages of five, seven, and ten to draw a square, a diamond, and a more complex design (Terman & Merrill, 1973) (see Figure 7.1).

Obviously, the child's physical and motor development are closely related, because the acquisition of many skills depends on development of the required musculature and on control of these muscles. The relationship of physical development to other areas of development is

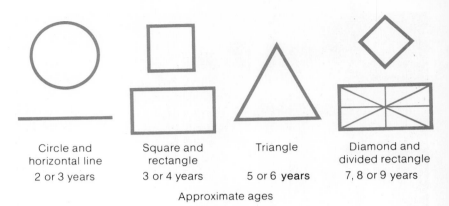

Figure 7.1
Usual order of difficulty for copying simple geometric designs reasonably well. Because of the close relationship between motor and intellectual development in early childhood, some intelligence tests for young children include items such as these.

Circle and horizontal line
2 or 3 years

Square and rectangle
3 or 4 years

Triangle
5 or 6 years

Diamond and divided rectangle
7, 8 or 9 years

Approximate ages

sometimes not so obvious, although no less real. For example, a child's play, particularly when it involves peers, is often influenced by motor skills, because various aptitudes are called for in different games. A child who is still incapable of jumping with both feet is not likely to be invited by older children to join in a game of jump rope; a child who cannot grasp marbles skillfully may be left out of the traditional spring marble games. Conversely, the child who is precocious in physical and motor development is likely to be the first one asked to participate in games—indeed, may be the one to initiate them. Clearly, physical and motor development may have an influence on the general social development of the child; game playing is one important means of socialization (see Chapter 8).

■ Cognitive Development

We do not expect our preschool children, much less our infants, to be completely logical. We are seldom surprised when our three-year-olds insist loudly that a small cat, identical to their small cat, must surely be theirs; we are not shocked by the four-year-old's apparent failure to realize that there really are not more candies in his sister's dish when they are all spread out; we express little dismay when our two-and-one-half-year-old calls a duck a chicken. For some reason, these instances of *ego-*

centric, perception-dominated, and *illogical* thinking simply amuse us; that is what we expect of young children.

But we would be surprised if our seven-year-olds continued to insist on calling all reasonably shaggy-looking pigs "doggy," if they refused to believe that six ounces of soft drink in a glass is the same amount as six ounces in a bottle, or if they thought that they could decrease the mass of a wad of gum simply by stringing it out and wrapping it around their ears! These illustrate some of the intellectual (or cognitive) differences that we expect between our preschoolers and older children.

This chapter looks at the cognitive development of the preschool child, primarily through the eyes of Jean Piaget, the psychologist most responsible for drawing our attention to this aspect of child development. Recall that in Chapter 5 we described the *sensorimotor* intelligence of the infant. This label describes the most prevalent feature of the child's interaction with, and understanding of, the world during that stage. The infant's intelligence involves immediate sensation and action.

Piaget's label for the next developmental period, one that spans the preschool years, is *preoperational*. In Piaget's theory, an operation is a thought characterized by some specific logical properties. Put very simply, an operation is a logical thought. Thus, the child who believes that he has more gum when he rolls it into a fat ball and

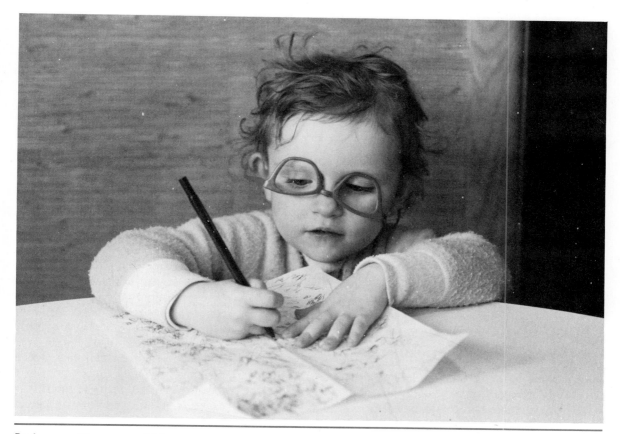

By the age of five, many children can copy a cross, a diamond, a circle, or a square reasonably well; most, like this bespectacled urchin, can also scribble and scratch.

less when he spreads it out like a thin pancake on his sister's pillow is not only engaging in punishable behavior but also is demonstrating *preoperational* thinking.

Piaget divides the preoperational period (ages two to approximately seven) into two subperiods: The first, lasting from two to four, is termed *preconceptual*; the second, from four to seven, is called *intuitive* (see Table 7.2).

Preconceptual Thinking

The major intellectual difference between the sensorimotor child and the preschooler is in the means

each has of representing the world and reasoning about it. The young infant's intelligence is initially rooted in sensation and action, but toward the end of the second year, and especially with the advent of language, infants begin to symbolize. They begin to represent their actions mentally and to anticipate their consequences before the action actually occurs, and they begin to develop some notion of causes—of actions as means to ends.

As children begin to symbolize, they develop the consequent ability to represent mentally (internalize) objects and events in the environment. Thus they develop **concepts**; these concepts, not as complete and logical as an adult's, are referred to as **preconcepts**. Despite their incom-

Table 7.2 Piaget's stages of cognitive development.

Stage	Approximate Age	Some Major Characteristics
Sensorimotor	0–2 years	Motoric intelligence. World of the here and now. No language, no thought in early stages. No notion of objective reality.
Preoperational Preconceptual Intuitive	2–7 years 2–4 years 4–7 years	Egocentric thought. Reason dominated by perception. Intuitive rather than logical solutions. Inability to conserve.
Concrete operations	7–11 or 12 years	Ability to conserve. Logic of classes and relations. Understanding of number. Thinking bound to concrete. Development of reversibility in thought.
Formal operations	11 or 12 to 14 or 15 years	Complete generality of thought. Propositional thinking. Ability to deal with the hypothetical. Development of strong idealism.

pleteness, they are nevertheless sufficient to permit the child to make the simple classifications necessary for identifying some of the objects of the world. Thus, children recognize a man because they have a budding concept that tells them that a *man* is whatever walks on two legs, has hair, wears pants, and speaks in a gruff voice. By noting their characteristics, children can identify dogs, birds, elephants, and houses. What they frequently cannot do, however, is distinguish among different individuals belonging to the same species. Piaget illustrates this with his son, Laurent, who pointed out a snail to his father as they were walking. "Régardez l'escargot," he allegedly said, in the polite manner of a Swiss child of the early 1920s. Piaget's reply to this observation is unrecorded, but he reports that several minutes later they came upon another snail, and the child exclaimed that here again was the snail. The child's apparent failure to recognize that similar objects can belong to the same class and still be different objects—that is, they can retain an identity of their own—is an example of a *preconcept.* A related example is the preschooler who steadfastly continues to believe in Santa Claus, even after seeing ten different Santas on the same day. For the child, they are all *identical* (Lefrancois, 1967).

One additional striking feature of the child's reasoning processes during the preconceptual period is subsumed under the imposing heading of **transductive reasoning**. *Transductive reasoning* makes inferences on the basis of particular instances or on the basis of single characteristics of objects. Such reasoning is in contrast to *deductive reasoning,* which proceeds from general to particular instances, or its converse, *inductive reasoning,* which begins with a number of particular instances and proceeds to a general statement. Reasoning from particular to particular occasionally results in a correct conclusion, but frequently it does not. (See *A Child's Reasoning.*) Consider the example:

A flies;   B flies;   therefore, B is A.

Clearly if A is a bird and B is also a bird, then A is a B and vice versa. If A is a plane and B is a bird, the same reasoning process leads to an incorrect conclusion. Thus a preschooler can unashamedly insist that cats are dogs and chickens are turkeys.

The period of *intuitive thinking* begins at about age four and ends at approximately seven. It is labeled *intuitive* because much of the child's thought is based on immediate comprehension rather than logical, rational processes. Children solve many problems correctly, but they do not always do so on the basis of logic. Piaget refers to a problem in which a child is shown three beads strung on a wire, which is then inserted into a hollow cardboard tube so that the child can no longer see them. The beads are blue, red, and yellow. At first, when the tube is held vertically, the child knows clearly which bead is on top. Then, the tube is turned a half rotation (180°), and the subject is asked which bead is now at the top. Alternatively, it may be turned a full rotation, one and one-half turns, two turns, and so on. Piaget found that as long as subjects could continue to *imagine* the position of the beads inside the tube, they could answer correctly, but they could not arrive at a rule concerning the relationship between the odd and even numbers of turns or half turns and the location of the beads. In other words, the solution to the problem was achieved through *intuitive* mental images rather than logical reasoning.

Intuitive thinking is also characterized by a limited ability to classify, **egocentric** thought, and a marked reliance on perception. Each of these qualities is illustrated here.

The preschooler's limited ability to classify is demonstrated in a classic series of experiments that present the child with a collection of objects made of two subclasses. The objects may consist of twenty wooden beads—fifteen brown ones and five blue ones—or of twenty-five flowers—nineteen roses and six tulips. The subject is asked what the objects are. "They are wooden beads"—a proud and intelligent answer. The experimenter then divides them into the two subclasses, brown beads and blue beads, and asks whether there are more brown beads or more wooden beads. The trick is obvious, you say! Not to the child at this stage of development. "There are more brown beads"— again a proud, though somewhat less intelligent, answer. The answer reflects the child's incomplete understanding of classes. It is as though breaking down a class into its subparts destroys the parent class. Markman (1979; Markman, Horton, & McLanahan, 1980) notes that even older children sometimes experience difficulty with problems involving class inclusion, although few would have difficulty with problems as simple as the wooden-bead exercise.

An experiment in which a girl doll and a boy doll are placed side by side on a piece of string illustrates the egocentric nature of the preschool child's thought. The experimenter holds the ends of the string in both hands and stands behind a screen that hides the dolls from the child's view. The child is asked to predict which of the dolls will appear first if the experimenter moves the string toward the right. Let us assume that the boy doll appears first. The experimenter then returns the dolls to their original position and repeats the

A CHILD'S REASONING

There are numerous examples of transductive reasoning in the preschooler's thought processes (also called semantic overgeneralization). A two-and-one-half-year-old girl exclaims over an animal during a picnic: "Kitty, Daddy. There's a kitty! There's a kitty! There's a kitty! Daddy! There's a kitty!" she says, once or twice, until her father eventually turns and looks at a lovely and wholly undomesticated skunk. The evidence of transductive reasoning is clear: Kitties have fur; that thing has fur; therefore that thing is a kitty. I would have enjoyed the illustration of transductive reasoning except that the girl was my daughter (I'll get you back, Denise).

same question, "Which of the dolls will now appear first if they are moved to the same side?" The procedure is repeated several times regardless of whether the child answers correctly. A normally intelligent child will answer correctly for every early trial. What happens in later trials is striking. The child eventually makes the opposite, clearly incorrect prediction. If asked why, one of the more common answers is that it is not fair that the same doll comes out first every time; now it is the other doll's turn. Children inject their own values, their own sense of justice, into the experimental situation, thus demonstrating their egocentric thought processes. Egocentrism refers to the inability of the child to take another person's perspective, cognitively. Hence, the term *egocentric* is not derogatory, but simply points out an excessive reliance

on the thinker's individual point of view coupled with a corresponding inability to be objective.

Egocentric thought is further demonstrated by the preschooler's inability to imagine what a mountain looks like when seen from another point of view—for example, the top or another side.

The preschooler's perception also dominates thinking, as seen in the conservation problems. When children decide that there is more modeling clay in the snake than there was in the ball from which the snake was formed, they are relying solely on the object's appearance rather than on any thought processes that might be more appropriate. In contrast, an adult faced with a conflict between perception and thought is more likely to rely on thought than perception. (See Figure 7.2 for illustrations of relevant experiments.)

Figure 7.2
Experiments concerned with preoperational thought.

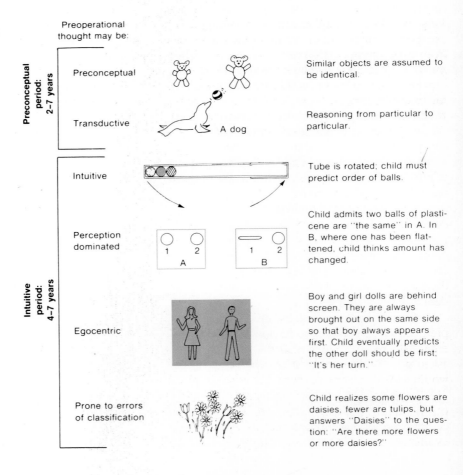

Preoperational thought may be:

Preconceptual period: 2–7 years

Preconceptual — Similar objects are assumed to be identical.

Transductive — A dog — Reasoning from particular to particular.

Intuitive period: 4–7 years

Intuitive — Tube is rotated; child must predict order of balls.

Perception dominated — A 1 2 — B 1 2 — Child admits two balls of plasticene are "the same" in A. In B, where one has been flattened, child thinks amount has changed.

Egocentric — Boy and girl dolls are behind screen. They are always brought out on the same side so that boy always appears first. Child eventually predicts the other doll should be first; "It's her turn."

Prone to errors of classification — Child realizes some flowers are daisies, fewer are tulips, but answers "Daisies" to the question: "Are there more flowers or more daisies?"

Research and Implications

Literally hundreds of studies have been conducted to investigate Piaget's description of the child's progression through stages of cognitive development. With a few exceptions, most have found that the *sequence* described by Piaget is valid not only in European and North American countries, but in many other parts of the world as well. For example, when Opper (1977) looked at the classification abilities of preoperational children in Thailand and Malaysia, she found that they, like Piaget's subjects, believed that a bouquet consisting of seven roses and two orchids contained more roses than flowers. Other cross-cultural research is in general agreement that the sequence described by Piaget is cross-culturally valid (Dasen, 1977). However, some evidence shows that Piaget's estimates of the ages of attainment are, in effect, underestimates for some North American and European children on specific tasks. This evidence typically comes from experiments that attempt to make it simpler for children to demonstrate knowledge of the concept or ability in question. Many of these studies, for example, concern Piaget's mountain problem, which illustrates the child's egocentricity.

In Piaget's original demonstration of egocentricity, children observe three mountains of unequal height, set on top of a table. They are allowed to walk around the display, thus becoming familiar with all sides of the mountains. Later they sit on one side of the table, a doll is placed on the other side, and they are asked to select photographs representing the doll's point of view. Piaget found that children in the preoperational period usually indicated that the doll would see the same things they themselves saw, a finding that he interprets as evidence of egocentricity.

When Piaget's mountains task is made simpler, the child sometimes responds quite differently (Borke, 1975; Bower, 1974). Liben (1975) asked preschoolers to describe what a white card would look like from their point of view and from the experimenter's point of view, under a number of different conditions that involved wearing colored glasses. In one condition, for example, the experimenter would wear green-tinted glasses, and

the children, no glasses. In this case, a correct, nonegocentric response would be that the card would look green to the experimenter. Liben found that almost half the three-year-olds answered correctly, and most of the older children had no difficulty with the questions. Similarly, when Hughes (reported in Donaldson, 1978) presented preschoolers with a situation where they had to determine whether a "policeman" could see a boy doll from a vantage point quite different from the child's, subjects had little difficulty determining what the policeman's point of view would actually be (see Figure 7.3).

Do these studies mean that Piaget's conclusions with respect to the preoperational child's egocentricity are invalid? The answer is no. Donaldson (1978) points out that all these studies present the child with problems that are really very different from the problem of the mountains. The child who can accurately predict whether or not a policeman can see into an area, when the policeman is on the *opposite* side of the table from the child, should not be expected to be able to describe what the physical array would look like to the policeman. Among other things, doing so would

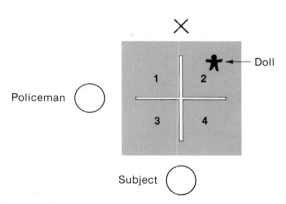

Figure 7.3
Arrangement for the Hughes experiment. Subjects had to determine whether a doll hidden in 1, 2, 3, or 4 could be seen by the policeman. In a later part of the experiment, a second policeman was placed at X. The child now had to decide where the doll would have to be hidden so it would not be seen by either policeman. Preschoolers had little trouble answering correctly.

require that the child be able to reverse left and right (so that the child realized that the policeman's left is the child's right)—a task that is sometimes difficult even for adults, as those of us who have occasionally been surprised by our movements in mirrors can testify.

What these and related studies most clearly point out is that the egocentricity and other characteristics of children's thinking are far more complex than had been suspected. We have only begun to explore that complexity. The preoperational period has often been described in terms of what children cannot do rather than in terms of their cognitive achievements. This approach results as much from the nature of the theories that have traditionally been employed to organize our child development "facts" as from the facts themselves. Piagetian theory, for example, describes preschoolers largely by contrasting them with children in the period of concrete operations. Thus preschoolers are described as intuitive, egocentric, perception dominated—in short, as *preoperational*.

Although this description of preschoolers is to a large extent valid, it is also misleading. As Gelman (1978) notes, our preoccupation with what preschool children cannot do has blinded us to their achievements. Research has only recently begun to recognize that preschoolers are not egocentric in all situations, do have considerable understanding of numbers, and can classify and make logical inferences under a variety of circum-

PRESCHOOL EDUCATION

All of children's experiences from birth to school age compose their preschool education. The language they hear, the people who serve as models for their behavior, those who control some of their rewards and punishments, television programs, books, stories, movies, visits to different places, the activities in which they engage—all of these are teachers. Life is the curriculum; adaptation is the major objective; development becomes the teaching process; and the child is the learner at the center of the process.

The most striking feature about preschoolers' environment is its haphazard, unstructured nature, yet the strides they make from birth to school age are phenomenal. If children can learn as much as they do from teachers as unskilled as parents and from a curriculum as unsystematic and frequently unstimulating as parts of their lives, one might suppose they could certainly learn better from the more organized efforts of people trained in the schooling of young children. Indeed, this reasoning underlies many preschool education programs.

Research comparing children exposed to various preschool programs with children who remained in their homes has not always supported the belief that preschool education enhances cognitive, social, or emotional development (Bronfenbrenner, 1977b). Some early studies found that after participation in a preschool program, experimental children are superior in one or more

ways, but the initial differences disappear with the passage of time. These findings need not mean, of course, that preschool education is undesirable. The failure of children in experimental groups to maintain their gains might mean that the programs were not sufficiently effective; that the instruments employed to gauge the effects of preschool education have not been sensitive enough, have not measured the right things, or have done so inaccurately; or that the child's later school experiences have been less than optimal.

Later research suggests that perhaps a combination of these explanations is most valid. For example, measuring instruments have typically been intelligence tests, yet we know that it is extremely difficult to bring about significant changes in intelligence test scores. More recently, a number of studies have measured more specific abilities; for example, the Illinois Test of Psycholinguistic Ability (Kirk & McCarthy, 1961) yields scores for a number of different language abilities. In addition, researchers have looked at social development and adjustment as well as at cognitive development. General results of much of this research are far more optimistic. There is little doubt that preschool education can have markedly beneficial effects on the cognitive, social, and emotional development of children (see, for example, Belsky & Steinberg, 1979; Bronfenbrenner, 1979; Schweinhardt & Weikart, 1977).

stances. In short, preschoolers are a tremendous cognitive distance from sensorimotor children. And, as we have known for some time but have not always emphasized, their language development is nothing short of phenomenal. Its development, to which we turn next, presents a fascinating study.

■ Language and Communication

Language, despite its tremendous power, is not essential for **communication**. Animals that do not have language can communicate, sometimes remarkably effectively. The reflexive communication of danger (Hebb, 1966) is the simplest level: white-tailed deer wave their tails; pronghorn antelope bristle their rump patches; ground squirrels whistle shrilly; nesting crows pierce the air with raucous cries. These signals communicate danger to other members of the same species. Barnett (1967), in his studies of the behavior of some monkeys, has observed a similar, but more advanced, phenomenon. Baboons and other subhuman primates often mingle with herds of gazelles, apparently because the gazelle has much better vision and probably a better sense of smell than most baboons. The signals of danger that the gazelle emits are clearly meaningful for the baboon also.

In addition, there is evidence of communication between humans and lower animals. An animal trainer who instructs his dog to roll over is communicating with the animal (at least when the dog obeys—and perhaps even when the dog does not obey). The animal can also communicate with its master, as dogs frequently do when they are displeased, hungry, or otherwise agitated. As I wrote, "A dog who looks at his master, walks to his dish and barks, looks at his master again, and then begins to growl is not only dangerous but is also communicating very effectively" (Lefrancois, 1982, p. 173). This communication, however, is a far cry from that made possible by language. Even the parrot that has learned one hundred words and can say whole sentences on occasions, when those sentences are clearly appropriate, is still incapable of using language. For language involves the use of *arbitrary* sounds with established and accepted referents, either real or abstract, that can be arranged in sequence to convey different meanings. The parrot who can say "Polly wants a cracker" is not only boringly conventional but is also probably incapable of saying "Polly does not want a cracker, heh, heh," with the intention of conveying a different meaning. The parrot merely mimics; it does not communicate.

■ A Definition of Language

But a child learns to speak in time. And the learning involved is incredibly complex. To begin with, what is spoken language? We have already stated that it involves the use of arbitrary sounds that have accepted referents and that can be arranged in different ways to produce different meanings. This definition includes what R. Brown (1973) describes as the three essential characteristics of language: displacement, meaning, and productiveness.

Language involves displacement by making it possible to represent objects and events that need not be immediate—hence, that are displaced in both time and space. One of its primary functions is the communication of meaning (semanticity). Unfortunately, the meaning of the concept "meaning" is by no means clear (Clark & Clark, 1977). The meaning of a verbal expression might relate to the objects or events for which it stands, to the mental images that are evoked, to the defining characteristics of the things to which it refers, to the emotional reactions associated with its referents, or to any combination of these aspects. Although psycholinguists do not always agree about the best definition for meaning, we, in our ordinary conversations, tend to agree much more than disagree. Indeed, it is because you and I have similar meanings for words and sentences that we can communicate as we are now doing.

The third characteristic of language, productiveness, is implicit in the notion that—given a handful of words, a set of mutually accepted rules concerning the manner in which they can be combined, and agreement concerning the significance

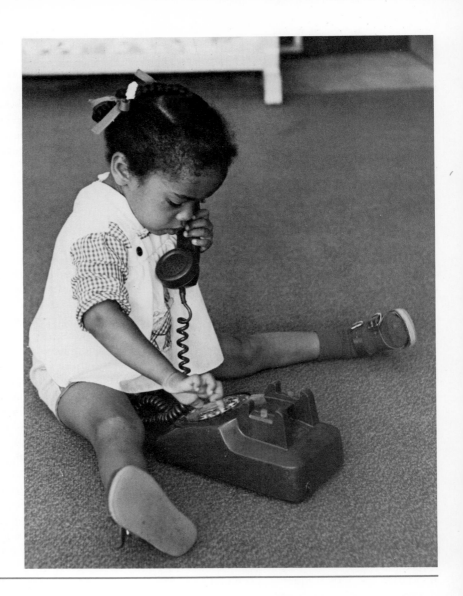

Providing we have similar meanings for sequences of voice-produced sounds, we can communicate at great distances, even with our eyes closed.

of the various pauses, intonations, and other characteristics of speech—we can, in a sense, produce meaningful language almost forever. Language presents so many possibilities for meaningful combinations that almost every day of your life you will say something that no one else has ever said in exactly the same way. Language makes you creative.

■ Elements of Language

The simplest unit of language is the **phoneme**: a single sound such as that represented by a consonant or word. There are forty-five phonemes in the English language. Phonemes can be combined to form **morphemes**, which are the units of meaning in language. Children cannot form morphemes until they can first pronounce the phonemes. Further, simply making the sound is insufficient; they must be able to make it when they intend to do so. In addition to the ability to utter words (single morphemes and morpheme combinations), the child must also acquire the ability to combine these in units. That is a large step, for there is a world of difference between being able to say "daddy," "mommy," "teddy," and "my," and turning with wide-open arms to a beaming parent and saying "my mommy" or "my daddy." Organizing words into meaningful sentence units requires an intuitive knowledge of **syntax**—or grammar, the rules governing the combinations of words that will be correct for the speakers of that language. As children practice and master phonemes, morphemes, and syntax, they must also practice **prosody**; they must learn the manners of expression, the intonations, the accents, and all the subtle variations that give different meanings to the same morphemes. Phonemes, morphemes, syntax, and prosody are the elements of language. Most of us have acquired these elements in an amazingly painless, effective, and efficient way, without really being conscious of what we were doing.

■ Language and Nonhumans

The statement has often been made that language is a uniquely human characteristic, that although animals can communicate, as was shown earlier, they do not possess language. And we have generally assumed as well that they are incapable of learning a language.

Dolphins and whales have been prime candidates for the speculation that certain mammals capable of relatively complex and varied sounds may have developed a language that we cannot understand—indeed, that we cannot even identify as a language. But extensive research now indicates that they actually have a very limited range of calls, used primarily for locating objects (including other whales and dolphins) and perhaps as unlearned expressions of a small number of emotions. There is no convincing evidence that these

calls are used in anything remotely resembling a conversation (Wardhaugh, 1976).

If any animal can learn a language, our closest biological relatives would seem most likely to do so. Early attempts to teach chimpanzees to speak were totally unsuccessful (Hayes & Hayes, 1951; Kellogg, 1968; Kellogg & Kellogg, 1933). It now seems clear that nonhuman primates are not likely to learn to *speak* a language, given the limitations of their vocal apparatus. But might they not be taught to "speak" a sign language? Perhaps—and perhaps not. (See *"Speaking" Chimpanzees?*)

■ The Development of Language in Children

Early studies of language acquisition in children concentrated on counting the number of words children had in their vocabularies at a given age. Psychologists soon found that children's passive vocabularies far exceed their active vocabularies; that is, in the early stages of language learning, children can invariably understand many more words than they can use in their own speech. It is as if knowledge were always far ahead of capabilities—and perhaps it continues in that manner throughout life.

Tables of vocabulary size provide a relatively simple guide for comparing the progress of different children, but attempting to determine the vocabulary of an individual child requires caution. Most tables are based on estimates of the child's passive vocabulary, rather than on active vocabulary, and it is exceedingly difficult to arrive at an accurate estimate of the number of words that a child knows and understands. Table 7.3 shows the average passive vocabulary of different children from the age of eight months to six years (from Smith, 1926). Smith obtained data for his study by including both the words that the children could speak and those that they showed evidence of understanding. A number of other estimates of vocabulary have been considerably higher. Smith (1941), for example, in establishing norms for the Seashore-Eckerson Vocabulary Test, found a vocabulary range between 6,000 and 48,800 words for first-grade students. The average vocabulary for this sample was 23,700 words—approximately ten times greater than the most often cited norms.

A second way of approaching early language development is by examining the *quality* of the language acquired, rather than by estimating vocabulary size at different ages. Landreth (1967) has observed that contemporary linguists treat the developing child as a fellow linguist; they examine the progression of children's knowledge of each of the elements of language, not only to learn how the child acquires the ability to use language but also to learn more about language itself.

Prespeech Stage

For convenience, language learning is frequently divided into two major stages: the prespeech stage and the speech stage; logically, the second stage follows the first. The prespeech stage involves the gradual development of meaningful speech sounds; the speech stage is best described in terms of a progression from sounds to words to grammar (Gurney, 1973).

The prespeech stage lasts from birth to about the end of the first year or the early part of the second and terminates with the utterance of single words. During this first stage, children engage in

"SPEAKING" CHIMPANZEES?

In 1966, the Gardners came up with the idea of teaching sign language to chimpanzees. They chose American Sign Language (ASL), which is used extensively by the deaf. One form of this language, that which spells out words, would obviously be very difficult for chimpanzees. A second form, however, uses various gestures, movements, and positions of the hands as symbols for words and concepts, and seems much more suitable.

Washoe, a female chimpanzee, was the first subject (Gardner & Gardner, 1969). She was kept in a trailer in the Gardners' backyard, exposed to all manner of enriching stimulation and experiences, and "spoken" to extensively in ASL. Through a combination of operant conditioning procedures that relied heavily on tickling as a reinforcer (Washoe became a tickling addict) and a "molding" technique involving physically "shaping" Washoe's hands, she succeeded in learning 38 signs in her first two years. Thus the sign for *dog* also became a sign for a picture of a dog or the sound of a bark. A year later, Washoe had mastered 85 signs, and by the age of five, she had a "vocabulary" of 160 separate signs. By then, her use of signs apparently involved a number of novel combinations, many of which appeared to have identical meanings for her. For example, when faced with a locked door, she made the signs for all of the following on different occasions: more key, gimme key, open key, gimme more key, gimme key more, open gimme key, in open help, help key in, and key help hurry (Gardner & Gardner, 1969).

Is Washoe a rare and gifted chimpanzee, capable of feats beyond the dreams of other nonhuman primates? Perhaps beyond their dreams, for we do not know of what our distant cousins dream, but maybe not beyond their capabilities. Fouts (1973) and some student volunteers taught four other chimpanzees ten ASL signs. All four learned all ten signs, although there were impressive differences in the ease with which each chimpanzee learned. The "brightest" required an average of 54 minutes per sign, the "dullest," 159.1 minutes.

Other languages are also being taught to chimpanzees. The Premacks (1972) developed a series of plastic shapes that stand for objects as well as for abstract notions such as "same as" or "different." Sarah, their chimpanzee, apparently mastered them easily. Similarly, Rumbaugh (1977) has taught a chimpanzee, Lana, to use a computer keyboard on which a number of arbitrary word characters correspond to various objects and activities. Even gorillas have entered the language-learning fray. Francine Patterson (1978) borrowed a young female gorilla, Koko, from the San Francisco Zoo and, with a number of deaf assistants who spoke only ASL, taught this gorilla more than 200 signs in twenty-nine months. By then, Koko could apparently invent new combinations for unfamiliar objects (for example, "eye hat" for mask and "white tiger" for zebra). In addition, she "talked" to herself constantly while she played.

Have these anthropoids actually learned language? Or are they like my grandmother's parrot or my cat?

three different speech-related behaviors: They cry (sometimes a great deal), they develop a repertoire of gestures, many of which are intended to communicate desires, and they practice **babbling**. (See *Universal Communication.*)

The roots of language are found in the infant's babbling; indeed, all the phonemes of every language in the world are uttered in the babbling of an infant (even in the babbling of deaf children, Lenneberg, 1969). Prior to the age of six months, the child's babbling appears unsystematic and erratic. But there is evidence that, even before the age of six months, infants can discriminate among simple sounds (Moffitt, 1971).

After the age of six months, infants' babbling becomes more systematic and more controlled. They repeat the same sounds more frequently, sometimes convincing parents and grandmothers that they can talk. "Listen to little Norbert. A child prodigy. A lot like his father," says a proud mother when she hears her son say "bah," as she hands the little tyke a new purple ball. What mother might not have noticed is that little Norbert, who is eight months old, has been practicing "bah" all afternoon.

Babbling, defined as the practicing of single sounds, is a necessary first step to acquiring language. Osgood (1957) describes the process as a circular reflex that results when children become

You see, my grandmother's parrot does not talk; it does not even communicate. It merely imitates French words that might be colorful had we not heard them so many times, always delivered in that same grating voice. Edgar, my cat, communicates exceedingly well. He rubs doors that he would like to have opened; he stares pathetically at the refrigerator when he is hungry; and when he has reason to be annoyed with the contemporary state of affairs at two o'clock in the morning, he comes leaping through the air, screeching horribly, and lands abruptly, all claws extended, on my stomach or on some other delicate part of my sleeping person. But he cannot imitate the violent French that ensues; nor can he imitate any ASL whatsoever, in spite of my most valiant efforts.

Can chimpanzees and gorillas, more gifted perhaps than our cats and parrots, actually learn and use language? The Gardners, Francine Patterson, Roger Fouts, the Premacks, and others assure us that they can. Terrace (1979a, 1979b, 1980), the Sebeoks (1979, 1980), and others say no.

Terrace, initially very impressed with ape-language research and convinced that they were capable of language, spent five years teaching a young chimpanzee ASL. He named this chimpanzee Nim Chimpsky (after the famous linguist, Noam Chomsky—himself not a believer in the language capacities of nonhuman primates). Nim, like his predecessors, quickly learned a large number of signs. But in the end, Terrace was no longer at all impressed. It appears that over 90 percent of Nim's "utterances" were direct imitations. What might otherwise have been interpreted as being sentences were, in effect, nothing more than sequences of imitations. And a careful examination of videotapes of other chimpanzees using ASL revealed that they too relied almost exclusively on direct imitation. In Terrace's words, "I could find no evidence confirming an ape's grammatical competence, either in my own data or those of others" (1979b, p. 67).

Terrace is not alone in his conclusions. Sebeok and Umiker-Sebeok (1980) present a devastating criticism of ape-language claims, arguing that ape language is almost entirely direct imitation and that what has been interpreted as evidence of humor or teasing is simply erroneous. Most of the ape's sequences of signs are nonsensical rather than meaningful. Both the Sebeoks and Terrace argue that the sole purpose of the chimpanzee's signing is not to communicate meaning but to obtain a reward that cannot be obtained another way. What the chimpanzee has learned is not language, but a relatively elaborate series of imitations that, on the whole, might not be much more impressive than the bar-pressing of the hungry Skinnerian rat or the fridge-door rubbing of my Edgar.

The ape-language controversy remains a controversy; it cannot be resolved here. If apes can learn a language, we might learn about language from them. If they cannot, then the ape-language studies might not reveal much.

Table 7.3 The early growth of vocabulary in children.

Age (years–months)	Average Number of Words
0–8	0
0–10	1
1–0	3
1–3	19
1–6	22
1–9	118
2–0	272
2–6	446
3–0	896
3–6	1,222
4–0	1,540
4–6	1,870
5–0	2,072
5–6	2,289
6–0	2,562

From M. E. Smith, An investigation of the development of the sentence and the extent of vocabulary in young children. *University of Iowa Studies in Child Welfare*, 1926, Vol. 3, No. 5.

capable of responding to their own vocalizations. Children emit a sound, hear it, and repeat it because they hear it; as they repeat it, they hear it again and are again moved to repeat it. Thus, the babbling of young children is a monotonous repetition of the same sound, with occasional accidental variations—but it is through this repetition that children acquire control over the sounds that compose the language they must master. Whether this circular process is the manifestation of a primitive tendency to imitate, or whether there is some reinforcement involved in the process, or both, remains unclear.

The foregoing description illustrates the problem of determining when infants say their first word. Such expressions as "bah," when they come to *mean* something for the child, may be considered words (termed *holophrases*). However, most infants repeat a sound such as "bah" many times before it becomes associated with an object. The point at which the sound "bah" ceases to be babble and becomes a *word* (*ball*, for example) is nearly impossible to determine. Somewhere near the age of one year, children do utter their first meaningful

words, frequently created by repeating two identical sounds, such as in "mama," "dada," or "bye bye." The appearance of the first word is rapidly followed by new words that the child practices incessantly. But even prior to acquiring this facility with single words, infants have begun to show signs that they understand much more than they can say—words that will not be part of their active vocabulary for some time, as well as entire sentences. "Stick out your tongue," a child is told by a proud parent, and out comes the tongue. "Show daddy your hand," and the hand appears. "Can you wink?" Sure can. Two eyes, though.

Children continue to acquire words during the second year, but the range of syllables available to them is limited. Many of their words are one- or two-syllable words, which often repeat the same syllable in different combinations. For example, the child says "mommy," "daddy," "baby," "seepy" (sleepy), "horsy," and "doggy." Even when it is incorrect to do so, the child may frequently repeat the syllable in a one-syllable word, as in "car car" or "kiss kiss." In a comic, unintelligent, and frequently unconscious attempt to communicate with their children, parents sometimes exaggerate the trivial errors committed by their infants in the course of learning to speak. The result is occasionally something like, "Wou my itsy bitsy witta baby come to momsy womsy?" But there is no evidence that parental models of this type hinder the acquisition of language. In the early stages, the warmth of the interaction may be more important than the nature of the language employed.

Most of an English-speaking child's first words are nouns—simple names for simple things. Verbs, adjectives, adverbs, and prepositions are acquired primarily in the order listed, with the greatest difficulty usually having to do with pronouns, especially the pronoun *I*.

Speech Stage

The space between the appearance of the first meaningful speech sound and the production of adultlike sentences involves what might seem to be an overwhelming amount of learning. Yet it is

UNIVERSAL COMMUNICATION: SMILES AND TEARS

We have noted that nonhuman animals communicate, although they do not use language. We are more gifted; we employ language to communicate. But could we communicate if we had no language?

Probably. And interestingly, if we were to communicate without language, I might find it considerably easier to let a Bedouin or a Hindu know that I am happy, displeased, ashamed, or angry than is now the case. Eibl-Eibesfeldt (1974) and Morris (1977), two of a number of researchers currently investigating the emerging field of ethology (the study of innate behavior patterns), provide evidence to support this notion. They identify a wide range of human expressions and gestures that are common across cultures (they have identical meanings in these cultures) and that, consequently, are probably largely unaffected by learning. Crying, smiling, frowning, raising the eyebrows, bowing the head, kissing, and laughing are but a few of these. Everywhere and at all times, smiling signifies happiness or agreement; crying signifies sorrow or hurt. We need no language to use and to understand these symbols. Indeed, Eibl-Eibesfeldt reports that children born deaf and blind make use of these same gestures, although they can never have observed them. Blind children, for example, have been seen covering their faces with their hands when embarrassed.

accomplished relatively easily by almost all children and in the short space of two or three years. Adults who are initially without language do not fare nearly so well, an observation that has led to the belief that there is a "sensitive" period for language acquisition highly reminiscent of the critical periods that govern the development of attachment behaviors and imprinting among some animals and birds.

The development of speech and the acquisition of grammar have been extensively investigated in recent years, not only by linguists and semanticists, whose primary concern is with language itself, but also by psychologists, whose concerns include the role of language in intellectual functioning—hence the term *psycholinguistics*.

For convenience, the acquisition of language is described here in terms of the six sequential stages suggested by Wood (1976; see Table 7.4).

The Sentencelike Word   Some time after the sixth month (usually around the age of one), children utter their first meaningful word. This word's meaning is seldom limited to one event, action, or person, but may mean a great variety of different things—hence the term *holophrase*. Furthermore, besides being a word that might have many meanings, it also appears to function as many different parts of speech: nouns, verbs, or entire phrases. McNeill (1970) suggests that children's knowledge of grammar is innate, that they have notions of grammar long before they arrive at an understanding of how to express different grammatical forms in adultlike ways. Thus, although most holophrases refer to nouns, they are not used simply for naming. When a child says "milk," she might mean, "There is the milk." She might also mean, "Give me some milk," "I'm thirsty," or, "Are you finally going out to milk the cow?" A simple preposition such as "on," employed as a holophrase by my youngest linguist, meant "Turn the light on," "Pick me up," "Put me on the chair," "Dress me," "Daddy is nice," and many other things.

Modification   Not surprisingly, the progression of speech development is from one word to two, then three, and more (Boyd, 1976). By the age of eighteen months, single-word holophrases begin to merge as two-word sentences. Bloom (1973) suggests that this process begins slowly, with the relatively hesitant combining of familiar words, but that their use increases very rapidly once the child begins to understand the number of meanings that can be conveyed with two-word sentences. Speech at this stage is sometimes described as being telegraphic, since it eliminates

Table 7.4 Six stages in children's syntactic development.

Stage of Development	Nature of Development	Sample Utterances
1. Sentencelike word	The word is combined with nonverbal cues (gestures and inflections).	"Mommy." "Mommy!" "Mommy?"
2. Modification	Modifiers are joined to topic words to form declarative, question, negative, and imperative structures.	"Pretty baby." (declarative) "Where Daddy?" (question) "No play." (negative) "More milk!" (imperative)
3. Structure	Both a subject and predicate are included in the sentence types.	"She's a pretty baby." (declarative) "Where Daddy is?" (question) "I no can play." (negative) "I want more milk!" (imperative)
4. Operational changes	Elements are added, embedded, and permuted within sentences.	"Read it, my book." (conjunction) "Where is Daddy?" (embedding) "I can't play." (permutation)
5. Categorization	Word classes (nouns, verbs, and prepositions) are subdivided.	"I would like *some* milk." (use of "some" with mass noun) "Take me *to* the store." (use of preposition of place)
6. Complex structures	Complex structural distinctions made, as with "ask-tell" and "promise."	"Ask what time it is." "He promised to help her."

From Barbara S. Wood, *Children and communication: Verbal and nonverbal language development.* © 1976, p. 148. Reprinted by permission of Prentice-Hall, Inc., Englewood Cliffs, New Jersey.

a great many parts of speech while still managing to convey meanings. "Dog allgone" is a two-word utterance "telegraphed" from the lengthier adult equivalent, "The dog is not here right now."

Whether or not precise grammatical functions can be accurately assigned to these two-word utterances is a matter of some debate. The functions of the words *fish* and *eat* in the two-word utterance "fish eat" are, in fact, dependent upon the intended meaning. But since the child does not employ number agreement (for example, "fish eats" to mean "the fish eats" and "fish eat" to mean "I eat fish") or order ("eat fish" versus "fish eat") to signal meaning, the psycholinguist can never be certain that children at this stage are aware of grammatical functions (Clark & Clark, 1977).

Structure In time, children move from two-word combinations to multiple-word sentences. This typically occurs around the age of two to two and one-half. "Allgone dog" becomes "Dog is gone" and eventually "The dog is gone" or "My dog is gone." The significance of this transition from a linguistic point of view is that it requires the use of complete subjects and predicates. The grammatical sophistication of three- or four-word combinations, as they are employed at this stage, far outdoes that of earlier two-word combinations.

There is evidence of inventiveness as well in the child's use of speech at this stage. Carlson and Anisfeld (1969) report the case of a twenty-nine-month-old boy who deliberately and playfully manipulated phonemes in songs and rhymes. To the tune "the bear went over the mountain," he sang "Da de de doder da doundin," and for "I've been working on the railroad," he sang "I pin purkin' on a pail poad." Indeed, examples of inventiveness abound in the speech of many children, as in that of my middle linguist who, having learned that "pitch black" is very black, insisted that other things can be "pitch clean," "pitch empty," or "pitch big."

Operational Changes   Between the ages of two and one-half and three or four, children begin to acquire some of the more complex aspects of syntax. In particular, they develop the ability to make meaningful *transformations*. These typically take one of three forms: *conjunction, embedding,* or *permutation* (Wood, 1976). Simple conjunction is illustrated by the addition or combination of the two sentences "Where?" and "We go" to form a third sentence, "Where we go?" Embedding involves inserting. For example, the word *no* may be embedded in the sentence "I eat" to form a sentence with quite a different meaning: "I no eat." Permutation involves altering the order of words in sentences in order to change their meaning. Initially, children make use of inflection rather than permutation. For example, the sentence "I can go" may be a simple declaration when the "I" or the "can" is inflected, but becomes a question when "go" is inflected. A simple permutation from "I can go" to "Can I go?" achieves the same meaning with considerably less ambiguity.

Categorization   As children begin to manifest an understanding of various adult-accepted rules for transforming sentences, they also behave as though they had an implicit understanding of the grammatical functions of various words and phrases. That is, they employ nouns as nouns and not as verbs, adjectives are no longer treated as verbs, and nouns are further categorized as plural or singular. Evidence of children's understanding of this type of categorization is provided by their appropriate use of verbs and of such determiners as *that, the, those,* and *these.* For example, the child will now say "That box is empty"; an earlier error might have taken the form of "This boxes is empty."

Complex Structures   The further refinement and elaboration of speech requires mastery of countless subtle and intricate grammatical rules that we all employ unconsciously (termed **phrase structure** and **transformational rules**). For example, we know the distinction between "I asked him to go," "I told him to go," and "I ordered him to go." The younger child does not. Much of this learning occurs in the first elementary grades.

Phrase structure rules govern the arrangement of words in meaningful expressions; they specify what is and is not grammatically acceptable and meaningful. Transformational rules are the grammatical rules that permit us to transform the structure of phrases, to combine them, and to make a variety of meaningful statements. A transformational rule is what allows us to transform a passive sentence into an active one ("The dog was bitten by the man" to "The man bit the dog") or a negative to a positive ("I did not go" to "I went").

■ Explanations of Language Development

Each of us uses language as though we had a complete, albeit unconscious, understanding of a great variety of phrase structure and transformational rules. Initially, children have no understanding of these rules and speak as though they had none. But in an amazingly short time, they acquire functional knowledge of an incredibly complex grammar. We have been able to describe some of the details of the sequence of language acquisition, but can we explain how and why children learn language?

Learning Theory

A behavioristic model of language acquisition was quite popular at one time (Skinner, 1957). In essence, this theory maintains that language learning comes about through reinforcement of the child's spontaneous verbal utterances and through imitation. The simple observation that children acquire the speech patterns, idioms, accents, and other language characteristics of the models that surround them lends direct support to this theory. But a number of observations cannot easily be explained employing a behavioristic model. For example, Lenneberg (1969) found that children of deaf and speechless parents babble in much the same way and in the same general sequences as other children. He also reports that he has found no cases of these children not developing standard

English in much the same way as normal children. His studies of human sounds in groups of children whose mothers were deaf and comparisons of these children with others whose mothers were normal led him to the conclusion that the early appearance of human sounds is unaffected by parental influence. Note, however, that this conclusion applies to the *earliest* development of human sounds, not to the development of an understanding of the language.

Imitation and reinforcement theories are most clearly inadequate as explanations for the child's acquisition of syntax. As Chomsky (1972) notes, children make few grammatical errors that they could have learned through direct imitation, but they make a great many that are not only novel but predictable. When children say "I dood," "I runned," or "I eated," it is not because the adults around them make those errors, but because of a budding understanding of grammatical rules. These errors provide far more impressive evidence of the child's linguistic capabilities than they would if they were based entirely on imitation. This, of course, does not mean that imitation is not involved in language learning, but it does indicate that imitation does not provide an entirely adequate explanation.

LAD: Language Acquisition Device

Chomsky (1957, 1965) has advanced a theory to account for the child's acquisition of syntax—a theory that has attracted a great deal of attention but has not been verified or disproved. Partly because of children's incredibly rapid acquisition of grammatical rules during their third and fourth years, and partly because none of the conventional explanations of learning seem to account adequately for this acquisition, Chomsky has suggested that children are born with a previously established neurological something (labeled a **Language Acquisition Device**, LAD, or an Acquisition Machine) that corresponds to grammar. Because this something is already present, it facilitates learning grammar and explains why children make only a fraction of all possible errors while learning syntax.

As noted earlier, children frequently make grammatical errors that they could not possibly have heard; imitation is therefore not an adequate explanation. Children may say, for example, "It doos" for "It does," because they have invented a rule that says adding the sound "s" to any verb makes it appropriate for a third-person subject—and the children's syntactical rule, clever little linguists that they are, admits of no exceptions. Similarly, they say: "I sayed," for "I said," "It goed" for "It went," and "I runned" for "I ran." In many ways, these young linguists are more consistent than the language. "Mistakes" are logical errors resulting from irregularities in the language rather than from the misapplication of rules (Slobin, 1972).

Whether LAD is responsible or whether there is another explanation, by the time children have reached the age of five, their intuitive understanding of the grammar of their language will be sufficient to handle any verbal situation. Given the complex structure of language, this understanding ranks among the higher accomplishments of our young humans.

A Theory of Mother-Infant Interaction

In Chapter 6 we speak of the bidirectionality of parent-child influence, noting that although it may be quite obvious that what a mother does influences her infant, it is no less true that what the infant does influences the mother. Bruner (1977, 1978) supplies evidence of bidirectionality of influence in the development of language as well. It seems fairly clear that imitation is involved in the acquisition of langauge. If this were not the case, we would be as likely to learn Ilocano or Karelian rather than the langauge of our parents. What has not been clear until recently is that the infant's level of language comprehension and use has subtle but marked effects on the behavior of parents. In this connection, Bruner (1978) refers to a "fine-tuning" theory of mother-infant interaction. His observations of mothers and their children lead him to the conclusion that virtually all mothers alter their speech patterns in accordance with the understanding of their children. It is as

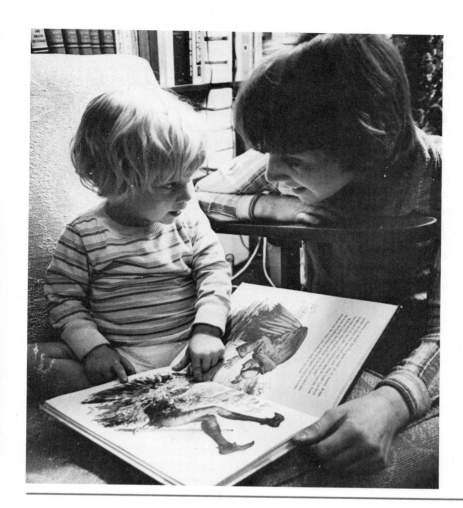

Parents become teachers, often unconsciously, by fine-tuning their questions and responses to their child's interests and level of understanding.

though the mother becomes a teacher, not because she consciously intends to be but because she "fine-tunes" her responses and behaviors to the immediate demands of her child. Furthermore, the mother's altered speech patterns are consistent and regular. One mother typically employed four sequential types of statements when reading to her young son. First she would say "look": an attention-getting utterance. Next she would pose a standard question—"What is that?"—pause, and provide a label: "It's an X." Finally, following the child's response, she would say, "That's right." Additional evidence of fine-tuning occurred whenever the child

responded earlier in the sequence. If, for example, he said "truck" as the page turned, the mother would go immediately to her final response: "That's right."

In later stages of language development, the role of the mother as a sensitive, fine-tuned teacher becomes even more apparent. Boyd (1976) notes that the language that mothers employ when talking to their children is quite different from what they would normally employ when speaking with adults. Thus mothers tend to use simpler, shorter, and more repetitive utterances. In other words, they *reduce* (by simplifying and repeating). On other occasions, mothers *expand* the child's expressions. For example, a child might say, "Daddy gone," to which the mother might reply, "Yes, Daddy is gone."

There are other, perhaps more subtle, ways in which the speech of the mother (or other caretakers, as well as siblings) is influenced by the presence of infants. Moskowitz (1978) describes typical caretaker speech as simpler and higher pitched than normal and characterized by exaggerated intonation, short sentences, and a higher than normal percentage of questions. In addition, the speech of caretakers with their infants is almost always concerned only with the here and now and seldom with the past or future, almost as though they knew, with Piaget, that the young infant's world is a world of the *here and now*. Accordingly, as Goodwin (1980) suggests, we would expect that most of the child's first words would deal with things that are immediate and directly perceivable. This expectation is supported by Bloom's (1970) observation that early vocabularies consist primarily of words that deal with physical properties of objects (big, small, heavy), with reward and punishment (bad, good, careful), and with actions (open, give).

In the absence of caretaker-infant verbal interaction, language is unlikely to develop as it normally would. Moskowitz (1978) reports the case of a normal child whose parents were deaf but who spent a considerable amount of time watching television. At the age of three, this child could understand and speak sign language but neither spoke nor understood any English.

In summary, growing evidence suggests that the mother (or father) plays a crucial role in the development of language and that this role goes well beyond that of providing a suitable model of the family's language. Unconsciously, parents modify their speech and become teachers—perhaps far better teachers than they could possibly be trained to be. As Moskowitz (1978) observes, the level of a mother's language usage appears to remain relatively constant at a stage very close to six months in advance of where the child is. From birth, there is an "interpersonal synchrony" (Schaffer, Collis, & Parsons, 1977) between mother and infant;

research has scarcely begun to explore the nature and dimensions of this synchrony. (See *Additional Findings in Language Development*.)

■ Partial Summary

If we summarize all available knowledge about the child's acquisition of language, we merely have the suggestion of the beginning of an answer. We have succeeded (we do not know how accurately) in counting the number of phonemes, morphemes, words, and sentences that a child knows at every age; we have described the specific characteristics of these elements of language; and we have noted reassuring regularities in the sequence in which different children (even from different cultures) acquire language (Slobin, 1970). In the process we have discovered that children appear to reinvent the grammar of language as they learn it, because ample evidence shows that they do not learn syntax through imitation. At the same time, their reinvention of grammar appears to have shortcuts for, as Chomsky points out, they make many fewer errors than we might expect. The greatest mystery of the intrinsically mysterious process of acquiring language is our inability to explain how children make such extraordinary progress, particularly between their second and fifth years. How do they invent grammar? Is Chomsky's conjecture of a prewired, neurological mechanism (Language Acquisition Device) correct? Or do patterns of grammar fall from heaven?

Table 7.5 presents a summary of language development to age four. Lenneberg (1967) describes the normal sequence of motor development as parallel to language acquisition. He deliberately juxtaposes the two to convey the close relationship between the development of motor capabilities and acquisition of language—a relationship that some have interpreted as evidence of a biological basis for language learning. Lenneberg, Nichols, and Rosenberger (1964) support this interpretation, based on their examination of the language and motor development of sixty-one Down's syndrome children, aged two to twenty-two years. One of their striking observations was

ADDITIONAL FINDINGS
IN LANGUAGE DEVELOPMENT

Psychological and psycholinguistic research is replete with isolated findings in language acquisition. Some of the more interesting and potentially useful of these are listed briefly here.

Sex Differences In a number of investigations, girls appear to have a slight edge in learning language. For example, it has been reported that they learn to speak at an earlier age than boys (Templin, 1957) and that they frequently articulate better and have fewer speech defects (Johnson, Brown, Curtis, Edney, & Keaster, 1948). These observations have been explained by the assumption that a girl has more intimate interaction with her mother than a boy; because fathers are frequently away from home more than mothers, it is reasonable to expect that girls would be slightly accelerated in learning language. The supposed linguistic superiority of girls has been widely reported in psychological literature and is frequently employed as one example of a clear male-female difference (Maccoby & Jacklin, 1974). However, research results in this area are often contradictory; observed differences are often so slight as to be totally insignificant, and a careful analysis of available evidence strongly suggests that no reliable sex differences in language exist (Macaulay, 1977).

Twins Evidence indicates that twins are sometimes retarded in language development (McCarthy, 1954). First, they do not receive as much individual attention from their mother as would a single child; in addition, twins seem to develop a private jargon and a gesture vocabulary; hence they have less incentive to invent syntax or to learn vocabulary.

Stuttering Stuttering in young children is not abnormal; it is highly common among three- and four-year-olds. It is generally accepted that, throughout most of the early years of language acquisition, children's cognitive ability is somewhat ahead of their language facility (Petretic & Tweney, 1977; Sachs & Truswell, 1978). Therefore, they frequently want to say things that they cannot quite articulate or find that their words come more slowly than they wish. This is particularly evident when a child becomes tense or excited. Bloodstein (1960) notes that if parents are patient and accept the child's behavior without drawing undue attention to it, the stuttering will eventually disappear completely.

that when the children were still crawling, regardless of age, they were usually at the babbling stage in their language development. And when they had begun to walk, they had also begun to talk. For these children, as for normal children, simple motor development and language development seem closely allied. This provides additional support for the belief that various aspects of biological and intellectual development, including the learning of language, may be influenced by genetic principles. In short, the sequence and the nature of locomotion and language learning in humans appear to be highly predictable. But here, as elsewhere in child development, there are exceptions to the average behavior ascribed to the non-existent average child.

■ Language and Thought

The significance of language acquisition for children is in many respects obvious. Not only does language allow children to direct the behavior of others in accordance with their wishes (as when children ask for something), it also provides a means for acquiring information that would otherwise be inaccessible (as when children ask questions, listen to stories, or watch television). In addition, there is considerable evidence that language is closely implicated in logical thought processes, although the exact relationship between thinking and language remains uncertain. One extreme position, first elaborated by Whorf (1941, 1956) (and therefore labeled the Whorfian hypothesis),

Table 7.5 Milestones in motor and language development.

At the Completion of	Motor Development	Vocalization and Language
12 weeks	Supports head when in prone position; weight is on elbows; hands mostly open; no grasp reflex.	Markedly less crying than at eight weeks; when talked to and nodded at, smiles, followed by squealing gurgling sounds usually called *cooing*, which is vowel-like in character and pitch-modulated; sustains cooing for fifteen to twenty seconds.
16 weeks	Plays with a rattle placed in hands (by shaking it and staring at it); head self-supported; tonic neck reflex subsiding.	Responds to human sounds more definitely; turns head; eyes seem to search for speaker; occasionally some chuckling sounds.
20 weeks	Sits with props.	The vowel-like cooing sounds begin to be interspersed with more consonantal sounds: labial fricatives, spirants, and nasals are common; acoustically, all vocalizations are very different from the sounds of the mature language of the environment.
6 months	Sitting; bends forward and uses hands for support; can bear weight when put into standing position, but cannot yet stand with holding on; reaching; unilateral; grasp; no thumb apposition yet; releases cube when given another.	Cooing changing into babbling resembling one-syllable utterances; neither vowels nor consonants have very fixed recurrences; most common utterances sound somewhat like *ma, mu, da,* or *di.*
8 months	Stands holding on; grasps with thumb apposition; picks up pellet with thumb and fingertips.	Reduplication (or more continuous repetitions) becomes frequent; intonation patterns become distinct; utterances can signal emphasis and emotions.
10 months	Creeps efficiently; takes sidesteps, holding on; pulls to standing position.	Vocalizations are mixed with sound play such as gurgling or bubble blowing; appears to wish to imitate sounds, but the imitations are never quite successful; beginning to differentiate between words heard by making differential adjustment.
12 months	Walks when held by one hand; walks on feet and hands—knees in air; mouthing of objects almost stopped; seats self on floor.	Identical sound sequences are replicated with higher relative frequency of occurrence, and words (*mamma* or *dadda*) are emerging; definite signs of understanding some words and simple commands.
18 months	Grasp, prehension, and release fully developed; gait stiff, propulsive, and precipitated; sits on child's chair with only fair aim; creeps downstairs backward; has difficulty building tower of three cubes.	Has a definite repertoire of words—more than three but less than fifty; still much babbling but now of several syllables with intricate intonation pattern; no attempt at communicating information and no frustration for not being understood; words may include items such as *thank you* or *come here*, but there is little ability to join any of the lexical items into spontaneous two-item phrases; understanding is progressing rapidly.
24 months	Runs, but falls in sudden turns; can quickly alternate between sitting and standing: walks stairs up or down, one foot forward only.	Vocabulary of more than fifty items (some children seem to be able to name everything in environment); begins spontaneously to join vocabulary items into two-word phrases; all phrases appear to be own creations; definite increase in communicative behavior and interest in language.

Table 7.5 *(continued)*

At the Completion of	Motor Development	Vocalization and Language
30 months	Jumps up into air with both feet; stands on one foot for about two seconds; takes few steps on tiptoe; jumps from chair; good hand and finger coordination; can move digits independently; manipulation of objects much improved; builds tower of six cubes.	Fastest increase in vocabulary, with many new additions every day; no babblings at all; utterances have communicative intent; frustrated if not understood by adults; utterances consist of at least two words, many have three or even five words; sentences and phrases have characteristic child grammar—that is, they are rarely verbatim repetitions of an adult utterance; intelligibility is not very good yet, though there is great variation among children; seems to understand everything that is said to him or her.
3 years	Tiptoes three yards; runs smoothly with acceleration and deceleration; negotiates sharp and fast curves without difficulty; walks stairs by alternating feet; jumps twelve inches; can operate a tricycle.	Vocabulary of some one thousand words; about 80 percent of utterances are intelligible even to strangers; grammatical complexity of utterances is roughly that of colloquial adult language, although mistakes still occur.
4 years	Jumps over rope; hops on right foot; catches ball in arms; walks line.	Language is well established; deviations from the adult norm tend to be more in style than in grammar.

From Eric H. Lenneberg, *Biological foundations of language.* Copyright 1967 by John Wiley & Sons, Inc., New York. Used by permission of John Wiley & Sons, Inc.

maintains that language is necessary for thinking. This position is based on the assumption that all thinking is verbal and that thought is therefore limited to what is made possible by language. Given ample evidence of thinking in nonverbal animals as well as in infants, however, this extreme position is not tenable. Nor is the opposite extreme plausible: namely, that thought precedes language and is necessary for it. The best conclusion at this time is probably that thinking and language are extremely closely related and often interdependent (see de Villiers & de Villiers, 1978).

Numerous experiments and observations link language and thought. For example, my grandmother was amazingly gifted when it came to identifying cows. She knew all her cows (and their genealogy) as well as the neighbors' cows, but she was completely incapable of learning to distinguish among the various pigs that roamed about the place. Indeed, she could not even tell the difference between her pigs and pigs that belonged to other farmers, a shortcoming that occasionally got her into difficulty. Now cows come in greater variety of sizes, shapes, and conformations than do pigs. Furthermore, they frequently sport a great many colors. Pigs, however, seem to come in fewer sizes and shapes, and most of them have been endowed with the same uninteresting color. All of this should make it considerably easier to distinguish among cows than among pigs.

As it happened, however, most of the cows with whom my grandmother was so familiar were ordinary black cows—that all seemed to me to be almost the same size. In contrast, there were indeed big pigs, small pigs, black pigs, reddish pigs, spotted pigs, and ordinary tan pigs. Add all the possible combinations of size and color and there were a large number of very different-looking pigs. Grandmother suspects that the cows could be distinguished because they had names. How in heaven could one mistake Bessie for Rosie? And how could a body be expected to know that the large black boar belonged to Old Man Taylor, despite the fact that he was the only one who owned black pigs?

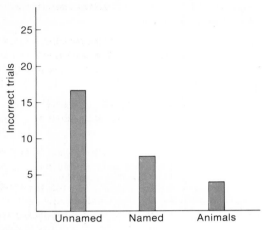

Figure 7.4
The median number of incorrect trials before choosing the correct stimulus four consecutive times. The results illustrate that verbalization facilitates learning. (Based on data provided by Marjorie Pyles Honzik, Verbalization as a factor in learning. *Child Development*, 1932, *3*, 108–113. Copyright 1932 by The Society for Research in Child Development. Used by permission of The Society for Research in Child Development and the author.)

Grandmother was probably right, as Pyles Honzik (1932) has demonstrated. She presented eighty children, aged two to seven, with the simple task of learning to differentiate among five objects, just as grandmother had successfully learned to discriminate among a large number of cows (although she had been unsuccessful in learning to distinguish a smaller number of pigs). All the children had to do was to select the correct object to obtain the toy hidden under it. In one situation, the stimuli were five familiar animal forms, each labeled appropriately by the experimenter. The second variation employed five unnamed and unfamiliar forms (corresponding to the pigs). In the third variation, the objects were also unfamiliar but were named (corresponding to the cows, and with names that were almost as meaningful as the names of most cows I have known: Mobie, Kolo, Tito, Gamie, and Bokie). The subjects were shown each of the three variations until they chose the correct stimulus object four consecutive times, thus

showing evidence of having "learned," or until twenty-five trials were completed.

The results of the experiment support my grandmother's hypothesis (see Figure 7.4), demonstrating clearly that learning was much easier with familiar objects whose names were already well known by the subjects. Also, giving names to unfamiliar objects greatly increases the ease with which these can be distinguished from one another. Thus only 54 percent of the sample successfully solved the unfamiliar-object, no-name condition, whereas 72 percent of the subjects chose the correct stimulus when the objects were given names. Pyles Honzik (1932) concludes from this study that verbalization facilitates learning.

Bernstein (1958, 1961), who attributes the inferior school achievement of children from disadvantaged homes to their language, also links language and thoughts. Following extensive studies of speech patterns of children, Bernstein (1958) concluded that some parents use what he terms **restricted**, as opposed to **elaborated, language codes.** Hypothetical examples of each are given below:

Restricted Language Code

Mother:	*Clean your feet.*
Child:	*Why?*
Mother:	*Because.*
Child:	*Because what?*
Mother:	*I said clean your feet, that's why.*
Child:	*But why clean my feet?*

Elaborated Language Code

Mother:	*Blow your nose, Henry. It is about to drip on the carpet.*
Child:	*Why you don't want it to drip on the carpet, Mom? Why, Mom? Why you don't want it to drip?*
Mother:	*Because it's messy, Henry, and we must keep the carpet clean for when Daddy comes home, because Dad doesn't like to have nose drips all over the carpet.*

In summarizing his findings, Bernstein (1958) observed that restricted language has the follow-

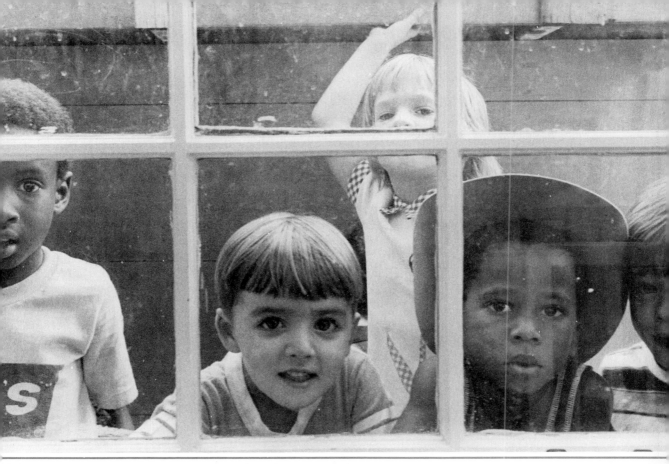

Language is the great binding force of all cultures, but children are more concerned with simple communication than with binding cultures.

ing characteristics: It is employed to control or to express emotion rather than to rationalize or to express information; it tends to be less personal despite the use of the first person; it is global and imprecise; it tends to be liberally sprinkled with idiom and colloquialism; sentences are typically exceedingly short, frequently grammatically incorrect, and often incomplete; and gestures and other forms of communication are frequently used in place of language. To the extent that this analysis is accurate, it is little wonder that children whose homes are characterized by restricted language codes often find themselves at a disadvantage in school. For the first time in their lives, they are required to use increasingly precise and gram-

matically correct forms of expression, and they are placed in a situation in which they inevitably begin by performing less well than those who have been more fortunate in their early language experiences. Perhaps before they have had a chance to catch up, they will find themselves so far behind that they will feel it is hardly worth trying.

■ Communicating and Conversing

Language is more than a collection of sounds, combinations of which refer to objects and actions, and the expression of which conveys our meanings. It is also more than a means by which we think and express our thoughts. More than all this, language is the means by which we draw information from past generations, record our own small contributions, and pass them on to generations that will come later. It is the great binding force of all cultures.

But the infant, newly learning language, is not concerned with its great cultural contributions. The first concern is with communicating. No more. And the first communications are simple assertions (that dog; see daddy; my ball) or requests (milk! more candy) (Clark & Clark, 1977). And the second concern is with conversation.

A conversation is an exchange typically involving two or more people, although some people do talk to themselves. It is generally verbal, although it can consist of a combination of gestures and verbalization, or it can consist entirely of gestures, as in the case of ASL. Genuine conversational exchanges begin at around the age of two. Initially, they are highly telegraphic, as is the child's speech; there are not a great many variations possible when one's sentences are limited to a single word. A short excerpt from an intelligent conversation with one of my own illustrates this:

Him: *Fish.*
Me: *Fish?*

Him: *Fish!*
Me: *Fish? Fish swim.*
Him: *Fish! Fish! (the conversation becomes more complex)*
Me: *There are fish in the lake. (an original thought, meant to stimulate creativity)*
Him: *Fish. (pointing, this time, in the general direction of the lake—I think)*

From this primitive, repetitive conversation, children progress to more complex expressions and begin to learn the importance of subtle cues involving intonation, accentuation of words, rhythm of sentences, tone, and accompanying gestures. And they learn, as well, about the implicit agreements that govern our conversations—the well-accepted rules that determine who shall speak and when, whether interruptions are permissible and how they should occur, the information that must be included in our conversations if we are to be understood, and what we can assume is already known. In other words, they learn, as Krauss and Glucksberg (1977) put it, the rudiments of *social* as opposed to *nonsocial* or egocentric speech.

Thus, more or less, does the infant progress from a sound to a word, from one word to two, from an expression to a conversation, from a conversation to a book. . . .

■ MAIN POINTS

1 Piaget describes the preschool period in terms of two substages of the preoperational period: the first, from age two to four, is labeled *preconceptual;* the second, from four to seven, is termed *intuitive.*

2 Preconceptual thinking is marked by the inability to understand simple classification and by transductive reasoning.

3 Intuitive thinking is characterized by egocentricity, by a limited ability to classify, and by a marked reliance on perception.

4 Life is children's only curriculum until they reach school age; they learn to adapt through their experiences.

5 Research on the effects of preschool education with respect to the cognitive, social, and emotional development of children is not always clear, given the short-term nature of some of the programs as well as measurement problems. In general, however, these results are positive.

6 Language is not necessary for communication, as evidenced by the behavior of many animals. However, it helps a lot.

7 Language may be defined in terms of three characteristics: <u>displacement, meaning, and productiveness.</u>

8 The simplest units of language are *phonemes;* meaningful sounds are termed *morphemes. Syntax* describes the rules that govern the production of meaningful sequences of sounds (in other words, grammar). Meaning is also a function of *prosody* (intonation, inflection, pauses) as well as of context.

9 Chimpanzees and gorillas have not been successfully taught to speak English (or any other spoken language), but they are being taught some aspects of American Sign Language (ASL). There is some controversy about whether they have actually learned a language or whether they have simply learned to imitate.

10 Children say their first words somewhere between nine and fifteen months of age—some sooner, some later.

11 The child's early babbling is usually unsystematic. After the age of six months, however, there is more controlled repetition. By the age of one, babbling declines rapidly and soon disappears.

12 There is evidence that children reinvent the grammar (syntax) of their language as they learn it.

13 The acquisition of syntax is incompletely explained by theories of learning or imitation. Chomsky, McNeill, and others believe that we are genetically predisposed to learn a language.

14 The mother plays an important role as language teacher, her speech patterns being strongly influenced, sometimes in subtle ways, by the presence of an infant.

15 There appears to be a close relationship between language and thinking.

■ FURTHER READINGS

The following three references discuss Piaget's description of the preschool child. The first is a highly comprehensive description of Piaget's work. The second and third present somewhat simpler accounts of Piaget's theoretical formulations:
Falvell, J. H. *The developmental psychology of Jean Piaget.* New York: Van Nostrand, 1963.
Ginsberg, H., & Opper, S. *Piaget's theory of intellectual development* (2nd ed.). Englewood Cliffs, N.J.: Prentice-Hall, 1978.
Singer, D. G., & Revenson, T. A. *How a child thinks: A Piaget primer.* New York: New American Library, 1978.

For an excellent collection of (mostly) highly readable articles covering the effects of early experiences and ranging from descriptions of children reared in isolation to preschool intervention programs, see:
Clarke, A. M., & Clarke, A. D. B. (Eds.). *Early experience: Myth and evidence.* London: Open Books, 1976.

For an analysis of the relationships between thought and language, see:
Greene, J. *Thinking and language.* London: Methuen, 1975.

The early development of language in infants is well described in:
Bloom, L. *One word at a time: The use of single word utterances before syntax.* The Hague: Mouton, 1973.
Brown, R. *A first language: The early stages.* Cambridge, Mass.: Harvard University Press, 1973.

Studies of mother-infant interaction are presented in the following collection of readings. Five selections deal specifically with communication:
Schaffer, H. R. (Ed.). *Studies in mother-infant interaction.* London: Academic Press, 1977.

Two textbooks currently representative of the field of psycholinguistics provide considerably more detail than is possible in a single chapter:
Clark, H. H., & Clark, E. V. *Psychology and language: An introduction to psycholinguistics.* New York: Harcourt Brace Jovanovich, 1977.
de Villiers, P. A., & de Villiers, J. G. *Early language.* Cambridge, Mass.: Harvard University Press, 1979.

The importance of language for the cognitive development of the preschool child is highlighted in Bruner's introduction to the following book and in several of the articles:
Bruner, J. S., Olver, R. R., & Greenfield, P. N. *Studies in cognitive growth.* New York: John Wiley, 1966.

8

SOCIALIZATION, PLAY, AND THE FAMILY IN EARLY CHILDHOOD

I had cherished a profound conviction that her bringing me up by hand, gave her no right to bring me up by jerks.

Charles Dickens
Great Expectations

There is only one service station in Vilna. In front of it a single metal sign, bent and rusted, hangs precariously from the last of what, at one time, must have been a pair of bolts. Unpretentious, it says only Garage. The building is old, barn shaped. Its back stoops delicately and it leans a wee bit to the east, where the prevailing west winds have slowly coaxed it. It looks like it was there long before I was born. Perhaps even before my grandmother was born. It also looks like its doors have not been opened for a long time.

We pull back onto Highway 28. The spare tire still holds, but I feel faintly uneasy.

"We'll get it fixed in Ashmont," I announce. Paul informs me that I will never get a good tire in a small town like Ashmont—or that if I do I will pay both of the proverbial limbs. I try to tell him that little towns have many things, some of which are very good; that life in large cities can sometimes rob us of far more than little towns are interested in taking. He disagrees. He knows better. He is a city dweller. I realize immediately that nothing I say will change his mind.

"I like little towns," Denise informs us. "They freak me. They freak me green." Nothing she says is likely to change his mind either.

The pavement is grayer now. At first I think my eyes must be getting tired or that there is simply less tar in the asphalt, but then I realize that fluffy white clouds have begun to shroud the sky. Heat waves still shimmer hazily over the road; it may storm later.

I marvel again at how different they are, my three children. Yet they were all brought up by the same people and in the same place—and only slightly separated in time. Why are they so different? Is it just age and sex? Or are they really so different? Would a complete stranger find them remarkably alike?

The brown pickup that was behind us earlier this morning—the one that turned off into Fort Saskatchewan—is now in front of us. It weaves gently between the shoulder and the center line like an old horse whose equilibrium is uncertain. A single elbow protrudes from the driver's window; nothing from the right. But the back now holds a lump of bodies, some apparently sleeping, others reclining on straw bales. One orange-socked foot dangles in the wind over the edge of the box. I wonder who they are. Sometimes I wonder who we are as well. Mostly, though, I wonder *why* we are what we are. That, in large part, is why I am telling the tale of the lifespan. For in it are many clues that might help to sort these great puzzles. Quickly, therefore, let us return to the tale, for the pickup may lead us too quickly to Ashmont, no matter how uncertain its weaving tracks.

■ Socialization

Socialization is the process by which children learn behaviors that are culturally appropriate for people of their sex and age; it transmits culture. But *culture* is an inclusive term not easily defined. It is accurate, for example, to say that a culture is the sum of all the mores, traditions, beliefs, values, customary ways of behaving, and implicit and explicit rules that characterize a group of people. It is also accurate to say that the trappings of a culture are its schools, its religions, and its laws. More specific definitions of culture might include child-rearing practices, chief occupations, principal leisure activities, taboos, and modes of behavior considered especially worthwhile.

Understandably, those aspects of the human condition most clearly determined by genetic factors are the least variable across cultures. People ordinarily have two legs, two arms, a single head, and a single navel; these we assume result primarily from heredity. In contrast, humans speak some 5,000 different languages, and social rules, moral beliefs, and sex-related behaviors sometimes vary dramatically from one culture to another; these variations are assumed to be related to environmental factors. And they are all aspects of culture. In light of what is known about the influence of environment on human development, consider for a moment how different the lives of Eskimo children might have been had they been born in your home—and how different your life might be had you been born in theirs.

The ways in which culture is transmitted from one generation to another are of central importance to a study of child development; they define the process of socialization, which occurs through such agencies as schools, churches, television, and the family. In the end, the results of socialization are manifested in our beliefs and in our behaviors; they are apparent in our sex roles and in our stereotypes; and, in the main, they reflect our backgrounds. These are the topics we look at here and in the next chapter.

■ Group Pressure

The effect that the opinions, the feelings, the exhortations, or the behavior of groups can have on the behavior of an individual is more difficult to illustrate in the complex, impersonal societies that have produced you and me than in the simple, highly personal cultures sometimes called "primitive." In a small and personal society, all members are intimately aware of the behavior of every individual in the group; the transgressions as well as the good acts of each can have serious repercussions on everybody. Accordingly, the pressure to conform to accepted and desirable codes of conduct is immediate and strong.

There is less pressure to conform in our society for two reasons: First, there is no single code of approved conduct in our complex culture; second, the pressure that the group can bring to bear on an individual is much more remote in our very large and often impersonal society. The feelings of abandonment and alienation assumed to affect increasing numbers of people in our culture (C. R. Rogers, 1951, 1969) are partly the result of the anonymity that results from living in societies in which the community has become so large that the individual is lost. Although this anonymity provides relief from social pressure, it also complicates an examination of the role of social pressure in development. Nevertheless, there are numerous instances of clearly discernible effects of social pressure on the beliefs and the behavior of individuals. Advertising techniques that appeal to consumers on the grounds that all their peers are using a particular brand are only one example; the tremendous similarities in our dress, our behaviors, our accents, and our use of slang are others.

The effects of social pressure are dramatically illustrated in Asch's (1955) study of conformity in group situations. In a series of studies, he demonstrated repeatedly that individuals can be made to behave in direct contradiction to their beliefs as a result of group pressure. The typical situation involves six or seven confederates who have been instructed to answer incorrectly for a number of simple perceptual problems. For example, subjects are shown three lines of different lengths that they are asked to compare to a standard (Figure 8.1). The task requires that they select the line equal in length to the standard—a task that is simple enough for almost any subject to answer correctly when not subjected to any contradictory pressures.

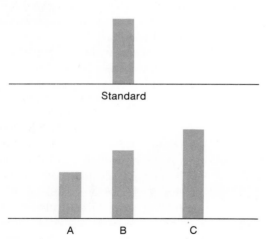

Figure 8.1
In Asch's investigation of the effects of social pressure, subjects were required to indicate whether A, B, or C is equal in length to the standard. B is the correct answer, but one-third of the time subjects agreed with confederates and answered incorrectly.

A single uninitiated subject is then introduced among the confederates, who are seated in such a way that they will always answer first. For the first several items the confederates answer correctly; afterward, they consistently answer incorrectly, and they *agree* on the incorrect answer. Presumably, this situation leads to considerable social pressure: The subject knows what the correct answer is and wonders about the answers of the other subjects. Approximately one-third of the time, during the study, the pressure was great enough for the subject to agree with the confederates and answer incorrectly. Is it any wonder that we comb our hair in similar ways and usually eat with knives and forks rather than with sharp sticks or our fingers?

For the developing child, social pressure includes the parents' influence, the influence of the school, pressure applied through various peer groups, and possible pressure from religious standards. Unfortunately, little research clarifies the role of social pressure in childhood. Nevertheless, bear in mind its significance as an environmental influence.

■ Social Imitation

Numerous explanations for social learning are based on the belief that culture is transmitted through a process of **imitation** (for example, Bandura, 1977; see Chapter 2). Again this is more apparent in primitive societies than in complex technological societies, partly because a society at a low level of technical development can usually provide its children with miniature *working* replicas of the tools it uses. In addition, parents, who are the chief agents for transmitting cultural information, demonstrate adult activities in the presence of children. Bandura and Walters (1963) describe child-rearing practices among the Cantalense people, a Guatemalan subculture. Cantalense parents provide their young children with the tools that are employed daily (for example, a miniature broom or a corn-grinding stone), and they are also constantly with the children. From their earliest years, children are exposed to models of the behaviors in which they will engage once they have matured. This cul-

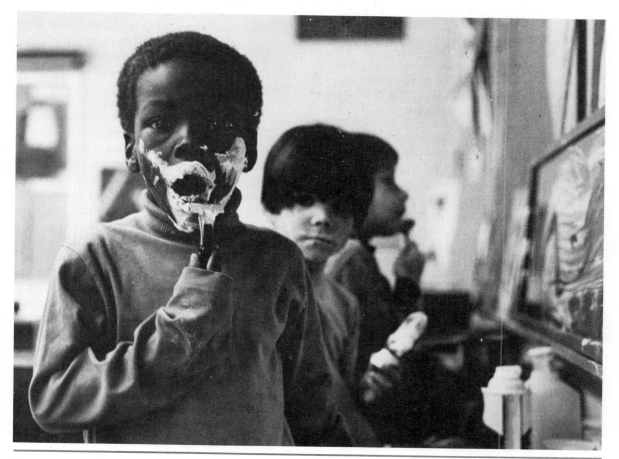

There are certain important things that we do not know how to do naturally—nor are we always given precise and detailed instruction. That we can imitate helps.

ture has little direct tuition—that is, the parents do not tell the child "This is how you must hold a broom, and this is how you must move it to sweep the cockroaches out of the house." There is obviously no need for such instruction; the learning demanded of the child is simple enough that it will occur simply through observation.

The Canadian Ojibwa Indians are another instance of social imitation; their livelihood is based mainly on hunting and trapping, and their culture is transmitted from one generation to the next mainly through observational learning. From the time he can walk well enough to keep up with his father, the young Ojibwa boy follows him around

his trapline to the lakes and streams where the father fishes, and he simply watches. Very early he is given his own traps, which he sets as he has seen his father set traps, in the manner of the grandfather and of the great-grandfather. Similarly the young Ojibwa girl learns how to prepare cooking fires and to make meals and clothing from the provisions of the woods and streams simply by observing her mother engage daily in these activities.

Observational learning, although not as evident in our culture, is no less prevalent. A model need not be a particular person whose behavior is copied by another, as in the illustrations just described. Anything that serves as a pattern for behavior may be considered a model: literature, movies, television programs, verbal and written instructions, religious beliefs, or folk heroes. Frequently models are **symbolic** rather than living people; indeed, these are the most prevalent models in a technological society. As we saw in Chapter 2, their effects are manifested in a variety of ways in the behavior of adults as well as children. And one of the most powerful of these symbolic models may well be your television set, a piece of equipment whose influence we have experienced considerable difficulty in clarifying (we look at this topic in detail in Chapter 9). Is it good, or is it bad? How good? How bad? How much more research do we need before we can leave our uncomfortable positions on the fence and play on the other side of the fence where the grass is always greener?

■ Play

The games that children **play**, unlike the games that adults play, are fun games. They are not designed to impress, to persuade, to deceive, or to annoy; they are played for the playing. And that, in a nutshell, is the difference between work and play: Play is designed for no end but its own enjoyment. **Work**, however, may consist of exactly the same activities as play, but it is engaged in not for the sake of pleasure, but for what may be gained as a result. A game is not necessarily play, and work is not necessarily work, but play is indeed play.

If the preceding paragraph confuses you, do not yet despair. I am playing—that is, I am writing simply for the enjoyment, although it looks like work to my neighbors who prefer to stay at home in the evenings and fight with their wives or watch television. Thus work is not necessarily work. Still, an acceptable distinction between work and play is difficult, because many pleasurable activities lead to productive ends other than simple enjoyment; at the same time, numerous activities that apparently have no purpose are also not enjoyable. We frequently play cards in friendly neighborhood groups. It is a game, but it is not play. Adults are

often confused about work and play—only children are not, for almost all they do is play.

If you persist in asking what importance play has, the psychologist must answer that because everything the child does is play, then play must be important for almost every aspect of the child's development. To accept this at the outset will prevent my making a lengthy series of platitudinous statements similar to those frequently found in textbooks of human development with section headings like "The Importance of Play for Learning," "The Importance of Play for Motivation," "The Importance of Play for Mental Health," and "The Importance of Play for Bingo." Or even "The Importance of Play for Survival," for Aldis (1975) has reported on extensive investigations of play among nonhuman animals and has concluded that it serves useful adaptive functions related to the development of motor skills necessary for survival. Having accepted that play is a fundamental and necessary part of the child's activities and that it is fundamentally involved in the processes of socialization, we move directly to an examination of the three general categories of play: sensorimotor, imaginative, and social.

Sensorimotor Play

Sensorimotor play involves the manipulation of objects or the performance of activities simply for the sensations involved. This type of play is engaged in most frequently by infants, for it is the only type of play of which they are capable during the early stages of development, when they have not yet developed the imagination necessary for other forms of play. Sensorimotor play may consist of motor activities such as creeping, crawling, walking, running, skipping, hopping, waving a hand or a foot or any other part of the anatomy that is wavable. It also includes manipulating objects, people, or anything else that is manipulatable. It is evident in countless solitary games of young children, such as moving the hand along the steep precipice of the table edge and roaring deep in the throat, in a manner of a well-tuned motorcycle, "*rrrrrr*"; running around a room with arms spread wide, sputtering like a badly tuned airplane, "*abrabrabrabrabr*"; or jumping up and down on the couch and repeating rhythmically "*upupup-upupupup.*" But these last activities are not simply sensorimotor; they can also be described as imaginative play.

Imaginative Play

Imaginative play includes the multitude of make-believe games that are made possible when, at around the age of two, the child can make objects, people, and activities *be* things that they actually are not (Gardner, 1982). These make-believe games become increasingly prevalent throughout the preschool years. Thus children who run about the room frightening their grandfathers with the sound of an airplane motor are engaging not only in a sensorimotor game but in one that is imaginative as well—they are no longer themselves, they are airplanes. And their voices are no longer simply voices but the roar of incredibly powerful airplane engines. The worn carpet has been transformed into fluffy clouds, and the bread crumbs on it are tiny houses and people far below our heroic aviators.

For children the world of make-believe is almost real. It is so close and so easily accessible, all they need do is pretend. Unhappily, this art is lost somewhere during the process of becoming an adult; it is sadly lacking among adults who pride themselves on a hard-nosed awareness of what is real and what is imaginary—we who have a troubling fear of one day mistaking the imaginary for the real. The fear is well founded, for adults who mistake the imaginary for the real soon find themselves incarcerated in institutions that we euphemistically call mental hospitals, or even more euphemistically, institutions. Indeed, those institutions are filled with people who cannot distinguish between the world in their minds and the world on the other side of their senses. That, by adult definition, is madness. But children who run about wailing like deranged baboons, transform-

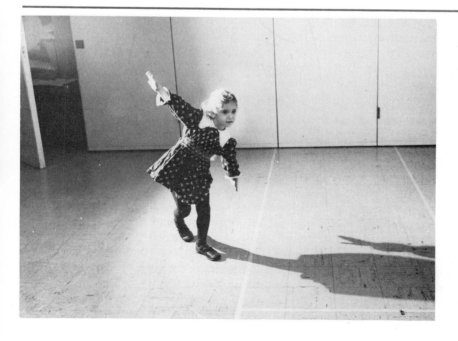

Imaginative sensorimotor play. Is she a ballet dancer, a tightrope walker, a seagull, or an airplane?

ing their world into the dense and terrifying jungles of an equatorial coast to be prowled in search of enemies, are not insane. They are simply children.

The child's imaginative play includes a variety of related activities. There is play in which children imagine that they are someone or something else: Batman, a dog, or a whale. There are related games in which they imagine that the activities they undertake are something other than what they really are or that the objects with which they play are something different (as illustrated by the airplane).

A type of imaginative play that becomes increasingly prevalent as the preschooler ages is daydreaming. Unlike the first two types of imaginative play, in which the child actively engages in fantasy, daydreaming simply involves the imagining without the activity. Greenacre (1959) reports that daydreaming becomes more prevalent when children reach school age. Prior to that time, their activity-oriented behavior did not lend itself to unlimited daydreaming.

Another type of imaginative play, related to daydreaming, involves the imaginary playmate—constant companion and friend to approximately half of all preschool children (Pines, 1978). These imaginary friends, complete with names and relatively stable personality characteristics, are spoken to, played with, loved, and hated by their creators. They are given names, forms, and places, and the young preschooler will seldom admit their imaginary nature.

The Implications of Imagination

In the play behavior of young children we find the first manifestations of imagination—manifestations that occur largely in the fantastic, the unreal. And fantasy has not always been encouraged by students of childhood or by grandparents. In a less enlightened age, daydreaming might have been feared as one possible manifestation of lack of contact with reality. Imaginary playmates would have been feared even more and seldom invited in to dinner or even to tea. Wertham (1954) included fairy tales among those aspects of fantasy that would

surely be harmful to young children, and Hurlock (1964) cautioned against the possibly deleterious effects of daydreaming, claiming that children who daydream excessively suffer physically from the resulting inactivity and also suffer psychologically from an eventual overreliance on daydreams to romanticize a self with which they are not happy.

Research and theory should do a great deal to relieve any leftover fears of fantasy that we might have. Freyberg (1973) describes in some detail the *constructive* role that imaginative play exercises in the development of cognitive skills, a position also elaborated by Piaget, who views imaginative (symbolic) play as the means whereby the child progresses from sensorimotor to more advanced forms of thought. And, contrary to what we might otherwise believe, imaginative play appears to be much more common among children whose biological and psychological needs are reasonably well satisfied (Freyberg, 1973). As Pulaski (1973) notes, fantasy play is not compensatory (the Freudian view) but is essentially constructive (the Piagetian view). That is, children do not fantasize to make up for emotional deficits or to overcome anxieties; instead, their fantasies are one of the means by which they progress to more advanced forms of thinking.

One of the few variables that successfully predicts later creativity is the presence of an imaginary playmate in childhood (Schaefer, 1969). College students who recall an imaginary playmate tend to be more creative than those who do not. But later creativity is not all that the imaginary playmate is associated with. In a study of 141 three- and four-year-olds, approximately half of whom had imaginary playmates, Singer (1973) and his associates found marked differences between those with personal fantastic friends and those without (see also Pines, 1978). Children with imaginary playmates watched less television (and selected fewer violent programs when they did), were less aggressive, smiled more, were less bored, and were more advanced in their language development. These observations are in close agreement with Singer's findings that children who were less prone to make-believe play appear also to be at a disadvantage in school achievement, particularly in areas that

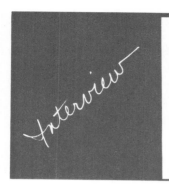

Subject: Male; age seven.

Question: "How do you play this game?" (a miniature portable video game)

See here. You press this button. This one. And a little guy comes out. You have to jump over the barrels and go up here. This way, then up here. If the barrel hits you, your man is dead. You have to rescue the girl. Darn, he got me!

require high verbal skills, and are also less adept in social situations, especially if these require self-control. Other studies show a relationship between *very low* predispositions to fantasy play and anti-social behavior or susceptibility to delinquency (see Singer, 1973).

Although none of these studies or observations is direct evidence that imaginative play *causes* healthy social and cognitive development, the relationship appears to be obvious. And cognitive development theories such as that of Piaget give us some reason to believe that imaginative play *might* be causally implicated in healthy development.

Daydreams, imaginary playmates, and even the fairy tale have been returned to the child. (See *Horton: An Imaginary Playmate.*) Bettelheim (1978), in his moving book *The Uses of Enchantment*, speaks of the potential benefits of frightening symbols in fairy tales. "If our fear of being devoured takes the tangible form of a witch, it can be gotten rid of by burning her in the oven." The fairy tale allows children to examine their monsters, gives substance and form to their anxieties, and provides methods for getting rid of them. Fraiberg (1968) attributes much the same function to the imaginary playmate, citing the case of a two-year-old child who had recently been frightened of dogs and whose imaginary playmate took the form of an animal, "Laughing Tiger," who neither roared nor bit; he simply laughed. As Fraiberg

explains, the girl chose to meet her enemy (the dog) in her imagination, where she could deal with him. And in the end she was no longer frightened of dogs.

Cobb (1977) describes the "genius of childhood" in terms of its imagination. And it is "the imagination of childhood from which all later creative activities evolve" (p. 18).

Social Play

It is true (though vastly oversimplified) to say that the child's developing motor skills owe a great deal to sensorimotor play and that cognitive development owes a great deal to imaginative play. By the same token, some of the roots of the child's personality and interpersonal skills lie in social play.

Social play frequently takes the form of games with rather precisely defined rules, which may or may not be followed by the players, depending largely on their understanding and their level of development. Although children may play together prior to the preschool period, the nature of their games is frequently described as "parallel" rather than truly social (Parten, 1932); that is, children play side by side but do not interact, do not share the activities involved in the game, and do not employ any mutually accepted rules. Parallel play is nevertheless social play of a primitive sort, because it involves two or more children who apparently

HORTON: AN IMAGINARY PLAYMATE

My young daughter's imaginary playmate, Horton, began to live with us when she was four. We paid scant attention at first; he took little room at the dinner table, usually just wanting to sit on her lap. And he ate only small tidbits from her plate. Later he sometimes required his own chair. And one night it was necessary to place a large turkey drumstick on his plate, where it sat, sadly becoming colder, while we ate our meal. "He doesn't really like turkey," our daughter informed us, "and I don't either."

But, generally, Horton was no great bother. He spent most of his time sitting in a chair, always close to his friend, where she could talk to him—which she did at great length and with sometimes breathless intimacy. And whenever we went anywhere, he always came with us. Often we had to wait for him; he had the annoying habit of not being ready on time. Whenever this hap-

pened, our daughter would rush back to get him from her bedroom, or sometimes from the bathroom, for he too needed to use that facility on occasion. She would drag him out then, complaining and scolding so severely that I sometimes felt sorry to see him so humiliated in front of his family.

Near her seventh birthday I asked her about Horton. "What do you mean?" she said. I told her what I thought I meant. "He likes chocolate and he wears different clothes," she answered. "Is he real?" I inquired. She looked up rather sadly. "No, he isn't. He's imaginary." But despite this, she continued to interact with him for some time longer, although she brought him out publicly less often. She no longer insisted that he come with us wherever we went. I have not seen him for some time now.

---

prefer to play together, even though they do not yet interact. This is a transitional period between the solitary play of early infancy and the cooperative play of the later preschool period.

In a detailed investigation of the development of play and games in children, Piaget (1932) arrived at a classification of games by the *structures* that underlie them. This classification includes the *practice* game, games that use *symbols*, and games that have *rules*. In effect, the first type is the sensorimotor game to which we referred earlier; the second (games with symbols) is the imaginative play of children; the third is the social game. These games develop sequentially as well, beginning with the simplest and culminating with the most complex. Practice games, for example, are engaged in by animals and young infants (Piaget suggests a kitten batting a ball around and chasing it). Symbolic games do not develop until the final substage of sensorimotor development, for they require imagination, and the ability to symbolize emerges during this stage. Rule-regulated games begin to appear between the ages of four and seven, but do not become common until after the age of seven.

Sex Differences in Play

There are a number of relatively consistent findings among studies that have looked at sex differences in play behavior. To begin with, there is little evidence of any greater predisposition toward fantasy (imaginative play) in either girls or boys (Singer, 1973). But there is repeated evidence of sex typing with respect not only to the toys that are given boys and girls but also to the toys they choose to play with when there is a choice (Fein, Johnson, Kosson, Stork, & Wasserman, 1975). Not surprisingly, boys are given what we consider to be male-typed toys: trucks, airplanes, boats, soldiers, and guns. Girls are given dolls, plastic dishes, cooking utensils, and doll houses (Rheingold & Cook, 1975). And both typically select toys according to their sex, although girls from homes with higher educational backgrounds tend to select male-typed toys more often than girls from lower educational backgrounds (Wesley & Wesley, 1977).

Additional sex differences with respect to play behavior are evident in the observation that boys employ more physical space in their play, play out-

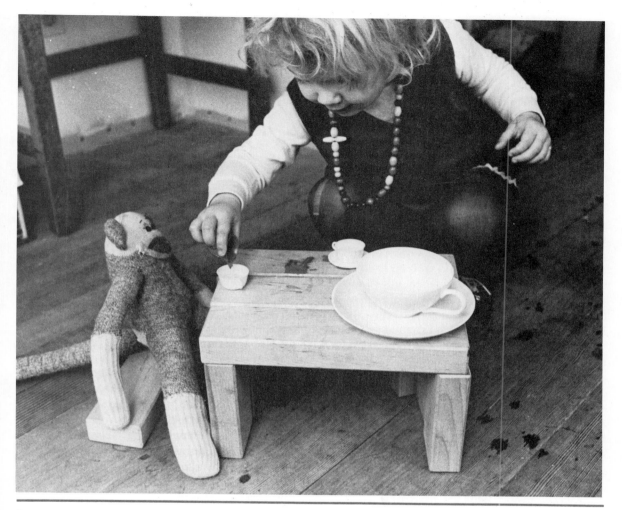

Sex typing in selection of toys and in play activities is often evident at a very early age.

doors more (Cramer & Hogan, 1975), and are more prone to overt expressions of joy when they play (Pulaski, 1973).

Differences between the sexes go far beyond the toys children might play with or their expressions of joy while playing. They include a wide range of behaviors that are deemed to be appropriate for boys and girls—in other words, that are considered masculine or feminine. These behaviors, together with the attitudes and personality characteristics associated with them, are what define **sex roles**. The learning of sex-appropriate behavior, or sex-roles, is referred to as **sex typing**. We look at these topics in Chapter 12; the remainder of this chapter deals with one of the most powerful influences on the lives of most of us: our families.

■ Origins of the Family

It is interesting to speculate about the origins of the family, particularly because few of our phylogenetic precursors seem to have developed a **nuclear family** (mother, father, and children). Even the apes and monkeys that have been extensively studied ordinarily live in groups consisting of unrelated members. In addition, their sexual conduct (which, incidentally, is much more restrained than is commonly believed) gives no evidence of any permanent attachment between a male and a female or between a male and a group of females (or vice versa in a hypothetical world of liberated female monkeys or apes). Much less have they developed **extended families** (parents, children, grandparents, and other relatives). Early sociologists, such as C. Lloyd Morgan (1894, 1896), assumed that the social organization of early humans was parallel to that of apes and monkeys. Morgan believed that bands of men and women lived apart and that the men visited the women only when the urge to rape them became overpowering. Engels (1902) also thought that primitive humans did not live in family groups, but in a communistic tribe where sexual relations were indiscriminate and matter of fact.*

Whatever the origins of the family, in societies such as ours many people live in relatively cohesive family groups ordinarily consisting of one or more parents and their young children. These family groups occasionally extend to include other relatives as well.

■ The Contemporary Family

The nuclear family was once North America's most prevalent family; only a few years ago, over 85 percent of all children lived in families consisting of two parents and approximately half of one sibling, this latter phenomenon made possible solely through those statistical manipulations that revealed the average family size to be around 3.5—and dropping (Keniston, 1975). In contrast, a majority of the world's societies have traditionally been characterized by extended families—parents, immediate children, grandparents, uncles, aunts, cousins, and various other assorted relatives.

But all was not well with the nuclear family. Bronfenbrenner (1977a) warned us that it was rapidly "falling apart." Not only had the extended family almost disappeared from the contemporary American scene, the number of one-parent families had increased dramatically as well. Whereas only one child in fourteen (under the age of six) was brought up in a one-parent family in 1948, by 1973 the proportion had doubled to one child in seven (Keniston, 1975); now, estimates are that somewhere between 40 and 50 percent of all children born since 1970 will spend an average of six years living in a one-parent family (Glick & Norton, 1978). Almost 90 percent of one-parent families are headed by a mother.

The decline in the proportion of nuclear families, with the corresponding increase in one-parent families, is due to a number of factors. Although the number of unmarried women having babies and keeping them has increased and the number of widowed parents has also increased, neither of these facts account for many one-parent families. The single most important contributing cause is clearly a dramatic rise in divorce rates—a rise of more than 700 percent during the current century.

Although the nuclear family continues to be one of the most common child-rearing institutions in North America, most of our recent research in this area has focused on the impact of divorce on children (as well as on their parents), on the effect of being brought up in a one-parent family, on the effects of day-care facilities or other substitute caretakers, and on the effects of the absence of the father. These topics are examined in the following sections.

Day Care Versus Home Care

In the old days, most North American children spent their preschool years in intimate contact with their mothers, a situation that many people might consider an ideal child-rearing arrangement. Today, an ever-increasing number of children are cared for during the day by others. As many as 25 percent

---

*Some professional cynics believe that contemporary American society may be reaching the beginning of the cycle again.

of four-year-olds are recipients of day care; a smaller but growing number of infants are in the same position (Bronfenbrenner, Belsky, & Steinberg, 1977).

The growing number of children in day-care facilities is due not only to an increase in the number of one-parent families where the parent must work but also to the large number of families where both parents work—sometimes because of financial need, often for other reasons.

Day care takes a variety of forms, ranging from situations in which families can afford to hire a private caretaker to substitute for the mother during her absence, with the caretaker in the child's home, to institutionalized centers involving large numbers of children and a number of caretakers. Research and speculation have been less concerned with day care in private homes than with centralized day care. What are the effects of day care on children?

Bronfenbrenner, Belsky, and Steinberg (1977) reviewed several dozen studies, most of which attempted to compare day-care and home-care children in terms of social, intellectual, and motor development. Cognitive differences were seldom significant. A number of studies found a slightly greater tendency for day-care children to interact with others (both peers and adults), and several reported somewhat more aggressiveness among day-care children. Blehar (1974) found that children in day-care institutions reacted with more distress at separation from their mothers and displayed more anxiety and ambivalence upon reunion than did children whose mothers stayed home. Kagan, Kearsley, and Zelaza (1977) found few important differences between a group of thirty-three infants who attended a day-care center and comparable children who were kept at home by their mothers. On a battery of measures administered on eight occasions—and including assessments of attentiveness, language development, confidence, memory, and maternal attachment—day-care and home-care infants performed equally well.

We are not yet in a position to arrive at a final evaluation of the social, cognitive, and emotional effects of day care in general. Most of the available research has looked at children from middle- or upper-class backgrounds, where day care is often provided by university-affiliated centers. These centers are typically more development oriented, both in cognitive and social areas, than are the larger and often more custodial institutions to which a great many working mothers take their children. (See *Finding Quality Day Care*.) In general, however, available evidence suggests that day care does not have detrimental effects on young children. Competent day care might actually have noticeably beneficial effects on certain children (those from impoverished backgrounds, for example) but would have no measurable effects on those from more advantaged backgrounds. More research is needed.

■ Family Influences

Although the family can easily be described in terms of its composition (mother, father, children), it is not at all easily described as a unit of social influence. To begin with, the family is a dynamic rather than a static unit—dynamic in the sense that it changes with the addition of new members (and sometimes the loss of old ones) and in response to external and internal pressures. That is, the family exists as a relatively isolated unit within society, but at the same time it responds to pressures from its social, political, religious, and educational environment. This is clearly evident in changes that have occurred in child-rearing styles through history, many of these changes being reflected in the advice given parents by society's experts (to breast-feed or not, to be permissive or strict, to spank or not to spank, to toilet train early or late).

In addition to being responsive to outside influences, the family functions as a network of dyadic (paired) relationships: mother-child, father-child, mother-father, child-child. And, as we saw in Chapter 6, it also involves more complex relationships that define family systems (marital relationships, parenting styles, and their complex interrelationships in the triadic system of mother-father-child) (Belsky, 1981). These relationships change constantly as parents and children grow. And, as we have seen earlier, the nature of influence in these relationships can probably never be considered as operating in only one direction. Parents change because of their children, even as parents change their children, a process that we have frequently and understandably overlooked, since children are clearly the more influenced and the more changing of the two groups.

Given the highly dynamic nature of the family as a social unit, it has proven extremely difficult to isolate particular characteristics of parents and to assess their influence on specific characteristics of children. In addition, since the family has traditionally been a highly private unit, researchers have seldom had access to the most intimate aspects of its functioning except, occasionally, in cases of pathology or crime. Most of the research data have therefore been limited to what could be obtained from interviews or observation by a third party. Unfortunately, each of these methods has drawbacks. Data from interviews are subject to errors resulting from intentional or accidental distortion, the weaknesses of human memory, the inadequacy of questions asked, and the occasional reticence of interviewees. Observations by a third party, even when accomplished through an impersonal camera, must always take into account the possibility (and sometimes the probability) that the presence of the observer will influence the behavior of the observed.

Parent-Child Relations

The effects of the parent-child relationship on the development of the child's personality is of considerable practical interest. Although much research has been devoted to examining this question, it is still not completely answered. Researchers have found it difficult to describe the relations that exist between parents and children and to ascertain precisely what the personality of the child is. It is particularly difficult to determine, for example, whether a permissive approach to child rearing develops independent or dependent children, when the nature of parental permissiveness is no easier to define than the dependent or independent child

is to identify. To further confuse the issue, parents' and children's behavior is inconsistent in different situations. For example, Hatfield, Ferguson, and Alpert (1967) observed mothers and their children in a playroom setting and found their behavior highly inconsistent from one session to another. Under such circumstances, the nature of the mother-child relationship is puzzling at best.

Despite these difficulties, there is no lack of general conclusions about parent-child relations in psychological literature. These deal primarily with the effect of such qualities as parental permissiveness, dominance, warmth, and rejection on the child's independence, self-control, masculinity or femininity, assertiveness, and so on. One study (Baumrind, 1967) investigated preschool children who were identified as belonging to one of three personality groups: The first group consisted of children described as buoyant, friendly, self-controlled, and self-reliant; the second group had discontented and withdrawn children; and the third group's children lacked self-reliance and self-control. Parents of the children in the first group were significantly more controlling, demanding, and loving than parents of either of the other groups. Parents of the discontented and withdrawn children also exercised much control, but were detached rather than warm and loving, whereas parents of the children who lacked self-reliance (had low self-esteem) were warm but highly permissive. This study is representative of a number of other studies demonstrating that children of relatively demanding but loving parents tend to be better adjusted, more independent, and more self-reliant. The investigation by Getzels and Jackson (1962) of creative children revealed that the more highly creative children in their sample had parents who expected more of them at an earlier age (controlling and demanding) but who were nevertheless warm and loving.

Does this mean that parents who are loving but demanding cause children to be creative, self-reliant, controlled, friendly, and a host of other good things? Not really. Although this might well be the case, the kind of research to which we are presently limited is hardly likely to provide us with the kind of evidence needed to make this asser-

FINDING QUALITY DAY CARE

Working parents make arrangements in a variety of ways for the care of their young children. A few, mostly the very wealthy, hire private "nannies" and tutors; the vast majority leave children in their own homes with relatives, friends, or neighbors; and an increasing number turn to day-care facilities. Some children are simply not cared for—they are left alone, sometimes on the street and sometimes at home and in school. Among these are the *latch-key children*—so-called because their parents sometimes hang keys around their necks so that they can let themselves into their empty homes when the schools discharge them.

Of those who are placed in day-care facilities, the majority are found in what is termed *family day care*—that is, in private homes where one woman or several look after a number of neighborhood children. Parents often select family day care when they have a choice, because they assume that these are more likely to provide the type of experiences and care for their children that they would themselves provide in their own homes. In addition, family day care is generally more convenient and less expensive than what is termed *center day care*.

Although research reviewed in the text indicates that day care in general does not usually have detrimental effects on young children, there is evidence that *good* day care might have decidedly beneficial effects; conversely, *bad* day care might have the opposite effects. How can parents determine what is likely to be good or bad day care?

In a highly practical little book, Endsley and Bradbard (1981) present some advice. They suggest that although it is difficult to evaluate different day-care programs, those that are very bad may have a number of characteristics in common and those that are excellent might also. Among characteristics of poor programs are the following (Endsley & Bradbard, 1981, pp. 32–33):

1. Unsanitary and unhealthy physical surroundings
2. Obvious physical hazards
3. Excessive overcrowding both in terms of the available space and too many young children for the available supervising adults (for example, adult-child ratios that exceed one-to-twenty or, in the case of infants, one-to-ten)
4. Lack of activities and materials that are interesting and challenging to young children
5. Staff, usually untrained, who are at best thoughtless and insensitive and at worst reject and abuse young children
6. Disregard for parents' feelings about child rearing. (p. 32)

In contrast, characteristics associated with high-quality programs include:

1. The financial resources to design and equip a special environment for their children
2. The time, freedom, motivation, and physical energy to work only with their children for six-to-ten hours each day
3. The training necessary to organize experiences and activities to develop optimally their children's understanding of themselves and the world about them. (p. 33)

In agreement with this assessment of *quality* day care, Kagan (1978) stresses that what appears to be important in day care is that the ratio of staff to children be kept low, that staff be reasonably knowledgeable with respect to child development, and that children be given ample opportunity to exercise social, cognitive, and language skills. How does a parent assess day-care facilities with respect to these characteristics? Not by paying a great deal of attention to the Yellow Pages or to newspaper advertising but through personal references and, perhaps most important, by visiting the centers, observing them in operation, and talking with the people in charge. And to facilitate evaluations, Endsley and Bradbard provide detailed checklists of what to look for and what questions to ask.

Ironically, however, most of us are likely to spend more time looking, comparing, and obtaining references when buying a car than we are when finding someone to care for our children.

tion. Other explanations for these observed relationships might well be equally plausible. For example, the most important *causal* factors may be genetic rather than social. In other words, parents who are themselves demanding, controlling, and achievement oriented might have a greater *genetic* probability of producing creative, self-reliant, friendly children.

Another explanation that should not be overlooked relates to what we know and suspect about the bidirectionality of parent-child influence—about what Klein, Jorgensen, and Miller (1978) call *reciprocal causality*. Is it not possible that strong, self-reliant, creative, well-adjusted children should encourage loving and somewhat demanding behavior in their parents? And would it not also be likely that children who are discontented, withdrawn, and highly dependent should foster a colder, more rejecting relationship with parents? Given these possibilities, what sort of advice are the child experts most likely to give parents today?

Child-Care Advice

Two important models have dominated most of our thinking about the importance of parents in the development of the child (Skolnick, 1978). Both stress the malleability and vulnerability of the child. On the one hand, the Freudian model asserts that children are extremely sensitive to the emotional experiences of their early lives and most especially to their relationships with their parents (LeMasters, 1977). On the other, the behavioristic model emphasizes the plasticity of children in response to the rewards and punishments of their environments.

If these models are accurate, their usefulness resides primarily in the advice relevant research might provide concerning specific experiences that should be provided for children, or in whatever cautions such research might provide concerning experiences to which they should not be exposed. Much of the parent-child research of the past fifty years may be viewed as an attempt to provide information of this type. How successful have we been as dispensers of child-care advice? Perhaps not very successful.

Although retrospective studies with delinquent and otherwise disturbed adolescents and adults have generally found that their childhoods were marked by a variety of traumas, sometimes associated with "broken" homes, alcoholic or abusive parents, poverty, authoritarianism, rejection, and a variety of other factors, nonretrospective studies have not always corroborated these findings. When researchers attempted to predict which children would later be maladjusted and which would be happy and adjusted, on the basis of considerable information concerning their home lives, they were unsuccessful two-thirds of the time (Skolnick, 1978). Indeed, some very brilliant, well-adjusted, and successful individuals had childhood environments that might be generously described as poor. It seems that predicting the effects of child-rearing practices is far more difficult than explaining these effects after the fact. And what this indicates most clearly is that our after-the-fact explanations might have been entirely wrong in the first place.

One of the most painstaking studies of parent-child influences was conducted in the early 1950s by Sears and his associates (Sears, Maccoby, & Lewin, 1957). They interviewed 379 mothers of kindergarten children, rated each on more than one hundred child-rearing practices, and looked at the relationships between these practices and the personalities of their children. In general, the observed relationships were unimpressive and the findings ambiguous. And even if they had been less ambiguous, they would still have been tentative, given that the characteristics of the children were based on their mothers' descriptions rather than on direct observation or measurement. Nor could the study answer the question that underlies most of this research: Do styles of child rearing make a difference in the end?

McClelland, Constantian, Regalado, and Stone (1978) suggest that it probably does not. He and his associates tracked down seventy-eight subjects from the original Sears study—subjects who had been children at the time of the original interviews, but who were now thirty-one years of age. These subjects were interviewed in depth, and forty-seven of them were brought into a clinical setting for a series of psychological tests. The conclusion

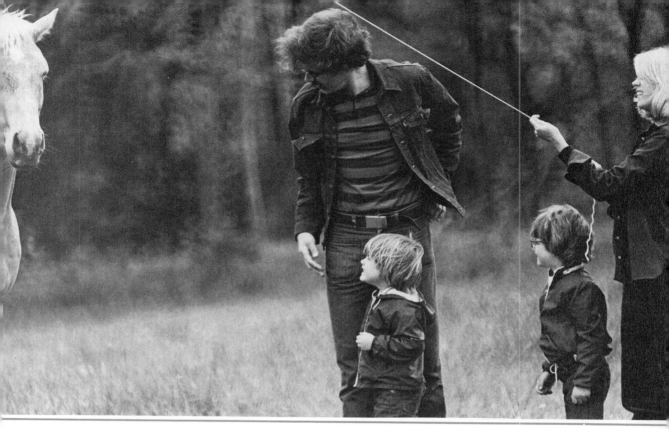

A dynamic social unit, the nuclear family. At left, not a member of the family, is a horse.

of McClelland and his associates is particularly striking when considered in relation to our model of child vulnerability and plasticity: "Wide variations in the way parents reared their children didn't seem to matter much in the long run. Adult interests and beliefs were by and large not determined by the duration of breast-feeding, the age and severity of toilet-training, strictness about bedtimes, or indeed any of these things" (1978, p. 46).

Does this mean that parents do not really matter? No. The researchers are quick to point out that one variable appears to be related to adjustment and maturity: *love* (McClelland et al., 1978). Parents who genuinely care for their children are most likely to do the right things, whatever those are. And there is increasing evidence that there are no *specific* right things.

Baumrind (1977), who has conducted extensive investigations of the relationships between behavior and characteristics of parents and the personalities of their children, concluded that there is no one best way of rearing children. Like McClelland, Bronfenbrenner, and a host of contemporary researchers, she presents the argument that no specific child-rearing practices should be advocated rather than others (regarding breast-feeding and toilet training, for example), but some general characteristics of parents, reflected in their behaviors toward their children, might have highly positive effects—and negative ones, too. She found, for example, that parents who were firm and directive were more likely to have children who would be responsible (as opposed to socially disruptive and intolerant of others) and active (as opposed to passive). Her position has been widely interpreted as advocating authoritarianism and firm discipline. And although she does not dispute the interpretation, she presents the important proviso that the parent who is firm and demanding should also be warm, nurturing, and loving.

In addition, Baumrind presents an argument against permissiveness that was ushered in and justified by what is sometimes termed the "Spock" era of child rearing. She suggests that the advocacy of permissiveness is based on a number of false assumptions. These assumptions relate to our belief that firm feeding habits, toilet training, spanking, and other forms of punishment are unquestionably bad and that unconditional love is good. She points out that punishment is effective and does not rupture attachment bonds between parents and children, provided it is reasonable punishment by a loving parent; that unconditional love is likely to lead to the development of selfish and "obnoxious" children; and that no good research evidence supports a belief that toilet training or insisting on regular feeding habits is inadvisable.

Kagan (1978), an eminent child psychologist, has also criticized the belief that all parents need to do to protect their young from the misery of maladjustment and failure is to love them. He traces the history of our belief in the absolute necessity of parental love for the well-being of the child, uncovers numerous cultures and ages where parental behavior would be described as cold, rejecting, and sometimes cruel by present standards, and finds no evidence that clearly links these parental behaviors with developmental problems in children (or adjustment problems in the adults that later result). However, a strong word of caution is in order. The argument being presented here applies to *unconditional* love—that is, to the kind of unquestioning love that is given to the child in such a way that it becomes meaningless. Unconditional love does not depend on anything. Accordingly, it provides children with no information concerning the rightness or desirability of their behaviors; it presents no guidance and no direction.

In summary, although there is some reason to question the venerable assumption that all children are highly fragile and that the development of their personalities and their consequent social adjustment and happiness are entirely in the hands of their parents, it would be highly misleading and not a little foolish to insist that parents do not make a difference. They do. And so do other members of the family.

Birth Order

Among the intriguing observations in connection with studies of the family and its role in child development are those relating to **birth order**. Galton (1896) was among the first to note the effects of birth order when he observed that there was a preponderance of firstborn children among great British scientists. Koch (1955) studied 360 five- and six-year-old children extensively and concluded that firstborn children have an advantage in several areas of development. For example, Koch found that firstborn children spoke more articulately than those who were born second, that they scored higher on measures of intellectual performance, and that they were more responsible and better planners than their siblings. Other research has been no less kind to the firstborn. In comparison to their younger siblings, firstborns have a higher **need to achieve** (Sampson, 1962), perform better academically (Altus, 1965, 1967), are more curious (Altus, 1967) and more competitive (Koch, 1955), and are more likely to prefer the novel or complex (Eisenman, 1967). The probability that a firstborn child will attend college is usually higher than that for other siblings (Bayer, 1966), and their scores on measures of intelligence are higher on the average (Melican & Feldt, 1980; Page & Grandon, 1979). And, for what it is worth, their probability of going into space is also higher. Of the seven original astronauts, two were only children and the remaining five were firstborn sons; of the first twenty-three astronauts to travel in space, twenty-one were either only children or firstborn (*Newsweek*, 1969). Of the remaining men, one had an older brother who died as an infant; the other was thirteen years younger than his older brother.

The meaning of birth order data is not completely clear, depsite the rather impressive agreement among the conclusions derived from various studies. The most redundant and most often investigated finding is that firstborn children appear to excel in scholastic achievement (Zajonc & Markus, 1975). It is also generally agreed that firstborn children develop language more rapidly, as do only children. Twins and triplets show retarded language development, not only in comparison to firstborns but also in comparison to children who have no twin (Davis, 1937). Blatz (1937), for example, found that the Dionne quintuplets were much slower in language development than the average child.

These last observations offer some possible explanations for the observed effects of birth order. Generally, these effects are not due simply to being firstborn or lastborn, but to the type of social interaction most characteristic for firstborn as opposed to children born later (Grotevant, Scarr, & Weinberg, 1977). It is not surprising that children from multiple births develop more slowly than children from single births, because they are almost necessarily in much closer contact with their twin and, at the same time, have less individual interaction with the parents. Similarly, it is reasonable to attribute most of the observed differences between firstborn and later-born children to the more intensive and stimulating interaction that firstborn children enjoy with their parents before succeeding children arrive. Certainly birth order alone explains little, although, as the evidence shows, it may be of value in predicting some of the child's characteristics. Some of these observed differences may have physiological bases. For example, the prenatal environment of firstborn children may be different from that of later-born children. In light of the plausible social explanations that have been advanced, however, it is unlikely that physiological explanations will contribute much to the intriguing phenomena associated with the order of birth.

Family Size

The smallest family interesting to a developmental psychologist is one with only one child—a condition often thought to be injurious to the healthy development of that child. Research does not support this ancient belief. Davis (1937), for example, reports that only children consistently develop more rapidly than children with siblings, particularly in language development. Faris (1940), McCurdy, (1957), and Velandia, Grandon, and Page (1978) provide evidence of superior intellectual achievement and greater eminence among only children. In addition, no conclusive evidence shows that being an only child has any ill effects on the child's personality. These results clearly agree with the findings about birth order. The superior achievement of only children may be explained in the same way as the attainments of firstborn children: Each firstborn is an only child for some period of time; consequently, each is favored with a greater degree of parent-child interaction in the formative years.

The effect of belonging to a large family has not been investigated as thoroughly as the effect of ordinal position within the family, partly because the topic is at least superficially more sociological than psychological. Therefore, much of the research is sociological, consisting more of descriptions of life in large and small families than of reports of measured differences among the children produced by each. Bossard and Sanger (1951) and Bossard and Boll (1956) report that larger families seem to be more authoritarian than smaller families and also less overprotective, less overindulgent, and less intrusive. From their interviews with members of one hundred families of six or more children each, Bossard and Boll have made a variety of generalizations concerning the authority structure, the discipline, and the typical personality types of large families. Although their research is interesting and provocative, it is not designed to identify the different effects that family size might have on children.

More recently, research has looked at the effects of family size on intellectual development. In this connection, a number of researchers have found consistent evidence of lower intelligence test scores among members of larger families (Grotevant et al., 1977; Zajonc, 1976). In explaining these findings, Zajonc has argued that the *intellectual climate* in homes with large families is, on the average, less conducive to cognitive development than the climate characteristic of homes with smaller families. However, here as elsewhere, we cannot easily separate the effect of family size from the effects of social class, religion, or rural versus urban environment.

Siblings

Birth order and family size appear to be clearly implicated in the development of children's personality characteristics. In addition, sex and age of siblings also influence the child, particularly with respect to the adoption of sex roles. Traditionally, these roles have dictated that boys will be more aggressive and more achievement oriented than girls and that girls will be more emotional and more passive than boys. These distinctions between sex roles continue to be culturally valid, despite indications that they are becoming less pronounced (see Chapter 12).

Strauss (1959) reports that girls with male siblings but no sisters tend to adopt an extreme sex role. On the one hand, they may be excessively "feminine," exaggerating the differences between their behavior and interests and those of their brothers and, in a sense, expecting recognition and praise for their femininity. Alternatively, such girls may adopt many of the characteristics of their brothers, becoming "tomboyish." Girls with a single older brother tend to be more aggressive and more dominant than girls without older brothers (Sutton-Smith, Roberts, & Rosenberg, 1964). Similarly, boys who have an older sister tend to be more passive and more "feminine" than would otherwise be expected. Not surprisingly, girl-girl dyads tend to produce highly "feminine" girls; boy-boy dyads tend to produce highly "masculine" boys.

■ One-Parent Families

As noted earlier, close to half of all American children are spending (or will spend) an average of six years in a family with only one parent, and in more than 90 percent of these families, the single parent is the mother. The large majority of these one-parent families result from separation or divorce; a smaller proportion result from the death of a parent or are the result of bearing children out of wedlock (Bane, 1976).

The impact of the one-parent family on the social and emotional welfare of children has been a subject of considerable recent research. A great deal of this research has focused on the significance of the father's absence, so that observed effects have often been attributed to the lack of a father. Unfortunately, the situation is not so simple as this analysis might imply. Some of the effects of one-parent families can at times be attributed to changes that occur in the family itself, after the father has left, rather than to the lack of a father as a source of psychological influence. The child has to cope not only with the absence of the father but also with a husbandless mother. In addition, the economic conditions of the one-parent home are, on the average, considerably less advantageous than those of the two-parent family, a phenomenon that has led to what is sometimes referred to as the *feminization of poverty* (Friedan, 1983).

In summary, then, absence of the father could affect children either because the roles traditionally fulfilled by the father would no longer be fulfilled (or might be fulfilled less adequately by the mother, who must also continue to carry out her own roles) or because the absence of the father has an effect on the mother, who then interacts with her children differently. These traditional fatherly roles are, on the one hand, economic and, on the other, psychological. Freudian theory suggests, for example, that the presence of both parents is especially crucial during the phallic phase of development (ages four to six), when children resolve their Oedipus or Electra complexes, identify with the like-sexed parent, and begin to develop appropriate sex roles. Accordingly, the absence of a father should be more harmful for boys than for girls. But the provision of a male model for young girls is also of considerable importance in Freudian theory, and the absence of a father should therefore have noticeable consequences for them as well. Presence of the male model is important, not only because it provides some indication of what men should be like when girls begin to date but also because of the role a loving and accepting father plays in the development of a daughter's self-esteem. Similarly, the absence of a mother, an increasingly common situation, might be expected to have different effects on boys than on girls.

Children in One-Parent Families

A great deal of research has linked delinquency (particularly among lower-class children), emotional disturbance, and other developmental problems with the absence of a father (see Lynn, 1974). Almost all this research is retrospective; that is, researchers have looked among populations of "disturbed" adolescents and adults, matched them with control groups of "normals," and looked at family backgrounds. Frequently, members of the "disturbed" group were significantly more likely to be the products of one-parent families.

Caution should be exercised in generalizing the results of studies such as these. Not only do they provide no proof of causation but they are also inapplicable to individuals as opposed to groups. That is, although there might be a higher incidence of maladjustment among children of one-parent families, the notion that one-parent families cause maladjustment is clearly untenable. If that were the case, then all children of one-parent families would be maladjusted (and perhaps none from two-parent families would be).

Investigations of the effect of one-parent families have not been limited to attempts to discover whether they are associated with maladjustment. Hetherington (1972) conducted a comprehensive examination of the effects of one-parent families on adolescent girls. Three different groups participated in the study: girls from intact families, girls whose fathers had died, and girls whose parents had separated or divorced.

Part of the study involved interviewing the girls in a recreation center. Four chairs were placed in the interviewing room. The interviewer (male on one occasion and female on the other) sat in one chair, with the other three chairs at varying distances from the interviewer. The girls therefore had a choice of sitting close to the interviewer, far away, or at an intermediate distance. Daughters of divorced mothers sat closest to male interviewers; daughters of widowed mothers sat in the most distant chair. When the interviewer was female, the groups displayed no consistent patterns of chair selection.

This observation, interpreted as indicating that girls of divorced mothers are more likely to seek the company of males and that daughters of widowed mothers are more likely to avoid male company, is corroborated by other findings of the study. Daughters of widows engaged in less eye contact with male interviewers, sat "properly" with their legs together and their postures rigid, and reported less heterosexual activity (dating). In contrast, daughters of divorced women engaged in significantly more eye contact, sprawled loosely in their chairs ("open leg and arm posture"), and reported more heterosexual contacts. However, neither of these groups had as many male contacts, or attitudes as positive toward males, as did girls from intact families.

One additional finding from this study is noteworthy. Loss of the father before the age of five usually had a more pronounced effect than if the father was lost later. An earlier study with boys (Hetherington, 1966) found much the same thing, with loss having more damaging consequences if it occurred early.

A second comprehensive and careful series of studies is summarized briefly here. The studies involved sixty middle-class, relatively affluent, recently divorced families (Wallerstein & Kelly, 1974, 1975, 1976). A team of researchers studied each child during a six-week period, shortly after the divorce occurred and again a year later, and, in addition, obtained access to school records. Results are summarized for children divided into groups according to ages.

The early effects of parental separation for the youngest group (two- to three-year-olds) included regression manifested in loss of toilet habits, bewilderment, and clinging behavior directed toward strangers. In some cases, development still appeared to be retarded one year later. Three- and four-year-old preschoolers exhibited loss of confidence and self-esteem and were prone to blame themselves for the departure of the father.

The next age group (five- and six-year-olds) was less affected developmentally, although some of the daughters tended to deny the situation and to continue expecting that their fathers would return. The seven- and eight-year-olds were understandably frightened by the divorce and intensely saddened, many of them missing their fathers constantly. Many of these children also lived in fear of making their mothers angry, perhaps imagining that she too might leave them.

Nine- and ten-year-olds initially reacted with apparent acceptance, many of them trying to understand why the divorce had occurred. But their outward calm covered feelings of anger, sometimes intense hostility toward one or the other parent (or both), and shame (Wallerstein & Kelly, 1976). A year later, half of these children seemed to have adjusted, with resignation and some lingering sadness, to their new situation. However, half suffered from varying degrees of depression, low self-esteem, poorer school performance, and poorer relationships with peers.

In summary, divorce undoubtedly has a tremendous immediate impact on the majority of affected children. There is evidence as well that the effects may be manifested later in problems of adjustment at school, with peers, and with adults. Hetherington (1979), following a careful review of research, reports findings very similar to those described by Wallerstein and Kelly. Separation and divorce are emotionally upsetting for the great majority of children. The child's first reaction is most likely to include a combination of anger, fear, depression, and guilt and is likely to be affected by the child's age, personality, and sex (Hetherington, 1979). In general, children who have previously had emotional or adjustment problems are most likely to be adversely affected. In addition, children who are subjected to a series of additional stresses (illness, for example) cope less well with their parents' divorce. Sex differences in adjustment to divorce are also striking, with boys being more adversely affected than girls (Hetherington, Cox, & Cox, 1979; Tessman, 1978). Whereas emotional and adjustment problems suffered by girls have typically disappeared within two years, those experienced by boys are often manifested in adjustment problems (truancy, delinquency, and so on) considerably later (Magrab, 1978). Among the possible reasons for this finding, Hetherington (1979) suggests that lack of a male model to imitate, stress associated with loss of the father, and the divorced mother's tendency to relate less well to sons than daughters immediately following divorce might all be important.

Several dangers are implicit in interpreting studies such as these. One is that we might inadvertently stress either the negative or the positive aspects of divorce. Although there appears to be little doubt that divorce is almost invariably a trying time for children, living in conflict (and sometimes with physical and mental abuse) can also be very trying. Divorce often is the best solution, both for parents and for their children. In addition, we also have to be careful not to mistakenly assume that what might be true *on the average* must also be generally true. We might mistakenly conclude, for example, that divorce is always detrimental to the welfare of children and that intact families are always good. This is clearly not the case. It bears repeating that some loving single parents can effectively overcome whatever trauma might be associated with the loss of one parent and that there are countless two-parent families in which parenting is inadequate and love is seldom if ever manifested.

■ Child Abuse

Do parents always love their children? And if they do, are children always treated as though they are loved? DeMause (1975) traces six stages in the treatment of children. In antiquity, infanticide was a prevalent mode of dealing with millions of children; the Middle Ages were characterized by abandonment rather than murder; the Renaissance was marked by an ambivalent attitude toward children; this ambivalence gradually gave way to control

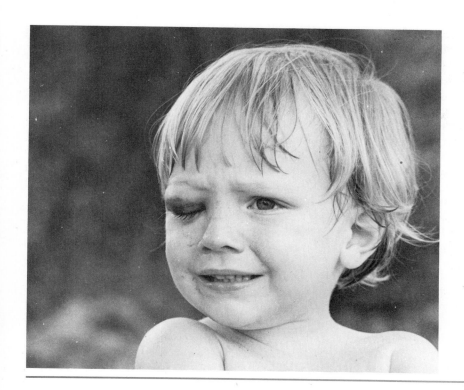

Sadly, child abuse is far more common than we might think.

during the eighteenth century; the nineteenth century heralded increasing social concern over the plights and the rights of children—a concern that applies to the present as well; finally, we are, according to DeMause, at the threshold of a deep-seated helping attitude toward children.

Unfortunately, although this may be history, it is not all past. Infanticide, abandonment, and scarcely believable instances of child abuse are shockingly prevalent in contemporary society. Estimates are that as many as 250,000 children are sufficiently abused in the United States each year to require the help of protective agencies (Bakan, 1971). Given the difficulty of obtaining information from parents and even from doctors in cases of child abuse, this figure probably represents a very conservative estimate (Stolk, 1974). In a national survey of child abuse in the United States, Gil (1970) found that an average of 9.3 children per 100,000 had suffered *reported* physical abuse

in 1968; the figure was 8.4 in 1967. In a more recent survey, Gelles (1979) found that 58 percent of a sample of 1,146 parents had used some form of physical violence on a child at least once during the past year. An astounding 2.9 percent admitted to having used a knife or a gun on one of their children at least once in their life—small wonder that one out of every four murders in North America is committed among immediate family members in their own home (Gelles & Straus, 1979).

The Nature of Child Abuse

The nature of child abuse is described, perhaps overly dramatically but effectively, by Bakan (1971, p. 4):

Children have been brought into hospitals with skulls fractured and bodies covered with lacerations. One parent disciplined a child for presumptive misbehavior with the buckle end of a belt, perforating an intestine and killing the child. Children have been whipped, beaten, starved, drowned, smashed against walls and floors, held in ice water baths, exposed to extremes of outdoor temperatures, burned with hot irons and steam pipes. Children have been tied and kept in upright positions for long periods. They have been systematically exposed to electric shock; forced to swallow pepper, soil, feces, urine, vinegar, alcohol, and other odious materials; buried alive; had scalding water poured over their genitals; had their limbs held in an open fire; placed in roadways where automobiles would run over them; placed on roofs and fire escapes in such a manner as to fall off; been bitten, knifed, and shot; had their eyes gouged out.

More representative perhaps is Gil's (1970) finding that the majority of children who were reported victims of abuse suffered from bruises and welts (67.1 percent); abrasions, contusions, and lacerations (32.3 percent); bone fractures and skull fractures (10.4 and 4.6 percent, respectively); burns and scaldings (10.1 percent); and wounds, cuts, and punctures (7.9 percent). (See *Sexual Abuse* for another type of child abuse.)

Who Is Abused

Contrary to some research and thought, physical abuse of children is less prevalent among very young children than among older children. In Gil's sample, more than three-quarters of all abused children were two years old or more; more than half were six or older. Not surprisingly, however, young children tended to be more seriously injured than older ones.

Among young children, more of those abused are boys than girls; this is no longer true in early adolescence. Parents appear to punish young male children more violently than older male children. In contrast, young girls receive physical punishment less frequently than older girls. Gil (1970) suggests that parents' anxieties concerning their daughters' sexual behavior may be a contributing factor in the physical abuse of older girls. Mothers tend to abuse more often than fathers, although mothers are not often as extreme in their abuse (Blumberg, 1974; Gelles, 1979).

In the United States, nonwhite children are abused more than whites. This higher incidence appears to be related to a variety of socioeconomic factors, including poverty and lower educational levels of parents (Garbarino & Crouter, 1977). The absence of the father from the home or the presence of a father substitute is related to child abuse. In addition, children from large families (four or more children) are more likely to be victims of abuse than children from smaller families.

It would be misleading to suggest that the probability of being an abused child is linked solely to social and economic characteristics of the home, sex of the child, and personality characteristics of the parents. There is mounting evidence that certain children are much more likely than others to be victims of abuse (Martin, 1976). Such children are frequently the products of difficult births and often suffered from postnatal complications, a fact that might be related to the absence of a strong parent-infant bond, particularly if the child was hospitalized for some time following birth. In addition, children who are abused are sometimes characterized by extreme irritability, feeding problems, excessive crying, and other behaviors that are annoying to parents. Sadly, many of these children are abused in their homes, although none of their siblings are, and continue to be abused when placed in foster homes.

Who Abuses

Child abuse is not solely a lower-class phenomenon, although parents of abused children tend to be from lower socioeconomic levels and have lower educational achievements; they also are more likely to be unemployed and to be recipients of social aid. A relatively small number may be classified as psychotic or as suffering from some other personality disorder (Boisvert, 1972). A number of abusive parents have themselves suffered abuse as children (Oliver & Taylor, 1971).

Although it has not been widely believed that any parent is capable of child abuse, research indicates that most parents might be. Mulhern and

Passman (1979) found, for example, that punitiveness tends to increase in parents as a consequence of the child's behavior. Specifically, if punishing a child leads to desirable behavior, attempts to obtain desirable behavior in the future may involve progressively higher levels of punishment.

Not unrelated to this, Passman and Mulhern (1977) conducted an experimental investigation of the effects of stress on mothers' punitiveness. They found that, with increasing stress, mothers tended to increase levels of punishment, a finding that provides experimental corroboration for the hypothesis that parental stress is sometimes directly implicated in child abuse (see, for example, Knutson, 1978; Parke & Collmer, 1975).

■ What Can Be Done

Although it is unlikely that child abuse can be completely eliminated, particularly since physical force is a widely accepted child-rearing technique in contemporary societies (Gelles, 1978), a number of things can be done. For example, Gil (1970)

SEXUAL ABUSE

A girl, aged seventeen, mother of a one-year-old child, presented herself for help (Bogopolsky & Cormier, 1979). Her complaint? Incest. For the past six years, her father had been having sexual relations with her. In the end, she had become pregnant. And a year ago, she had given birth to a child—of an unknown father, she told her mother, who accepted this explanation and began to raise the child as though it were her own.

The father, now also a grandfather, continued to force his attentions upon his daughter who, desperate, turned to her thirteen-year-old sister for help. Once the youngest sister had been told the story, she exposed it. The father's reaction? Denial. The mother's? Negation as well. And a sixteen-year-old brother, extremely intelligent and successful? Abject disappointment with his father.

An uncommon occurrence? Perhaps. Given the extreme social taboos that surround all forms of incest, especially father-daughter incest, we have no way of knowing how common it is. Estimates have typically been based on cases reported to courts or other legal jurisdictions, or on those that come to light in the course of mental health treatment (Meiselman, 1978), and are probably gross underestimates. Research cited by Herman (1981) suggests that approximately 10 percent of all women have been forced into some sexual experience with a relative and that as many as one in a hundred are victims of father-daughter incest.

Research on father-daughter incest (and on other forms of incest as well) is scarce; it consists largely of psychiatric case studies or collections of informal reports. In one study, a group of forty psychiatric patients who had had incestuous relationships with their fathers were compared with twenty other psychiatric patients whose fathers behaved seductively but who had not had directly incestuous relationships with them (Herman & Hirschman, 1981). In this study, incest is defined as any physical contact between father and daughter that has to be kept a secret. Genital fondling, masturbation, and oral-genital contacts as well as actual intercourse were the most common forms of incest. Other behaviors such as showing a daughter pornography, describing sexual conquests, or asking for detailed descriptions of the daughter's sexual behavior were classified as *seductive* rather than *incestuous* providing they did not involve physical contact.

Results of this study indicate that some broad characteristics might serve to identify families where incest is most likely to occur. First, fathers in incestuous families were far more likely to resort to violence to maintain authority. Frequently, however, persons toward whom violence was directed included the mother and other siblings but not the favored daughter. A second finding was that mothers in incestuous families were often ill, disabled, alcoholic, or battered. A third notable finding is that girls whose fathers abuse them sexually have a higher incidence of running away, attempted suicides, adolescent pregnancies, and emotional disorder. It is not a pretty picture.

suggests three separate approaches that might reduce its frequency and seriousness. First, systematic educational efforts should be directed toward changing our contemporary permissive attitudes toward the use of physical punishment. Second, because poverty and its related ills appear to be related to the incidence of child abuse, efforts to relieve poverty should be redoubled. Finally, preventive and therapeutic agencies should address themselves directly to problems related to child abuse.

What can be done and what is actually being done are not identical. As Starr (1979) notes, most child abuse programs have focused on treating parents who abuse as well as on protecting victims of abuse; relatively few have been concerned with prevention. And estimates of the effectiveness of child abuse treatments vary considerably, ranging from a high of 80 percent improvement (Kempe & Kempe, 1978) to a low somewhere around 40 percent.

Among the most optimistic of prevention strategies are those that have attempted to discover ways of *predicting* which parents or children are most likely to be involved in child abuse, so that corrective action can be undertaken before the problem occurs. Unfortunately, several large-scale and well-controlled investigations have identified few consistent differences between children who are most likely to be abused and those less likely (Starr, Dietrich, & Fischhoff, 1981). Similarly, a systematic investigation of abusive and nonabusive parents found no consistent patterns of differences between the two groups (Starr, 1982). Thus, although we know that certain racial, economic, and social factors are involved in child abuse, we cannot reliably predict who is most likely to be abused (or abusive). Hence prevention based on prediction remains difficult, costly, and susceptible to considerable error involving false identification.

Other preventative strategies that might be highly effective in the long term include Gil's suggestion that we change contemporary society's attitudes toward corporal punishment, as well as Starr's (1979) suggestion that we make wider use of parent training programs. However, dramatic changes in parental attitudes are likely to be difficult if not impossible to effect. Nor can social agencies attempt to identify and label potential abusers without running the risk of unfair and discriminatory practices, slander, and invasion of privacy. The problem is not simple, nor is its solution.

■ MAIN POINTS

1 Culture, family, peer groups, and activities such as attending school and watching television constitute powerful influences on the child's behavior and development.

2 *Culture* may be defined as the sum of the mores, beliefs, customs, traditions, accepted behaviors, and implicit rules that characterize a people. The trappings of a culture are its language, its religion, and its schools.

3 The pressure to conform, which appears to be less powerful in our society than in the intensely personal groups that typify primitive societies, can nevertheless be powerful enough to lead people to believe (and say or do) things that contradict their rational inclinations or beliefs.

4 Socialization is the process whereby culture is transmitted from one generation to the next. A widely accepted theory of socialization is premised on the notion that much social learning takes place through imitation.

5   There are three broad categories of children's play: sensorimotor games such as practicing to run, skip, or stick out one's tongue; imaginative games in which the actor, the actions, or the objects acted upon are treated as something other than what they really are; and social games that involve interaction between two or more children.

6   Evidence suggests that daydreaming, imaginary playmates, and other forms of fantasy are constructive. Children prone to fantasy play appear to be more creative, more verbal, happier, and less aggressive than children who engage in less fantasy play.

7   Sex differences are not readily apparent in imaginative play, although boys tend to play more physically and more loudly than girls. The toys that boys and girls are given, and the toys they select, are stereotypically different.

8   A nuclear family consists of mother, father, and children. Extended families also include a variety of other blood relatives.

9   There has been a dramatic increase in the number of one-parent families.

10 The family is a highly dynamic social unit; it changes as a function of external pressures and as a result of internal events. Here, as elsewhere, influence is bidirectional.

11 Our predominant psychoanalytic-behavioristic model of parent-child influence stresses the sensitivity, vulnerability, and malleability of the child. The model exaggerates all three of these characteristics.

12 It is difficult to predict future adjustment and personality characteristics of children on the basis of what might be known about the child-rearing practices of their parents.

13 Parents do make a difference. But that difference may relate more to their attitudes toward children and child rearing than to specific child-rearing practices.

14 Evidence suggests that firstborn and only children are more achievement oriented than other children; in addition, they are more likely to go to college, to achieve eminence, to score higher on tests of intellectual performance, and to develop language facility sooner.

15 Children from larger families *on the average* do less well than children from smaller families on measures of intellectual performance; this finding might result as much from any of a number of social variables as from family size itself.

16 Some of the effects of one-parent families on children may be due to the lack of a father; they may also result from altered economic conditions or from having to cope with a husbandless mother.

17 The relationship between delinquency and other manifestations of maladjustment and one-parent homes has not been demonstrated to be causal; hence one cannot predict that children from one-parent homes will be maladjusted.

18 Daughters of widowed mothers are less likely to seek contact with males than are daughters of divorced mothers. Neither of these groups has attitudes toward men that are as positive as those of girls from intact homes.

19 The emotional effects of divorce depend on the age of the child, on sex, and on the child's previous adjustment. The reactions of different children vary widely.

20 Reported instances of child abuse may represent the tip of a rather frightful iceberg.

21 More older than younger children are physically abused; in the United States, more nonwhites than whites are included in this group. Abusers are sometimes disturbed in a clinical sense, although they often are not; many of those who abuse their children have themselves been abused when young.

■ FURTHER READINGS

A highly poetic and thoughtful look at imagination in childhood is provided by:
Cobb, E. *The ecology of imagination in childhood*. New York: Columbia University Press, 1977.

Singer's book presents a great deal of theory and research relating to make-believe, as well as some convincing arguments for the importance of encouraging fantasy in children:
Singer, J. L. (Ed.). *The child's world of make-believe: Experimental studies of imaginative play*. New York: Academic Press, 1973.

The biological significance of play is the focus of this highly interesting book, concerned primarily with play among nonhuman animals:
Aldis, O. *Play fighting*. New York: Academic Press, 1975.

The following is an excellent collection of articles relating to child development. In particular, Part 6 contains six articles that address themselves directly to such topics as parent-child relationships, child-rearing practices, one-parent families, and child abuse.
Cohen, S., & Comisky, T. J. (Eds.). *Child development: Contemporary perspectives*. Itasca, Ill.: F. E. Peacock, 1977.

Two books by Lynn present a comprehensive attempt to collect and interpret research relating to families and children. The first is concerned specifically with the role of the father, and the second with daughters; both deal extensively with the family.
Lynn, D. B. *The father: His role in child development*. Monterey, Calif.: Brooks/Cole, 1974.
Lynn, D. B. *Daughters and parents: Past, present and future*. Monterey, Calif.: Brooks/Cole, 1979.

Two sources of information on child abuse are:
Bourne, R., & Newberger, E. H. (Eds.). *Critical perspectives on child abuse*. Lexington, Mass.: D. C. Heath, 1979.
Martin, H. *The abused child*. Cambridge, Mass.: Ballinger, 1976.

An optimistic description of the problems and possibilities of single parenthood that could be valuable to single parents is:

Knight, B. M. *Enjoying single parenthood.* New York: Van Nostrand, 1980.

A moving, first-person account of father-daughter incest, told by the daughter, is presented in:

Brady, K. *Father's days: A true story of incest.* New York: Seaview Books, 1979.

Those interested in a guide to the selection of day care for their children—or those interested in establishing quality day care might consult:

Endsley, R. C., & Bradbard, M. R. *Quality day care: A handbook of choices for parents and caregivers.* Englewood Cliffs, N.J.: Prentice-Hall, 1981.

9

COGNITIVE AND SOCIAL DEVELOPMENT IN MIDDLE CHILDHOOD

Instruct them how the mind of man becomes
A thousand times more beautiful than the earth
On which he dwells.

William Wordsworth
The Prelude

No problem. Have it fixed in an hour or so," the man says. "You folks in a rush, you oughta keep goin' 'n get it fixed in Bonnyville."

It seems as though there should be no rush. I say so. We leave the car, the front half inside the garage's only stall, the back protruding dangerously into the lane. I can drive no further; a half-disassembled engine, an anvil, miscellaneous tools, and a sleeping dog block my way.

"It'll be all right. Nobody much drives down this alley."

We walk across the street to Ashmont's only restaurant. There is a large splotch of shade across the schoolyard at the far end of the street and another partly covering the restaurant and the adjoining billiard hall. I walk through the edge of the shade and into the restaurant. Two men in dusty overalls slurp coffee from cups that look too small in their hands. Their voices are low and quiet.

A sad-eyed waitress shuffles over, shoulders and hair drooping. Sundaes, milkshakes, french fries, and other assorted delicacies; my tribe orders all. I order nothing. I have no hunger. I have had no hunger for a long time now. I know it is a bad sign.

I leave money. It seems that I am always leaving money. Paul and Denise immediately get most of it changed into quarters and rush to the video games, Marcel hot on their heels. Grandmother sits, knitting something large and green.

"Eat something," she says. She looks worried.

"Not hungry. I'll just go next door for a bit. Call me when they're ready to go."

"Don't . . ." she begins, but doesn't finish. I don't ask her to. We both know what she was going to say.

When I first walk in, the pool hall seems empty. It has a deserted feeling. There are no souls here, I think wryly.

Then I see him. A large man sitting behind the counter, close to his cash register, staring out the window. He wears a white T-shirt, badly stained over his distended belly—worse yet, under each arm. A large, mostly blue tattoo covers his left forearm—a snake coiled around a banner. On the banner, in faded red, there is a single word: Mother.

He turns and studies me for a moment.

"Shoot pool?" It's half question, half statement.

"A bit." I'm noncommittal. Cool. I sense the familiar surge of adrenaline, the excitement. I breathe deeply, savoring the smell of pool chalk and leather. It's been a long time. Too long. "Sometimes." Still cool.

"Shoot you a game," he offers. His voice is low, almost menacing. "You name the stakes." The challenge is like an order. I repress a smile. This is almost too easy. I can feel the effects of the first adrenaline rush receding. I try to hold the feeling just a bit longer.

What should I say? I don't want to frighten him off by making the stakes too high, but they need to be high enough.

"Fifty," I answer.

"Fifty cents?" he jeers, turning back to the window.

"Dollars." I have his attention. He comes around the counter, his cue already in his hand. "Eight ball," I continue, only momentarily uneasy. "Call shot. Scratch on the eight or miss it and you lose. One game, fifty dollars."

"Put your money on the counter," he says. Is there a hint of a smile?

"You too."

I chalk up. The wood feels light, smooth, made for my hands. I glance at the money on the counter, and I know that it's really not the money. I have been told often enough that it's not the money. Still, there must always be money.

He breaks; the balls scatter well. An easy table, I survey it almost casually. Four ball, side pocket, low right-hand English, shape up for the six. Six straight in, upper corner, strong draw coming off the cushion for the seven. I love that shot. The seven, now, a long gentle cut to the lower corner, cue ball once off the right cushion and in perfect shape for the three ball. I straighten up, chalk my cue again, and glance at my opponent. Is he still looking out the window?

The three and one, in rapid succession into the side, followed by a moderately difficult shot on the five—a single bank to the corner. Now an easy two and, finally, only the eight. The whole game riding on a single shot, adrenaline coursing sweetly through my veins. I have an open field to the eight!

I glance at my opponent, perhaps wanting to savor his discomfort. He no longer stares out the window. Instead, he grins at me widely, revealing a huge toothless space, upper front. I look again at the table. Understanding floods over me; there is no open pocket for my eight ball. All are covered by my opponent's unspent balls. I hide my momentary confusion behind a thin smile, knowing that I will get another shot. One more is all I need. I nudge the eight ball delicately into the center of the table, where it will be most vulnerable when next I shoot.

My opponent approaches the table, casually it seems. His hands are too large; there is no grace in his movements. He holds the cue too tightly and stands too straight. I will have no problems with him.

"Let's go, dad. I can see he's got the tire back on the car." Paul is at the door, Denise behind him. They both look anxious.

"Just one more shot. And then maybe just one more real quick game."

They now look scared.

"Okay. Just one more shot. I'll just finish this game." My opponent has now sunk four of his seven balls. His stance is still terrible, his grip clumsy. He continues to grin.

Two more balls. Quickly. They roll into the pockets, dead center, smoothly and earnestly. I am amazed because he plays so badly.

Another ball, now, a long, delicate slice to the far corner. The eight ball lines up perfectly to the short side. He scarcely hesitates, before tapping it gently in. Dead center again.

"Another?" he asks, stuffing my bills into his pants.

I begin to nod. I can beat him because I am a better player.

"We've got to go!" There is a note of hysteria in Denise's voice. Grandma now stands behind her. She looks sad. Reluctantly, I leave.

The silence in the car is awkward. I break it. "How'd you make out with your games?" All three begin to answer at once, excited and animated; all are video addicts. How different their childhoods from mine. Will their vices also be different? And their virtues?

Perhaps we can come closer to some answers in this, the ninth chapter of our tale—a chapter that continues to deal with social and intellectual development at a point very close to where the last chapter left off.

■ Middle Childhood

The period that concerns us in this chapter spans the years referred to as **middle childhood**. Its boundaries are somewhat arbitrary: It begins near the age of six, a convenient age because the preschool period stops there, and it ends at approximately age twelve.* Because this stage terminates with the beginning of pubescence, and pubescence occurs at different ages for males and females and for different individuals of the same sex, its upper boundary is indefinite. (See *Capsule Views of Ages Six and Twelve*.)

■ Physical Development

During the years from six to twelve, children become taller and heavier. The parallel growth that existed for boys and girls prior to this period is not maintained throughout middle childhood. Although girls tended to be slightly shorter and slightly lighter than boys from birth to the end of the preschool period, the growth curves for each were almost identical; that is, both gained at approximately the same rate. Table 9.1 summarizes height and weight data for boys and girls

---

*Many authors end middle childhood at age ten and insert another period between there and adolescence, labeled *late childhood* or *preadolescence*.

from the ages of six to twelve. An examination of these norms reveals that although the average girl is three-fourths of an inch shorter at the age of six, she has caught up with and surpassed the average boy by the age of eleven and is still slightly taller at the age of twelve. With respect to weight, girls are close to two pounds lighter at the age of six

and do not catch up with boys until the age of eleven. Between the ages of eleven and twelve, however, there is a sudden spurt of weight gain for girls that puts them three pounds ahead of boys in the course of a single year. Chapter 11 points out that not until the age of fourteen and one-half do boys overtake girls in weight, and at

CAPSULE VIEWS OF AGES SIX AND TWELVE

Physically, six-year-olds are characterized by a relatively adultlike distribution of forty-eight pounds set upon a frame that stretches just a little under four feet (forty-six inches). Their vocabulary includes several thousand words, and they have pretty well succeeded in mastering the grammar of their language and in developing a symbolic (verbal) representation of their world. Despite this, they continue to engage in a great many sensorimotor games—games that require no symbolization and no abstract reasoning. Also, they still frequently represent reality in concrete mental images. The reasoning of six-year-olds abounds with contradictions, although they will attempt, and occasionally solve, problems that a two-year-old would not begin to understand. According to Piaget, their thinking is dominated by sense perception and is intuitive and egocentric.

In the Freudian view, six-year-old children have probably been successful in overcoming some of the sexually based conflicts that beset them from infancy. If the child is a boy, he has renounced his overpowering attachment to his mother and has begun to identify with his father. If the child is a girl, she has abandoned her unconscious desire to have a baby by her father and has overcome the consequent jealousy of her mother; she is now ready to identify with her mother. Both the boy and the girl will enter a period of sexual latency, during which there is no dominant source of sexual gratification and interest in the opposite sex is at its lowest ebb.

In contrast to the typical six-year-old, consider the twelve-year-old. The average twelve-year-old boy weighs eighty-four pounds and is almost five feet tall (fifty-nine inches). The vocabulary of twelve-year-old children is incredibly larger and includes many frequently used idiomatic and slang expressions of their particular peer group. Their immediate family has diminished in importance, and the influence of peer groups has increased. They attend school, have learned to read and write, and have refined their powers of concentration, abstract

thinking, and problem solving. According to Piaget, they have developed a fairly sophisticated logic, sufficient to handle all types of concrete problems. They can classify and deal with seriation, and they understand the concept of number. They no longer make the errors that characterized their earlier attempts to solve conservation problems. These problems have become so easy for them that they may be embarrassed by their simplicity. The thinking of twelve-year-old children is symbolic, although usually related to real objects or to situations that they are easily capable of imagining. Just as their thinking has become more refined, so has their verbal skill.

From the Freudian view, twelve-year-old children are about to emerge from the period of sexual latency, during which they avoided heterosexual contact, much preferring to consort with members of their own sex. They have developed notions of sex-appropriate behavior as a result of identification with the like-sexed parent and also from having spent much time with like-sexed peers. Peer groups are particularly prone to reinforce their members for sex-appropriate behavior and to extinguish all other behavior, both by not reinforcing it and by drawing attention to its inappropriateness through ridicule, ostracism, or some other form of punishment. A sometimes difficult transition from this period to the final stage of psychosexual development marks the termination of middle childhood and the beginning of adolescence.

By the age of twelve, children are ready to move from concrete to more abstract thought processes; from a period of sexual latency to the genital phase of development, when members of the opposite sex begin to assume the importance that they maintain throughout most of the individual's life; from the last period of development that can still be called childhood to one that must now be interpreted as at least the beginnings of adulthood.

thirteen and one-half they exceed girls in height. The weight and height of average men continue to exceed those of women until the end.

Another trend of physical growth that continues throughout middle childhood is a gradual decrease in growth of fatty tissue, coupled with increased bone and muscle development. Muscle development is generally more rapid in boys, whereas girls tend to retain thicker layers of fat longer. This fatty tissue is distributed so that girls have rounder, smoother, and softer contours and frequently retain a babyish appearance (resulting from plumpness) longer than boys.

The growth spurt in height and weight during this period occurs approximately two years earlier for girls than for boys. For this reason, it is probably fortunate that boys and girls usually choose to associate with members of their own sex during the growth spurt, because the obvious physical differences that exist not only between the sexes but also between members of the same sex are frequently a source of acute embarrassment for children. At a time when children are very sensitive to peer approval, it is a great misfortune to be either precocious or retarded in physical development. It is humiliating for a boy to suddenly find that his younger sister has become taller than he; the humiliation is often accompanied by the fear that he will continue to be short. It is probably equally uncomfortable to be the tallest boy or the tallest girl in the class and to live with the secret fear of being a tall, skinny freak.

Nature usually compensates for initial discrepancies. The tall girl finds that she was an early bloomer; she ceases to grow at the time when her peers begin their growth spurts, and in a short time she finds herself surrounded by equals. The short boy discovers that he was merely a slow starter; when his seemingly more fortunate friends have nearly reached their adult heights, he suddenly stretches skyward.

Motor Development

Children's muscular control continues to develop during the years from six to twelve. Early in this

Table 9.1 Height and weight at the fiftieth percentile for American children.

Age	Height (inches)		Weight (pounds)	
	Girl	Boy	Girl	Boy
6 years	45½	46¼	46½	48¼
6½ years	47	47½	49½	51¼
7 years	48	49	52¼	54
7½ years	49¼	50	55¼	57
8 years	50½	51¼	58	60
8½ years	51½	52¼	61	63
9 years	52¼	53¼	63¾	66
9½ years	53½	54¼	67	69
10 years	54½	55¼	70¼	72
10½ years	55¾	56	74¼	74¾
11 years	57	56¾	78¾	77½
11½ years	58¼	57¾	83¼	81
12 years	59¾	59	87½	84½

Adapted by the Health Department, Milwaukee, Wisconsin; based on data by H. C. Stuart and H. V. Meredith, prepared for use in Children's Medical Center, Boston. Used by permission of the Milwaukee Health Department.

period their control of large muscles is considerably better than their control over smaller muscles (an explanation for the inelegant writing of first- and second-grade children). By the end of middle childhood, control of the large muscles has become nearly perfect and control over the small muscles is much improved.

The changes in locomotor skills, agility, coordination, and physical strength are particularly interesting, not only because they demonstrate such marked differences between the sexes but also because they may be significant in explaining the child's interests. Perhaps this partially explains why boys are more interested in physical activity than girls. For example, throughout middle childhood the boy's physical strength (measured in terms of grip strength) is superior to the girl's, even though the average girl is taller and heavier than the boy (Keogh, 1965). However, these physical differences may not explain different interests at all; the physical differences (greater grip strength, for example) may result from different activities—in short, from the greater interest that boys initially have in activities requiring grip strength.

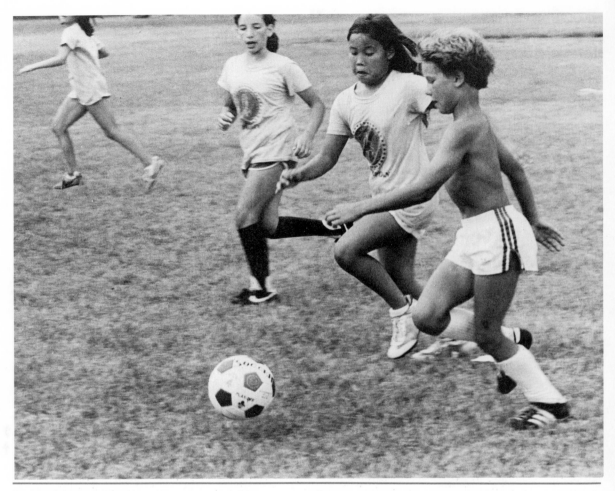

Participation in activities requiring greater skill becomes possible as children's motor control, strength, agility, and coordination increase. Such activities contribute significantly to social as well as physical development.

On a number of other locomotor indexes, boys typically surpass girls. Johnson (1962) provides data on the average height that the child can jump from a standing start, summarized in Figure 9.1. Boys consistently outreach girls after the age of seven. This finding is assumed to indicate that boys' leg power and arm-leg coordination for jumping are better than those of girls. Johnson also found that boys did better than girls in tests of kicking, throwing, catching, batting, and zigzag-

ging. This last test involved four chairs aligned six feet apart, with the first chair six feet from a starting line and the last chair six feet from a wall. The subject was instructed to run around the chairs, alternating sides (zigzagging), to touch an X that had been drawn on the wall, and to return to the starting line by the same route. Figure 9.2 presents the results of this test for boys and girls from grades one to six.

Other measures of motor performance show

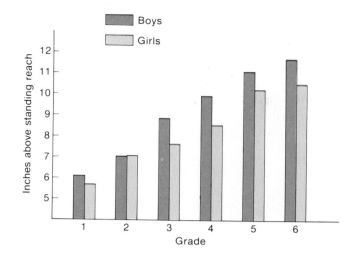

Figure 9.1
Number of inches above standing reach jumped by boys and girls from grades one through six. (Based on data in Robert D. Johnson, Measurements of achievement in fundamental skills of elementary school children. *Research Quarterly*, 1962, *33*, 94–103, p. 97. Copyright 1962 by the American Association for Health, Physical Education and Recreation. Used by permission of the American Association for Health, Physical Education, Recreation and Dance.)

that boys jump significantly farther than girls on a broad jump (Keogh, 1965), that boys perform better with hurdles (Cowan & Pratt, 1934), and that they are more adept at hopping on alternate feet (Keogh, 1968, cited by Cratty, 1970). Boys also run faster and throw a ball farther. However, girls do surpass boys in a limited number of motor skills during the middle childhood period (but rarely afterward). These skills include cable jumping—jumping over a cable or rope that the jumper holds in the hands. In addition, Cratty (1970) reports that girls sometimes surpass boys in tasks involving rhythmic movements, such as those in hopscotch and rope skipping.

Reaction Time

Reaction time, defined as the length of time between the presentation of a stimulus and the initiation of a response, is one of the variables that plays an important role in the development of the child's motor abilities. Whiting (1969) reports that the reaction time of a five-year-old child is approximately twice as long as that of an adult. He argues that the child's initial difficulty with such tasks as catching a ball is due largely to slow reaction time. It is not clear whether the child is physiologically incapable of reacting more rapidly, or whether the child simply takes longer to decide to react or how

to react. In any case, rapid games are very difficult, if not impossible, for the young child. Different reaction times and different levels of motor skills (which are probably related to some extent) also make it likely that children of different ages will seek peers of similar ages to play with, because they not only share similar interests but also bring more compatible skills to their games.

■ Intellectual Development

When we left children's minds early in Chapter 7, it was not because their minds had ceased to develop, while they continued to advance physically and socially, but because the minds of authors and sometimes of readers are not always adept at rendering lucid a subject as complex as the child's total development. We pick up the thread of intellectual development once more, keeping in mind that as their intellect is developing, children are also growing in other ways. Our guide again is Jean Piaget, and the period through which we are moving is labeled **concrete operations.** The child approaches this period by way of the sensorimotor period (birth to two years) and two preoperational subperiods: preconceptual thought (two to four years) and intuitive thinking (four to seven years). The child's thinking toward the end of the intuitive

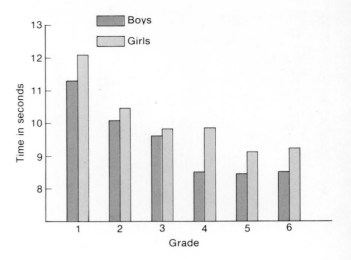

Figure 9.2
Time in seconds required by boys from grades one through six to run a zigzag course. (Based on data in Robert D. Johnson, Measurements of achievement in fundamental skills of elementary school children. *Research Quarterly*, 1962, *33*, 94–103, p. 97. Copyright 1962 by the American Association for Health, Physical Education and Recreation. Used by permission of the American Association for Health, Physical Education, Recreation and Dance.)

stage is egocentric, perception dominated, and intuitive. Consequently, it is marked by contradictions and errors of logic. With the beginning of the period of concrete thought, many of these deficiencies will disappear and be replaced by more logical thinking.

Transition from the intuitive stage to concrete operations is marked by the acquisition of one or more *conservations*—and these are at once the most widely researched, the most interesting, and perhaps the most significant manifestations of the child's thinking investigated by Piaget.

The Conservations

Conservation refers to the fact that the quantitative aspects of objects do not change unless something has been added to or taken away from them, despite other changes in the objects. In Chapter 7, for example, we described a situation where a child is presented with two equal balls of modeling clay and asked whether there is still as much clay in each after one has been rolled out into something like a snake. The preoperational child's belief that there was more clay in the snake than there had been in the ball (presumably because it was now longer and therefore *looked* as though it had more) is an example of the inability to

conserve. The eventual realization that the transformed object does not have more or less substance than it previously had marks not only the acquisition of concepts of conservation but also the transition between preoperational thought and concrete operations.

The significance of the acquisition of conservation is not so much that children cease to be deceived by a problem but rather that they have now developed certain fundamental logical rules, evident in much of their thinking. These rules make it possible for children to overcome many of the errors that characterized their thinking during the preoperational period. In a sense, they free the child from reliance on perception and intuition; like some of us, children can now rely on *logic*. Put another way, they can rely on *operations* (thought processes governed by rules of logic) rather than on *preoperations*.

Three rules of logic that are highly characteristic of concrete operations, and particularly important for the acquisition of conservation, are **identity, reversibility**, and **compensation**. Each can be illustrated by reference to the simple conservation of quantity problem described earlier, in which children are presented with two identical clay balls. They admit the balls contain the same amount of modeling clay. One is then elongated while the other is left unchanged. Each subject is

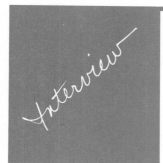
asked whether the deformed object still contains the same amount of clay as the unchanged object, or whether it has more or less. If they say that it has an equal amount (conservation), they may be reasoning in one of three ways. They may think that nothing has been added to or taken away from the elongated object and that it must therefore be identical to what it was *(identity)*. Or, they might reason that the sausagelike shape can be reformed into the original ball, in which case the sausage and ball must contain the same amount *(reversibility)*. A third assumption might be that the elongated object appears to have more material because it is longer but also appears to have less because it is thinner. The two dimensions therefore compensate each other and the changes are canceled *(compensation)*.

More formally, *identity* is the notion that for every operation (internalized act or thought) there is an operation that leaves the product unchanged. In other words, amount does not change if nothing is added or taken away. *Reversibility* means that every operation can be undone (reversed or unthought) and that certain logical consequences follow from this possibility. Thus, even a very ugly clay sausage can be made back into a ball resembling the original ball. *Compensation* specifies that several operations can be combined in different ways to yield the same result.

How general are these logical rules? That is, once the child has learned about identity, compensation, and reversibility, do these rules apply

to all thinking? The answer is no. Consider, for example, that there are many different kinds of conservation—about as many as there are characteristics of objects that can vary in quantity. Thus, in addition to conservation of amount (or mass, involving liquids or solids, or discontinuous material like beads, beans, or baubles), there is conservation of number, length, area, volume, and so on. If the rules of logic that make these conservations possible were completely general, they would all be acquired at the same time. That is, when children realize that the amount of clay does not change when a ball is flattened, they should also realize that the amount of water does not change when it is poured from a tall thin vase into a shallow wide bowl. But, as Figure 9.3 shows, approximate ages at which the various conservations are acquired span a number of years. (See also *Acceleration of Conservation.*)

Additional evidence that the rules of logic of a child at the concrete operations stage are not completely general is derived from a series of *extinction* studies. In these studies, children who have already acquired a specific conservation are provided with actual evidence that their reasoning is incorrect. The argument is that if a conserver truly believes that conservation is a logical and *necessary* consequence, there should be strong resistance to *extinction* of that logic. To simplify, consider a typical extinction experiment in conservation of weight. First, subjects are presented with two identical clay balls. Each agrees that both

1. Conservation of substance (6–7 years)

A

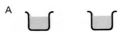

The experimenter presents two identical plasticene balls. The subject admits that they have equal amounts of plasticene.

B

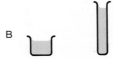

One of the balls is deformed. The subject is asked whether they still contain equal amounts.

2. Conservation of length (6–7 years)

A

Two sticks are aligned in front of the subject. The subject admits their equality.

B

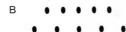

One of the sticks is moved to the right. The subject is asked whether they are still the same length.

3. Conservation of number (6–7 years)

A

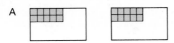

Two rows of counters are placed in one-to-one correspondence. Subject admits their equality.

B

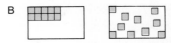

One of the rows is elongated (or contracted). Subject is asked whether each row still has the same number.

4. Conservation of liquids (6–7 years)

A

Two beakers are filled to the same level with water. The subject sees that they are equal.

B

The liquid of one container is poured into a tall tube (or a flat dish). The subject is asked whether each contains the same amount.

5. Conservation of area (9–10 years)

A

The subject and the experimenter each have identical sheets of cardboard. Wooden blocks are placed on these in identical positions. The subject is asked whether each cardboard has the same amount of space remaining.

B

The experimenter scatters the blocks on one of the cardboards. The subject is asked the same question.

Figure 9.3
Some simple tests for conservation with approximate ages of attainment.

ACCELERATION OF CONSERVATION

One of the questions that American researchers and educators were fond of asking Piaget went something like this: "If we can accurately describe some of the important capabilities that children develop and the sequence in which these appear, might it not also be possible to accelerate their appearance by providing children with appropriate experiences? And could we not, by so doing, speed up the developmental process, increase children's cognitive capabilities, and perhaps even make them more intelligent?" But Piaget did not have a direct answer for this question based on his own research. His concerns had always been more with the description and explanation of cognitive development than with attempts to change its ordinary course. However, an impressive number of other researchers have attempted to answer. And the majority of these have looked at the possibility of accelerating the development of concepts of conservation—concepts that are simply defined, easy to measure, and highly significant with respect to general cognitive development. The general assumption is that if the acquisition of concepts of conservation is truly important in the child's cognitive development, and if it can be accelerated through training, then it might be possible to design school programs that might be far more beneficial for cognitive growth than those presently in vogue.

Many of the early studies designed specifically to teach conservation to young children before they would be expected to acquire it naturally were not successful. A task as apparently simple as teaching a child that the amount of modeling clay in an object does not change unless material is added or taken away seemed almost impossible (Smedslund, 1961a, 1961b, 1961c, 1961d, 1961e)—almost, but not quite; a number of systematic and detailed training procedures were sometimes at least partly successful in teaching conservation (for example, Lefrancois, 1968; Travis, 1969). In the Lefrancois experiment, subjects were given systematic practice in identifying relevant qualities of objects (length, width), as well as practice with situations where the amount was increased or decreased by actually adding or subtracting material. Similarly, Gelman (1969) succeeded in teaching conservation, using training procedures emphasizing that distracting perceptual changes in conservation problems are irrelevant. She suggests that, to be successful, conservation training programs must provide the child with an opportunity to work with and handle relevant materials in a variety of forms and that they must be provided with frequent information concerning whether their estimates relating to size, number, quantity, and so on are accurate.

Other research in the area of acceleration of conservation has continued to report mixed success. A variety of approaches have been employed. Siegler and Liebert (1972), like Gelman, accelerated acquisition of liquid conservation by providing children with rules and with information concerning the accuracy of their responses. Rosenthal and Zimmerman (1972) employed a conserving child as a model. Many nonconserving subjects subsequently demonstrated knowledge of conservation on related but not identical tasks. But when these investigators used instruction in relevant rules rather than models, they were unsuccessful in accelerating conservation. And Kuhn (1972), who also employed a modeling procedure, failed to increase conservation behavior appreciably in subjects.

In summary, the conclusion that development can be altered easily and significantly through short-term training programs in specific areas is not warranted by the available evidence. Conservation can be accelerated, but training programs, especially if the children are still some distance from acquiring conservation naturally, need to be detailed and systematic (see Furth, 1980; Gelman & Gallistel, 1978). And whether such efforts, when successful, contribute significantly to intellectual development—or to happiness and self-esteem—remains unclear.

weigh an equal amount and continues to maintain that this is the case, even after one or both of the balls have been deformed or broken into little pieces. At this point, however, the experimenter asks subjects to verify their conservation response by means of a balance scale. Alas, the scale is "rigged," so that one of the "balls" now weighs more than the other.

More than twenty-five extinction experiments have been conducted (Miller, 1981). And in a majority of them, subjects believe evidence that contradicts their original conservation response,

	Mangy coyotes	Healthy coyotes
Fat coyotes	Fat, mangy coyotes	Fat, healthy coyotes
Skinny coyotes	Skinny, mangy coyotes	Skinny, healthy coyotes

Figure 9.4
How many kinds of coyotes are there if there are fat ones and skinny ones and mangy ones and healthy ones? An illustration of the classification abilities of the concrete operations child.

and that, by the same token, also contradicts the logical rules that underlie that response. Thus, young conservers (and sometimes older ones) do not always behave as though they believe these rules of logic to be *necessarily* true in all relevant cases. However, further questioning of subjects reveals that they do not doubt the certainty of the logical rule but that they are simply not always clear about when to apply the rule. Miller's (1981) research indicates that even young children realize that social rules, for example, are arbitrary and uncertain, but that Piagetian rules of logic are more universal. However, the rigged balance scale presents a real-life problem rather than a problem in logic. Specifically, in this situation, the child is not deciding whether or not the logical rule is correct (she knows it is) but whether or not the scale is correct.

Other Abilities

In addition to acquiring various conservations, children acquire three distinct abilities as they enter concrete operations. First, they learn to deal with classes, achieving the capacity to understand class inclusion and to reason about the combination and the decomposition of classes. An eight-year-old child, for example, would be unlikely to make a mistake when asked to decide whether there are

more roses or more flowers in a bouquet consisting of fifteen roses and five tulips. At this level, children typically understand that roses make up a subclass of the larger class of flowers. Similarly, they would have little difficulty multiplying two classes in the problem that follows: If there are fat coyotes and skinny coyotes, and some are mangy and some are healthy, how many kinds of coyotes are there? The classes they must multiply are fat and skinny coyotes by mangy and healthy coyotes. The answer is illustrated in Figure 9.4.

During the period of concrete operations, the child comes to understand the concept of **seriation**—that is, the concept of ordering in sequence. Piaget developed a problem to demonstrate the lack of seriation during the preoperational period; this same method can be employed to demonstrate its presence during concrete operations. The child is presented with two ordered series of objects—for example, a group of dolls and a group of canes, each a different length so that the objects might easily be arranged from longest to shortest. Figure 9.5 illustrates the arrangement desired, easily and quickly produced by the child in concrete operations, even when both series are presented in random order. The child at the stage of intuitive thinking, however, is ordinarily incapable of responding correctly even with a single series. A typical response is to place several of the dolls in order while ignoring the fact that others may fit in between those that have already been positioned. If the next doll the child selects is too short to be placed where the child intended it to be (at the upper end), it is placed without hesitation at the other end, even though it might be taller or shorter than the doll that is already positioned there. The child fails to make an inference that signals complete understanding of seriation. This understanding is almost essential to the solution of the problem: If A is greater than B, and B is greater than C, then must A also be greater than C? Understanding this concept eliminates the necessity for making all the comparisons that would otherwise be necessary.

Once children understand classification and seriation, they can also understand the concept of

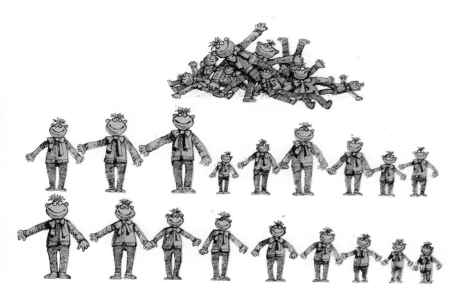

Figure 9.5
A test of a child's understanding of seriation. The elements of the series are presented in random order and the child is asked to arrange them in sequence of height.

number. Although they might have previously learned to recite numbers in the appropriate order and they might appear to associate collections of objects with particular numbers, their concept of number is still incomplete. Children must comprehend both the ordinal (the ordered sequence or succession of numbers) and the cardinal (quantitative) properties of number; the first concept involves seriation; the second relates to classification. That is, a number involves classes because it represents collections (classes) of different, or increasing, magnitude (the cardinal property of number); a number involves seriation in the sense that numbers are ordered in relation to other numbers of greater or lesser magnitude (the ordinal properties of number).

Note that Piaget's estimates of the ages of acquisitions during concrete operations are often underestimates, as are his estimates of when preoperational and sensorimotor children achieve certain things. In particular, Gelman and Gallistel (1978) draw attention to the fact that many preoperational children have a far more complete understanding of number concepts than Piaget's theories indicate.

Summary of Concrete Operations

An *operation* is a thought that is characterized by rules of logic. Because children acquire conservations early in this period and because these concepts are manifestations of operational thinking, the period is called *operational*. It is also termed *concrete*, because children's thinking deals with real objects or those they can easily imagine. Children in the concrete operations stage are bound to this world; they do not yet have the freedom made possible by the more advanced logic of the formal operations stage—freedom to contemplate the hypothetical, to compare the ideal with the actual, to be profoundly unhappy and concerned about the discrepancy between this world and that which they imagine possible.

■ Social Development

But physical and intellectual development do not occur in isolation from each other nor in isolation from other aspects of human development. Even as the child is stretching and expanding both in

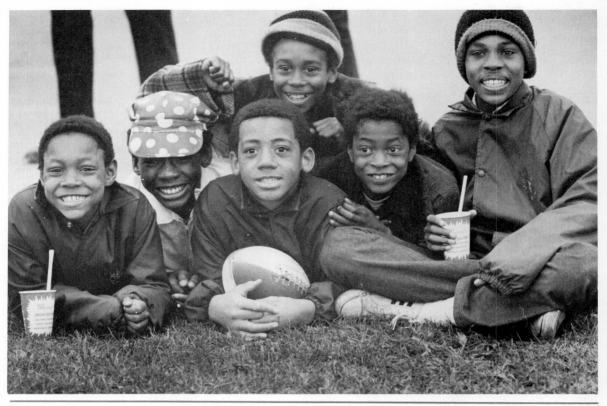

Every boy in this picture will be influenced by the others, his peers, who will play a part in determining his values, beliefs, goals, and ideals.

mind and body, so too are there social and emotional changes. In the remaining pages of this chapter, we look at three important forces involved in these changes: peers, the school, and television.

■ Peer Groups

A peer group is a group of equals. Most individuals in our society have a peer group, excluding hermits, whose peers, by definition, are also isolated and therefore of little consequence to their development. Actually, most people have a number of peer groups: individuals whose occupations bring them into frequent contact with one another and

individuals who are related by virtue of common causes, similar ambitions, identical avocations, geographical accident, or the whims of fortune. Each of these groups elicits specific behavior from its members, more or less different from that elicited by other groups, and each is somehow influential in determining a person's values, beliefs, goals, and ideals.

Characteristics

The peer group is both a product of culture and one of its major transmitters, particularly during middle childhood and adolescence. During the years of middle childhood (appropriately called the latency period by Freud), the peer group typically consists of like-sexed children. (See *One Peer Group*.) In addition, because of the disparate abilities, capacity for understanding, and varied interests among the different ages spanning this period, the peer group usually consists of peers close in age. During adolescence the peer group may be enlarged to include members of both sexes and a wider range of ages.

Increasing Influence

Very young children do not ordinarily have peer groups that are of great psychological importance to them, because they remain dependent upon their immediate family during most of their early years and because they are not ordinarily brought into extensive or prolonged contact with other children until later in life. Piaget (1951) has observed that, prior to the age of three or four, children do not interact with other young children except in a transitory and superficial manner. The play behavior of several three-year-olds, even in the same room and with similar toys, is usually egocentric rather than social—that is, it is concerned primarily with the self rather than with others and makes no use of mutually accepted rules. Sears, Maccoby, and Lewin (1957) maintain that until children are five or six, the family is the primary socializing force in their lives—the source of positive reinforcement or the source of punishment. After this first stage, however, children turn gradually to peer groups, whose influence eventually supersedes that of parents in importance in the middle and later years of childhood.

Research conducted by Prado (1958) clearly illustrates the shift in allegiance from family to peers during the transition from middle childhood to adolescence. Prado selected two groups of boys, all of whom had indicated that their father was their favorite parent. One group consisted of boys between eight and eleven years of age; the second group contained boys between fourteen and seventeen. For the experiment, a boy and his father were brought to a laboratory, along with the boy's best friend—a boy of similar age who had been selected as the "best friend" on the basis of interviews and questionnaires. The friend and the father were asked to throw darts at a target. The target was arranged so that the boy could not see the exact scores made by his father or his friend. His task was to estimate their performance.

The results of the study reveal that both the younger boys and the adolescents were almost equally accurate in their estimates. However, the younger boys consistently overestimated the scores made by their fathers and underestimated those made by their friends. In contrast, adolescents tended to underestimate their fathers' scores and overestimate their friends' scores. The evidence strongly suggests that from middle childhood to adolescence there is a marked decline in the importance of parents and a corresponding increase in the importance of peers.

In connection with the influence of peer groups on the child, studies have shown the harmful effects that the absence of contact with peers seems to have on the young of other species. Harlow and Zimmerman (1959) report that infant monkeys reared in isolation are frequently unable to achieve mature social relations when finally brought into contact with their peers. Such monkeys, particularly males isolated for a prolonged period, are typically incapable of normal sexual activities. The females fare better, because their sexual role is passive rather than active; consequently, they occasionally become pregnant and bear young. But it is both striking and potentially significant that these monkey mothers fail to display the maternal attachment typical of mothers reared under more normal conditions. In fact, some monkey mothers raised without peers torture their own offspring mercilessly (Harlow, Harlow, & Suomi, 1971).

Despite this research, relatively little is known about the peer group's role in developing an individual's ability to interact socially with others. Although it is possible to isolate young monkeys to observe the effects of this isolation on their later behavior, most of the research reported has nec-

ONE PEER GROUP: SAM'S GANG

When Sam Bellott, temporarily passing through sixth grade, was assigned the task of writing about himself and his friends as homework due tomorrow, he presented his teacher with a page that could have been torn from a smallish book. Presumptuously, perhaps even then sensing an urge to become a king or a leader, he entitled it "Sam's Gang." It is reproduced here with Sam's permission.

Sociologists typically define a *gang* as a group that forms spontaneously, that interacts on a face-to-face basis, and that becomes aware of its group membership through *conflict* with some other group or, perhaps more often, with some representatives of established society (Cartwright, Tomsom, & Schwartz, 1975). A gang may consist of different numbers of individuals from a wide variety of backgrounds and locales, although it typically has a fairly homogeneous group of individuals who at least live close to one another and who often attend the same

October 25, 1935

Dear Diary,

Here I am again, Diary. Loney and Bill and George and Jim and Guy and Me had a great time last night, Diary. We all met near Old Man Wists' barn and I gave the secret word which I said I would never write in my diary cross my hart and hope to die and so I cant tell you what our secrit word is but it sure is a good one. When I said the word my best friends, Loney and Bill said the answering word which is a secrit too so I cant tell you that one either. Then George and Jim came and said the word and we let them in through the broken board into the stall where we keep all our treasures. I have to steal a candle, Dear Diary, because we burned our last one last night and Bill stole one last time so its my turn. I would steal anything for the Packrats. And you know what happened last night? When Guy came he forgot the secret password. Hes not my best friend cause he's kind of dum. We wouldn't let him in for the longest time and he was going to start crying if we didn't say it was ok and tell him what the word was so we let him in and he memorized the word all night. When we grow up me and my gang are all going to go into business or something together and none of us are ever going to get married but we are going to live in a fine house along a river where there's lots of fish, and we'll have secret passwords and sentences even and we won't let anybody in who doesnt know them, except maybe our dads when they come to visit us to go fishing. Loney and Bill sure are my very best friends, goodbye Diary because I have to go and steal that candle while Mom is in the bathroom.

essarily involved maternal isolation, and the possibility that the mother is more closely connected with the development of intimate relationships than are peer groups is quite likely (Harlow, McGaugh, & Thompson, 1971).

Peer Acceptance or Rejection

The characteristics of children most likely to be accepted as peers vary, depending on age and sex. In general, children who are friendly and sociable are more easily accepted than those who are hostile, unsociable, withdrawn, or indifferent (Tuddenham, 1951). Similarly, children who are intelligent and creative are more acceptable than those who are slow learners or retarded (Gallagher, 1960). Size, strength, athletic prowess, and daring are particularly important characteristics for membership in boys' peer groups; maturity and social skills are more important for girls, particularly as they approach adolescence.

The most common technique for assessing the nature of peer acceptance or rejection is called **sociometry**. It involves the use of a questionnaire or an interview to determine patterns of likes and dislikes in a group. For example, the investigator might present each of the children with the pictures or names of all the other children in their class and ask them to sort them according to the ones they would most like to be with or those whom they like the best. The investigator might also ask children to discuss those children whom they like the least and would least like to be with. Alternative methods involve asking children to select the most popular boy or girl in the room and the smartest child or the dumbest one (see, for example, Hartup, 1975). The data gathered in this way are frequently interpreted through pictorial or graphic representations in a **sociogram** (see Figure 9.6).

A sociogram is valuable as a source of potential insights about social relationships in the classroom—relationships about which the teacher might be totally unaware. However, its reliability is frequently limited. The sociogram shown in Figure 9.6 reveals that Bob and Sam are the best-liked boys—not surprising if the teacher already knows that they are among the best athletes, the most intelligent, and the most friendly and outgoing. Similarly, the most popular girls are Joan and Marie; that too, given their buoyant personalities and their intelligence, is not particularly surprising. But there is also a message of sadness and loneliness in this sociogram. There is a shy and retiring child who admires the two most popular boys but who is liked by no one in return—Guy. There is a little girl not overly endowed by nature and to whom nurture has not been kind, either. Her name is Rose, and she, like Guy, is liked by no one. There is something terribly tragic and poignant about young children whose only source

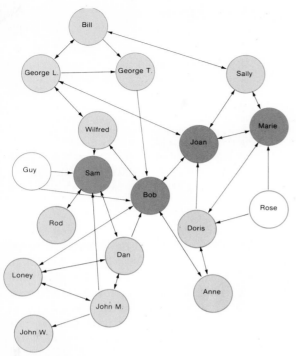

Figure 9.6
A sociogram of a fourth-grade classroom. The popular children are Sam, Bob, Joan, and Marie. The unpopular are Rose and Guy.

of friendship is their dog (if their parents will permit that friend). Perhaps a sensitive and concerned teacher can help such children. (See also *Social Isolation*.)

Friendship Patterns

By definition, peers are groups of equals. And, as we noted, each of us can have a variety of peers—of equals—depending on circumstances. Thus we have peers at work, church peers, social peers, peers in our communities, and so on. In addition to the important social relationships that most of us have with our various peers, the great majority also have closer, more intimate, relationships with a small number of individuals. These more intimate relationships define our friendships.

Friendships are of paramount importance in the lives of children. Not only do they provide the

child with intimacy, encouragement, and support, but they might also be important in the development of the capacity to form meaningful and lasting emotional relationships in adulthood (Sullivan, 1953).

Investigations of the formation of friendships among children indicate that most children have a number of close friends, rather than only one "best" friend (Berndt, 1981), and that they are more likely to do favors (behave in prosocial ways) for their close friends than for others who are simply classmates. It is interesting, however, that close friends also seem to be motivated to compete against one another. Thus, in competitive situations, where doing a best friend a favor means losing out personally, close friends often behave selfishly.

Berndt's (1981) systematic investigations of friendship and helping among school children also found that girls tended to have slightly fewer friendships than boys but that these were generally more intimate—that is, they involved more self-revelation and more close sharing. Like boys, most girls have two or three close friends rather than only one best friend. And for the large majority of children from kindergarten to eighth grade, friendship patterns appear to be highly mutual. That is, if one child indicates that a second is a best friend, the second child will very likely also have chosen the first as a best friend.

A second sex-difference with respect to friendship patterns concerns the extent to which friends will compete or cooperate with each other. In one of Berndt's (1981) experiments, pairs of friends were given a timed coloring task where each would be rewarded on the basis of the number of squares colored correctly on a pattern but where only one crayon of the appropriate color was provided. In one experimental condition, the child who first has the crayon does not *have* to share with the friend but *may* do so. Although experiments such as these tend to show that friends will compete under these circumstances (some friends never share the crayon), there is generally less competition (more cooperation) among girls than boys. This finding provides additional evidence that boys are often more competitive (more aggressive) than girls (Knight & Kagan, 1977).

As we mentioned earlier, as children age, parents become less important, and peers and friends, more important. Accordingly, it is not surprising that research has generally shown an increase in intimacy of friendships with increasing age (Bigelow & LaGaipa, 1980). However, this increased intimacy is typically not reflected in a greater willingness to cooperate with friends rather than with others who are simply class peers (Newcomb, Brady, & Hartup, 1979).

We can only speculate about the ultimate importance of childhood friends. About their immediate importance, there is far less doubt—as I am reminded daily as my young daughter ties up the telephone with long hours of breathless conversation with Sherri and Lana.

Functions of Peers

During the first years of school, children's peer groups have several important functions, some of which have been implied earlier. First, the child's need for acceptance and approval is satisfied mostly

SOCIAL ISOLATION

We are not all equally loved and sought after by our friends. Indeed, not all of us have friends. Some of us are *social isolates*.

Two separate definitions of social isolation are often used in studies of this phenomenon. One looks at frequency of interaction among peers and defines social isolation in terms of scarcity of interaction; the socially isolated are those who do not often interact with peers or even with adults. The other looks at the nature and extent of peer acceptance and defines the socially isolated as those who are seldom selected as "best friend" by anyone but who might often be chosen as "someone I don't really like very much." And evidence suggests that these two measures are, in fact, different (Gottman, 1977). Some children are liked and accepted but do not interact much with their peers; at the same time, some children are very low on everybody's list of "my best friends" or "who I would most like to be with" or "who I would most like to be like," but they nevertheless interact frequently with peers.

In an attempt to investigate these definitions and to arrive at a clearer description of social isolation, Gottman conducted a study involving 113 preschool children enrolled in Head Start classrooms. Each of these children was observed at length by three different observers. Observations were based on a time-sampling procedure and involved detailed recordings of peer-peer and peer-teacher interaction, as well as observations when the child was alone. Time samples involved twelve separate three-minute observations for each child. In addition, a "picture" sociometric technique, described by Hartup, Glazer, and Charlesworth (1967), was em-

ployed. It involved presenting each child with a random arrangement of classmate photographs, making sure the child recognized each of the photographs, and asking for three positive choices (find someone you especially like at school) and three negative choices (now find someone you do not like as much).

Analysis of Gottman's data led him to describe five distinct categories of children. *Sociometric stars* include those who are consistently "especially liked." *Sociometric rejectees* are those who are consistently "not liked as much." A third group, the *teacher negatives* is typically in conflict with teachers. These students might or might not be low on measures of peer acceptance. *Mixers* are those observed to interact most with peers. These too might be high or low on measures of acceptance. And the *tuned out* are those who are frequently not involved with what is going on—who are tuned "out" rather than "in."

Two of these categories describe specific examples of social isolation: rejectees and the tuned out. The principal difference between the rejectees and the tuned out is that, rather than being strongly rejected by peers, the tuned out are simply ignored. These are the shy, withdrawn, and inattentive children whose behaviors might generally be described as immature. They are more likely to pout, cry, have their eyes shut, suck their fingers, shuffle, fall, flinch, be chased, crawl, whine, or use baby talk (Gottman, 1977). And, as Gottman suggests, it might be very important for parents and teachers to know more about these socially isolated children. How do they become that way? What are the implications of social isolation? What can be done to help social isolates?

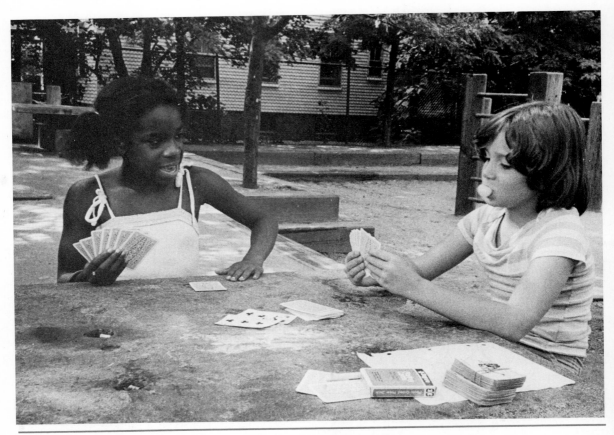

Studies of friendship patterns indicate that girls tend to have fewer close friends than boys, but girls' friendships are often more intimate, involving more self-revelation and more sharing.

by the peer group. Children also need to develop a favorable self-concept (Murray, 1938)—to achieve self-esteem—and the concept of the *self* is directly related to how children think others perceive them. G. H. Mead (in Strauss, 1964) has developed a philosophical theory based on the development of self, asserting that the *self* that adults eventually come to possess is a conglomerate of the ways they think the significant others in their lives perceive them. Psychological research supports this position. Horowitz (1962), for example, found that children who were rated unpopular by their peers tended to have negative self-concepts; these children were most likely to be dissatisfied with what they were

and to want to become like the other children whom they thought more popular. Coleman (1961) has corroborated these findings with studies of high school children (see Chapter 12 for a discussion of the importance of self-esteem).

Second, peer groups are important for the formation of sexually appropriate values and attitudes. Ample evidence indicates that prolonged membership in a group makes its members more similar, by bringing their values and attitudes into closer correspondence. Campbell and Yarrow (1958) found that racially integrated summer camps significantly reduced feelings of social tension and distance among children. Similarly, Coleman (1960) found that the predominant academic values of a school were transmitted via peer groups. With the passage of time, freshmen's estimates of the importance of the school's predominant values tend to increase. More precisely, with continued exposure to a group with relatively defined values, the individual's values gradually approach those of the group.

■ The School

Perhaps it is presumptuous to attempt to describe the effects of the school on children, not only because some of these effects vary widely from one student to another but also because the major effects are so inclusive that they are too obvious to be worthy of mention and, at the same time, too indeterminate and general to be analyzed easily. Consider, for example, six-year-old children entering school. Although they have already learned the language of their people and might have begun to acquire some of the skills necessary if they are to have access to even a fraction of the cumulative wisdom of humanity, it is the school (in most cases) that will make that wisdom accessible. In this age of accelerating technological and theoretical progress, it is no longer possible for parents to transmit more than the merest hint of culture; the schools are our monolithic disseminators of culture.

Throughout this book we have referred to the average child and the normal course of development, despite frequent reminders that these have been invented for the sake of convenience; now we invent the average school and examine the average effect it has on the average student. And we begin, of course, by asserting that none of these is real but simply the requirement of conceptual simplicity.

The average school, monolithic culture machine, opens its smiling jaws to the incoming hordes of six-year-olds every September; although it may appear to disgorge them every afternoon and to swallow them again the following morning, resting only on weekends, during holidays, floods, and bomb scares, it does not really free them. The culture machines detain their charges until they reach adolescence; their influence pervades the child's life.

In school, children learn the basic skills and acquire knowledge fundamental to their understanding of, and effective interaction with, this complex world. Also through the school, children develop the social skills and public personality that will characterize them throughout life, for it is in school that they find themselves in situations demanding interaction with people other than their immediate family. There is virtually nowhere for frightened first graders to run—their parents have abandoned them. Although parents continue to love them, to wash their clothes, to cook for them, and to sympathize with their expressions of joy and sadness, they are far away at work and at home and children are here alone. They have discovered that the world stretches beyond the circle of home and family, that it is necessary to adjust to this world, and that the adjustment is sometimes painful.

The School and Minority Groups

If adjustment to school is not always easy for the well-fed, well-stimulated, healthy child from the typical middle-class home, imagine how much more difficult it is for the disadvantaged child. It is no myth that the child from a minority group (frequently disadvantaged in one or more ways) fares less well in school than the more advantaged majority student. Numerous reasons have been advanced for this unhappy state of affairs. Crossland (1971) lists verbal handicaps, the middle-class orientation of school examinations, inferior teachers and school facilities in deprived areas, and various motivational deficiencies as contributing factors. To this list of disadvantages facing the child from a lower-class home can be added another factor—the effect of the teacher's expectations on the student.

Teacher Expectations

Rosenthal and Jacobson (1968a, 1968b) report a study that has tremendous implications for our understanding of how teachers' expectations affect the behavior of their students. The investigation involved students in a lower-middle-class school. Each student was administered an intelligence test in the spring of the school year. Teachers in the school were not informed that the measures were of aptitude; they were told instead that the experimenters were attempting to validate a new test designed to identify academic "bloomers." Teachers were also advised that students frequently show a sudden spurt in performance at some time during their academic career. For some children this spurt comes very early; for others it occurs later. The experimenters had ostensibly developed a test that would enable them to predict which students would most likely "bloom" during the following school year.

The following September, a number of students were chosen at random from the school and designated as the experimental group; they represented approximately 20 percent of the school's population. The experimental treatment consisted of casually informing teachers that these were students who had been identified as "late bloomers" the previous spring. No other treatment was undertaken. Hence, the only difference between the experimental group and the remainder of the students in the school was that their teachers had some reason to expect better performances from them during the year. Most teachers did observe the level of performance that they expected. The experimental group not only scored higher on measures of achievement but even scored better than the control group on a general measure of intelligence. Equally interesting is the observation that younger students seemed to improve most, which suggests that younger children are perhaps more malleable, more subject to the subtle influences of a teacher's expectations.

Studies of the effects of teachers' expectations on schoolchildren may help us understand the lower achievement of minority-group children: Teachers frequently expect less of a lower-class or minority-group child than they do of a middle-class child. On the average, this expectation is proven. Thus, part of the inferior performance of minority-group children may be due precisely to the teacher's lower expectations for them.

The Rosenthal and Jacobson studies have been criticized extensively. In particular, Barber and Silver (1969a, 1969b) have examined many of the studies with which Rosenthal and Jacobson support their hypothesis, contending that few of these studies clearly demonstrate the effects of teachers' expectations. Rosenthal's (1969–1970) replies to these criticisms are equally adamant in maintaining that the studies do indeed support his conclusions. Although it is too early to resolve the mild controversy surrounding the **Rosenthal effect,** failure to replicate the original findings does not necessarily invalidate the conclusion that, at least in some cases, the expectations that teachers have for their students may dramatically affect the social and intellectual development of the students. In addition, several subsequent studies have also found a Rosenthal effect. For example, Rubovits and Maehr (1971, 1973) manipulated teacher expectations with respect to black and white students and found not only that teachers gave preferential treatment to students identified as "gifted" but also that they were more likely to do so for white than for black students.

Self-Expectations

We have known for some time that teacher expectations might have a significant effect on the performance of individual students. We might also have suspected, had we thought about it, that the individual's personal expectations might have an even more profound influence on performance.

Research in this area has recently focused on what is generally called *attribution theory*. An attribution is an assignment of cause (or blame or origin). If I think my stupidity is due to my having hit my head on a low branch, then I *attribute* my stupidity to that event. Thus, attribution theories look for predictable regularities in the ways in which we attribute causes to the things that happen around us (or to us).

Attribution theories, although relatively new

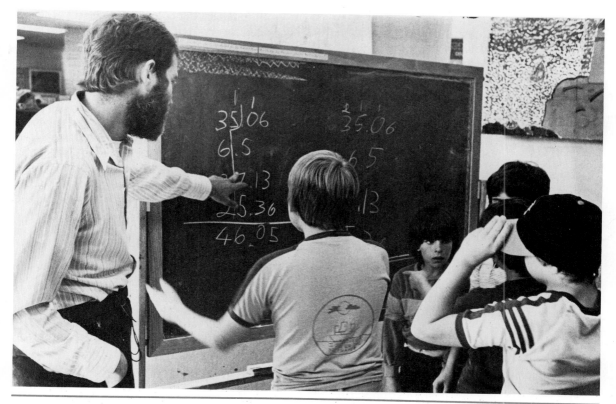

School has a tremendous impact on the emotional, social, and cognitive lives of children; its effects are so vast and so complex that they cannot easily be analyzed or described.

(see Weiner, 1979, 1980a, 1980b), have already produced a number of findings that may prove to be important. Among them is the observation that people appear to be very different in terms of the ways in which they typically assign responsibility for their successes or failures. In general, there appear to be two kinds of people (with many falling in between these two classifications). On the one hand, there are those who accept personal responsibility for the consequences of their behavior; they are *internally oriented* (Weiner, 1980) or, using Dweck's (1975) labels, *mastery oriented*. On the other hand, there are those who are prone to attribute successes and failures to circumstances or events over which they have no control; these

are *externally oriented* individuals (Weiner, 1980). In Dweck's terms, these individuals are characterized by *helplessness* rather than by a mastery orientation.

Differences between mastery-oriented and helpless children are often highly apparent. Mastery-oriented children are the ones most likely to attribute their successes to ability or effort (factors that are personal or over which they at least have personal control); in contrast, helpless children are more likely to attribute their failures or successes to luck or the difficulty of the task (that is, it was too hard or too easy), factors over which they have no personal control—in other words, factors in the face of which they are helpless.

Table 9.2 Why did you fail or succeed? Your reasons reveal something about your personality and achievement motivation.

External	Internal
Difficulty (task easy or too difficult)	Ability (intelligence, skill, or lack thereof)
Luck (bad or good)	Effort (Hard work, industriousness, self-discipline, or laziness, distraction, lack of time)

Several important findings show differences between children who can be classed as helpless and those described as mastery oriented. One is that mastery-oriented children tend to be much more highly achievement oriented (Thomas, 1980; Uguroglu & Walberg, 1979). A second is that mastery-oriented and helpless children react very differently to successes and failures. When Diener and Dweck (1980) arranged a problem so that all children would experience an unbroken sequence of eight successes, helpless children predicted that they would not do well if they had to repeat the eight tasks. In contrast, mastery-oriented children were confident that they would continue to perform equally well. In other words, children who see themselves as being helpless find it difficult to interpret success as indicating that they are capable. Thus, even after succeeding, they not only continue to underestimate the number of likely future successes, but they also overestimate the number of likely future failures. In contrast, when mastery-oriented children were given a series of failures, they continued to see themselves as capable and to predict future success.

A number of crucial questions remain unanswered. Perhaps the most important of these concerns the origins of helplessness. Although the majority of researchers think it is learned (see Seligman, 1975) and that it can therefore be unlearned, the issue is still not clear. In addition, *helplessness* has been implicated in physical and psychological disorders, as well as in achievement and adjustment problems, but its precise contribution to these has yet to be established.

In summary, the influence of the school clearly goes well beyond simply imparting intellectual skills. It provides the child's first opportunity for meaningful and prolonged interaction with other significant adults and peers. Perhaps most important, along with the family and other socializing influences, it is centrally involved in the development of morality, prosocial behaviors (sharing, cooperating), and antisocial behavior (aggression). Each of these developments is examined in Chapter 11. We now turn to another aspect of the child's environment that might also have a profound influence on the development of morality as it is manifested in prosocial and antisocial behavior: television.

■ Television

There is a fear in the hearts of many adults that mass media will taint their still tender and highly corruptible young. First to be feared were fairy tales, few of which have happy endings and even fewer of which are without violence. But the force of attacks on the Brothers Grimm and on Hans Christian Andersen never reached the passionate intensity with which the finger waggers went after the comic book, whose primary characteristics have been described as "violence in content, ugliness in form and deception in presentation" (Wertham, 1954, p. 90). (Fairy tales actually rarely involve fairies and comic books are usually not comic.) In a stinging indictment documented with numerous case studies, Wertham ascribes many of the ills that beset young children to their addiction to comics, which, he maintains, are replete with unexplained, unjustified, and often unpunished violence, sadism, and other forms of criminal perversion. He claims that comics qualify neither as art nor literature, that they are antieducational, and that they demonstrate that the greatest evil is not crime but the stupidity that allows the criminal to be apprehended. His book is aptly titled *Seduction of the Innocent*.

Arnold (1969) presents an equally scathing attack on comic books, objecting primarily to the models of violence they present young readers. But comics are only one of the mass exponents (and proponents) of violence; there are also books, toys, and television—the latter being the most widespread and perhaps the most powerful.

Federal Communications Commissioner Nicholas Johnson (1969) reported that of the sixty million homes in the United States in 1969, over 95 percent had television sets. Murray (1973) points out that 99 percent of homes with young children have television sets. Moreover, the average male viewer between the ages of two and sixty-five will watch television for almost nine full years of his life (each year consisting of 365 twenty-four-hour days). Before they reach the age of eighteen, children spend approximately twenty-two thousand hours watching television. First graders watch television for an average of two to three hours a day, and as many as 25 percent of sixth graders in one sample were still watching television at 11:30 at night during the school week (Lyle & Hoffman, 1972). Given these inordinate amounts of time spent in front of television sets, it is important to consider the influence of television on a child's development.

For some time now, prophets of doom have been decrying the influence of television on children. Their primary claims, based on personal

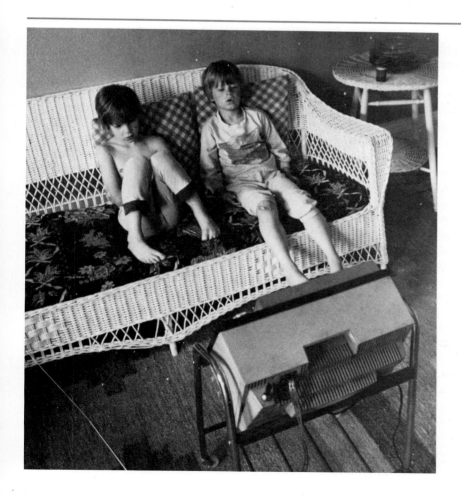

Is television producing a generation of passive individuals who are content to watch the world go by? Is it contributing to a society with a high tolerance for crime and violence? Or is it producing a generation that is itself violent?

opinion rather than experimental data, are that television is producing a generation of passive people or, alternatively, that the violence that pervades many television programs will produce a generation of violent people. (See *Violence and Aggression*.) Critics ordinarily adopt one or the other stance, because the two are essentially antithetical. Furthermore, claim the critics, television has a deleterious effect on family relationships, on social development, and on sports, reading, and playing bingo. Although the evidence is incomplete, sufficient research exists to provide a partial response to these criticisms and to present a more balanced impression of the actual influence of television on the lives of children.

Aggression and Antisocial Influences

First, it cannot be denied that many television programs contain aggression and even violence in one form or another: sometimes verbal, frequently physical, and occasionally symbolic. It is not as clear that such aggression has a discernible effect on the attitudes or the behavior of children. Himmelweit, Oppenheim, and Vince (1958) found that approximately one-fourth of the boys and one-third of the girls in a sample of 1,000 young television viewers reported that they were frightened by violence on television. The same study, however, failed to find any higher frequency of maladjustment, delinquent behavior, or aggression among television viewers than among nonviewers.

In contrast to these findings, Bandura, Ross, and Ross (1963), Bandura and Walters (1963), and Bandura (1969) consistently show an increase in aggressive behavior as a result of exposure to aggressive models. This behavior appears to be relatively independent of whether the model is a live person or a film depicting either cartoon characters or real people. The typical experiment involves having children view models (live or filmed) who engage in aggressive acts with inanimate objects such as inflated rubber clowns. The child is then allowed to play with the objects against which the aggressive acts were directed and is observed at play, usually through a one-way mirror. Young children typically respond aggressively when placed in this situation, *after* viewing an aggressive model; children who have not been exposed to an aggressive model, or who have seen a model who sits quietly or interacts with the toy in a nonaggressive manner, typically respond less aggressively.

It is probably unrealistic to generalize from studies such as these to real-life situations. The findings of Himmelweit, Oppenheim, and Vince contradict those of Bandura and his associates, but the contradiction is largely resolved when the differences between the situations are considered. First, the aggression presented in an ordinary television program is directed against people rather than inanimate objects, and children learn early in life, through socialization, that aggression against people is normally punished. Next, the experimental situation generally requires that the child be exposed to the *same* objects as were employed by the model, *immediately* after observing the model or very shortly afterward. A child who watches a violent scene on television is rarely presented immediately with an object (or person) similar to the one upon whom the televised violence was inflicted. Finally, to assume that striking a rubber clown with a mallet, kicking it, or punching it is evidence of aggression is to suggest a redefinition of the term as it is ordinarily employed by those who condemn television because of its violence. After all, inflated rubber clowns are designed to be punched, kicked, and otherwise abused; the object in the experiment was provided for that purpose.

The findings of Himmelweit and her associates are also relevant to the passivity that television is expected to produce in children; they indicate that television viewers have a wider range of interests than nonviewers. In a related study, Schramm, Lyle, and Parker (1961) found that American children who watch television read as many books as nonviewers, and they read fewer comic books. Commercial television is reputed to accelerate the development of language skills, although this effect is most pronounced among young children of deprived backgrounds (Himmelweit, Oppenheim, & Vince, 1958; Schramm, Lyle, & Parker, 1961).

VIOLENCE AND AGGRESSION

In the vast body of literature that looks at the influence of television on children, the terms *violence* and *aggression* are used not only as though they mean exactly the same thing but also as though everybody knows exactly what it is that they do mean. Not so. The terms mean slightly different things, are manifested in rather different behaviors, and are not understood in exactly the same way by everybody.

The more general of these two terms is *aggression*, which may be defined as "hostile or forceful action intended to dominate or violate" (Lefrancois, 1983, p. 504). It includes a wide range of behaviors, beginning with insistence, assertiveness, or perhaps intrusion at the one end and culminating with anger and *violence* at the other. Thus, violence is simply an extreme form of aggressiveness. Violence implies physical action or movement and possible or actual harm to people or objects. It is well illustrated in episodes where people are kicked, beaten, shot, or knifed, or where rocks and other objects are dropped on their heads from great heights.

Aggression is clearly not always undesirable; the totally nonaggressive are unlikely to succeed in ways that the more aggressive might. Indeed, human survival, as well as that of many other animals, was very likely related to aggressiveness. That, of course, does not necessarily mean that we still need to be as aggressive as many of us now are.

Moyer (1976) describes six forms of aggression that are commonly observed among animal species. *Predatory* aggression is common among hunting carnivores and is associated with hunger rather than with anger. It typically occurs *between* rather than within species, with the exception that some predators will occasionally eat the young of their own species. *Intermale* aggression is also quite frequent among a variety of animals and is most often related to mating or disputes over territory. *Sex-related* aggression is evident in a number of animal species, including rhesus monkeys, where the males become highly aggressive when sexually aroused. It may also be evident in instances of rape among humans. *Fear-induced* aggression may be seen in some captured or cornered animals and is typically related to self-protection. *Maternal* aggression is manifested by females of many species when their young are attacked or threatened. *Irritable* aggression, unlike other forms of aggression, does not occur in specific circumstances (mating or defending the young) or against specific individuals or objects but is instead a general aggressive reaction to irritation. Irritation might result from frustration, deprivation, or pain. It appears to be far more common among humans than among other species.

Similarly, the amount of general information to which the child is exposed prior to coming to school has increased dramatically with television.

Given the frequently inconclusive and contradictory results of research on the influence of television and given continued concern that the content of television programming might have a negative effect on the young child, a massive series of studies was undertaken in the United States under the auspices of the Surgeon General. Following the allocation of a one-million-dollar research fund in 1969, twenty-three separate research projects were undertaken. Resulting reports and papers were then examined by the Surgeon General's Advisory Committee on Television and Social Behavior, and a five-volume report was published three years later (Rubinstein, Comstock, & Murray, 1972). The report focuses on three questions: What is the nature of television programming? Who watches what? What are the potential or real effects on viewers?

Answers to the first two questions are straightforward and reliable. Violence, defined as "the overt expression of physical force against others or self, or the compelling of action against one's will on pain of being hurt or killed," is the dominant theme of television. In fact, programs designed especially for children abound in violence. One study reports that more than 98 percent of all cartoon programs contain violent episodes; the frequency of violence in children's programs is six times greater than that in adult programs (Gerbner, 1972)

Viewing patterns are also relatively clear cut. Three separate age groups spend the greatest amount of time viewing television: young children, young adults, and elderly people. A number of studies suggest that, of these, young children spend the greatest amount of time in front of television sets (Lyle & Hoffman, 1972). Young children tend to prefer cartoons. As they get older, preferences shift to situation comedies and to action-adventure programs. And although some researchers have argued that young children become mesmerized by the succession of sights and sounds on television, regardless of its content (for example, Mander, 1978; Singer & Singer, 1979), this does not appear to be the case. Evidence suggests that young children watch those parts of television programs that are understandable for them (Anderson, 1979).

Questions concerning the impact of television violence cannot be answered as easily. To begin with, researchers have experienced tremendous difficulty locating children who have not been exposed to television and who can therefore serve as control groups (Pingree & Hawkins, 1980). It is unfortunate, but true, that the great majority of studies included in the Surgeon General's report involve children with a wide and uncontrolled background of television experiences. Many of the contradictions among the results of these studies might stem from this simple fact.

A study that does not suffer from this limitation is one conducted by Joy, Kimball, and Zabrack (1977). Spanning two years, it involved several small towns where television-viewing history was well known. When the study began, for example, television was just being introduced in one of the towns, whereas another still remained without television. All were highly comparable socially, educationally, and economically. And children in each of these towns appeared to be equally aggressive at the beginning of the study. Two years later, however, children in the town where television had been brought in manifested a significant increase in aggressive behavior.

A related study (Liebert & Baron, 1972) made use of an experimental device—children were free to press buttons that would ostensibly either help or hurt another child. The buttons were actually nonfunctional. Prior to being placed in this situation, children were shown segments of violent programs (from "The Untouchables") or of neu-

tral programs. Those children who had been exposed to the violent programs, particularly if they were younger, showed a greater tendency to press the "hurt" button than did children exposed to neutral programs.

Although these studies and a number of others successfully demonstrate some short-term, though rather undramatic, effects of television violence (Liebert & Schwartzberg, 1977), few studies have attempted to look at its possible long-term effects. Clearly, there are methodological problems involved in doing so. Such a study would have to be longitudinal. Subjects would need to be matched on all relevant variables at an early age, their viewing patterns monitored periodically, and their eventual behaviors, attitudes, and interests compared some considerable time later. One of the reasons why a cross-sectional approach could not easily be employed is that it would now be extremely difficult to find a group of children who are not exposed to television while growing up, yet are not significantly different from other children reared in homes with television.

Lefkowitz, Eron, Walder, & Huesmann (1972) report one longitudinal study that examined children's preferences for violent television programs and their aggressive behavior and attempted to relate these variables to the same children's preferences and manifest aggressive behavior ten years later. Although results indicate that preferences for violent programs are significantly related to aggressive and delinquent behavior ten years later (at age eighteen), particularly for boys, the study cannot establish that viewing violent television programs was a cause of this aggression. It may well be that children who initially preferred violent programs would have been more aggressive and more prone to delinquency than other children, even if they had not been exposed to these programs.

A Conclusion   The Surgeon General's report concludes that there is evidence of short-term *causation* of aggressive behavior as a function of exposure to televised violence. Lefkowitz et al. (1972) similarly conclude that violence on television *causes* viewers to behave more aggressively.

These conclusions may well be valid, but given the correlational nature of the studies upon which they are based, they are not fully warranted (see Chapter 1). At best, some uncertain relationships between televised violence and actual behavior have been observed, but that these are *causal* relationships has not been established.

Singer (1982) observes that there are more published studies that link television and aggression than there are studies that did not find this connection and concludes that the connection between the two exists but is modest. Nor is the nature of the connection clear. Perhaps televised violence causes aggression; perhaps, too, aggressive tendencies determine which children view which programs. Despite these many studies, there are still insufficient data to arrive at a final conclusion regarding the long-term antisocial effects of television on children. And perhaps many of these effects will have far less to do with violence and aggression than was at first suggested. As Singer suggests, "The problem with heavy television viewing is not so much that it may or may not stimulate aggression, but that it may interfere with the development of the social skills and mental capacities that children need to acquire the socially approved, successful behaviors they need to get what they want without resorting to aggression" (1982, p. 60).

Prosocial Effects

The most popular area of television research, particularly in the early 1970s when television research was at its height, has been concerned primarily with television's potential antisocial effects, especially with its contribution to aggression. Comstock (1978) reports that antisocial research outnumbers prosocial research in this area by a factor of four to one. Unfortunately, in the rush to demonstrate television's harmful effects, its *prosocial* influences have tended to be overlooked. At present, only a relatively small number of studies are concerned with the benefits of television. In the main, their results are encouraging. Baran, Chase, and Courtright (1979) found that cooperation could

be increased in young children after exposure to an episode of "The Waltons" that dealt with cooperation in problem solving. Similarly, research with "Sesame Street" programs, with episodes from "Mister Rogers' Neighborhood," and with a number of other deliberately prosocial programs provides strong indication that prosocial behavior can be positively affected (Ahammer & Murray, 1979; Collins & Getz, 1976; Gorn, Goldberg, & Kanungo, 1976). Among the *prosocial* behaviors that have improved following television exposure are friendliness, cooperation, creativity, empathy, and racial tolerance (see Roberts & Bachan, 1981).

Why Is Television Influential?

Three models are currently resorted to by those who are concerned with the impact of television violence on children: a cathartic model, a catalytic model, and an imitation model (Felsenthal, 1976). Presumably, these models would be as valid for explaining television's *prosocial* effects, since the processes underlying prosocial and antisocial effects would probably be similar.

A *catharsis,* in Freudian theory, is a behavior or event that serves as a release for pent-up emotions. For some individuals, painting might serve as a catharsis for aggressive impulses that cannot be acted upon for moral reasons; others might try to kick their cats. Accordingly, the cathartic model of television influence maintains that exposure to television violence may serve as a release for pent-up hostility, aggressive urges, and other antisocial tendencies. To the extent that this model is valid, it would follow that television violence might result in a decrease in violent behavior. Similarly, prosocial themes on television might occasionally result in a decrease in prosocial behavior.

In contrast to the cathartic model, the catalytic model predicts that exposure to television violence will serve as a *catalyst*, initiating or at least facilitating the manifestation of violence among viewers. Following a 1966 telecast of *The Doomsday Flight*, which involved attempted extortion from a major airline by means of a bomb placed on board a plane, several airline companies received telephone calls similar to that depicted in the movie (Pember, 1977). Similarly, airing information concerning contributions during a fund-raising television program tends to result in an increase in donations.

The imitation or modeling hypothesis, extensively investigated by Bandura and Walters (1963), among others, maintains that television serves as a model for prosocial or antisocial behavior among viewers, or that it often serves simply as a cue that elicits related behavior in the viewer, rather than as a model that leads to the learning of new behavior. This hypothesis, too, has received its share of support.

To these three models might be added a fourth: the *no-effect* model. It predicts that exposure to television violence will have no effect on viewers. This model is also frequently supported by the evidence we now have.

A Conclusion

There is little doubt that television can have both beneficial and harmful effects. That it has had more of one than the other still remains uncertain and will be difficult to determine. Further clarification depends upon longitudinal, carefully controlled studies in which the characteristics of viewers as well as the characteristics of programs are carefully identified and adequate control groups are available. There is already some indication that not all portrayals of violence have the same effects. Singer (1982), for example, suggests that comedies with slapstick violence and violent cartoons are too unrealistic to serve as powerful models of violence. In contrast, realistic portrayals of violence, violence perpetrated by "good guys" in their attacks upon "bad guys," and violence that appears in ad hoc fashion unrelated to the plot produce more real-life violence among viewers.

It is perhaps unfortunate that the potentially beneficial effects of television—contributing to prosocial behavior, language development, moral development, and increases in general information—have tended to be overlooked in the rush to demonstrate its harmful effects. Perhaps the most important implication of the Surgeon General's report is not its attack on violence in television but its appeal for more prosocial content.

■ MAIN POINTS

1 Middle childhood spans the ages from six to twelve; the last two years of this period are frequently included in late childhood or preadolescence.

2 Although boys are normally heavier and taller than girls throughout their lives, there is a brief period late in middle childhood when girls become heavier and taller than boys. It is a momentary reflection of different growth timetables.

3 Boys surpass girls in most motor activities, except those involving rhythmic movements and balance, such as playing hopscotch. Boys can usually reach higher, jump farther, and run faster than girls.

4 Reaction time for young children is considerably slower than for adults.

5 The transition to concrete operations is marked by the child's acquisition of concepts of conservation, a process that reflects the acquisition of important rules of logic (identity, reversibility, compensation). In the beginning, these rules are not completely universal.

6 Attempts to accelerate the acquisition of specific conservations have met with mixed success but have demonstrated that acceleration is possible, given systematic training programs.

7　In addition to conservations, children acquire abilities relating to classification, seriation, and number during the period of concrete operations.

8　During the school years, peers become increasingly important as a socializing influence. They are considerably less important in the earlier preschool years.

9　Research with nonhuman primates indicates that absence of contact with peers can have harmful effects on social and sexual development.

10　Sociometry, a common technique for assessing peer acceptance and rejection, suggests that children who are friendly, sociable, and intelligent are better liked than those who are hostile, withdrawn, or indifferent.

11　Peer groups are of particular importance in developing positive self-concepts, as well as in the formation of sexually appropriate values and attitudes.

12　Friends are of great importance to the school-age child. Most children tend to have more than one "best" friend; although they want positive outcomes for their friends, they also are likely to compete with them at the same time. Girls are slightly more likely than boys to have fewer "best" friends but to share a deeper intimacy; at the same time, they are less likely to compete than are boys.

13　The school is a particularly powerful socializing influence, explicitly charged with many of the functions that might otherwise be the responsibility of parents.

14　Research on the effects of teacher expectations may provide one additional basis for understanding the performance of minority-group children, as well as of children who are labeled for other reasons.

15　Student self-expectations are also important. Some children appear to be *mastery* oriented; they accept personal responsibility for the outcomes of their behaviors (intelligence or effort, for example) and are encouraged by success but not overly discouraged by failure. Others are *helpless*; they attribute their successes and failures to factors over which they have no control (luck or task difficulty, for example) and tend not to change their estimates of their capabilities when presented with success.

16　There is evidence that television may lead to antisocial behaviors, as its critics have predicted. There is also evidence that television may lead to prosocial behavior, if the content is appropriate. Unfortunately, violence is a predominant theme in children's programming.

17　Three models may be employed to explain the effects or noneffects of television: the cathartic model (violence on television provides release of aggressive urges), the catalytic model (violence on television triggers violence in some individuals), and the imitation model (violence on television provides a specific pattern for violent behavior).

■ FURTHER READINGS

One of the clearest and most comprehensive descriptions of the child's motor and perceptual development is provided by Cratty. Particularly interesting are the detailed descriptions of motor development in children of different ages and sexes.

Cratty, B. J. *Perceptual and motor development in infants and children*. New York: Macmillan, 1970.

The following two books summarize some of Piaget's theorizing and give particularly good accounts of the development of conservation in the schoolchild:
Donaldson, M. *Children's minds*. London: Fontana/Croom Helm, 1977.
Ginsberg, H., & Opper, S. *Piaget's theory of intellectual development* (2nd ed.). Englewood Cliffs, N.J.: Prentice-Hall, 1978.

The following are two of many articles relating to the acceleration of conservation in children:
Gelman, R. Conservation acquisition: A problem of learning to attend to relevant attributes. *Journal of Experimental Child Psychology,* 1969, 7, 167–187.
Lefrancois, G. R. A treatment hierarchy for the acceleration of conservation of substance. *Canadian Journal of Psychology*, 1968, *22*, 277–284.

Comprehensive reviews of research on peer groups and the significance of peer interaction from infancy to adolescence are provided by:
Lewis, M., & Rosenblum, L. A. (Eds.). *Friendship and peer relations*. New York: John Wiley, 1975.
Shaffer, D. R. *Social and personality development*. Monterey, Calif.: Brooks/ Cole, 1979.

The powerful effects of social pressure are dramatized in Golding's fictional account of the lives of a group of school boys marooned on an island. Is fact stranger than fiction?
Golding, W. *Lord of the flies*. New York: Coward, McCann & Geoghegan, 1962.

The effect of teacher expectations, as well as the sometimes disconcerting tendency for prophecies to fulfill themselves, are examined in:
Rosenthal, R., & Jacobson, L. *Pygmalion in the classroom: Teacher expectations and pupils' intellectual development*. New York: Holt, Rinehart & Winston, 1968.

The preceding should probably be tempered by following it with this highly critical review:
Barber, T. X., & Silver, M. J. Fact, fiction and the experimenter bias effect. *Psychological Bulletin Monographs Supplement*, 1969, 70, 1–29.

A fascinating account of the potential effects of learned helplessness is presented in:
Seligman, M. E. P. *Helplessness: On depression, development, and death*. New York: W. H. Freeman, 1975.

A large-scale American investigation of the effects of television on children is reported in five volumes (the Surgeon General's research program of 1972) and is partially summarized in simple form in:
Murray, J. P. Television and violence: Implications of the Surgeon General's research program. *American Psychologist*, June 1973, pp. 472–478.

A more recent summary of research that has looked at the effects of television viewing is the following:
Comstock, G., Chaffee, S., Katzman, N., McCombs, M., & Roberts, D. *Television and human behavior*. New York: Columbia University Press, 1978.

10

INTELLIGENCE, CREATIVITY, AND EXCEPTIONALITY

Du sublime au ridicule il n'y a qu'un pas.
(It is but one step from the sublime to the ridiculous.)

Napoleon Bonaparte

We slip quickly, quietly, through Bonnyville. I scarcely notice the sprawling, vacant commercial subdivisions, the empty windows down the main street, the "For Sale" signs—all relics of an oil boom that never quite happened.

Highway 28 curls slightly coming out of town, then heads straight east through small fields and poplar groves. The clouds have become thicker, darker, and the afternoon air seems heavy. But the car streaks smoothly on its repaired tire, rapidly eating the last Alberta miles; Saskatchewan is only minutes away.

We play a word game now—Marcel's idea. Each, in turn, must think of a word that begins with the last letter of the preceding word.

My turn: "Hippopotamus."

"Snake," Denise returns.

"Elephant," Grandma maintains the theme.

Paul replies quickly: "Tusk."

And Marcel, just as rapidly, "Kangaroo."

"Freak me green! You're super intelligent!" Denise informs him. Grandma, knitting something green, chuckles. We all think he's super intelligent. He can add 5,000 and 5,000 almost as quickly as 2 and 2. He plays Monopoly and unerringly subtracts 15 or 25 from 100 or 500. He can spell words so long they don't easily fit in his six-year-old mouth.

Is he really so intelligent? Was he born different from those who might appear less intelligent? Or is he different simply because he has a brother a decade older than he, an enthusiastic sister, and a multilingual grandmother who finds life gently amusing?

Now, before Beaver Crossing and the Saskatchewan border, we will take time to ponder these questions. First, we look at the nature of intelligence and creativity; then we turn and look at the exceptional, not only in terms of intellectual development but also in terms of social and physical characteristics.

■ Intelligence

"Intelligence is what the tests test," Boring (1923, p. 35) informed us. This, perhaps the simplest available definition of what is not a simple concept, is a useful and not entirely tongue-in-cheek definition. Weight is not a simple concept either. Yet to say that weight is what a scale measures is, in fact, useful and accurate. A butcher need not understand or know the scientific definition of weight in order to make proper use of the scales. Perhaps a psychologist or a teacher need not know what intelligence is in order to make use of the results of intelligence tests. In this case, however, it might be useful to know what intelligence is, and especially what it is *not*, so as not to *misuse* intelligence tests. Unfortunately, it appears that many who use intelligence tests also misuse them (see Gould, 1981).

An intelligence test is really quite different from a scale. A *scale* measures weight with an accuracy never yet attained in psychological measurement. In addition, a scale, if it is a good one, measures relevant weights and nothing else. The same cannot be said of an intelligence test. In other words, a scale is **valid** (measures what it is supposed to measure) and **reliable** (measures consistently). Intelligence tests typically produce different results for the same individuals when administered at different times—hence they are not perfectly reliable. In addition, there is little doubt that they measure many things not always included in definitions of intelligence. They are less than perfectly valid, frequently reflecting such factors as the subject's mood, the effects of fatigue or anxiety, and the influence of other preoccupations.

Numerous other definitions of intelligence have been advanced. Perhaps among the best known are Wechsler's (1958, p. 7): "The global and aggregate capacity of an individual to think rationally, to act purposefully, and to deal effectively with his environment"; Hebb's (1966, p. 332): "The innate potential for cognitive development"; and Binet's (Terman & Merrill, 1973, p. 6) description of "intelligence in action" as involving "direction, adaptation, and self-criticism."

Controversies concerning whether intelligence is a single fixed quantity or quality or whether it consists of a number of separate abilities and disagreements concerning the best ways of measuring this quality (quantity) are common in psychological literature. Although no universal agreement has yet been reached, a number of intelligence tests are widely employed in sometimes useful and intelligent ways by individuals not overly concerned with the precise nature of whatever it is that they are attempting to measure. Perhaps it has no precise nature in any case. A large number of tests are also employed by many individuals in ways less wise and less useful. Many of these individuals have inadvertently fallen prey to one or more of a number of myths and misconceptions surrounding the IQ (intelligence quotient: a numerical expression of measured intelligence whose average is preset at 100). Some of these myths are discussed briefly here.

Some Misconceptions

It is frequently assumed that all individuals have "an IQ," as though this "IQ" were a fixed something possessed in lesser or greater quantities by everyone. In fact, the IQ is simply a mathematical expression based largely on an individual's ability to perform in prescribed circumstances. It does not reveal mystical, hidden qualities that would otherwise be known only by clever psychologists who have dedicated their lives to the pursuit of the hidden truth. Given the questionable validity of intelligence tests, even if intelligence were a fixed, detectable, and measurable quality of human performance, we have not yet developed the tools required to detect and measure it accurately.

It is also widely believed that IQ is highly related to success, particularly in school. And measured intelligence does correlate moderately highly with performance in school. But numerous studies have shown that previous success correlates even more highly with present or future success than does IQ (Cohen, 1972). Although IQ is important, it is perhaps not all that important.

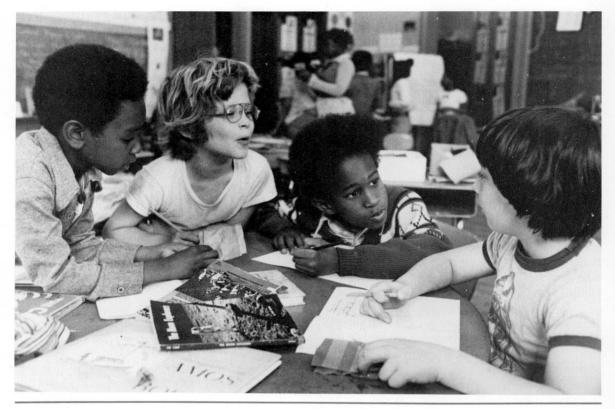

Intelligence tests are often culturally biased and rarely measure interpersonal skills, creativity, and other important traits. When used wisely, however, they can provide useful information.

Two additional weaknesses of traditional measures of intelligence should be noted. Intelligence tests typically do not measure a wide variety of interpersonal skills, athletic ability, creativity, and many personality variables that are of considerable importance to the individual. Perhaps most important for our purposes, many (though by no means all) intelligence tests are culturally biased; they penalize children whose backgrounds are different from the dominant white, middle-class majority. They are culturally biased because they are constructed with the middle-class child in mind and because they are usually standardized on samples of middle-class children. It is almost inevitable that children from minority groups will do less well on these tests than their like-aged, middle-class, white counterparts. (See *Culture and Intelligence* for an alternative test.)

Despite the many weaknesses of intelligence tests, they are extremely widely used, particularly in schools. Unfortunately, they are not at all widely understood. Psychologists, educators, and parents all too often behave as though IQ were fixed, measurable, and so important that it must be shrouded in secrecy, for some have more and others less; some are bright and others stupid. And would it not be thoroughly unfair and perhaps even a little undemocratic to make public such important knowledge?

The key point is that the knowledge may not be nearly so valid or important as we have assumed it to be. We are still measuring something that we cannot define and not measuring it very accurately in any case. Furthermore, our tests are often unfair, not only because they are intrinsically unfair for certain children but also because we use them unfairly. We base some of our most important educational decisions on numbers that represent an unknown, that bear a moderate and sometimes unimpressive relationship to school success, and that are sometimes highly inconsistent (unreliable).

The foregoing should not be construed as an argument for the abandonment of intelligence testing, although it has been abandoned in numerous jurisdictions—usually at the insistence of parent groups. Rather, the argument is for the restrained and intelligent use of information derived from tests. In effect, this would mean that no important decisions should be based on a single test and that considerable additional information about the individuals concerned should affect our decisions.

CULTURE AND INTELLIGENCE: THE CHITLING TEST

Many of the tests traditionally used to measure aptitude in American schools have been designed with the white, Anglo-Saxon, middle-class majority in mind. And many of these tests are consequently less than completely fair for children whose backgrounds are significantly different from that of this majority. In a semi-serious reaction to these tests, black sociologist Adrian Dove presents the Dove Counterbalance General Intelligence Test—dubbed the "Chitling Test." It draws freely from black language and culture of the late 1960s. And a low score on this test might indicate a "reverse" type of cultural deprivation.

1. A "handkerchief head" is: (a) a cool cat, (b) a porter, (c) an Uncle Tom, (d) a hoddi, (e) a preacher.

2. Which word is most out of place here? (a) splib, (b) blood, (c) gray, (d) spook, (e) black.

3. A "gas head" is a person who has a: (a) fast-moving car, (b) stable of "lace," (c) "process," (d) habit of stealing cars, (e) long jail record for arson.

4. "Down-home" (the South) today, for the average "soul brother" who is picking cotton from sunup until sundown, what is the average earning (take home) for one full day? (a) $.75, (b) $1.65, (c) $3.50, (d) $5, (e) $12.

5. "Bo Diddley" is a : (a) game for children, (b) down-home cheap wine, (c) down-home singer, (d) new dance, (e) Moejoe call.

6. If a pimp is uptight with a woman who gets state aid, what does he mean when he talks about "Mother's Day"? (a) second Sunday in May, (b) third Sunday in June, (c) first of every month, (d) none of these, (e) first and fifteenth of every month.

7. "Hully gully" came from: (a) East Oakland, (b) Fillmore, (c) Watts, (d) Harlem, (e) Motor City.

8. If a man is called a "blood," then he is a (a) fighter, (b) Mexican-American, (c) Negro, (d) hungry hemophile, (e) Redman or Indian.

9. Cheap chitlings (not the kind you purchase at a frozen-food counter) will taste rubbery unless they are cooked long enough. How soon can you quit cooking them to eat and enjoy them? (a) forty-five minutes, (b) two hours, (c) twenty-four hours, (d) one week (on a low flame), (e) one hour.

10. What are the "Dixie Hummingbirds"? (a) part of the KKK, (b) a swamp disease, (c) a modern gospel group, (d) a Mississippi Negro paramilitary group, (e) deacons.

11. If you throw the dice and seven is showing on the top, what is facing down? (a) seven, (b) snake eyes, (c) boxcars, (d) little Joes, (e) 11.

12. "Jet" is (a) an East Oakland motorcycle club, (b) one of the gangs in "West Side Story," (c) a news and gossip magazine, (d) a way of life for the very rich.

13. T-Bone Walker got famous for playing what? (a) trombone, (b) piano, (c) "T-flute" (d) guitar, (e) "Hambone."

Correct answers: 1. (c), 2. (c), 3. (c), 4. (d), 5. (c), 6. (e), 7. (c), 8. (c), 9. (c), 10. (c), 11. (a), 12. (c), 13. (d).

Among the most widely used and respected intelligence tests are the Stanford-Binet and the Wechsler. Both are individual intelligence tests; that is, they can only be administered to one child at a time and only by a trained tester. They yield a richer picture of intellectual functioning than do group tests—tests that can be administered to a large group at one time and that are commonly of a paper-and-pencil variety. The Lorge-Thorndike Tests and the Otis-Lennon Mental Ability Test (1967) or the Otis-Lennon School Ability Test (1979) are among the group tests most commonly used with schoolchildren.

The Stanford-Binet   The Binet Scales originated with the work of Alfred Binet and Theodore Simon in 1905 and were later revised at Stanford University to become the Stanford-Binet. It originally consisted of items arranged by age levels. For example, all items that 67 to 75 percent of five-year-olds could pass were placed in the five-year level (Reisman, 1966, p. 68). Five-year-olds who could answer questions at the four-year level were deemed to have a mental age of four. The IQ would then be computed as 4/5 of 100, or 80 (Mental Age/

Chronological Age $\times$ 100 = IQ). A five-year-old who passed items at the six-year level would have an IQ of 6/5 $\times$ 100, or 120. Later revisions of the test, in 1937, 1960, and 1973, make use of large standardization samples and of the deviation IQ— a mathematical function with a mean (average) of 100 and a standard deviation (a measure of variation from the mean) of 16 (Terman & Merrill, 1973). Figure 10.1 presents the distribution of IQs.

The Stanford-Binet is presently in wide use, particularly with young children (ages three to eight), although it is also designed for use with children as young as two and with adults. A highly verbal test, it tends to correlate relatively well with school success but is highly sensitive to experiential deficits, particularly to the extent that these deficits are reflected in language development.

The Wechsler Tests   The Wechsler tests yield a composite IQ score closely comparable to that obtained with the Stanford-Binet. The tests differ in several important ways, however, the most important of which is that the Wechsler Scales also yield separate standardized scores for a variety of subjects, as well as a verbal IQ and a performance IQ (in addition to the composite IQ). Deficiencies in language background are frequently apparent

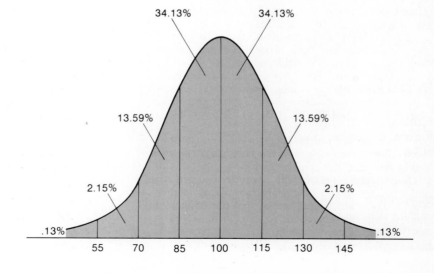

Figure 10.1
A normal curve depicting the theoretical distribution of IQ scores among humans. Note, for example, that the average score is 100 and that 68.26 percent of the population scores between 85 and 115. Only 2.28 percent scores above 130.

Table 10.1 The Wechsler Intelligence Scale for Children Revised (WISCR).

Verbal Scale	Performance Scale
1. *General information.* Questions relating to information most children have the opportunity to acquire.	1. *Picture completion.* Children indicate what is missing in pictures.
2. *General comprehension.* Questions designed to assess children's understandings of why certain things are done as they are.	2. *Picture arrangement.* Series of pictures must be arranged to tell a story.
3. *Arithmetic.* Oral arithmetic problems.	3. *Block design.* Child is required to copy exactly a design with colored blocks.
4. *Similarities.* Child indicates how certain things are alike.	4. *Object assembly.* Puzzles to be assembled by subjects.
5. *Vocabulary.* Child gives meanings of words of increasing difficulty.	5. *Coding.* Child pairs symbols with digits following a key.
6. *Digit span.* Child repeats orally presented sequence of numbers in order and reversed.	6. *Mazes.* Child traces way out of mazes with pencil.

in differences between verbal and performance scores.

Among the various forms of the Wechsler tests are the Wechsler Adult Intelligence Scale (WAIS, for ages sixteen to seventy-five), the Wechsler Intelligence Scale for Children Revised (WISCR, for ages five to fifteen), and the Wechsler Preschool and Primary Scale of Intelligence (WPPSI, for ages four to six and one-half). The various subtests of the Wechsler Scales are described in Table 10.1.

IQ Constancy

Although "intelligence" as a general quality of human functioning is generally assumed to be relatively constant, experimental evidence does not always support this assumption. Intelligence tests given to infants are particularly suspect. Most of the research that has attempted to predict later intelligence on the basis of measures of infant intelligence have found very low relationships between the two (Thorndike & Hagen, 1977). This,

of course, does not mean that intelligence is unstable and highly variable; it might simply indicate that intelligence is difficult to measure accurately, particularly in very young children.

Bloom (1964) summarizes a large amount of research that has examined the constancy of IQ scores for older children. He concludes that there is a substantial correlation, particularly with advancing age. An IQ score at the age of nine, for example, is a fairly good predictor of measured IQ at the age of fifteen. Note, however, that while correlations tend to be high when groups are considered, longitudinal studies have demonstrated marked individual variations in measured IQ. In other words, although children who score high on intelligence tests at the age of seven tend to score high at the age of fifteen, numerous individuals will show opposing trends. Some high-scoring seven-year-olds will be low-scoring fifteen-year-olds. In short, although measured intelligence may appear to be relatively constant, individual variations are sufficient to warrant only very cautious predictions on the basis of tests given in childhood.

Piaget-Based Measures

As yet there are no widely used *standardized* scales of intellectual development based on Piaget's theories. Uzgiris and Hunt (1975) have developed a scale of sensorimotor development that will undoubtedly be of considerable value in research. Whether this scale will be a useful diagnostic tool, or whether it will serve as a predictor of later intellectual development, remains to be seen. These questions can only be answered following longitudinal studies. The most ambitious attempt to develop an intelligence scale paralleling Piaget's description of cognitive development began several decades ago (Pinard & Laurendeau, 1964). The test is still being developed and standardized (Pinard & Sharp, 1972).

Studies that have looked at the relationship between specific Piagetian tasks and mental age or IQ have generally found little or no relationship between IQ and the Piagetian tasks but have found some relationship between mental age and the tasks (see Baer & Wright, 1974). There is evidence, however, that IQ may be associated with qualitative differences in performance on Piagetian tasks rather than with specific Piagetian stages (Little, 1972). In other words, the relationship between IQ and Piagetian tasks might become more apparent when the quality of the child's verbalizations are taken into account instead of looking simply at whether the responses are correct or incorrect.

A common practice in the development of intelligence tests is to validate new tests by comparing them with old ones. Thus, if a new intelligence test correlates highly with previously used tests, we assume that the new test is valid and useful. By the same token, if a new test bears little or no relationship to "established" measures, it tends to be dismissed. In fact, this procedure is not easily justifiable, particularly because we do not know clearly what our intelligence tests are measuring or that the numbers we derive from them have more than limited predictive and diagnostic value. "Intelligence" scales based on Piaget's findings may not correlate at all highly with IQ tests but may nevertheless contribute in important and as yet unknown ways to our understanding of children and to the teaching-learning process. At this point, it would be highly inappropriate to judge their worth on the basis of evidence derived from comparisons with other tests.

■ Creativity

Although creativity has long been prized, it has only recently found its place as a respectable subject of study in psychological investigations. And relatively little is yet known with certainty about this, one of the most elusive properties of humans.

Creativity is generally considered to involve the capacity for innovation and may involve intellectual functions that are in some respects different from those most often tapped by conventional measures of intelligence (Guilford, 1959). Torrance (1962) reports that attempts to identify creatively gifted individuals on the basis of intelligence tests alone would eliminate from consideration approximately 70 percent of the most creative. High intelligence (as measured by tests) does not imply high creativity, nor does low intelligence imply low creativity. One reasonable hypothesis is that a minimum of intelligence is required for creative functioning but that, given this minimum, other variables determine who is creative and who is not (Barron & Harrington, 1981).

One of the principal problems with research in creativity has been the tremendous difficulty experienced in attempting to define creativity. Part of the confusion stems from the fact that a number of researchers have been interested primarily in the personality characteristics of creative persons, whereas others have been interested in the processes involved in being creative. And others, most notably those with industrial concerns, have been concerned with the nature of creative products. Thus a complete definition of creativity must take into account the person, the process, and the product (see Lefrancois, 1982).

Measuring Creativity

Creativity is most frequently measured by means of open-ended tests, which require subjects to pro-

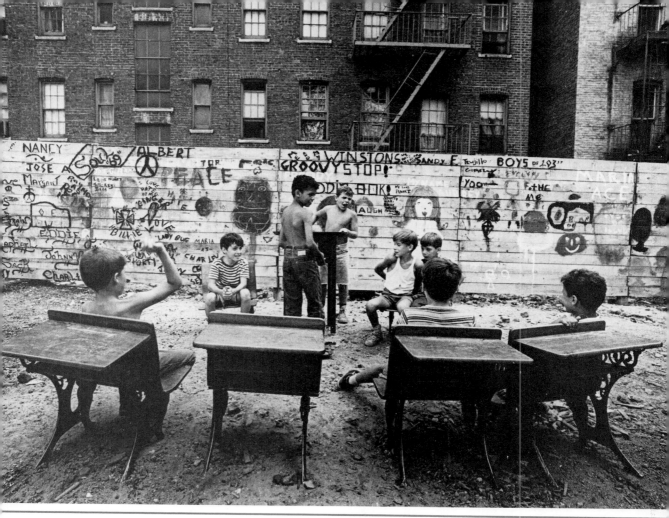

Creative play, manifested in a mock courtroom. Will one of these children grow up to be a Clarence Darrow, a Perry Mason, or an Agatha Christie?

duce a variety of different responses. The intellectual ability involved is defined as *divergent thinking*. Individuals think divergently when they produce a number of different solutions for a single problem. In contrast, measures of intelligence typically present items that require *convergent thinking*—the production of a single correct response. Table 10.2 presents an example of an item common to measures of creativity together with one way of scoring the item for three factors assumed to be related to creativity. Most measures of creativity are based on Guilford's (1950) work,

elaborated by Torrance (1966). These measures do not yield scores comparable to IQs but are sometimes useful in comparing individuals within a single testing group. Unfortunately, however, creativity tests based on the work of Torrance and Guilford have been highly verbal and might not have tapped creative abilities that are unrelated to verbal skills. Thus, creativity tests given in early grades have not often been found to be highly related to evidence of creativity obtained later in life. (See *Creative Problem Solving* for some tasks that call for creative solutions.)

Table 10.2 Sample answers and scoring procedure for one item from a test of creativity.

Item: How many uses can you think of for a nylon stocking?

Answers:		
*		wear on feet
§*		wear over face
*		wear on hands when it's cold
†*		make rugs
*		make clothes
§†*		make upholstery
†*		hang flower pots
*		hang mobiles
§†*		make Christmas decorations
†*		use as a sling
†*		tie up robbers
§†*		cover broken window panes
§†*		use as ballast in a dirigible
†*		make a fishing net

Scoring:			
*	Fluency:	14	(total number of different responses)
†	Flexibility:	9	(number of shifts from one class to another)
§	Originality:	5	(number of unusual responses — responses that occurred less than 5 percent of the time in the entire sample)

Encouraging Creativity

Attempts to increase creativity in schoolchildren have often been based on techniques developed in industry. Best known of these is Alex Osborn's *brainstorming,* which involves a small group of individuals (six to ten), often with a wide variety of backgrounds, who are assembled and asked to think of as many solutions as they can for a specific problem. A brainstorming session operates according to four rules. The first, based on Osborn's (1957) principle of *deferred evaluation,* forbids any of the members to evaluate any of the ideas presented during the session. Among other things, this means that members can neither applaud nor laugh in derision, nor can they say good or bad. The second of Osborn's brainstorming rules specifies that wild and unusual ideas are to be encouraged, the third, that quantity of ideas is important, and the fourth, that modifications and combinations involving other ideas are also to be encouraged.

During the course of a brainstorming session, various aids might be employed to stimulate the production of creative ideas. Among these are checklists of ideas (for example, Parnes, Noller, & Biondi, 1977). The checklists encourage participants to think of ways of "combining," "reversing," "substituting," "rearranging," and so on.

Although specific programs designed to increase creativity among students often result in higher scores on the rather inadequate measures of creativity that we have so far developed (for example, Lefrancois, 1965), there is no evidence that these programs have any long-term beneficial effects. However, we have every reason to believe that creativity can be fostered, not only by teaching

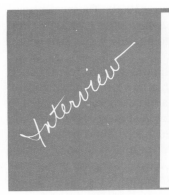

Interview

Subject: Male; age seventy-five; retired school teacher.
(referring to one of his sons, who is a writer)

He was probably always different . . . well, maybe not really *different.* What I mean is you sort of knew, even when he was just little, that he was going to *do* something or be famous. Not that he went out of his way to get people's attention. Just that he stood out. A lot of his teachers mentioned it one time or another. And it wasn't that his marks were that much better than anyone else's or that his writing really stood out that much. I'm not sure he was even interested in writing then. But he *was* independent and he liked to express himself. He liked to say what he thought. And he had a tremendous sense of humor even though he didn't seem to care that much to make other people laugh. He just found all sorts of things funny.

the skills that might be involved in the creative process and the knowledge required to recognize and appreciate creative products, but perhaps primarily by encouraging the kinds of personality characteristics most closely associated with creativity. These must surely include openness to new ideas, tolerance of ambiguity, willingness to experiment, and the courage to communicate—and sometimes to be wrong and perhaps to appear stupid and foolish.

CREATIVE PROBLEM SOLVING

A *problem,* we are told, is "an incomplete situation; a situation where certain elements are known but others must be found, discovered, provided, implemented, begged, borrowed, or stolen" (Lefrancois, 1983, p. 224).

Problems vary considerably in terms of their difficulty as well as in terms of the strategies that might be employed to solve them. Greene (1975), for example, describes six levels of problems:

Level 1: The solver already knows the solution. The problem is therefore simply one of retrieving from memory. (Example: What was your previous phone number?)

Level 2: The solution is unknown, but rules and procedures that will lead to the solution are known. (Find the square root of 1244.)

Level 3: The solution is learned in the course of dealing with the problem. (Find a way out of a forest—or a city.)

Level 4: Different possible solutions must be selected and evaluated. (Do a crossword puzzle.)

Level 5: The problem needs to be reformulated and analyzed, and the required solution will be a novel one. (Invent something.)

Level 6: The solver first needs to realize that a problem exists and is then required to generate new solutions or new procedures for arriving at solutions. (Invent a new fuel-saving carburetor.)

The lives of ordinary people probably are filled largely with lower-level problems. Indeed, the lives of most people might involve very few problems of the kind we are considering here. And when faced with such problems, a typical response might be: "If I don't know the answer, forget it!" But you, whose life is more extraordinary, might want to consider the following "creative" problems:

A. Take four oblong blocks or boxes and try arranging them so that: (a) every block touches every other, (b) one block touches one other, one touches two others, and one touches three others, (c) every block touches two others, and (d) each block is touching one other (based on de Bono, 1976).

B. Join all the dots in the following arrangement with no more than *four* continuous straight lines (that is, without lifting your pencil from paper):

```
•   •   •

•   •   •

•   •   •
```

C. Let us suppose that one day you walk from Pascal to Shell River. You leave at 8 o'clock in the morning, stop four or five times to rest, fish off the bridge for almost an hour at lunch time, and finally arrive at Shell River at four in the afternoon. Having spent the night in Shell River, you return the next day to Pascal, following exactly the same route and again leaving at 8 o'clock in the morning. But this time, you walk faster and reach Pascal by noon. Is it true that, at some point on your return trip, you will necessarily be at one place at exactly the same time that you were the day before?

D. Using only six matches of equal length, make four equal-sized triangles so that the length of each side is equal to the length of one match.

E. Two fathers and two sons went fishing and caught only three trout. Each took one home. How can that be?

F. Two trains hurtle toward each other, one traveling 100 miles per hour, the other going a mere 50 miles an hour. When the trains are only 75 miles apart, a deranged hummingbird flies from the front of one train directly toward the other at an incredible speed of 90 miles an hour. And when it reaches the other train, it turns immediately and flies back to the first again. And again it turns . . . and again . . . and again . . . flying back and forth between the two trains, always at 90 miles an hour, slowing down not a whit every time it turns. How far will this deranged hummingbird have flown by the time the two trains collide?

Solutions are in the next box.

There is something to be said for fools, too. Speaking of which, and at the risk of offending my grandparents, my parents, all of my uncles, several of my aunts, and approximately 143 first cousins, not to mention the remainder of my relatives, I will tell you of my cousin Reginald. He is the one about

whom we no longer speak. First, let me change his name to Robert to lessen the risk of offending.

Little can be said of Robert's early life in these respectable pages, if they are to stay respectable. Let me just mention that at the age of nine he confessed to having drowned more than one hundred flies by ingeniously inverting over the slop pail a glass half full of sweetened water and half full of flies. Only a short time later, four of my

CREATIVE SOLUTIONS

A. Solutions to the block problems are straightforward, although sometimes surprisingly difficult. Our solutions are often hampered by what psychologists call "set"—a predisposition to respond in certain ways.

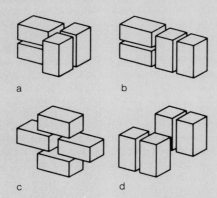

a   b

c   d

B. Set might also have affected your ability to solve the nine-dot problem (if you had any difficulty with it). Most people who have never seen this problem assume that the lines must all be *within* the boundaries of the nine dots. As the solution shows, that is not the case.

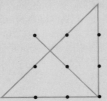

C. You will, indeed, be at exactly the same place and time on your way back from Shell River. This is easy to explain (and understand) if you consider what would happen if one person left Shell River and the other Pascal at the same time and on the same day. It makes no difference how fast each goes; providing they follow the same route, they must meet (that is, they must be at the same place and time on one occasion). The problem described earlier is identical to this one; you are simply "meeting" yourself on a different day.

D. If you had trouble with this one, it is probably because of "set" again. You likely tried to lay the matches flat on some horizontal surface. The solution, illustrated below, requires a shift from horizontal to vertical.

E. The problem is a bit of a "trick." Two fathers and two sons need not be four people; it might, as it obviously was in this case, be only three: a grandfather with his son and grandson—hence two fathers and two sons!

F. The problem sounds far more complex than it is. The two trains, since their speeds are constant, will collide in exactly 30 minutes, because they cover 150 miles in one hour (one travels 100 miles and the other 50), and they start out 75 miles apart. And the crazed hummingbird, no matter that it turns back and forth faster and faster as the trains approach each other, can only travel 45 miles in 30 minutes, since it is always going 90 miles an hour.

uncle's pigs drowned while trying to swim across the lake behind his barn—a mystery that few of the people who matter have solved even to this day.

At the age of ten, my cousin Robert nailed our teacher's shoes to the floor. Naturally, he did this not while the good nun was standing in them, but while she rested her feet, weary from pacing back and forth between my desk and Robert's. When she later slipped her feet back into her shoes, she would surely have pitched forward onto her nose had I not jumped up immediately to help her. What none of us could later figure out was how Robert managed to nail the back of her habit to the floor at the same time as he pried her shoes loose.

It is largely because of his later misbehaviors that we no longer speak of Robert. I dare not tell you why he was put away the last time. He is still away, entertaining his fellows.

They bought him a grand piano three Christmases ago. They say that on Sunday nights when he plays in the big hall, the great steel bars resonate with the fullness of his music, and all the birds, of which there are always many around prisons, stop and listen. And grown men, hardened criminals who have without emotion torn limbs from men and decapitated babies and wives, exult at the joy of his music—and weep at its sadness. There is no pianist in the world like my cousin Robert.

■ Exceptionality

My cousin Robert is not the average person whose development is the stuff of most of this text. He is an *exceptional* person but exceptional only in relation to the average or the "normal." Hence we need to understand the average if we are also to understand the exceptional.

Popular usage has confounded the term *exceptional* with *outstanding, gifted,* or *specially endowed.* But these words describe only one dimension of exceptionality. The other dimension, which has received far more attention both in research and in education, describes those individuals whose development is handicapped for any

of a number of reasons. In short, there are two types of exceptional individuals: those to whom nature or nurture (or, very often, both in interaction) has granted special gifts in the form of talents, predispositions, or abilities and those to whom fortune and other circumstances have been less kind. In addition, there are others whose exceptionalities are more complex—who, for example, may be exceptionally gifted in one area but deprived in another.

Dimensions of Exceptionality

Our discussions of the child have centered on three important areas of development: physical, social-emotional, and cognitive. We have dealt in some detail with the forces that influence development in each of these areas, with the processes that might account for their influence, and with the resulting products as they are manifested in physical characteristics, personality, interpersonal qualities, and intellectual performance. And although our emphasis has generally been on the optimal development of the individual child, we have paused on occasion to note how nature and nurture sometimes conspire, often in little-understood ways, to bring about atypical development.

In the remaining pages of this chapter, we look specifically at exceptionality in those three areas that have been our concern throughout: physical, social-emotional, and cognitive development. And in each of these areas, we look at both dimensions of exceptionality: the gifted or talented and the deprived or disturbed (see Figure 10.2).

Defining Exceptionality

Here, as elsewhere in psychology, there has been considerable historical disagreement concerning the most useful and the most valid ways of defining *exceptionality* in different areas. But here, more than elsewhere, there has also been a far greater need to arrive at relatively precise, or at least widely accepted, definitions. The reason that definition is

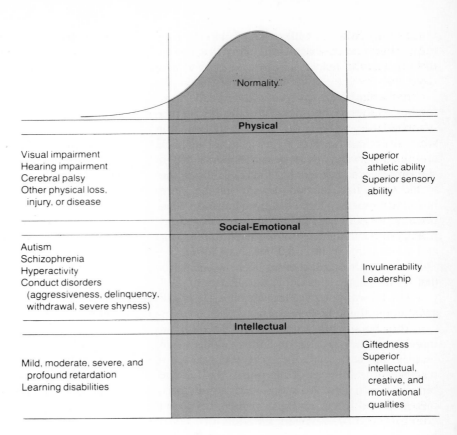

"Normality."

Physical

Visual impairment
Hearing impairment
Cerebral palsy
Other physical loss,
  injury, or disease

Superior
  athletic ability
Superior sensory
  ability

Social-Emotional

Autism
Schizophrenia
Hyperactivity
Conduct disorders
  (aggressiveness, delinquency,
  withdrawal, severe shyness)

Invulnerability
Leadership

Intellectual

Mild, moderate, severe, and
  profound retardation
Learning disabilities

Giftedness
Superior
  intellectual,
  creative, and
  motivational
  qualities

Figure 10.2
The dimensions of excep-
tionality discussed in this
chapter.

so important in regard to exceptionality relates directly to the needs that exceptional children have for *special* medical, educational, and sometimes institutional services. Without adequate definitions, not only would it be extremely difficult to determine which exceptional children should be provided with which services, but communication among involved personnel and the advancement of theory and research would also be greatly impeded. Unfortunately, definitions and classifications often continue to be vague and changing. Nevertheless, there is general agreement that exceptional children include all children "who require special education and related services if they are to realize their full human potential" (Hallahan & Kauffman, 1978, p. 4). The crux of the problem does not lie with this definition, however; it lies instead with the difficulty of determining

which children require special education and what services will be optimal for them.

One additional problem in this area deserves special mention. It concerns the potentially misleading nature of the categories often used to describe exceptional children. Exceptionality is seldom as clear cut as our categories might lead us to believe. In fact, many children who are exceptional do not suffer from a single problem but from a variety of related problems. (My cousin, alias Robert, is a case in point.) For these children, no single category adequately describes exceptionality. Nevertheless, it is useful and even necessary to simplify our description by means of categories or classes. Without these categories it would be difficult to provide the services that exceptional children require. However, these should not be interpreted as labels to conveniently place on an individual child for automatic insight concerning that child's condition. Indeed, there is currently a strong reaction against the use of categories as labels, not only because of the social stigma often associated with the labels but also because educators have too often adjusted their expectations and their behaviors unfairly in reaction to these labels. Partly for this reason, labels have undergone numerous euphemistic changes, especially in the area of **mental retardation**, where such terms as *imbecile*, *idiot*, and *moron* have largely been abandoned in favor of less negative terms such as *educable mentally retarded* or *mild, moderate, severe*, and *profound* to indicate degrees of retardation.

■ Physical Exceptionality

Although physical exceptionality is often defined as including only nonsensory problems, in this section we look as well at sensory impairments involving vision and hearing. The treatment presented in this chapter is no more than an introduction to a vast and complex area. Consult the further readings annotated at the end of the chapter for more detailed information.

Prevalence

Estimates of the prevalence of physical disabilities vary a great deal. The U.S. Office of Education (1975) estimates that perhaps 5 children out of 1,000 are physically handicapped. The number that would be considered "exceptional" in terms of our earlier definition would necessarily be considerably lower, since not all these children would require special education or special services. However, this figure does not include visually handicapped or hearing-impaired children. The number of "legally blind" individuals in the population is estimated at between 1 and 5 per 1,000. Again, however, many of these people are not functionally blind. That is, they are able to see well enough to be mobile and often to read large print with or without magnifying equipment. Estimates of hearing impairment indicate that approximately 5 out of 1,000

school-age children have hearing impairments and that 1 out of these 5 may be considered deaf (U.S. Office of Education, 1975). Approximately 1 out of every 1,400 babies is born with a *severe* hearing loss (Jaffe & Luterman, 1980).

Nonsensory Physical Problems

Physical problems that fall under the rubric of exceptionality include a variety of health problems, as well as physical handicaps or impairments. A number of these are congenital (present at birth or appearing shortly thereafter). This does not mean that the problems are genetic, because many congenital defects are related to problems at birth, to malnutrition of the mother, and to diseases, drugs, and infections during the prenatal period.

Cerebral Palsy   The condition labeled *cerebral palsy* is a collection of symptoms (a *syndrome*) that includes motor problems, psychological problems, convulsions, or behavior disorders (Cruickshank, 1976). An alternate label for this condition is *significant developmental motor disability* (Abroms & Panagakos, 1980). Associated with brain damage, it varies in severity from being so mild that it is virtually undetectable to being sufficiently serious that it is manifested in paralysis.

Total or partial paralysis of limbs is sometimes a concomitant of cerebral palsy; the majority of people who are paralyzed are hemiplegic (35–40 percent). Paralysis of one (monoplegia) or three (triplegia) limbs is rare. The following terms describe five types of paralysis:

Monoplegia	one limb
Paraplegia	both lower extremities
Hemiplegia	both extremities, on the same side
Triplegia	three extremities
Quadriplegia	four extremities

Cerebral palsy is a congenital condition: It is present at birth and would therefore not result from brain damage occurring later in life, even though many of the same symptoms might result. Estimates of its prevalence are highly uncertain; many of the milder cases are not reported, partic-

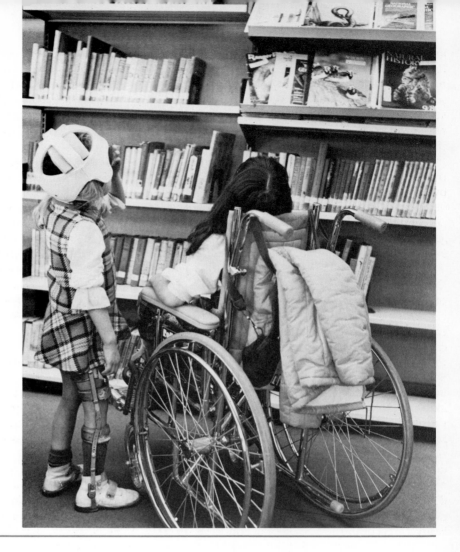

Although as many as 5 out of 1000 children are physically disabled, the number of those actually requiring special education is much smaller.

ularly since there is no cure for the condition. Estimates cited by Abroms and Panagakos (1980) vary from 1.63 to 7.5 cases for every 1,000 live births.

The causes of cerebral palsy include all factors that are capable of producing brain damage in the fetus or at birth. Some of these factors, many of which are described in Chapter 4, include maternal infections and diseases, X-rays, premature birth, difficult delivery, anoxia (oxygen deprivation), or a direct blow or injury to the brain.

Although cerebral palsy is generally considered to be a motor disability, there is increasing evidence that it may also involve a variety of emotional and cognitive problems that are generally discussed under different headings (Cruickshank, 1976). Indeed, the effects of cerebral palsy are highly variable, as are its causes (Denhoff, 1976).

Epilepsy   Also a neurological impairment, epilepsy does not usually lead to problems in school and is therefore mentioned only in passing in this section. It is essentially a seizure disorder whose causes are unknown. Seizures, which may take a variety of forms, involve abnormal electrical activity of the brain. The more serious forms of epilepsy (sometimes termed *grand mal*, as opposed to *petit mal*) can often be controlled with drugs. Petit mal seizures, which only last between one and thirty seconds, are manifested in a momentary "absentness" of the child and are often accompanied by rhythmic, fluttering movements of both eyelids (Abroms & Panagakos, 1980). These seizures may occur frequently and are sometimes interpreted by parents or teachers as a sign that the student is deliberately not paying attention. In more than 70 percent of all cases, petit mal seizures cease altogether by the age of eighteen (Sato, Dreifuss, & Penry, 1976).

Other Physical Problems   A large number of other physical problems sometimes require special education or services. These include such diseases and conditions as muscular dystrophy, cancer, asthma, diabetes, and the absence of one or more limbs, as well as paralysis, to name but a few. Some are congenital, some are caused by infections, and others result from accidents of various kinds. In many cases, serious emotional and social problems are associated with them; many of these problems are related to difficulties the child experiences in being accepted by others and in developing a positive self-concept. Hence a great deal of what special education programs, parents, and therapists can do for physically exceptional children relates to their emotional and social well-being.

Visual Impairment

Those who can see at twenty feet what a "normal" person can see at twenty feet are said to have 20/20 vision (or normal vision); those who can see at 20 feet what normal people see at 200 feet are said to have 20/200 vision and are classified as legally blind if their *corrected* vision in their better eye is no better than 20/200. Accordingly, a large majority of individuals who are classified as legally blind do, in fact, *see*; this is one reason why the term *visually impaired* is highly preferable to *blind*. Approximately half of all legally blind children can read large type or print with the help of magnification. For the special education teacher, it is especially important to determine whether a child will be able to learn to read visually or will have to learn to read by touch. For those who can read visually, the "special" qualities of education might not need to go beyond providing magnifying equipment or large type, unless there are other problems involved. Multiple handicaps, as mentioned earlier, are not uncommon (Donovan, 1980).

Special classrooms and special teachers for visually impaired children are much less common now than they once were; many of these children are now being educated in regular classrooms, a practice termed *mainstreaming* (about which more is said later in this chapter). Those who must learn to read Braille, however, require special equipment and teachers (Nolan, 1978).

Hearing Impairment

Although there are a number of different ways to define *deafness,* the most useful for our purposes are those that distinguish between prelinguistic and postlinguistic deafness—in other words, between loss of hearing that occurs prior to learning a language and that which occurs later. Unfortunately, loss of hearing is most often congenital, so that fewer than one child in ten who is deaf lost hearing after the age of two. In effect, *deafness* is the inability to hear sounds clearly enough for the ordinary purposes of life. The *hard of hearing* are described as those who suffer from some hearing loss but who can function with a hearing aid and sometimes without one.

In terms of cognitive development, deafness generally presents a far more serious handicap for the child than does visual impairment, largely because of the severe difficulties it presents for learning to understand and to speak—hence the historical, but no longer popular, expression "deaf and dumb" or "deaf-mute." There is little evidence that the visually impaired are intellectually handicapped as a result of their blindness, but the same is not true of those who are hearing impaired. Although there is considerable controversy concerning whether deaf children are as intelligent as children with normal hearing (see Wiley, 1971), their academic achievement often lags behind, a problem that can be attributed largely to language deficiencies. Furth (1973) points out that only a very small percentage of deaf individuals ever progress far enough in their development of language skills that they can read a college-level text with understanding. This, of course, applies to the prelinguistically deaf and not to those whose loss of hearing occurred after they have already learned a language.

In addition to the academic problems often associated with deafness, there are frequently a number of emotional and social problems as well (Meadow, 1975). These problems probably result from lack of social interaction, resulting from impaired abilities to communicate through language. Meadow notes that these emotional problems are frequently manifested in marital and occupational problems, for example, rather than in severe emotional disturbance.

The education of the deaf generally requires specially trained teachers and most often occurs in institutions. Understandably, the principal emphasis is on the acquisition of language. The two separate approaches to teaching language to the deaf both have their passionate advocates; neither has been able to establish clear superiority on the basis of research evidence (Larsen & Miller, 1978). The *manual* approach teaches language by means of gestures and takes one of two forms: American Sign Language (ASL), where gestures stand for words and concepts, and finger spelling, where letters of the alphabet are signaled by positions of the fingers and combined into words. The manual approach was long the most popular method in schools for the deaf, but the *oral* approach may now be more popular (Silverman, 1971). It attempts to teach deaf children to speak and understand (often through lip reading, also called "speech reading") ordinary language so that they can converse with those who are not deaf. In general, the approach is more difficult than manual language, particularly if hearing loss is so severe that auditory discriminations are not possible. Attempts to employ a combination of manual and oral

approaches have also been advocated (Garretson, 1976). This combination is difficult as well, partly because the structures of ASL and spoken language are not always the same.

The education of children with only a partial hearing loss may also require special instruction, particularly if the loss is manifested in speech disorders. Although many children with partial hearing are capable of following conversations if they are at close range or sufficiently loud, they often experience difficulty in distinguishing among consonants for which there are no visual clues (for example, *p-b, t-d,* and *f-v*). Their own speech may consequently be affected. Special education for these children can often be implemented without removing them from regular classrooms, simply by providing special instructional sessions for them. Itinerant teachers are often used for this purpose.

The Physically Gifted

The predominant emphasis in the area of exceptionality has long focused on those individuals whose exceptionalities have placed them at a disadvantage relative to normal children. But there are exceptional individuals at the other end of the spectrum as well. Unfortunately, although increasing attention is being paid to cognitive giftedness, particularly in intellectual and creative talents, much less attention has been focused on systematically identifying those who possess exceptional physical skills and on providing special education programs so that these children might "develop their full human potential." Indeed, there is an increasingly noticeable lack of research on the emotional, social, and intellectual characteristics of the physically gifted and on how their development might be enhanced. But we do provide scholarships for those who are inclined toward competitive athletics.

■ Social-Emotional Exceptionality

Problems associated with social-emotional exceptionality are both varied and highly individualistic; hence they do not easily lend themselves to classification or even to definition. Terms that are frequently employed synonymously to refer to children with such problems are *behavior-disordered, emotionally disturbed,* or *socially maladjusted.* Each describes children who are troubled and who may also cause trouble for parents, teachers, peers, and others (Whelan, 1978).

Note that the labels employed to describe social and emotional problems serve only as descriptions, not as explanations. Thus children who are diagnosed as autistic are so labeled because they display a common set of behavioral and emotional symptoms; but the term *autism* serves in no way to explain these behaviors and symptoms.

Social-emotional maladjustment presents problems of identification that are far more difficult than those relating to physical exceptionality. Whereas reasonably competent individuals can usually arrive at an agreed-upon diagnosis with respect to visual or hearing impairments, for example, the same does not hold for the common social-emotional problems (for example, autism, childhood psychoses and anxiety disorders, and attentional disorders such as hyperkinesis).

Prevalence and Causes

Estimates of the prevalence of *emotional* or *behavior* disorders (the terms are used interchangeably in this section) vary considerably, depending on the criteria employed for identification and depending as well on whether estimates include mild and severe instances of disturbance. Kelly, Bullock, and Dykes (1977) report that these estimates range from 2 to 20 percent of the school population.

The assumed causes of emotional disorders also vary a great deal. These causes are often classified in one of two ways: predisposing versus precipitating or biogenic as opposed to psychogenic. *Predisposing* factors are conditions that increase the risk that a child will develop and manifest emotional disturbances. Genetic factors, poverty, parental abuse or rejection, physical handicaps, and racial and religious discrimination have each been implicated as predisposing factors (Morse, 1977).

Precipitating factors in emotional disturbance are limited to those events or situations that lead directly to the disturbance. Specific childhood traumas such as might be associated with the death of a parent, divorce, or an accident to the child might precipitate emotional disorders.

Whereas predisposing and precipitating factors are often employed as an explanation for the onset of a disorder, the specific *type* of disorder that is manifested has sometimes been associated with biogenic and psychogenic factors. *Biogenic* factors include genetic and biological forces that, in effect, predispose the individual toward emotional exceptionality. The presence of biogenic factors is most clearly evident in the case of the more severe emotional disturbances, such as childhood schizophrenia, which, as was mentioned in Chapter 2, sometimes has a strong genetic component. *Psychogenic* factors are related to the child's relationship with the environment and, in a Freudian sense, are often described in terms of conflicts that are assumed to exist within the child.

Given adequate knowledge of the child's biological history and environment, it is possible to identify children who may be described as being greater psychiatric risks than others. Anthony (1975; Anthony & Koupernik, 1974) has undertaken longitudinal research designed not only to identify factors that might be useful for predicting the probability of emotional disturbance in later childhood or even in adulthood but to prevent disorders as well. If we can accurately identify predisposing factors, then we might also be able to modify the environment in order to reduce the incidence of emotional disturbance. However, considerably more research is needed to identify not only those forces associated with emotional disorders but also those that might be associated with healthy development. We speak again of healthy development later in this chapter.

Classifications

As Ross (1980) notes, attempting to classify the psychological disorders of childhood presents some extremely difficult problems, many of them relating to lack of agreement concerning what it is that needs to be classified. In other words, experts have had considerable difficulty agreeing on what a childhood psychological disorder is, whether it is different from an adult disorder, and whether it should even be labeled in the first place. In the following sections, we look at several of the more common and severe manifestations of emotional disorders: autism and schizophrenia, hyperactivity, and conduct and personality disorders. We also look at social-emotional giftedness.

Autism and Schizophrenia

Among the most severe but least prevalent forms of early emotional disorders are autism and schizophrenia. Both of these conditions ordinarily require institutional care.

Autism develops within the first thirty months of life and is characterized by a lack of responsiveness to others, impaired or nonexistent communication skills, and various bizarre behaviors (Ross & Pelham, 1981). Autism in early infancy is sometimes evident in the refusal of the infant to "cuddle" or even to make eye contact and an unresponsiveness to language that is sometimes so complete that parents often incorrectly assume their infant is deaf.

Childhood schizophrenia is not always clearly distinguished from autism; many researchers believe that autism is simply an early form of schizophrenia (American Psychiatric Association, 1980). Ross (1980) suggests that they are distinctly different disorders. To begin with, schizophrenia does not start as early, often not becoming apparent until adolescence. Second, autism is characterized by extreme isolation or *aloneness*, manifested in a lack of verbal and physical contact, as well as by an apparently strong need to have everything remain the same. Autistic children frequently become very disturbed when anything is changed in their environment. Finally, the autistic child typically manifests grossly impaired or completely absent language development; such is not the case for schizophrenic children.

Goldfarb (1970) includes the following among the most common characteristics of childhood schizophrenia: aloofness, withdrawal, and other manifestations of abnormal interpersonal relationships; self-injurious and sometimes bizarre assaults on the child's own body; an abnormal attachment to objects; unusual responses to sensory stimulation, sometimes manifested in a complete insensitivity to pain or an exaggerated sensitivity to pain; poor coordination and balance, sometimes accompanied by repetitive body motions such as rocking or twirling; and general intellectual retardation.

Clinicians do not always try to differentiate between autism and childhood schizophrenia, particularly if the condition appears to be severe and if the child is still very young. Regardless of the label employed, treatment approaches would be virtually identical. A number of different treatments might be employed. For example, tranquilizers and antipsychotic drugs are often used. Although there is little evidence that they are very effective in alleviating the condition, they are useful in making patients more manageable. The use of psychotherapy—psychoanalysis, for example— also has not been demonstrated to be particularly useful. However, behavior therapies beginning early in the child's life and sustained over a long time are sometimes beneficial (see Rincover & Koegel, 1977). But as Ross and Pelham (1981) note, none of these therapies, including the behavior therapies, are likely to make autistic children act normally.

Follow-up studies of children diagnosed as having childhood psychoses (autism or schizophrenia) have not provided much reason for optimism. Combining several long-term studies that looked at these children between five and ten years after initial diagnosis, DeMyer et al. (1973) found that only 1 to 2 percent would recover sufficiently that they would later be classified as normal. Another 5 to 15 percent would be almost normal, 16 to 25 percent might be classified as "fair," and more than half would be in poor condition. In one study, only five out of sixty-three autistic and schizophrenic children were in ordinary schools or in occupational settings ten years later (Rutter & Lockyer, 1967).

Hyperactivity

The American Psychiatric Association (1980) describes *hyperactivity* as an *attentional deficit disorder with hyperactivity*. It is commonly called hyperactivity (or hyperkinesis), largely because its most obvious symptom is excessive physical activity. However, hyperactivity is only one of the symptoms of this condition.

Estimates are that as many as 3 percent of current elementary school children suffer from varying degrees of hyperactivity (American Psychiatric Association, 1980). Some of these children experience considerable difficulty adjusting to school and home; many are considered to be relatively serious problems. The syndrome itself is often characterized by restlessness, inability to sit still, purposeless and disorderly behavior, impulsiveness, short attention span, and poor performance in school even when the children are of average intelligence. It is small wonder that hyperactive children are treated as psychological and medical problems. One of the most common treatments for these children involves the use of drugs to sedate them.

Research involving twins suggests that hyperactivity has a genetic component. Willerman (1973) found that if one member of a pair of twins was hyperactive, the other was much more likely to be hyperactive than another sibling. Similarly, Morrison and Stewart (1973) found that hyperactive children had more biological relatives who had also been hyperactive than did children who were not hyperactive. Additional evidence that hyperactivity is at least partly genetic is implicit in the observation that far more males than females are hyperactive (between 80 and 90 percent are male; Wesley & Wesley, 1977). Other evidence suggests that hyperactivity is to a large extent a maturational problem involving the central nervous system. This explanation is supported by the observation that many hyperactive children tend not to display the same symptoms of hyperactivity after adolescence and that the activity level of hyperactive children is often similar to that typical of children four or five years younger. However, more recent evidence suggests that not all children "outgrow" their hyperactivity at adolescence (see Ross & Pelham, 1980).

Other explanations for hyperactivity have sometimes implicated neurological impairment or brain damage and dietary or vitamin-linked causes. However, there is little evidence that neurological impairment or brain damage is involved in the majority of cases diagnosed as hyperactive. With respect to dietary factors, the conclusion is the same. Whereas Feingold (1975a, 1975b) suggests that certain food additives contribute to hyperactivity, more carefully controlled research has not found this to be the case, at least for most children (for example, see Hallahan & Heins, 1976; Spring & Sandoval, 1976). There is some reason to believe, however, that between 5 and 10 percent of hyperactive children react badly to certain food dyes and that these children might therefore be helped through dietary means (Ross, 1980).

Conduct and Personality Disorders

A number of sometimes serious behavior disorders of childhood cannot easily be classified. Many of these involve problems of socialization and are manifested in aggressive, hostile, and essentially antisocial behavior; alternatively, conduct disorders might be evident in withdrawal, social isolation, or extreme shyness. Not surprisingly, aggressive and hostile behaviors (delinquency, vandalism, and so on) are likely to be dealt with—or at least punished. Social isolation and extreme shyness are much more likely to be ignored.

Other social disorders may be manifested in lying, stealing, inability to form close relationships with others, temper tantrums, disobedience and insolence, extremely negative self-concepts, and related behaviors and attitudes.

Treatment of children exhibiting conduct and personality disorders depends largely on the severity of the disturbance. In cases of moderate or mild disturbance, teachers and parents can often cope adequately; with the occasional help of professional personnel, they can sometimes do much more than cope. More severe disturbances may require therapeutic and sometimes judicial intervention.

Social-Emotional Giftedness

Here, as elsewhere, exceptionality has two dimensions: the disadvantaged, among whom are the autistic, psychotic, hyperactive, and those exhibiting personality and conduct disorders, and the advantaged, to whom we have paid little special attention. Nevertheless, it is possible to identify two groups of gifted children in recent literature. One group, variously labeled "superkids" or "the invulnerables" (see Pines, 1975, 1979), has been identified in research originally designed to investigate psychiatric risk among children. One of the observations that intrigued researchers was that a significant number of children whose biological and environmental histories suggested that the likelihood of emotional disorder was extremely high did not become psychological casualties. Quite the contrary: Not only did some of these children appear to be invulnerable to the emotional disorders that would surely claim most other children in the same circumstances, but they also appeared to thrive on early adversity and to emerge unscathed and, in some ways, superior. Garmezy (1976) describes these invulnerables as exceptionally competent and at ease in social situations, highly capable in social interaction with adults, characterized by feelings of personal powerfulness (as opposed to helplessness or powerlessness), highly autonomous, and achievement oriented.

The importance of understanding why some children survive and even thrive in high-risk situations, and why others do not, is related directly to the possibility of "inoculating" children against risk or of ameliorating risk for those who are most vulnerable. Anthony (1975) suggests, for example, that exposure to a certain amount of adversity may be crucial for the development of resistance to disturbance. At the same time, exposure to too many stresses may have just the opposite effect. There may be a particular combination of personality characteristics or genetic predispositions that, in interaction with a stressful environment, produces a highly adjusted healthy person. The critical problem is to identify this combination of characteristics and environment in an effort to maximize the development of human potential. The emphasis is dramatically different from that focusing on identifying and treating disorders.

Exceptional social-emotional competence may be manifested not only in those who survive high risk but also in the development of exceptional individuals whose early lives and biological history present no unusual psychological threats. Walker (1978) suggests that among the socially gifted may well be found the leaders of tomorrow, and perhaps today's leaders were yesterday's socially gifted children.

How do we recognize these children? They are the intelligent, alert, talkative, inquisitive, autonomous, socially competent youngsters. Berkowitz (1975) cites research indicating that these, too, are the qualities of adults who are most likely to be leaders. Do we provide "special" education for the socially gifted?

■ Intellectual Exceptionality

Early in this chapter you were cautioned that the labels employed to categorize various types of exceptionality are descriptive rather than explanatory and that they are potentially misleading. Not only are specific instances of exceptionality often highly individual, but the application of any one specific label cannot, by itself, take into account the possibility that the individual so labeled may be atypical in a variety of ways—and also quite normal in others. Unfortunately, many children who might be described as mentally or intellectually retarded also manifest social-emotional and physical problems. The point might be made that, in the same way as there is no average "normal" child, there is also no average retarded child. Nevertheless, in the same way as the average children of earlier chapters had a great deal in common, so too do intellectually exceptional children.

Mental Retardation

The most obvious feature of mental retardation is a general depression in the ability to learn; a feature that may not be so obvious involves problems in adapting. These two characteristics are reflected in the widely accepted definition of retardation presented by the American Association on Mental Deficiency (AAMD): "Mental retardation refers to significantly subaverage general intellectual functioning existing concurrently with deficits in adaptive behavior, and manifested during the developmental period" (Grossman, 1973, p. 11). This is essentially the definition now adopted by the American Psychiatric Association as well.

In practice, mental retardation is most often identified and defined in terms of performance on intelligence tests, with some occasional, though limited, attention to adaptive behavior, a characteristic that is difficult to measure or define. Important distinctions are also made among four categories of retardation: mild, moderate, severe, and profound. These categories are defined rather precisely in terms of scores on intelligence tests (see Figure 10.3). Overlapping categories that are of more practical importance for special educators distinguish among educable, trainable, and custodial retardation.

Estimates of the prevalence of mental retardation vary. The normal distribution of intelligence in the general population suggests that between 2 and 3 percent of the population may be retarded (Scheiner & McNabb, 1980). If level of adaptation is taken into account, only 1 percent are actually retarded (Mercer, 1973).

The causes of mental retardation are also varied. They may be related to brain damage or to hereditary and environmental influences. Chromosomal aberrations and defects such as those manifested in Down's syndrome and phenylketonuria (see Chapter 3), maternal infections (such as rubella) drugs, radiation, infections, malnutrition, and other factors may be involved (Bruininks & Warfield, 1978). Although identification of causes may be of considerable importance, particularly for medicine and genetics, it is less important for

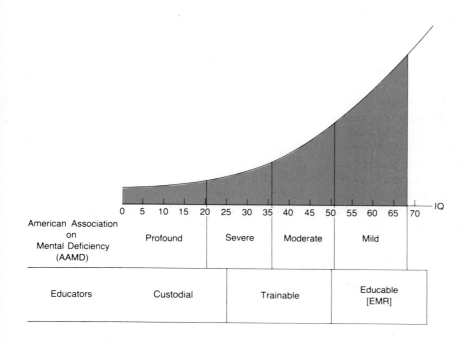

Figure 10.3
Two common classification schemes for mental retardation. Note that these classifications are based entirely on measured IQ. In practice, adaptive skills would also be taken into account. The AAMD classifications shown here are based on the Stanford-Binet or Cattell tests. The Wechsler Scales have a different distribution and therefore different "cutoff" points: 55–69 (mild); 40–54 (moderate); 25–39 (severe); below 25 (profound).

special educators and clinicians. Hence mentally retarded children are ordinarily described in terms of *degree* rather than cause of exceptionality.

The largest proportion of retarded children (approximately 75 percent) are only *mildly* retarded. Most of these children are not identified as being retarded until they enter school. Prior to this time, they ordinarily develop social and language skills and experience relatively normal motor development. In school, most are capable of academic achievement at approximately the sixth-grade level, although they do not normally reach this level until their teens. These children are described as the *educable mentally retarded*.

Children classified as moderately retarded compose another 20 percent of the retarded group and, along with some of the severely retarded, are often described as *trainable*. These children are capable of learning to talk during the preschool period; most will also learn to walk, although their verbal and motor skills are generally markedly inferior to those of normal children. Whereas a large number of mildly retarded children are educated in regular schools—in the mainstream, though often with special teachers and equipment—the majority of the moderately retarded are eventually placed in special schools. The emphasis in these schools is on developing skills that might later provide the individual with a measure of independence. Most are unlikely to achieve competence beyond the second-grade level.

Severe mental retardation is usually associated with poor motor development, few communication skills (although these sometimes develop slightly later in life), and a high degree of dependence throughout life. Profound mental retardation generally requires custodial care that is solely maintenance. Children who are profoundly mentally retarded frequently do not learn toilet or dressing habits; in addition, many do not learn to walk.

The largest group of mentally retarded children, the mildly retarded, are of special importance to the regular classroom teacher, particularly since mainstreaming requirements make it likely that many regular classrooms will also include a number of exceptional children. Some of their personality and intellectual characteristics are discussed briefly here.

To begin with, it is important to realize that many mildy retarded children are not noticeably different from other children in terms of their social and personality characteristics or in terms of their needs. But, by definition, they do experience more difficulty in learning and sometimes, as a result, develop less positive self-concepts and other personality problems. Note also that little evidence supports the once prevalent notion that they learn differently from normal children. Present evidence indicates that they go through much the same developmental and learning sequences, but at a slower rate (see Haywood, Meyers, & Switzky, 1982). The most consistent differences between the mildly mentally retarded and normal children relate to memory and attention span. In general, these children are less able to attend and attend for shorter periods of time (Mercer & Snell, 1977). With respect to memory, they appear to be inferior in terms of short-term memory skills. In other words, they have difficulty remembering items that have just been presented to them. Once they have learned, however, their long-term memories do not appear to be different from those of normal children (Robinson & Robinson, 1976). Their poorer short-term memories are most frequently explained in terms of an inability to make use of processing strategies such as organizing and rehearsing.

In addition to attention and memory problems that often characterize mildly retarded children, some have language deficits and inferior motor development. Evidence suggests that, contrary to popular opinion, they are not stronger, faster, or in other ways physically gifted, as though nature or nurture were compensating for a deficiency in one area by endowing the individual in another (see, for example, Bruininks, 1977).

One of the principal considerations in the education of the mildly retarded focuses on the development of healthy social and emotional characteristics. It is highly unfortunate that our cultural prejudices have placed such value on excellence and such a stigma on mental retardation that the emotional well-being of those who are intellectually disadvantaged is often unfairly threatened.

Learning Disabilities

In the absence of perceptible emotional or physical disturbances and without being mentally retarded, a significant number of children in schools experience serious learning difficulties in one or more areas. Such children have sometimes been described as suffering from hyperactivity, learning dysfunction, cerebral dysfunction, minimal brain damage, perceptual handicaps, dyslexia, perceptual disability, or simply as being slow learners. Each of these terms is relatively nonspecific, often confusing, and sometimes meaningless (Ross, 1976). In 1963, Samuel Kirk proposed a new term that would, in effect, include all of the conditions previously described by these and other labels: *learning disability*. It does not carry the stigma attached to such terms as brain damage or cerebral dysfunction, nor does it complicate our understanding with excessive categorization. (See Kirk, 1979.)

The term quickly became popular and is now widely used to describe a variety of conditions that have in common the following characteristics (Hallahan & Kauffman, 1976):

1. Academic retardation

2. An uneven pattern of development

3. The occasional presence of central nervous system dysfunction

4. Learning problems that are not due to environmental disadvantage, mental retardation, or emotional disturbance.

The National Advisory Committee on Handicapped Children (1968) further states that the academic retardation or learning problems characteristic of the learning disabled child may be manifested in disorders "of listening, thinking, talking, reading, writing, spelling, or arithmetic." Given the central importance of the language arts, the identification and remediation of learning disabilities is of paramount importance to elementary school teachers. The following are some of the many symptoms sometimes associated with learning disabilities, either singly or in various combinations (see Clements, 1966; Edmonton Public School Board, 1978):

Inattentiveness (short attention span)
Impulsiveness
Hyperactivity
Frequent shifts in emotional mood
Impaired visual memory (difficulty in recalling shapes or words)
Motor problems (difficulty in running, hitting a ball, cutting, writing)
Disorders of speech and hearing
Specific academic difficulties (reading, writing, spelling, arithmetic)

Unfortunately, the identification of learning disabilities is far from simple. Although a number of standardized tests are useful for diagnosing the nature of specific disabilities and sometimes for suggesting appropriate remedial procedures, initial identification (which must always be highly tentative) is difficult. In addition, final identification, diagnosis of the specific problem (or problems), and remedial suggestions are ordinarily beyond the expertise of the regular classroom teacher. These activities should involve a person specially trained in learning disabilities. Here perhaps more than anywhere else, given problems of definition and identification, teachers and others must be careful not to mislabel children.

The prevalence of learning disabilities is variously estimated at between 2 and 4 percent of the school population, depending on the criteria employed and the individuals responsible for identification (Johnson & Morasky, 1980). The literature on learning disabilities provides no consistent or simple methods for classifying learning disabilities (Little, 1978). In practice, however, learning disabilities often involve language or arithmetic and are labeled in terms of whether they involve oral or written speech, comprehension or production of speech, or particular problems in spelling or arithmetic. These classifications by no means exhaust all problems that are sometimes considered to be symptomatic of a learning disability.

What causes learning disabilities? There is, of course, no single cause for all manifestations of this condition but more often a complex interaction of causes. These might include brain damage or other neurological impairment, various diseases and infections, malnutrition, and other environmental or genetic factors.

Learning disabilities, as they are presently defined, are treated within the context of the regular classroom. That is, learning disabled children are usually enrolled in regular classrooms but may spend time in "special" classrooms. Alternately, learning disability specialists, many of whom specialize in reading or writing skills, may work with these children in the regular classroom. In a declining number of cases, they are given no "special" treatment.

Intellectual Giftedness

There are two related manifestations of giftedness in cognitive functioning: high intelligence and high creativity. Recall that mental retardation is typically defined not only in terms of performance on an intelligence test but also in terms of adaptive behavior. In much the same way, intellectual giftedness cannot easily be identified solely on the basis of scores on measures of intelligence or creativity; motivational and personality factors that are associated with the full development of apparent potential must also be taken into account. For this reason, Hallahan and Kauffman (1978) suggest that "gifted" individuals be defined in terms of a combination of three criteria: high ability (often measured by intelligence tests), high creativity, and high task commitment (defined in terms of motivation and persistence). They suggest, further, that to be truly gifted, individuals must surpass 85 percent of their peers on all three measures and 98 percent on at least one. In this connection, the classic studies of giftedness by Terman et al. (1925) indicate that, in the same way as disadvantaged

children are often handicapped in more than one area, the gifted are also often exceptional in many respects.

It is perhaps unfortunate that so few national or international organizations promote the special education of the academically, intellectually, or creatively gifted and lobby for additional funding for these exceptional people. The one notable exception is the National Association for Gifted Children in the United States and the various TAG (talented and gifted) groups that do lobby for special programs for the intellectually gifted. Nevertheless, the gifted individual often remains imprisoned in regular classrooms for as long a period as average students and is exposed to the same academic fare. There is no doubt we feel a tremendous social responsibility toward those less fortunate than we: the deprived, handicapped, and otherwise disadvantaged. There is also little doubt that we do not sense the same responsibilities for those more fortunate. Indeed, we do not always tolerate them gladly (as we might fools); social ostracism and the ridicule of faintly disguised jealousy are too often our reactions to the gifted.

Lest this paint too cynical a picture of the current situation with respect to gifted children, note that there are sensitive parents, dedicated teachers, and conscientious administrators who do what they can. It is not easy, and it is not always enough.

■ Trends and Controversies in Special Education

Among the related trends in the implementation of special services for exceptional children are a number of controversies associated with these trends. Some of these are apparent in the preceding pages of this chapter and are summarized briefly here.

One notable trend in special education involves a gradual shifting of the responsibility for exceptional children from organizations and institutions established specifically to deliver special services to the public school systems. This trend is, in part, a reflection of a growing recognition that children

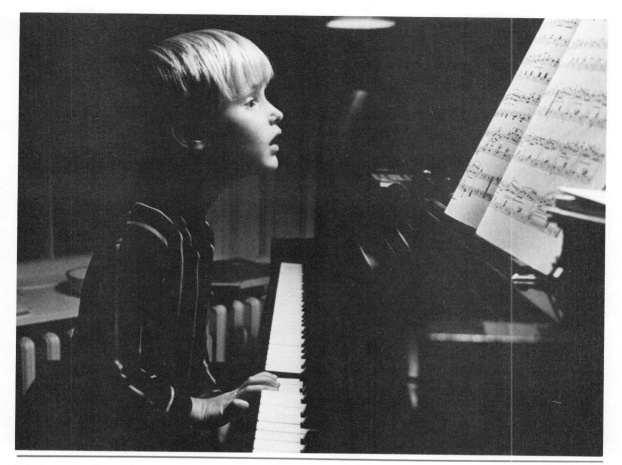

Giftedness usually involves more than exceptional ability or special talent. It requires creativity and, perhaps most important, a high degree of commitment and persistence.

who are exceptional in a disadvantaged sense should have an opportunity, whenever possible, to lead lives as nearly normal as possible. Deinstitutionalization and nonsegregation are the natural consequences of this trend, and perhaps nowhere is this more obvious than in the mainstreaming movement.

In effect, to mainstream is to place in regular classrooms those children who might otherwise be placed in special classrooms or even in institutions. Legislative action in a number of jurisdictions is largely responsible for the mainstreaming

movement. In California, for example, between 14,000 and 22,000 children previously classified as educable mentally retarded were moved into regular classrooms following the implementation of new legislation (Bancroft, 1976). Among other things, the effectiveness of special classrooms for mildly retarded children had been questioned by the results of studies (Dunn, 1968). A consensus seemed to be growing that mildly retarded children fared as well in regular classrooms, could perhaps avoid being labeled if they were mainstreamed, and could still be provided with special services in addition to their regular classroom experiences.

Other recent studies have not always confirmed earlier studies. Some children fare better academically in regular classrooms; some fare better in special classrooms with other retarded children. Some mildly retarded children develop more positive self-concepts in regular classrooms; others develop better self-concepts in segregated classrooms (see, for example, Budoff & Gottlieb, 1976). The controversy has not been entirely resolved.

A second controversy concerns the use of labels. Critics of the use of labels argue that they are unfair because (1) a disproportionate number of minority-group children are labeled (and perhaps mislabeled, given the biased nature of many tests), (2) the imposition of a label affects the child's self-concept, and (3) exceptional children are starting to be viewed as being quantitatively rather than qualitatively different from normal children. In spite of these objections, labeling has definitely not been abandoned, although there has been a concerted attempt to employ more euphemistic (less stigmatized) labels, to employ them more judiciously, and to avoid using labels as explanations. It has never been very helpful, for example, to label a child *autistic* and then to explain that the child is withdrawn and socially incompetent because of autism. Here, as elsewhere, labels name and classify; they do not explain.

■ MAIN POINTS

1 Intelligence has been defined in many different ways; there is relatively little agreement about any of these definitions. Perhaps it is nothing more than what the tests test.

2 What the tests test is represented as an IQ, an entity about which there are numerous misconceptions and considerable secrecy. Important decisions are often unwisely based on the results of single IQ tests.

3 Intelligence tests are individual (Stanford-Binet, for example) when they can be administered to only one child at a time and usually only by a trained examiner; group tests are administered to groups of children.

4 There is evidence that measured IQ is not constant from infancy through adulthood, but our measures become more stable with advancing age. This does not necessarily mean that intelligence itself is initially unstable, but it may mean that we commit fewer errors of measurement when testing older children. Besides, we do not know for certain what intelligence is or even that it *is*.

5 Creativity is often defined in terms of innovation or originality and may involve intellectual characteristics not ordinarily measured by intelligence tests.

6 A complete definition of creativity needs to take into account the characteristics of creative persons as well as qualities of creative products and processes.

7 Attempts to increase creativity often use Osborn's *brainstorming*, a group technique based on the principle of deferred evaluation and designed to encourage the production of wild and unusual ideas. Encouraging creativity among children would probably require encouraging the personality characteristics as well as the behaviors most closely related to creativity.

8 There are two types of exceptional individuals: those especially disadvantaged and those especially gifted. Most of our concern has been with the former.

9 Exceptional children are those who require special education and related services to realize their full human potential.

10 Physical and motor problems sometimes requiring special services include cerebral palsy, epilepsy, a variety of diseases, congenital physical problems, and physical problems resulting from accidents.

11 The majority of children who are classified as legally blind (corrected vision poorer than 20/200 in the better eye) can nevertheless see well enough to read large print, with or without magnification, and to function normally in society.

12 Hearing impairments often have far more social-emotional and academic problems associated with them than do visual impairments. This is largely related to the crucial role that hearing plays in the acquisition of language.

13 The two approaches to teaching language to the deaf are the manual approach (ASL or finger spelling) and the aural-oral approach (speech reading and verbalization). Sometimes the two are employed in combination.

14 The physically gifted may include professional tea tasters and perfume smellers, as well as outstanding athletes.

15 Causes of emotional disorders are sometimes described as predisposing or precipitating. In addition, distinctions are sometimes made between biogenic (genetic and biological) and psychogenic (psychodynamic) factors.

16 Knowledge of a child's biological and environmental history sometimes makes it possible to identify those who run a higher risk of emotional disturbance.

17 Autism and schizophrenia are two serious forms of emotional disorders in childhood, both of which require institutionalization.

18 Hyperactivity, sometimes termed hyperkinesis, is characterized by excessive activity without evidence of brain damage or neurological dysfunction. Hyperactive children frequently present behavior problems for parents and teachers and are sometimes treated with drugs.

19 Conduct and personality disorders are typically manifested in *misbehaviors* such as lying, stealing, delinquency, and aggression or social withdrawal and excessive shyness.

20 Those children who run a higher than average risk of emotional disorder yet survive and apparently thrive to become healthy, well-adjusted, bright children and adults are sometimes labeled "invulnerables" or "superkids."

21 Mental retardation is characterized by a general depression in the ability to learn and is defined in terms of subnormal performance on measures of intelligence and depression in adaptive behavior.

22 Mental retardation is currently classified in terms of the severity of retardation, regardless of cause: mild, moderate, severe, and profound. Educationally relevant labels, also corresponding to degree of retardation, are educable, trainable, and custodial.

23 Learning processes do not appear to be very different in mildly retarded and normal children. However, the attention span and short-term memories of the mildly retarded are inferior.

24 The term *learning disability* is currently employed to include a wide range of specific learning problems that are not associated with mental retardation or other physical or emotional disturbance. In other words, the label describes performance below expectation.

25 Intellectual giftedness is manifested in exceptional intelligence, exceptional creativity, and high motivation. Our consciences predispose us more easily toward helping the disadvantaged than the advantaged, in spite of our professed belief in the right of all children to be allowed to develop their "fullest human potential."

26 Recent trends in special education include deinstitutionalization, mainstreaming, and an antilabeling movement. Each is characterized by some controversy.

■ FURTHER READINGS

An excellent collection of articles on the measurement and development of intelligence is provided by:
Lewis, M. (Ed.). *Origins of intelligence: Infancy and early childhood*. New York: Plenum Press, 1976.

There are numerous outstanding sources of information regarding different methods of increasing or encouraging creativity. The books by de Bono are captivating accounts of some novel approaches to thinking and creative problem solving. Osborn's book is one of the classics in this area.
de Bono, E. *Lateral thinking: A textbook of creativity*. London: Ward Lock Educational, 1970.
de Bono, E. *Teaching thinking*. London: Temple Smith, 1976.
Osborn, A. *Applied imagination*. New York: Charles Scribner's, 1957.

The following are two excellent sources of general information concerning exceptionality and special education. The first is a particularly well-organized, clear, and comprehensive overview of the entire field. The second presents a collection of easily read chapters on exceptionality, each by a different author.
Hallahan, D. P., & Kauffman, J. M. *Exceptional children: Introduction to special education*. Englewood Cliffs, N.J.: Prentice-Hall, 1978.
Meyen, E. L. (Ed.). *Exceptional children and youth: An introduction*. Denver, Colo.: Love Publishing, 1978.

These three books should perhaps be required reading for teachers of exceptional children, particularly of the emotionally disturbed; all are moving and very well written:
Cottle, T. J. *Barred from school: Two million children*. Washington, D.C.: New Republic Book Co., 1976.
Hayden, T. L. *One child*. New York: G. P. Putnam's, 1980.
Rothman, E. P. *Troubled teachers*. New York: David McKay, 1977.

Among recent books dealing with learning disabilities and reading problems, Cruickshank, Morse, and Johns deal with a largely ignored area: learning disabilities beyond childhood. Johnson and Morasky provide a more comprehensive look at learning disabilities, together with numerous practical suggestions for remedial programs. O'Connor presents practical suggestions for teaching children with reading problems.

Cruickshank, W. M., Morse, W. C., & Johns, J. S. *Learning disabilities: The struggle from adolescence toward adulthood.* Syracuse, N.Y.: Syracuse University Press, 1980.

Johnson, S. W., & Morasky, R. L. *Learning disabilities* (2nd ed.). Boston: Allyn & Bacon, 1980.

O'Connor, K. *Removing roadblocks in reading: A guidebook for teaching perceptually handicapped children.* St. Petersburg, Fla.: Johnny Reads Inc., 1976.

The practical implementation of mainstreaming legislation and the controversies surrounding the movement are presented in:

Kreinberg, N., & Chow, S. H. L. (Eds.). *Configurations of change: The integration of mildly handicapped children into the regular classroom.* Sioux Falls, S.D.: Adapt Press, 1973.

O'Donnell, P. A., & Bradfield, R. H. *Mainstreaming: Controversy and consensus.* San Rafael, Calif.: Academic Therapy Publications, 1976.

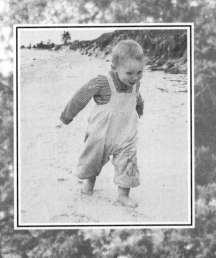

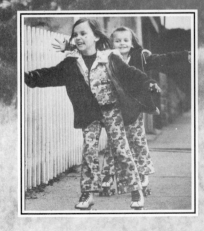

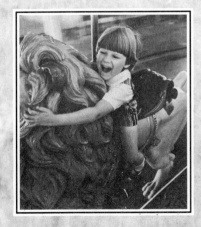

PART FOUR   ADOLESCENCE

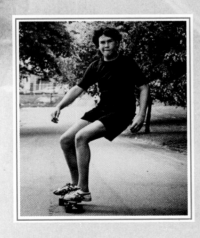

11

PHYSICAL, COGNITIVE, AND MORAL DEVELOPMENT

Gaudeamus igitur,
Juvenes dum sumus
Post jucundam juventutem,
Post molestam senectutem,
Nos habebit humus.
(Let us be happy while we are young, for after carefree youth and careworn age, the earth will hold us also.)

Anonymous student song

Near the Saskatchewan border, we stop for gas at a place called Cherry Grove. The name seems strange and inappropriate; the nearest grove of cherry trees is a huge distance from here. I mention this to the man who owns almost all of Cherry Grove.

"Lots of chokecherries, though," he chuckles.

There is very little in Cherry Grove: one service station-general store, one house, and what used to be a school. Its windows are all broken, grass grows through the cracks on the front step, and a rusted padlock holds the door. I stifle a twinge of nostalgia; all our windows will eventually break.

"Can I drive now dad?" Paul asks. His voice seems deeper, as though he has deliberately kept the pleading note out of it.

"I don't think so. We're in a bit of a hurry." I don't really want him to drive on this trip. I need to feel the wheel and the road—to know in my body as well as my mind that I am really going back.

"You never let me drive." The pleading note is clear now. I begin to tell him that I do let him drive. Rationally, I start to catalogue all the times that I remember him driving, beginning with a short trip to the store last night. But I see that he is upset and angry, and that my listing of his driving experiences will not change that.

"I'd rather you didn't drive today," I finish, lamely. I realize I have no strongly compelling reason to refuse.

"I thought you'd say that." He turns his back, pretending to study the sky. In the west, it has dropped low; it hangs just over the trees, blackish blue, threatening. I feel sad; I have no wish to hurt or upset him. It's just that sometimes he seems like he's an adult—almost a stranger—and other times, he's still a child. And I'm not always quite sure how to treat him.

"Okay. You drive before it starts to rain." He barely suppresses his excitement. For just a moment, he looks very much like a small child.

But in the driver's seat, his hands firm on the wheel, his entire concentration on controlling this large piece of equipment, he again looks a little like an adult stranger.

How do we know when our children have become adults? Is the transition irreversible? Are we, mature people, always adult?

Now, while I sit uncomfortably in the passenger seat, watching the poplars shoot past in streaks of white and green, I will tell you of the transition between childhood and adulthood.

■ The Passage

In Western culture the transition from childhood to adulthood requires passage through several years of adolescence, a period of life often described as the most troubled, the most stressful, and the most difficult of all stages of development. In numerous primitive societies, the passage from childhood to adulthood is marked by ritual and ceremony. These ceremonies are not always pleasant, but in most cases the result is the individual's certain knowledge that he or she is now an adult, with all the responsibilities and the privileges attendant upon being adult.

In contemporary Western culture there are no *rites de passage**. No one tells the child, "Today you are an adult, although yesterday you were a child. Yesterday you could play with children; today you must go to work, for you must now earn a living. You may also marry and behave as adults are permitted to behave. And you can vote, you can fight, you can be killed, you can have children, you can protest, you can become fat and lazy, and you can get drunk or otherwise dizzy. For today you are indeed an adult."

Because Western culture does not tell its children when they have become men and women, they must discover this for themselves. And the discovery is made particularly difficult because the culture training them is continuous—that is, there is no clear demarcation of passage from one state

to the other. The absence of such ritual is ironic when such events as birth and death are still observed by ceremony and ritual. These ceremonies are often every bit as elaborate and superstitious as the rituals of some primitive tribes. And for the individual who is most centrally involved in these ceremonies, they are quite meaningless (except perhaps for marriage). That is the irony of our ritualistic life.

Because our society is continuous rather than discontinuous, the passage from childhood to adulthood is much lengthier. In numerous treatments of this period, adolescence is divided into a series of stages. For example, Cole and Hall (1970) divide the period from eleven to twenty into three stages: preadolescence, early adolescence, and late adolescence. There is no easy way to determine the termination of adolescence, because there is no single criterion by which one may determine whether a person has achieved adult status; but its beginnings are somewhat more definite, although still variable.

■ Physical Development

Biologically, adolescence usually signifies the period from the onset of puberty to adulthood, though it occasionally designates the period beginning with pubescence and terminating with adulthood and sometimes simply indicates the span of the teen years (thirteen to nineteen). **Puberty** signifies sexual maturity; **pubescence** refers to the changes that result in sexual maturity. These changes occur in late childhood or early adolescence. Adulthood cannot easily be defined but may arbitrarily be considered to begin at the age of twenty. It would

---

*Exceptions include the Jewish ritual of Bar (Bat) Mitzvah, in which the Jewish boy (or girl) becomes an adult at the age of thirteen through a religious ceremony, and the "coming-out" party or debut in certain social groups.

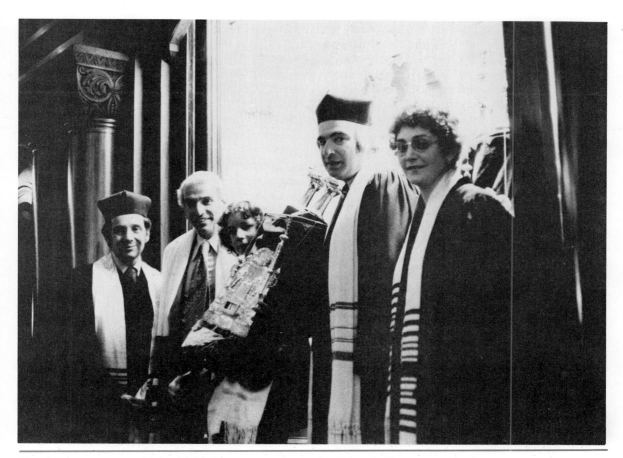

With a few exceptions, such as the Bar Mitzvah depicted here, children in Western societies receive no clear-cut indications of when they have become men or women.

be convenient for this text to say that adolescence begins at twelve, because we have included the earlier ages in preceding developmental periods. However, it is more accurate to say that the beginning of adolescence is variable and that age twelve simply serves as a general orientation.

Age of Puberty

Puberty defines sexual maturity—the ability to make babies—and is sometimes called *nubility* (Malmquist, 1978). As Jersild (1963) has observed,

prior to puberty individuals *are* children; afterward, they can *have* children. The problem in defining puberty in this manner is that it is almost impossible to determine exactly when a person becomes fertile. Past research has relied on information relating to the girl's first menstrual period (termed *menarche*) to discover the age at which puberty begins. Actually, however, a girl is frequently infertile for about a year after her first menstruation, so menarche is not an accurate index of puberty; nevertheless, it is a useful indication of impending sexual maturity. It is nearly impossible to arrive at a clear index for boys.

The generally accepted average age for sexual maturity is twelve for girls and fourteen for boys, immediately following the period of most rapid growth (the growth spurt). Consequently, the age of puberty may be established by determining the period during which the person grew most rapidly (Shuttleworth, 1939). The period of rapid growth may begin around the age of nine for girls, compared to eleven for boys. The actual range in age is wide, however—the start of sexual maturity for girls may range from as young as ten to as old as sixteen. Similarly, boys may reach puberty as young as twelve or as old as eighteen.

Research has revealed some interesting trends and differences in the age of menarche for different cultures and for different generations. Tanner (1955) reports that girls have been maturing earlier by as much as one-third or one-half a year per decade since 1850. In addition, adolescents are often taller and heavier than they were several generations ago. There is evidence that the trend toward earlier maturation is now slowing down (Frisch & Revelle, 1970).

Pubescence

Most signs of pubescence, the changes that lead to sexual maturity, are well known. Among the first signs in both boys and girls is the appearance of pigmented pubic hair, which is straight initially but becomes characteristically kinky during the later stages of pubescence. At about the same time as pubic hair begins to appear, the boy's testes begin to enlarge, as do the girl's breasts. The girl then experiences rapid physical growth, her first menstrual period, the growth of axillary (armpit) hair, the continued enlargement of her breasts, and a slight lowering of her voice. The boy does not experience anything comparable to the menarche. His voice changes much more dramatically; he too grows rapidly, particularly in height and length of limbs; he develops the capacity to ejaculate semen; he grows axillary hair, eventually develops a beard, and if blessed by the gods who determine (cultural) signs of masculinity, begins to grow a matting of hair on his chest.

Changes in Height, Weight, and Reach

The rapid changes in height and weight characteristic of pubescence have been described in Chapter 9. Table 11.1 shows average height and weight data for boys and girls from twelve to eighteen. By the age of eleven and one-half, girls often surpass boys in height and maintain a slight advantage until thirteen and one-half. Girls outweigh boys at approximately age eleven, but by fourteen and one-half, boys catch up to and surpass girls. An additional physical change, of particular significance to boys, is a rapid increase in the length of limbs. It is not uncommon for a boy to discover that his legs are suddenly several inches longer than they were a scant year ago and that he can reach an additional four or five inches. As a result of this growth, he acquires the gangling appearance so frequently associated with early adolescence, exaggerated by the fact that his rate of purchasing clothes is often considerably behind the rate at which he outgrows them.

Table 11.1 Height and weight at the fiftieth percentile for American children.

Age	Height (inches)		Weight (pounds)	
	Girl	Boy	Girl	Boy
12 years	59¾	59	87½	84½
12½ years	60¾	60	93¼	88¾
13 years	61¾	61	99	93
13½ years	62½	62½	103¾	100¼
14 years	62¾	64	108½	107½
14½ years	63	65	111	114
15 years	63½	66	113½	120
15½ years	63¾	66¾	115¼	125
16 years	64	67¾	117	129¾
16½ years	64	68	118	133
17 years	64	68½	119	136¼
17½ years	64	68½	119½	137½
18 years	64	68½	120	139

Adapted by the Health Department, Milwaukee, Wisconsin; based on data by H. C. Stuart and H. V. Meredith, prepared for use in Children's Medical Center, Boston. Used by permission of the Milwaukee Health Department.

Some Adolescent Concerns

Frazier and Lisonbee (1950) asked tenth-grade adolescents to indicate problems that concerned them and the degree to which they were worried about each. Items most frequently listed as the greatest worry for boys included the presence of blackheads or pimples, irregular teeth, oily skin, eyeglasses, and slight physical abnormalities such as noses that were too thin or too long, skin too dark, heavy lips, protruding chins, and so on. Girls, like boys, were most concerned about the presence of blackheads or pimples. In addition they were particularly concerned about freckles. Scars,

birthmarks, and moles were also a source of worry, in addition to the danger of being homely, having oily skin, and wearing glasses. Adolescents are very concerned with their rapidly changing physiques, to which they must learn to adjust.

The adolescent's physical appearance is of considerable importance to psychological adjustment as well, not only because of the part it plays in peer acceptance but also because of the way perception of the body affects self-concept. For example, it is obvious that a person who thinks she is a great orator is more likely to seek and to accept invitations to display her oratorical skills than is the individual who, because she stutters,

Physical appearance is of considerable importance to most adolescents and can greatly affect their psychological adjustment.

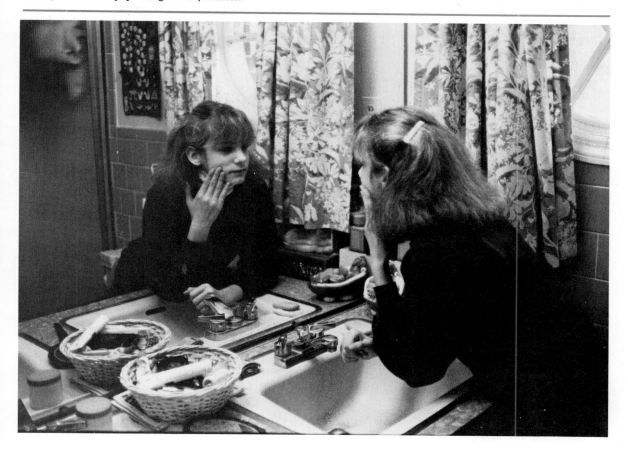

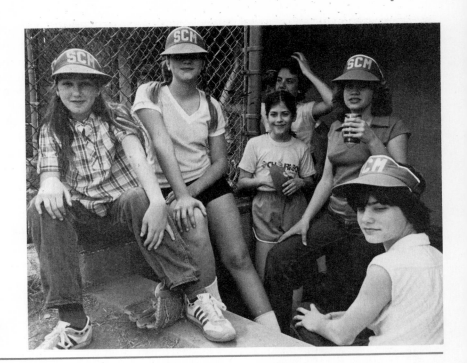

Although they are the same age, these adolescent girls will probably reach sexual maturity at different times, some as early as ten, others as late as sixteen.

believes that she is not gifted as an orator. Similarly, an adolescent who thinks he is attractive to the opposite sex because of his charm, his wit, and his irresistible good looks is more likely to expose himself to that sex than another who believes that he is decidedly unattractive. In this connection, it is not surprising that the preferred body type for adolescent males is athletic—neither obese nor thin (Lerner & Korn, 1972).

■ Early and Late Maturation

The average adolescent is no more real than the average child; both are abstractions, inventions designed to bring some semblance of order to our understanding of an incredibly complex subject. Hence, although the average adolescent matures at twelve or fourteen, depending on sex, some mature considerably earlier and some considerably later. Given that maturity tends to be judged

in terms of physical appearance, the age at which the physical changes of adolescence take place may be very important to the child.

In general, early maturing boys suffer fewer psychological problems than those who mature later, largely because they often excel in those activities and abilities that are highly prized in the adolescent peer culture. Not only are they larger and stronger, and therefore more likely to excel in athletic activities, but they are also more likely to serve as leaders in heterosexual activities. Detailed longitudinal studies of early and late maturation in boys (such as those by Jones, 1957, 1965) have usually provided clear and consistent findings. Early maturing boys are typically better adjusted, more popular, more confident, more aggressive, and more successful in heterosexual relationships. In addition, they appear to have clear advantages with respect to more positive self-concepts (about which more is said in the next chapter). In contrast, adolescent boys who mature later

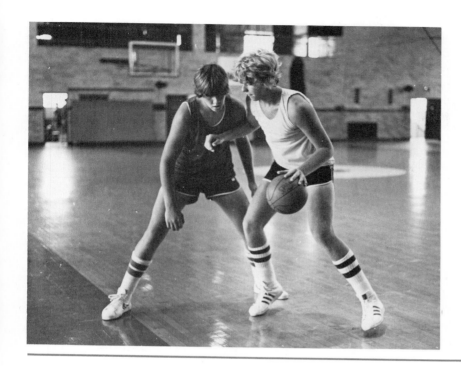

The long-term implications of early and late maturation are not nearly as clear as some of the immediate, short-term effects.

than average are, as a group, more restless and more attention seeking; they are also less confident and have less positive self-concepts.

Note that the apparent advantages of early maturation among boys are most evident *during* adolescence and that they apply primarily to social areas (adjustment, popularity, and leadership). In later life, the advantages of early maturation are not nearly so apparent (Clausen, 1975; Peskin, 1973).

Findings are less clear and less consistent with respect to girls. Jones (1949) reports that early maturing girls are at a disadvantage, a finding that directly contradicts the results of similar studies conducted with boys. In contrast, Douglas and Ross (1964) found that early maturing girls had some advantages over those who matured later. These contradictions may be partly explained by the possibility that the effects of early and late maturation in girls depend on their ages. Faust (1960), for example, reports that early maturation is a disadvantage in fifth or sixth grade, when most girls

have not yet begun to mature and when the early maturing girl is likely to find herself developmentally out of step with her peers and to be excluded from peer group activities. Because girls are also, on the average, two years in advance of boys with respect to physical maturation, the early maturing girl may well be four or more years in advance of like-aged boys, which would not contribute positively to her social life. However, starting around seventh or eighth grade, when most of her age-grade mates have also begun to mature, the early maturing girl may suddenly find herself in a more advantageous position. Her greater maturity is now something to be admired. The apparent contradiction may also be related to the years in which the studies were conducted. Being an early maturer may have been more of an advantage for a girl in 1960 than in 1949. In 1973, Peskin reported that early maturing might be slightly disadvantageous for girls to begin with, but that later in adulthood, early maturers were better

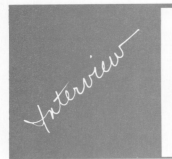
adjusted. It may be an even greater advantage now.

In summary, the effects of early and late maturation appear to be different for males and females and might also be importantly related to the adolescent's cohort (the current cultural and social conditions associated with being adolescent). (See *Anorexia Nervosa* for one type of maladjustment.) In addition, note that there are numerous individual exceptions to these effects. Not all early maturing boys will be characterized by the advantages of early maturation, nor will those who mature later all be equally affected.

■ Cognitive Development

We have traced the growth of the child's mind from birth to the beginning of adolescence, basing our account on the work of Jean Piaget and his associates. Let us briefly review the process. First were the fumbling attempts of infants to nourish themselves through the activation of their imperfect capacity to suck—the sucking scheme—followed by practicing and perfecting this and other schemes until the activities could be separated from the objects upon which they were performed and thought about. From these activities arose the ability to symbolize, and from this beginning there came speech and the dawning of a capacity to reason, at first fumbling and illogical—intuitive, ego-

centric, and qualified by perception. Children's thinking remained *preoperational* until their internalized actions (concepts) became influenced by rules of logic that allowed them to go beyond the sometimes misleading appearance of objects. At the age of seven or eight, with the appearance of reversibility, identity, compensation, and other rules of logic that could guide them in their interactions with the environment, children entered the period of concrete operations. And when we left Piagetian children at the close of Chapter 9, we left children who could classify, who understood seriation, who could deal with number, and who had consequently achieved a wide range of conservations. But children at the termination of the period of concrete operations are still some distance from late adolescence.

Consider the following problem that Inhelder and Piaget (1958) posed to a number of subjects of different ages. Five test tubes contain different unidentified chemicals; a combination of these chemicals will result in a yellow liquid. This phenomenon is demonstrated for subjects so that they know that one special tube, which is kept apart, is the catalyst for the desired reaction. What they do not know is which combination of the other four tubes is the correct one. They are asked to discover this for themselves and are allowed to experiment as necessary to solve the problem.

Typical ten-year-olds begin by combining two of the chemicals. Assuming that this combination

ANOREXIA NERVOSA

Karen Carpenter, a well-known singer, died at the age of thirty-two. Cause of death: heart failure due to a chemical imbalance that, in turn, was probably related to a medical condition for which she had been undergoing treatment. The medical condition: *anorexia nervosa*.

Translated literally, *anorexia nervosa* means loss of appetite as a result of nerves. It describes a complex and only partially understood condition that, although still relatively rare, appears to be increasing in frequency. It is far more common among females (more than 90 percent of all cases) than males and occurs most often during adolescence, although it can sometimes occur as young as nine or ten or even after the age of thirty (Bruch, 1973).

Anorexia nervosa is defined medically as involving a loss of at least 15 to 25 percent of "ideal" body weight, this loss not being due to any detectable illness (Yager, 1982). It almost always begins with a deliberate desire to be thin and consequent dieting and ends in a condition where the patient seems unwilling or unable to eat normally. Many affected females cease menstruating relatively early following initial dieting, and a significant number become excessively active and may continue to engage in strenuous exercise programs, even after their physical conditions have deteriorated significantly. Some become binge eaters, but typically follow their eating binges with prolonged fasts or, not infrequently, with voluntary vomiting or abuse of laxatives. Without medical intervention, anorexia nervosa is sometimes fatal.

The causes of anorexia nervosa are neither simple nor well understood. As Walsh (1982, p. 85) notes: "In anorexia nervosa, there are multiple psychological, behavioral, and physiological aberrations, suggesting that the central regulatory mechanisms which govern an individual's emotional and physical equilibrium are grossly disturbed." And although there is some evidence of endocrine imbalances in anorexia (Walsh, 1982), as well as some tentative indications that the disease may be genetically linked (Crisp, Hsu, Harding, & Hartshorn, 1980), the condition is acknowledged as being primarily psychological. Some speculate that anorexic individuals are typically those who do not feel that they are in control of their lives, but who discover that they *can* control their body weight; in the end, control becomes an obsession. Others suggest that a lack of positive self-image, coupled with the emphasis that society places on thinness (particularly among females), may be manifested in anorexia in those cases where the person attempts to obtain parental and social approval by dieting.

Anorexia nervosa is a particularly frightening and

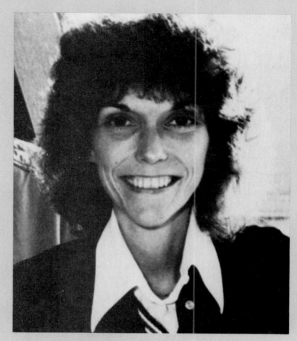

Karen Carpenter, who died of medical complications associated with anorexia nervosa.

baffling condition for parents. It is frightening because it can be fatal, and it is baffling and frustrating because it sometimes seems to parents that the anorexic adolescent *deliberately* and totally unreasonably refuses to eat. Neither pleas nor threats are likely to work. What is?

Since anorexia nervosa is not, in most instances, primarily a biological or organic disorder, its treatment is often complex and difficult. There are no drugs or simple surgical procedures that can easily cure it. In some instances, patients respond favorably to antidepressant drugs (Walsh, 1982), and it is sometimes necessary to force-feed anorexic individuals to save their lives. In the main, however, successful treatments have typically involved some form of psychotherapy. Among these, behavior therapy—the use of reinforcement or punishment in attempts to change behavior—has sometimes been dramatically effective (Davidson, 1976), as have approaches that treat the entire family as a *system* that affects each of its individual members (Minuchin, Rosman, & Baker, 1978).

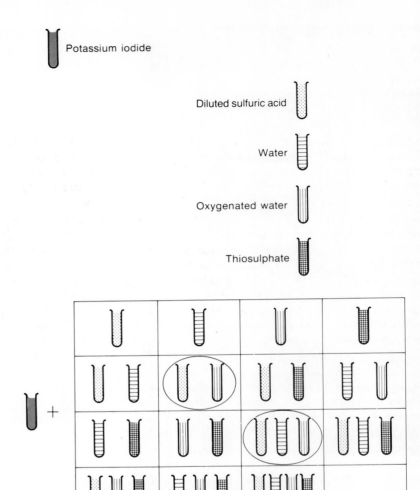

Figure 11.1
All possible combinations of the four test tubes to which the fifth can be added. The experiment requires the subject to discover the combination(s) that yields a yellow liquid when potassium iodide is added. The correct solutions are circled.

Potassium iodide

Diluted sulfuric acid

Water

Oxygenated water

Thiosulphate

does not provide any positive information, they might then combine another two chemicals, or perhaps they combine the first two test tubes with a third. They continue in this manner until, by chance, they arrive at a correct solution, whereupon they exclaim, "There, those two! That's the solution." If the experimenter then says, "Are there any other solutions—any other combinations that will also make a yellow liquid?" subjects will be forced to admit that they do not know yet but that they can try to find out. Their stategy changes little. They continue to combine pairs of liquids; they may even combine several groups of three, or perhaps all four, and to these they add liquid from the fifth tube. In the end they assert that they have tried them all and that there is but one solution. If they are less fortunate and less persistent, they may be incapable of discovering even one correct combination. Fourteen-year-olds behave in quite a different manner. Their solution, illustrated in Figure

11.1, involves systematically combining the tubes by twos, threes, and finally all four, thus yielding fifteen possible combinations. There is no doubt in their minds about whether or not they have found the only correct solution or whether there are others.

This experiment illustrates several of the principal differences between the child's thinking during the stage of concrete operations and thinking characterized by formal operations. First, ten-year-olds begin their solution by attempting actual combinations; their hypotheses are real behaviors. The fourteen-year-old, however, begins by imagining all the possibilities and then tries them. There is a fundamental difference in the orientations. The first reflects the concrete nature of the child's thought; the second reflects the hypothetical and deductive capacities of adolescent thinking.

Second, the experiment illustrates the *combinatorial* capacity of the adolescent's thinking. Because ten-year-olds consider every combination as a separate and unrelated hypothesis, and because they arrive at these combinations in a haphazard fashion, they are likely to overlook several possibilities in the process. In contrast, the adolescent first considers the range of possible combinations. The concrete logic that was sufficient to deal with classes and seriation is replaced by what Piaget terms the "logic of propositions." And this form of logic is a much more powerful tool than concrete logic for dealing with the hypothetical—with statements that need not relate to reality, but are simply characterized by the possibility that they can be true or untrue. (In fact, this is the definition of a proposition: a statement that can be true or false.)

Note that the changes in adolescent thinking implicit in the preceding discussion of Piaget's formal operations are potential changes but by no means always actual. Indeed, many individuals do not manifest formal thought between the ages of twelve and fifteen—or even later (Papalia, 1972; Rubin, Attewell, Tierney, & Tumolo, 1973). In the light of numerous recent studies that have not found formal operations among older adolescents and even adults, Piaget (1972) has conceded that this stage of thinking is not as general as was previously thought, and that social influences, partic-

ularly as they are manifested in different cultures, and individual interests and aptitudes are of considerable importance in the acquisition of formal operations (see Furth, 1980).

The consequences of the adolescent's newly acquired ability to deal with the hypothetical, to reason from the real to the possible or from the hypothetical to the actual, are reflected in a new, intense idealism. Children can suddenly contemplate states of affairs that do not exist; they can compare the ideal to the actual; and they can become profoundly disturbed at the failure of preceding generations to avoid the confusion that they observe around them. For some adolescents, this becomes a great source of frustration.

Adolescent idealism is further exhibited in some important changes in adolescent morality. It is not until children can reason about hypothetical states, becoming progressively concerned with the evils of the world and of the human condition, that they can begin to *internalize* rules of moral conduct. We look at the development of morality in childhood and adolescence later in this chapter.

■ Adolescent Egocentrism

As we noted earlier, in Piagetian theory, egocentrism is not a derogatory term, as it might be in ordinary usage. It refers less to a *selfishness* than to a cognitive and emotional *self-centeredness* and is apparent in children's inability to be completely objective in their understanding of the world and in their interactions with others. Recall, for example, that during sensorimotor development, egocentrism is evident in the infant's inability to differentiate between self and the physical world: Objects exist only when they are being looked at, tasted, felt, or smelled—a rather extreme egocentrism.

The egocentrism of the adolescent is perhaps not as extreme and certainly not nearly as naive as that of the infant. It involves an inability to differentiate between objects and events that are of concern to others and those of concern to the adolescent. This egocentrism is sometimes apparent in adolescent behaviors that seem to be motivated by the adolescent's self-consciousness or belief that everybody is watching and is terribly concerned.

Elkind (1967) clarifies the concept of adolescent egocentrism by reference to two separate notions that the adolescent creates as a result of this egocentrism. These notions, that of the **imaginary audience** and the **personal fable**, may be extremely useful in understanding some aspects of adolescent behavior and experience. Two additional notions, labeled *pseudostupidity* and *hypocrisy*, are also related to adolescent egocentrism, and they provide useful insights into what Elkind calls "troublesome" adolescent behaviors (Elkind, 1981).

LOCATING IMAGINARY AUDIENCES

Elkind (1967, 1981), Looft (1971), and a number of other psychologists, whose work is based largely on Piaget, suggest that one of the remarkable characteristics of adolescence is a kind of egocentrism to which we adults only infrequently fall prey. I fleetingly succumbed to it last night, when I accidentally dropped a tattered one-dollar bill while standing in line waiting to get into a hockey game. As I bent down to retrieve the dollar, I imagined that everybody there was looking at me, and I experienced a moment of acute self-consciousness. But when I straightened up and glanced surreptitiously around, I found nobody watching. Nobody really cared that I had dropped and retrieved a dollar. My audience was imaginary.

Theory has it that adolescent egocentrism also results in the creation of an imaginary audience—a belief "that others in our immediate vicinity are as concerned with our thoughts and behavior as we ourselves are" (Elkind & Bowen, 1979, p. 38). It leads, as well, to the elaboration of the *personal fable*—"the belief that we are special and unique, will not grow old or die, etc." (1979, p. 38).

How does research investigate beliefs such as these? How can psychology locate an imaginary audience? With an instrument—Elkind and Bowen (1979) have developed one—appropriately called the *Imaginary Audience Scale (IAS)*. It is based squarely on the assumption that individuals will be *self-conscious* to the extent that their behaviors are subject to examination by an imaginary audience. The scale attempts to measure two aspects of self-consciousness: those that are *abiding* or relatively permanent (labeled AS for *abiding self*) and those that are temporary or transient (labeled TS for *transient self*). One example of an *abiding* aspect of self is intelligence; a more transient characteristic is hair style or clothing.

Items for the IAS were selected from a pool of suggestions given by students who were asked to describe situations they might find embarrassing. The final scale consists of twelve items, the first four of which are reproduced here.

Elkind and Bowen administered the IAS to 697 students in grades four, six, eight, and twelve. Several findings from this study are especially noteworthy. First, young adolescents (eighth-grade students) were significantly more reluctant to reveal themselves to an audience than were younger children or older adolescents; this finding supports earlier beliefs concerning the imaginary audience and its relationship to the egocentrism of the adolescent. A second finding was that girls obtained higher scores than boys on the test. It seems that adolescent girls are perhaps more concerned with imaginary audiences than are adolescent boys, and that both are more responsive to these audiences than younger or older subjects.

Findings such as these have a number of practical implications, quite apart from what they might contribute to the elaboration of theory. In the first place, they might do a great deal to clarify the adolescent experience for us. And secondly, as Elkind (1981) suggests, they might contribute in important ways to our understanding of vandalism, teenage pregnancy, drug abuse, and other related behaviors. One of the important motives that might underlie these behaviors may relate directly to what the adolescent expects the reaction of the imaginary audience to be. Teachers, parents, counselors, and friends are all members of that audience. Mine is made up mainly of popes and presidents.

Imaginary Audience

The adolescent's *imaginary audience* is a collection of all who might be concerned with the adolescent's self and behavior, the *they* in expressions such as "they say . . ." or "they predict. . . ." Social psychologists inform us that each of us behaves as though "they" are watching and care. But the imaginary audiences of adults are much smaller, much less pervasive, and far less important than those of adolescents. (See *Locating Imaginary Audiences*.) Elkind suggests that this imaginary audience to which the adolescent is continually reacting explains why young adolescents are often very self-conscious. Because of this same audience, many become especially concerned with their hair, clothing, and

---

The Imaginary Audience Scale (IAS)

Instructions: Please read the following stories carefully and assume that the events actually happened to you. Place a check next to the answer that best describes what you would do or feel in the real situation.

TS scale
1. You have looked forward to the most exciting dress up party of the year. You arrive after an hour's drive from home. Just as the party is beginning, you notice a grease spot on your trousers or skirt. (There is no way to borrow clothes from anyone.) Would you stay or go home?
   _____ Go home.
   _____ Stay, even though I'd feel uncomfortable.
   _____ Stay, because the grease spot wouldn't bother me.

AS scale
2. Let's say some adult visitors came to your school and you were asked to tell them a little bit about yourself.
   _____ I would like that.
   _____ I would not like that.
   _____ I wouldn't care.

TS scale
3. It is Friday afternoon and you have just had your hair cut in preparation for the wedding of a relative that weekend. The barber or hairdresser did a terrible job and your hair looks awful. To make it worse, that night is the most important basketball game of the season and you really want to see it, but there is no way you can keep your head covered without people asking questions. Would you stay home or go to the game anyway?
   _____ Go to the game and not worry about my hair.
   _____ Go to the game and sit where people won't notice me very much.
   _____ Stay home.

AS scale
4. If you went to a party where you did not know most of the kids, would you wonder what they were thinking about you?
   _____ I wouldn't think about it.
   _____ I would wonder about that a lot.
   _____ I would wonder about that a little.

From D. Elkind and R. Bowen, Imaginary audience behavior in children and adolescents. *Developmental Psychology*, 1979, 15 (1), 38–44, p. 40. Copyright 1979 by the American Psychological Association. Reprinted by permission.

other aspects of their physical appearance. It is as though the adolescent believes that others are as deeply concerned about them as they themselves are and that these others constantly judge them.

Personal Fable

Adolescent egocentrism is reflected not only in the creation of an imaginary audience but also in the elaboration of fantasies, the hero of which is, not surprisingly, the adolescent. These fantasies, labeled *personal fables*, have a number of identifying themes, the most common of which are: "I am *special*," "Eagles and gods do not do untidy things upon me," "I will not get pregnant," "I will not become addicted to these drugs I take only for fun," "Mom, you just don't understand what real love is," "You don't either, dad!"

Elements of the personal fable run through the lives of most of us. We believe that we are somewhat different—just a little special. But these beliefs appear to be greatly exaggerated in adolescence and may account in part for the casualness with which adolescents will take risks that they know *cognitively* to be horrendous.

Pseudostupidity and Hypocrisy

Elkind (1981) suggests that some instances of apparent stupidity (pseudostupidity) and hypocrisy among adolescents are also manifestations of an adolescent egocentrism—an egocentrism that manifests itself not only in the creation of imaginary audiences and personal fables but that is apparent as well in what Piaget refers to as "naive idealism." This naive idealism often takes the form of an unrealistic belief in the power of ideas. It is well illustrated in the adolescent's frustrated and incredulous statement: "If they *know* that's what's going to happen, why don't they stop?"

The pseudostupidity of the adolescent is not limited to this unrealistic belief in the omnipotence of abstract ideas; it also reveals itself in the adolescent's occasional tendency to look at simple problems in inappropriately complex ways, as well

as to search for complex and perhaps devious motives for behaviors whose motives are very simple. In other words, *pseudostupidity* might result from an overreliance on the power of abstract thought, in the same way as *real* stupidity might result from an underreliance on thought processes.

Hypocrisy too might sometimes be related to adolescent egocentrism. A hypocrite's behavior contradicts expressed beliefs: One who speaks passionately in favor of nondiscriminatory hiring practices, but who refuses to hire left-handed Caucasians, is a hypocrite. In much the same way, adolescents who lament and ridicule the stupidities and excesses of their parents' generation while exercising their own right to be stupid and excessive are hypocritical; and those who disapprove of the materialistic commitments and values of their parents, but who ask for, expect, and use the resulting materials, are also hypocritical. As Elkind (1981) notes, the adolescent's hypocrisy stems from an egocentric confusion of ideals and pragmatics. It also reflects the egocentric notion that certain rules and beliefs need not apply to the "special" self of the adolescent's personal fable.

■ Moral Development

With the conviction that frequently accompanies intuition, most of us believe implicitly that people are good or bad in differing degrees, that goodness or evil is an intrinsic part of what we are—of our *selves*. Are we really *good* or *bad*? Or do we simply behave well some of the time and badly at other times? And if we are really good or bad, are we born that way, or do we become one or the other later? Furthermore, is being good in a moral sense the same thing as conforming to accepted social rules, or are the two separate?

Kohlberg (1964) discusses three aspects of morality: The first two are those to which we are most likely to respond when judging the relative "goodness" of people. The first is the behavioral aspect of morality, reflected in a person's ability to resist temptation; the second relates to the amount of guilt that accompanies failure to resist temptation; the third is the individual's estimate of the morality of a given act, based on a personal standard of good or evil. These dimensions of morality are not necessarily closely related. A person may repeatedly violate some accepted code of conduct—behave immorally, in other words—and yet feel a great deal of guilt. Another person may engage in exactly the same behavior and feel no guilt. Despite these differences, both may judge the act equally evil. Who has the stronger conscience?

What is a strong conscience? There are two classic approaches to answering this question. The psychoanalytic approach is based on the belief that the strength of the superego is the strength of conscience. It asserts explicitly that the stronger people's beliefs are about the immorality of an act, the less likely they are to engage in that act. Empirical evidence has not always supported this position. Several studies and reports (for example, Hendry, 1960) have indicated a low relationship between the strength of people's beliefs and actual behavior. Under some circumstances, it seems that the probability of behaving morally has more to do with anticipated reward and with the probability of getting caught than with conscience.

The second approach, a more religious one, is based on the belief that a good conscience is a manifestation of strength of character and good habits that have become engrained in the individual, usually through religious training. Kohlberg (1964) summarizes several studies that did not find a high relationship between religious training and actual behavior. Here, too, available evidence suggests that beliefs about right or wrong have less to do with children's behavior than the likelihood of their being caught or the gains to be derived from transgression. Other related factors are the individual's intelligence, ability to delay gratification (to choose long-range goals over short-range objectives), and self-esteem. Children who have favorable self-concepts apparently are less likely to engage in immoral behavior, presumably because they are more likely to feel guilty if they do. If this is correct, people who are involved with young children should find information about the importance of the children's self-concept useful in understanding and guiding their behavior.

Based on these findings, Kohlberg (1964)

argues that moral behavior is primarily a matter of strength of will (ego strength), rather than strength of conscience, superego, or character. In other words, morality is not a fixed behavioral trait, but rather a decision-making capacity. Furthermore, as Nucci and Turiel (1978) argue, morality is probably different from social convention. The learning of social conventions involves the learning of essentially arbitrary behaviors that are accepted or not accepted. Thus, in Western cultures, we learn conventions that have to do with eating. Specifically, we use knives and forks, we sit at tables, we eat from plates and bowls, and we try to refrain from belching and doing other things unmentionable in polite textbooks. Elsewhere, we might learn to eat with sticks while squatting on the ground, lapping food off rocks, and belching and making other fine noises with great gusto. Note that these behaviors are, in effect, highly arbitrary and that if different behaviors are substituted for them, we are not likely to be judged *evil*—foolish and disgusting, perhaps, but not truly evil. Morality, in contrast, is far less arbitrary. Specifically, it refers to behaviors and judgments relating to broad issues of human justice, such as the value of human life, the ethics of causing harm to others or to their property, and judgments concerning the place of trust and responsibility.

Morality, Rules, and Games

A close logical relationship exists between playing games that have rules and the development of **morality**. Indeed, Piaget's investigation of morality in children began with an examination of their progressive understanding of the rules of games, because *morality* may be defined as the internalization of rules. Whereas the regulations that govern game playing relate specifically to each game, the rules of morality govern life, and that too may be considered a game—not play, but a game nevertheless.

Children's understanding of the rules of games follows two frequently contradictory paths: (1) their verbalized belief about the nature of rules, their origins, and their permanence and (2) their understanding of rules as reflected in their actual behavior. Piaget (1932) reports that the actual play behavior of children reveals an initial stage, during which there is no adherence to rules (approximately until age three). This stage is followed by an intermediate period, during which children imitate rules but do not really understand them and consequently change them to conform to their interpretation of the game (ages three to five). By the time children are seven or eight years old, they have begun to play in a genuinely social manner, with rules that are mutually accepted by all players and that are rigidly adhered to. Not until the age of eleven or twelve is the true nature of rules understood—when children realize that rules exist to make games possible and that they can be altered by mutual agreement.

Parallel to children's demonstrated understanding of rules is their verbalization of this understanding. Piaget (1932) questioned a number of children about the origins of rules and about their characteristics. Their responses (or lack of responses) suggested the existence of three stages. The first lasts until the age of three and is characterized by no understanding of rules, which is reflected in their actual behavior as well. This initial stage is followed by a longer period, during which children believe that rules come from some external source (such as God), rules are timeless and immutable, and above all, children should not take it upon themselves to change them. This stage corresponds to the period in children's lives when their actual behavior in games is characterized by constantly changing rules. During the final stage of their actual behavior in games, they do not change rules, but gradually come to accept that rules are made by people and that they can be changed by the players if they so wish. Note the clear contradiction between their beliefs and their overt behavior, a contradiction that has been noted elsewhere as well. Hartshorne and May (1928–1930), for example, studied cheating in adolescents to discover the relationship between their understanding of moral rules and their behavior and arrived at the somewhat surprising conclusion that the probability of cheating is more affected by the likelihood of being caught than by any convictions about the relative evil of the act.

Piaget's observations concerning stages in the child's development of morality are derived partly from observing the manner in which children internalize rules of the games they play. In addition, he investigated children's notions of evil by telling them stories and asking them to make judgments about the goodness or evil of the characters. He employed a similar technique to investigate children's understandings of the nature of lies. For example, Piaget (1932) told a story of a child who accidentally breaks fifteen cups, asking the subject to compare this behavior to that of a child who deliberately breaks a single cup. From the children's responses to these stories, Piaget reached the general conclusion that there are two broad stages in the evolution of beliefs about guilt. In the first, lasting until about nine or ten years of age, the child judges guilt by the objective consequences of the act: The child who accidentally broke the larger number of cups is invariably considered more evil than the one who deliberately broke only one cup. After this stage, children's judgment becomes more adultlike—they are more likely to consider the motives behind an act.

As an aside, the moral judgment of adults frequently demonstrates the same characteristics as the child's earlier conception of guilt. My youngest son knew quite clearly, as I discovered on more than one occasion, that if he dropped a plate covered with great heaps of messy food face down on the floor, he was more likely to be reprimanded than if he dropped the same plate when it was empty, regardless of the fact that in both cases the act was apparently accidental. Adults frequently judge the transgressor's moral culpability by the absolute magnitude of the act; in contradiction, the person who commits a major felony is sometimes more admired than one who commits petty crimes. Witness the social hierarchy in a prison: Near the top of this structure is the embezzler who has stolen a million dollars; the petty thief is closer to the bottom rung.

Several other systematic investigations of the development of morality provide general support for Piaget's observations. Among these, the best known is probably that of Kohlberg, discussed in more detail shortly. Both Kohlberg and Piaget describe the evolution of morality as progressing from a simple, egocentric, highly unstable stage to a period of mutual cooperation and finally to a stage in which the legal aspects of rules come to be understood more clearly and are conformed to with religious devotion.

In addition to these investigations of the child's development of morality, there are numerous theoretical accounts of moral development. It is generally accepted that the rules of conscience that define morality are learned. It is not surprising, then, that learning models are sometimes used to explain the acquisition of these rules. For example, Bandura and Walters (1963) deal with the development of personality characteristics such as aggression and sex-appropriate behavior. Their explanation for moral development is based on the observed effects of imitation. Children are assumed to learn what is right and wrong not only through reinforcement or punishment for their behavior but also through observation of models presumably behaving in appropriate or inappropriate manners or through seeing models rewarded or punished for their behavior.

Kohlberg's Stages

Kohlberg (1969) has described three levels in the development of moral judgments, each consisting of two stages of moral orientation (shown in Table 11.2). The three levels are sequential, although succeeding levels never entirely replace preceding ones, making it almost impossible to assign ages to them. However, average children apparently progress from an initial *premoral* stage, in which they respond primarily to punishment or reward, through a rule-based, highly conventional morality, and finally to the stage of self-accepted principles (see Figure 11.2).

The progression of levels of moral development is interesting and informative. At the premoral level, the child's judgment of right and wrong

Table 11.2 Kohlberg's levels and types of morality.

Level I Premoral
Type 1 Punishment and obedience orientation
Type 2 Naive instrumental hedonism (behavior designed to obtain immediate pleasure and avoid pain)
Level II Morality of conventional role conformity
Type 3 Good-boy morality of maintaining good relations, approval of others
Type 4 Authority maintains morality
Level III Morality of self-accepted principles
Type 5 Morality of contract, of individual rights, and of democratically accepted law
Type 6 Morality of individual principles of conscience

takes one of two orientations. At this level, the child believes that evil behavior is that which is likely to be punished, and good behavior is based on obedience or the avoidance of the evil implicit in disobedience. Thus, the child does not evaluate right or wrong in terms of the objective consequences of the behavior or the intentions of the actor; judgment is based solely on the consequences to the child. Accordingly, the second moral orientation (Type 2) possible at this level is a hedonistic one, in which the child interprets good as that which is pleasant and evil as that which has undesirable consequences. At this level begins the reciprocity that characterizes morality at the second level, but it is a practical reciprocity. Children will go out of their way to do something good for someone if they themselves will gain by the deed.

The second level, a morality of conventional role conformity, reflects the increasing importance of peer and social relations to the developing child. Type 3, for example, is defined as morality designed to maintain good relations. Hence, moral behavior is behavior that receives wide approval from significant people—parents, teachers, peers, and society at large. Type 4, conformity to rules and laws, is also related to the child's desire to maintain a friendly status quo. Thus, conforming

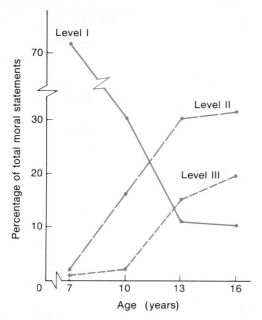

Figure 11.2
Mean percentage of moral statements of six moral types made by boys aged seven to sixteen. The chart illustrates the typical decrement from the first level of moral reasoning with advancing age and an increase to more advanced moral judgments. (From Lawrence Kohlberg, Development of moral character and ideology. In *Review of Child Development Research*, Vol. 1, edited by Martin L. Hoffman and Lois Wladis Hoffman. New York: Russell Sage Foundation, 1964, p. 403. Copyright 1964 by Russell Sage Foundation. Used by permission of Basic Books, Inc., Publishers.)

to law becomes important for maintaining adults' approval.

At the highest level, the child begins to view morality in terms of individual rights (Type 5) and as ideals and principles that have value as rules or laws, apart from their influence on approval. The person's individual notions of right and wrong (Type 6) begin to take precedence. (See *Moral Judgments*.)

Levels I and II are characteristic of older children: They are moral hedonists who conform to rules. Note as well that these two levels are also characteristic of most adolescents and adults. Although later childhood is still some distance from

the idealistic rejection of established order that adolescence makes possible, most adolescents and a great many adults continue to function at the lower levels of moral orientation.

Research and Kohlberg's Stages

It is unfortunate that people are seldom as simple as our theories. If they were, we would understand a great deal more than we actually do. Kohlberg's theories are a case in point. Some research suggests that moral development may not always be well reflected by Kohlberg's descriptions. Holstein (1976), for example, found that many subjects "skipped" stages, reverted to earlier levels of moral reasoning, or otherwise responded in ways that provided little evidence of stages. Kurtines and Greif (1974) have also subjected Kohlberg's findings to serious attack, noting, in particular, that with older subjects (even in Kohlberg's original samples) there are few distinguishable "advances" in moral orientation with the passage of time, with Type 4 judgments (authority-based morality) being predominant from late adolescence onward. In a study conducted by Fishkin, Keniston, and MacKinnon (1973), not a single subject out of a sample of seventy-five operated at the same stage for all five of the moral dilemmas presented to them.

In response to these criticisms, Kohlberg (1976) suggests that many of these inconsistencies and contradictions of his findings may be due to problems with the criteria employed for deciding at what stage subjects are operating. In addition, mounting evidence suggests that moral judgments are dependent not only on the age of subjects but also on a host of other variables, including the intentions of the transgressor and the damage that resulted in terms of social, material, or personal consequences (see, for example, Eisenberg-Berg, 1979; Suls & Kalle, 1979). In short, moral development is probably far more complex than our presentation of Kohlberg's stages would suggest. Nevertheless, this description has served as a basis for most of the research conducted in this area in the past several decades.

Implications of Research on Moral Development

Some of the most important implications of our current knowledge and beliefs about morality relate to the observation that individuals who operate at the lowest levels (hedonistic) are more likely to be delinquent than those who operate at higher levels (Fodor, 1972). Similarly, those who operate at the highest levels (self-accepted principles of conscience) are more likely to be politically or socially active (Haan, Smith, & Block, 1968). By the same token, altruism in children is highly related to the level of moral development. Specifically, children who are still at a hedonistic level (*good* things are those that lead to pleasant consequences) typically engage in less prosocial behavior (in this case, share less) than children at more advanced stages (Eisenberg-Berg, 1979). To the extent that these observations accurately describe reality, anything that schools, families, and other socializing influences can do to increase levels of moral orientation would apparently be beneficial.

What, precisely, can schools and parents do? Although suggestions must still remain relatively abstract, research deliberately designed to increase levels of moral judgment or behavior in adolescents indicates that this is possible. Kohlberg reports,

MORAL JUDGMENTS

Kohlberg identified levels of moral judgment in children by describing to them situations involving a moral dilemma. One example involves the story of a man whose wife is dying, but who might be saved if the husband steals a drug. Another concerns a doctor who is faced with a "mercy-killing" decision involving a terminally ill patient. Examples of responses corresponding to four stages of moral orientation are provided here:

Basis of Moral Worth of a Human Life*

Stage 1: Life's Value Based on Physical and Status Aspects—Tommy, Age ten: (Why should the druggist give the drug to the dying woman when her husband couldn't pay for it?) "If someone important is in a plane and is allergic to heights and the stewardess won't give him medicine because she's only got enough for one and she's got a sick one, a friend, in back, they'd probably put the stewardess in a lady's jail because she didn't help the important one." (Is it better to save the life of one important person or a lot of unimportant people?) "All the people that aren't important because one man just has one house, maybe a lot of furniture but a whole bunch of people have an awful lot of furniture and some of these poor people might have a lot of money and it doesn't look it."

Stage 2: Life's Value as Instrumental to Need-Satisfaction—Tommy at Age thirteen: (Should the doctor "mercy-kill" a fatally ill woman requesting death because of her pain?) "Maybe it would be good to put her out of her pain, she'd be better off that way. But the husband wouldn't want it, it's not like an animal. If a pet dies you can get along without it—it isn't something you really need. Well, you can get a new wife, but it's not really the same."

Stage 4: Life Sacred Because of a Social and Religious Order—John, Age sixteen: (Should the doctor "mercy-kill" the woman?) "The doctor wouldn't have the right to take a life, no human has the right. He can't create life, he shouldn't destroy it."

Stage 6: Life's Value as Expressing the Sacredness of the Individual—Steve, Age sixteen: (Should the husband steal the expensive drug to save his wife?) "By the law of society he was wrong but by the law of nature or of God the druggist was wrong and the husband was justified. Human life is above financial gain. Regardless of who was dying, if it was a total stranger, man has a duty to save him from dying."

*From "Development of moral character and ideology" by Lawrence Kohlberg, in *Review of Child Development Research*, Vol. 1, edited by Martin L. Hoffman and Lois Wladis Hoffman, New York: Russell Sage Foundation, 1964, p. 401. Copyright 1964 by Russell Sage Foundation. Used by permission of Basic Books, Inc., Publishers.

for example, that simply discussing moral dilemmas in the classroom typically leads to an increase in levels of moral judgment (advancing approximately one-third of a stage) (Kohlberg, 1978). And Arbuthnot (1975) reports an investigation in which older adolescents displayed higher levels of moral reasoning following role-playing situations involving specific moral dilemmas. In the Arbuthnot investigation, subjects played a role with a partner (opponent) who employed arguments at a level higher than that at which the subject had been assessed.

Modeling procedures have also been employed to increase morality (Hoffman, 1977). Religious training and other forms of indoctrination—teaching values directly by deciding what is right and wrong beforehand and presenting them as facts, rather than attempting to have children determine their own values—may be conducive to the development of higher levels of moral judgment and behavior (Sullivan & Quarter, 1972). Indeed, Kohlberg, who was initially opposed to indoctrination as a means of enhancing moral behavior, now suggests that it is necessary (1978, p. 84): "I no longer hold these negative views of indoctrinative moral education, and I now believe that the concepts guiding moral education must be partly indoctrinative. This is true by necessity in a world in which children engage in stealing, cheating, and aggression and in which one cannot wait until children reach the fifth stage in order to deal directly with their moral behavior."

Note that, in spite of what schools and educators might attempt to do, the values and behaviors of parents are highly instrumental in determining those of their children. Indeed, the values of adolescents typically resemble those of their parents rather than those of their peers (Reiss, 1966).

The recent upsurge of interest in morality is reflected in the schools, where a variety of "values clarification" and morality courses are being advocated and sometimes implemented. McPhail, Ungoed-Thomas, and Chapman (1972) have developed a teaching program for adolescents designed to foster empathy and caring. And an increasing number of researchers are arguing that the single most important attitude for fostering progression from lower to higher levels of morality is *caring* for others (for example, Peters, 1977; Sullivan, 1977).

More specifically, Hoffman (1976) suggests four different types of activity that might be conducive to the development of altruistic, caring behavior:

1 Situations in which children are allowed to experience unpleasantness rather than being overprotected

2 Role-taking experiences in which children are responsible for the care of others

3 Role-playing experiences in which children imagine themselves in the plight of others

4 Exposure to altruistic models.

In surprisingly logical fashion, we move then to altruism, cooperation, empathy, and related manifestations of prosocial attitudes and behaviors.

■ Prosocial Behavior

Closely related to investigations of morality are the various studies attempting to investigate cooperation, sharing, and other forms of altruistic behavior, as well as less altruistic forms of behavior: aggression, rivalry, and competition. Some of this research was clearly stimulated by a rash of newspaper reports in the early 1960s, describing various brutal murders, rapes, and other violent crimes where bystanders observed but carefully and deliberately did not intervene. One such report describes the murder of a young woman, later reported in the *New York Times* (Darley & Latané, 1968). Thirty-eight different individuals watched this murder that took a full half-hour to complete. Yet not a single one offered assistance or even phoned the police. Subsequent investigations of "altruism" revealed that a shocking majority of people are unwilling to become involved, even when clearly capable of coming to the rescue of people in serious trouble, particularly when they are only one of a number of others who could also intervene.

Several important questions suggest themselves for developmental psychologists: How is the tendency to help, to cooperate, or to share acquired? Can it be increased? Do sex, culture, or other factors account for prosocial behavior? Although no definite answers can yet be provided for most of these questions, research does offer some tentative conclusions.

It appears that prosocial behavior can be fostered through the use of models, as we saw in our discussion of the role of television (Chapter 9). For example, Paulson (1974) investigated the extent to which "Sesame Street" episodes designed to foster cooperative behavior had their intended effects. Thirty-six children who had watched all programs in the series were compared with forty-two children who had not been exposed to the programs. He found significantly more cooperative behavior among the first group, although this difference did not appear to transfer to testing situations that did not closely approximate the television content. Numerous other investigators (for example, Elliot & Vasta, 1970) have also found that cooperative behavior and sharing can be increased through modeling and reinforcement.

The literature with respect to sex differences does not lead to any clear conclusions (Cook & Stingle, 1974). Kagan and Madsen (1972) failed to find any sex differences in investigations of cooperative behavior; in contrast, McKee and Leader (1955) report that nursery school boys are more competitive (and less cooperative) than girls. Berndt (1981) found much the same thing with school-age children; here, too, girls are more likely than boys to cooperate with a "best" friend. Investigations of the relationship between age and cooperation have often reported that three- and four-year-old children do not cooperate in their play behavior, whereas six- and seven-year-old children show complete cooperation. This parallels Piaget's observation that very young children do not engage in social play and do not understand the nature of rules. Playing a game with mutually accepted rules does, in fact, require cooperation. Note, however, that although young children might not be sufficiently advanced *cognitively* to cooperate, they are nevertheless capable of altruistic behaviors at strikingly young ages. Yarrow and Zahn-Waxler (1977; Yarrow, Scott, & Zahn-Waxler, 1973) report that even before the age of two, some infants display highly altruistic behaviors. For example, a typical *altruistic* response to a picture of a sad-looking little girl surrounded by others who are all eating ice cream is "I would give her a lick." This research indicates that young children are *not* too egocentric to empathize with others and to offer assistance when they can. It indicates, as well, that there are marked individual differences in the altruism of different children, and there do not appear to be any significant increases (or decreases) in altruism between the ages of two and seven.

Investigations of *rivalry*—defined as competitiveness where an individual is willing to take a loss in order to ensure that the competitor will also take a loss—have shown that with increasing age there is a corresponding increase in rivalrous behavior (Kagan & Madsen, 1972). Both cooperative and competitive behavior appear to increase with age.

Cultural differences in prosocial behavior have also been documented. Research with Israeli children (typically kibbutz children) has repeatedly shown these children to be more cooperative than American whites (Shapira & Madsen, 1974). It has also been found that lower-class and rural children are less competitive than middle-class or urban children (Cook & Stingle, 1974). There is little doubt that various forms of prosocial and antisocial behavior are culturally influenced.

Role Taking and Empathy

Altruism and other forms of prosocial behavior imply caring and concern for the plights of others. They imply, as well, that those who care must be able to adopt the point of view of others. If not, they would not be able to care.

Research on role taking is relatively recent but plentiful. A great deal of this research has been concerned with perceptual problems, such as those described by Piaget, and has been designed to investigate the egocentricity that apparently characterizes the preoperational child. Recall, for example, the early inability of children to describe what a mountain would look like to a person viewing the mountain from a perspective different from that of the child.

Investigations of cognitive role taking have focused on the extent to which children are able to infer that other people may think differently than they do. Shantz (1975) summarizes this research in terms of four sequential stages that appear to characterize the development of cognitive role-taking skills. At the earliest stage, the child is unaware that another person is capable of having independent thoughts (or awareness). This realization seems to become general by the age of six and defines the second stage. During the third stage (around age eight), children realize that their own behavior may lead to inferences by others. The fourth stage, the ability to infer relatively accurately what other people are thinking, develops around the age of ten.

Obviously, a close relationship exists between emotional and cognitive role taking. Clearly, a child would be highly unlikely to make inferences concerning another's feelings prior to the realization that others are capable of independent and private thoughts. Studies of *empathy* (the ability to recognize and share the feelings of others) frequently ask children to recognize the emotion that would accurately reflect the reaction of a person in a story. One of the important and difficult problems with this type of research is that it is usually impossible to determine to what extent the child is accurately inferring emotional reaction and to what extent the emotion described is simply a projection of how the child would react in a similar situation.

Hoffman (1975) suggests that the ability to empathize follows a developmental progression paralleling the development of cognitive role-taking skills. Accordingly, it is not until later childhood that the child will empathize to the extent that the inferences made about the emotional reactions of others will be related to *their* experiences and not those of the child. However, Hoffman believes that very young children are capable of *empathy* before they can clearly separate themselves from others, a belief that would seem to be borne out by the Yarrow research on empathy in infants (see Mussen & Eisenberg-Berg, 1977; Pines, 1979). That is, an infant can empathize with another who has been hurt and might even cry as a result.

And it is precisely the development of empathy—of caring—that is fundamental to the development of altruistic behavior.

■ Antisocial Behavior

But we are not all altruistic; and even those of us who might claim an occasional selfless, self-sacrificing act might also have to admit to some degree of apathy. Indeed, there are those who are neither altruistic, nor even apathetic, but aggressive.

Aggression has a bewildering array of definitions. In general, however, it relates to behavior that is intrusive, assertive, and domineering. In its more extreme forms, it also involves physical damage to people or objects and is more properly referred to as violence.

Even as there are a number of definitions for aggression, so too are there a number of explanations. One of the oldest in psychological literature describes aggression as the inevitable consequence of frustration, where frustration is defined as the effect of being prevented from reaching a goal (Dollard, Doob, Miller, Mowrer, & Sears, 1939), or if it is not the *inevitable* consequence of frustration, it is likely to occur if the situation is appropriate (Berkowitz, 1965).

A second explanation, biological in origin, draws parallels between aggression in humans and in other animals. These explanations attribute aggressiveness to biological predispositions and maintain that, in certain circumstances (threat to one's children or one's person), aggression is the "natural" response.

A third explanation, described in some detail in Chapter 9, attributes aggression and other forms of social behavior to the influence of models. This social learning explanation has derived considerable support from studies of the effects of television on both aggressive and altruistic behavior in children.

A final explanation invokes physiology and attributes aggressiveness to such factors as hormones or the activity of specific brain structures. There is evidence, for example, that injections of testosterone increase aggressiveness in monkeys and that damage to certain areas of the brain's hypothalamus can increase or even trigger aggressive behavior.

Our present knowledge suggests that these explanations are complementary. Although we might well have some biological predispositions toward aggression in certain situations, and although some of our aggressive behaviors might be related to physiological factors, the *manifestation* of aggression is to a considerable extent under the control of environmental experiences such as frustration or modeling. There is considerable agreement that aggression is more characteristic of males than females. This can be attributed not only to our cultural biases and stereotypes but perhaps to physiological factors as well. In addition, models, the most highly researched of which are television

programs, are often implicated in manifestations of aggression.

It is important to understand that aggression, as a predominant way of behaving, is essentially antithetical to such forms of prosocial behavior as helping, sharing, and cooperating. And to the extent that care and concern for others (empathy) facilitates prosocial behavior, so too might its absence encourage aggressiveness. In this connection, it is highly encouraging to note that research emphases have shifted from investigations of aggression to a concern with prosocial behavior. Comstock and Lindsey (1975) conclude an extensive review of television-related research with the optimistic observation that the first priority for researchers in the area is prosocial behavior. Perhaps the fruits of theory and research will benefit generations to come in ways that we cannot yet imagine.

■ MAIN POINTS

1 Societies with clearly recognized boundaries between childhood and adulthood are termed discontinuous; those without boundaries are continuous. The continuity makes it difficult for some adolescents to determine when they cease to be children and become adults.

2 Puberty is sexual maturity. It results from pubescence—the period of change that includes the boy's ability to ejaculate semen and the girl's menarche, among other changes for both sexes.

3 The advantage that girls have over boys in height and weight during early adolescence is permanently lost before the age of fifteen.

4 Early maturation appears to be initially advantageous for boys but may be less so for girls; these early advantages (or disadvantages) are often lost or reversed in later life.

5 The intellectual development of the adolescent may culminate in thought that is potentially completely logical, that is inferential, that deals with the hypothetical as well as with the concrete, that is systematic, and that results in the potential for being idealistic. Then again, it may not.

6 Among other things, formal operations make possible a type of intense idealism that may be reflected in adolescent frustration or rebellion, as well as in more advanced levels of moral orientation.

7 Adolescent egocentrism describes a self-centeredness that often leads adolescents to believe that all others in the immediate vicinity are highly concerned with their thoughts and behaviors.

8 Egocentrism in adolescence may be manifested in the creation of the imaginary audience (an imagined collection of people assumed to be highly concerned about the adolescent's immediate behavior) and the personal fable (a type of fantasy whose themes stress the individual's invulnerability and uniqueness).

9 Piaget draws a parallel between the development of understanding rules governing games and moral development. Both proceed from an initial stage, where there is no understanding of rules, to a final stage, where rules are understood as being arbitrary, socially useful, and changeable.

10 Kohlberg describes the development of morality in terms of sequential progression through six stages, beginning with a preconventional, hedonistic orientation and culminating in a morality characterized by individually determined rules and principles.

11 Evidence suggests that progression through these six stages may not be sequential and that relatively few individuals ever reach the highest level.

12 Empathy and concern appear to be closely related to the development of higher levels of morality. They are also centrally involved in the development of attitudes that motivate prosocial behaviors such as helping and cooperating.

13 Role taking is involved in the development of empathy to the extent that it is difficult to care without also being able to adopt the emotional point of view of others.

14 Aggression has been explained by references to the effects of frustration and examples of models and to biological (ethological) and physiological observations.

15 Aggression and prosocial behavior are essentially antithetical.

■ FURTHER READINGS

An excellent account of contemporary adolescence, viewed against the backdrop of historical changes in adolescence, is provided by:
Kett, J. F. *Rites of passage: Adolescence in America, 1790 to the present.* New York: Basic Books, 1977.

The significance of biological changes in adolescence, and the nature of these changes, is well presented by:
Katchadourian, H. *The biology of adolescence.* New York: W. H. Freeman, 1977.

Insights into the differences between thinking in adolescents and children are found in the following book by Ault and in Piaget's short article:
Ault, R. L. *Children's cognitive development.* New York: Oxford University Press, 1977.
Piaget, J. Intellectual development from adolescence to adulthood. *Human Development,* 1972, *15*, 1–12.

Kohlberg has extensively investigated moral development, an area of considerable current interest. The following are two sources of information about these investigations:

Kohlberg, L. Development of moral character and moral ideology. In M. L. Hoffman & L. W. Hoffman (Eds.), *Review of child development research* (Vol. 1). New York: Russell Sage Foundation, 1964.

Kohlberg, L., & Turiel, E. *Research in moral development: A cognitive developmental approach.* New York: Holt, Rinehart & Winston, 1971.

An excellent recent examination of aggression, both in humans and in non-human animals, is contained in:

Moyer, K. E. *The psychobiology of aggression.* New York: Harper & Row, 1976.

A highly readable, short book that looks at prosocial behavior with emphasis on its causes is:

Mussen, P., & Eisenberg-Berg, N. *Roots of caring, sharing, and helping: The development of prosocial behavior in children.* New York: W. H. Freeman, 1977.

12

SOCIAL DEVELOPMENT

It's all that the young can do for the old, to shock them
and keep them up to date.

George Bernard Shaw
Fanny's First Play

Si jeunesse savoit; si vieillesse pouvoit.
(If youth had the knowledge; and if old age had the strength.)

Henri Estienne
Les Premices

Paul looks scared. I've been watching him since it started to rain. At first, when the drops where gentle, the sudden cool welcome, and the thunder distant like old memories, he smiled. But now the wind lashes great swirling gales of water across the pavement, thunder cracks sharply among blinding streaks and flashes of light, and the highway is a murky vision through the windshield.

"Pull way over on the shoulder. Up there where it looks wider." He obeys gladly.

Even with the car stopped and the motor shut off, the noise seems somehow louder, the gusting wind more fierce. Marcel has climbed onto my lap. He is completely absorbed, fascinated. And perhaps a little timid; I can scarcely remember the last time he sat on my knee.

"Nice storm," says Grandma. I know she loves it in the same way that she loves rainbows, winter, dragonflies mating, and countless other things. She smiles as she sits there, half covered in green knitting.

"Not so nice now," I answer. I see the first of the hailstones, tiny to begin with, pinging almost daintily on the car's surface, but rapidly growing until, large as the marbles Marcel calls "boulders," they pound a continuous, deafening, pulsing roar. I feel Marcel shiver, but it's not the cold. Perhaps we all shiver as we sit silent through this awesome display of forces almost beyond our imaginations.

Then it's over. As quickly as it started, the storm has passed, leaving a rapidly melting, sodden layer of hail in its wake.

"Well, freak me green!" Denise says, not for the first time.

"I'll drive, now. It might be slippery."

"I can handle it." I sense the hurt. He trusts himself and sees no reason why I shouldn't, and I am lost momentarily in the old conflict—a conflict more with myself than with him. It seems that I am always trying to protect my children from their own immaturity—that that is really what bringing up children is all about. But there needs to be a point where we recognize maturity, where we need to protect less.

"As soon as the hail is melted," I decide. "I've had some bad experiences on hail."

"Oh yeah?" The hurt has completely vanished. We change seats, and I, accustomed to center stage among my family, begin to tell them fascinating tales of horrendous happenings on icy roads in magical days before their short spans had even begun. But they interrupt repeatedly with their own small tales, and I realize again that my two adolescents have more than begun to grow up—that sometimes I scarcely know them. And I promise myself that I will spend more time with them before it's too late. Again that vague uneasiness—that old fear. Will it be too late, now that I'm going back?

I am not ready to think about that yet. We have other places to go, you and I, as we journey through the lifespan. Quickly, now, while we slosh our way gingerly toward Meadow Lake, we return to adolescence, specifically to the social and emotional developments of that period.

■ Social Development

Adolescence is marked by an increased emphasis on social skills. During this time, conversational talents that were previously more important for girls than for boys become important for both. Also during this period, relationships between males and females, as well as those between persons of the same sex, begin to assume a profound significance. Throughout adolescence, the influence of parents and family declines, and peer relations increase in importance.

For normal children, adolescence is a period of intense sociability. They awaken in the morning anxious to go to school primarily to see their friends and to practice their newly discovered roles as young men and women. And there is often some awkwardness and confusion about these roles. For these young people have not been initiated. No one has taken them to the ritual hut in the eerie light of some primitive, predawn morning; no one has sung the Songs of the People for them; nor have their uncles assisted with their Coming of Age. They must discover for themselves that they are adults, and they must also discover what it means to be adult.

Three Stages of Socialization

Although a gross oversimplification, the socialization of the adolescent may be described by three general stages, based on the changing roles of friends and parents. Early in adolescence, parents continue to be of considerable importance, socially, emotionally, and physically. Young adolescents are dependent on the family in a literal sense, not only for physical comforts but also for the psychological support they provide. It is clear, however, that the extent of this dependency is not nearly so great as it was in earlier periods of development.

Shortly after the onset of adolescence, children begin to move toward independence, and it is this progress that defines the second stage in adolescent socialization—a period of conflict both for the parents and for the children. Children find themselves torn between two forces: On the one hand, there is former allegiance to their parents, their continued love for them, and their economic dependence on them; on the other hand, there is a need to be independent and to be accepted by peers. Conflict between adolescents and their parents stems not only from their desire to associate more frequently and more closely with peer groups but also from a variety of other sources. Adolescents often list such causes of strife as parental interference with social life, lack of adequate financial assistance, parental intrusion about schoolwork or criticism of grades, the parents' failure to give information about sex, and their criticism of friends (Lloyd, 1954).

From a stage of high dependence on parents, the adolescent progresses through the intermediate stage of conflict just described and finally achieves the third stage—relative independence from parents. Independence does not imply that

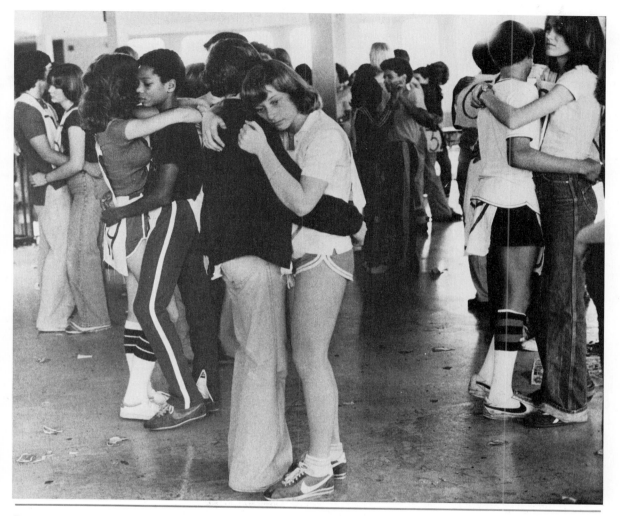

Dancing is only one of the many social skills that become important during adolescence. The drooping postures and expressions here are not characteristic of a new dance fad; this is around the twelfth hour of a twenty-one hour high school dance marathon.

children break all bonds with their family and tie themselves irrevocably to groups of peers but simply that they have achieved an independence allowing them to function in the milieu of peers that has become so important—an independence that frequently implies parental conflict. The generation gap is a cliché recognizing the significance (and indeed the existence) of the conflict between the reigning generation (the "establishment") and

the contemporary crop of adolescents from high schools to colleges, unemployed, employed, in love, out of love, or otherwise dead or alive. This gap is examined in more detail in a later section of this chapter.

The preceding discussion should not be interpreted to mean that parents and teenagers are typically in conflict but simply as information regarding prevalent sources of conflict. In an ambitious examination of parent-child relationships involving 1,278 high school boys, Meissner (1965) found that changes in parent-child interaction included both positive and negative aspects. Subjects felt that as they became older they were given more opportunity for socializing; consequently, they became more tolerant of parental authority and more grateful for parental guidance. At the same time, however, a number of adolescents reported increased unhappiness in the home, greater misunderstandings between parents and children, and increasing conflicts with parents over religion. Boys reported spending less leisure time at home than previously. Meissner concludes that although the pattern is clearly one of "gradual **alienation**" from parental control and a concomitant increase in rebelliousness, the data do not wholly justify rebellion as a general feature of adolescent-parent interaction.

The Nature and Importance of Peer Groups

Adolescent peer groups vary in size, interests, social backgrounds, and structure. They might consist of two or three like-sexed persons (buddies, pals, best friends), larger groups also consisting of like-sexed individuals, and a third group consisting of couples, usually of opposite sexes, who currently find themselves in the throes of romantic love. Yet another type of peer group contains persons of both sexes who "hang out" together. Most adoles-

cents belong to several groups at the same time. Membership in a closely knit peer group is not necessarily a mark of adolescent normality, for it is neither normal nor abnormal to behave as do the majority of people. However, an adolescent who is unable to establish the social relationships required for membership in peer groups, and who is rejected by peers, may be adversely affected. Effective adaptation in our culture requires a relatively high degree of social skill, as well as the ability to form and maintain personal relationships, thereby establishing the importance of the peer group. The person who, by choice or by circumstance, is isolated from peers is denied an important opportunity to develop the ability to interact socially.

Figure 12.1 illustrates the development of groups in adolescence as they progress from small groups of like-sexed members to interaction between groups of different sexes, leading eventually to the formation of what Dunphy (1963) calls the "crowd"—a large heterosexual group that has evolved from the smaller single-sex groups. In later stages of adolescence, the earlier cohesiveness of the groups gradually disintegrates because of the pairing of boys and girls into couples.

One of Dunphy's important observations was that adolescent peer groups tended to consist of individuals of relatively similar ages. Hartup (1978) suggests that age segregation is pervasive throughout development—that is, when children have a choice, they are most likely to select friends similar

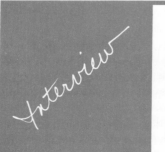

Interview

Subject: Female; age fourteen; ninth grade.
(concerning friends)

I have quite a lot of good friends. Lana is probably my best friend. And Sherri. The three of us always sit together in school and we go roller-skating. Jackie used to be with us too, but now she's going around with Phil. He's a hunk!

I have lots of other friends at band and at school, too. I think that's one of the most important things in life, is your friends. I would always be willing to do whatever I can for my friends and I'm sure they would for me, too. That's what being friends is about.

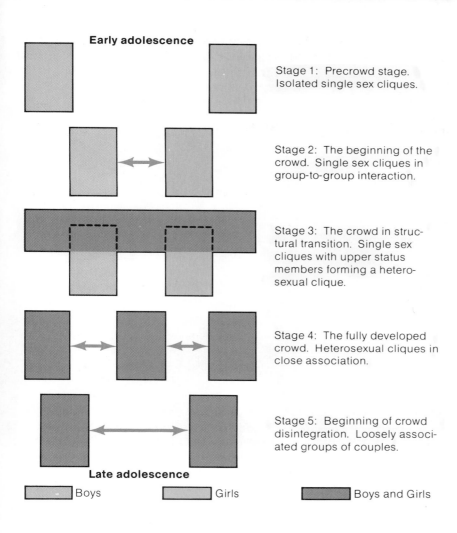

Early adolescence

Stage 1: Precrowd stage. Isolated single sex cliques.

Stage 2: The beginning of the crowd. Single sex cliques in group-to-group interaction.

Stage 3: The crowd in structural transition. Single sex cliques with upper status members forming a heterosexual clique.

Stage 4: The fully developed crowd. Heterosexual cliques in close association.

Stage 5: Beginning of crowd disintegration. Loosely associated groups of couples.

Late adolescence

Boys   Girls   Boys and Girls

Figure 12.1
Stages in peer group development during adolescence. (After Dexter C. Dunphy, The social structure of urban adolescent peer groups. *Sociometry*, 1963, *26*, 230–246, p. 236. Copyright 1963 by the American Sociological Association. Used by permission of the American Sociological Association and the author.)

to them in age (as well as ability and interests, both related to age). He suggests as well that age segregation is not necessarily good, a point also argued by Bronfenbrenner (1970) and others. These researchers maintain that it is extremely important for children to have significant contact with a variety of age ranges. They suggest, for example, that contact with young children might help prepare adolescents for parenthood; by the same token, contact with older people is important for the socialization of children and adolescents.

The extent to which adolescent groups are segregated by age has been investigated by Montemayor and Van Komen (1980). They observed a total of 513 subjects, of whom 403 were adolescents. Observations occurred in natural settings (parks, shopping centers, schools, playgrounds, and so on) and simply involved approaching groups of people containing adolescents and determining the relationships of the people in the group (for example, parents, friends, relatives). These researchers found considerable evidence of age segregation,

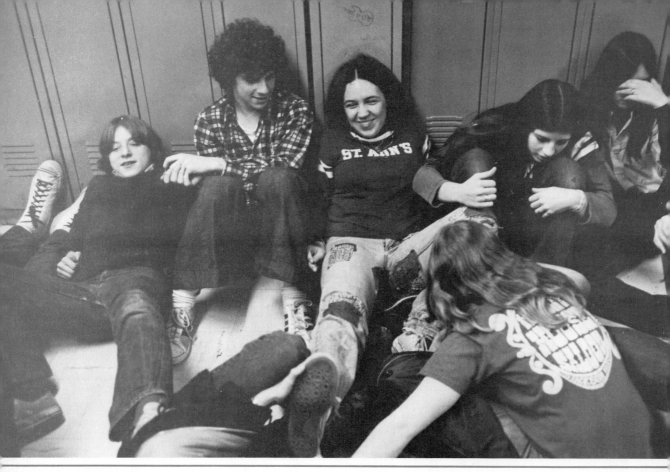

Adolescent groups tend to be highly age-segregated, probably because social skills, physical abilities, and interests are more similar among age-peers.

particularly in schools. Older adolescents were particularly likely to be found with same-sex, same-age peers; younger adolescents were sometimes found with people of different ages, most of these being relatives. In general, adolescents were found most often with other adolescents, rarely with younger children and also rarely with parents (especially fathers).

The characteristics of adolescents who are well liked by their peers are similar to the qualities of well-liked school-age children described in Chapter 9. Jersild (1963) reports a large number of studies indicating that students who like others are themselves well liked. Recall the studies

reporting that children who were friendly, sociable, and outgoing, as opposed to hostile, withdrawn, and unsociable, were most liked by their peers. In addition, adolescents tend to stress personality characteristics associated with happiness. The person who is sociable, cheerful, active, and fun loving is typically the most popular.

The importance of being accepted by peers is highlighted in a large-scale study reported by Gronlund and Holmlund (1958). A group of 1,073 sixth-grade children were asked to select five people with whom they would like to sit, work, or play. Based on these sociometric data, the investigators divided the entire sample into two groups, designated the *high-status* group and the *low-status* group. High-status children were those selected most often—twenty-seven or more times; low-status children were those selected fewer than three times. Seven years later, the records of some of the children in these groups were examined to determine how many had graduated from high school. It is significant that 82 percent of the high-status group, compared with 45 percent of the low-status group, had graduated, particularly because observed differences in intelligence between the two groups were, in the opinion of the authors, too small to account for the higher dropout rate of the low-status children. At the same time, however, the fact that the low-status children did score significantly lower on intelligence tests is further corroboration of the assumption that intelligence is an important factor in peer group acceptance. Such studies, however, cannot be interpreted as certain evidence that peer rejection is the causal factor in school dropouts, delinquency, or other forms of social maladjustment, for it is equally plausible to suppose that those factors responsible for maladjustment are the very factors that cause the child to be rejected by peers in the first place. In any case, the close relationship that exists between adjustment and acceptance demands further investigation.

■ Sex Roles

In Chapter 8 we pointed out some typical differences in the play behavior of young boys and girls. Not only is the play of boys frequently more boisterous, more aggressive, and more physical than that of girls, but the toys they select (and that parents select for them) tend also to be "sex-typed." But differences between the sexes go far beyond the toys children might play with or their expressions of joy and physical movements while playing. They include a wide range of behaviors that are deemed to be appropriate for boys and girls—in other words, that are considered masculine or feminine. These behaviors, together with the atti-

tudes and personality characteristics associated with them, are what define sex roles. (See *An Illustration of Cultural Forces*.) The learning of sex-appropriate behavior (of sex roles) is referred to as sex typing.

Sex Typing and Sex Roles

During their early years, children become increasingly aware of the behavior that their culture finds acceptable and desirable for their sex. In other words, they learn about sex roles. A *sex role* is simply a combination of behaviors, attitudes, and personality characteristics that are appropriate for one's sex. Sex roles are what define masculinity and femininity. The process of acquiring sex-appropriate behavior—in short, of learning sex roles—is referred to as *sex typing*. In our culture, for example, a boy learns to walk without undue buttock movement, to run fiercely with his arms swinging free, to sit with legs sprawled, to throw a ball with a full swing and a flexed wrist, and to wrestle and fight, or at least to be playfully aggressive. He may love sports, know the names of a thousand baseball, basketball, or hockey players, be able to play the trumpet, be interested in science and mathematics, and play bingo. The girl, however, learns to walk with a more exaggerated buttock movement, run with her elbows tucked into her ribcage and with limp-wristed hands, to sit with legs crossed properly at the knee and hands tucked neatly in her lap, to throw a ball with a little stiff-wristed pushing motion, and to sit quietly and demurely. Although less likely to learn the names of sports heroes, she plays the piano, is interested in art and books, learns to cook and sew, and plays bingo. (Bingo is the great meeting ground.)

There is evidence that the sexual stereotypes described in the preceding paragraph are slowly being eroded by the forces of female liberation movements. However, traditions die slowly. Boys and girls still have little difficulty in identifying personality characteristics that are stereotypically masculine or feminine. In fact, not only do they agree as to what boys and girls should be like, they also

AN ILLUSTRATION OF CULTURAL FORCES

Are men masculine and women feminine primarily because of the genes that determine sex? Or are masculinity and femininity largely the products of cultural forces? If the first notion is correct (genes determine sex roles), men and women from different cultures should be remarkably alike; but if the second is correct (cultures determine sex roles), we might expect men and women from different cultures to be very different.

Margaret Mead believed firmly that cultures determine personality. And some of her anthropological fieldwork provides dramatic evidence to support this belief. Particularly relevant are her studies of three New Guinea tribes: the Arapesh, the Mundugumor, and the Tchambuli.

Mead described the Arapesh as a culture in which both sexes were "placid and contented, unaggressive and noninitiatory, noncompetitive and responsive, warm, docile and trusting" (1935, p. 39). By contrast, among the Mundugumor both men and women "developed as ruthless, aggressive, positively sexed individuals, with the maternal cherishing aspects of personality at a minimum" (p. 190). Finally there were the Tchambuli, who lived principally for art, and where Mead found a "genuine reversal of the sex attitudes of our own culture" (p. 190). The approved personality characteristics in each of these tribes varied greatly, ranging from a society where "feminine" behavior is the norm for both sexes to a society where "masculine" behavior is the norm for each and, finally, to a group where males are "feminine" and females "masculine." It is revealing that the predominantly feminine Arapesh were an agricultural tribe that lived in the inhospitable and infertile mountain regions in the interior of New Guinea. The Mundugumor were a cannibalistic tribe, most of whom lived along the banks of the Sepik, a fast-flowing jungle river that they feared passionately but occasionally employed to approach the hamlets they raided periodically in search of victuals. The Tchambuli were an artistic and agricultural people. The men spent most of their time practicing elaborate dances that they sometimes performed for the women, devising new ceremonies, or experimenting with various art forms. The Tchambuli women spent most of their time gathering food for themselves and for the men.

Mead contends that personality traits such as masculinity and femininity are culturally determined; that because the qualities ordinarily associated with each are so clearly influenced by the cultural environment, there is no justification for believing them sex linked.

Is Mead correct? Perhaps. But her evidence appears somewhat flimsy. Not only is it highly subjective, but, in most cases, it is totally undocumented. In fact, Derek Freeman, following six years of research on Samoa, where Mead had done much of her important work on the role of culture in the socialization of adolescents, concludes that her observations were often inaccurate. Freeman (1983) suggests that Mead was so convinced of the importance of culture that she failed to notice all of the evidence that might have contradicted this view. As a result, the picture she paints of life on primitive islands is, according to Freeman, highly misleading.

Nevertheless, in view of the evident disparities in behavior and personality characteristics among different cultural groups, Mead's conclusions cannot be completely discounted. At the same time, however, caution should be exercised in interpreting and generalizing from evidence such as Mead's. The personality characteristics that she defines as the norm for each of the tribes are simply norms. It is almost inevitable that brief summaries of her work should make it seem that all Arapesh natives were feminine, that all Mundugumors were masculine, and that all Tchambulis had reversals of sex roles (employing our roles as standards). But a careful examination of Mead's writings reveals that these are personality characteristics "approved" by the culture and not necessarily possessed by all its members. In any culture, however small and cohesive, individuals vary considerably from the established norms. These general data can only illustrate that, through socialization, people who are brought up in the same culture will probably resemble one another more than they will resemble those who come from different cultures.

Note that traits such as masculinity and femininity are not only culturally determined but are also culturally defined—hence culturally relative. There is mounting evidence, for example, that some of the qualities that have long been associated primarily with males or females in this culture are no longer so exclusively descriptive of these categories (aggression among males and emotionality among females, for example). Despite this, there are numerous observable sex-role differences in contemporary society, the majority of which are imparted to the child at a very young age through various socializing agencies, not the least important of which is the family. Nor should we overlook the influence of heredity in determining sex roles. Certainly, at a superficial level, the probability that a child will be "masculine" or "feminine" is affected astronomically by anatomical sex.

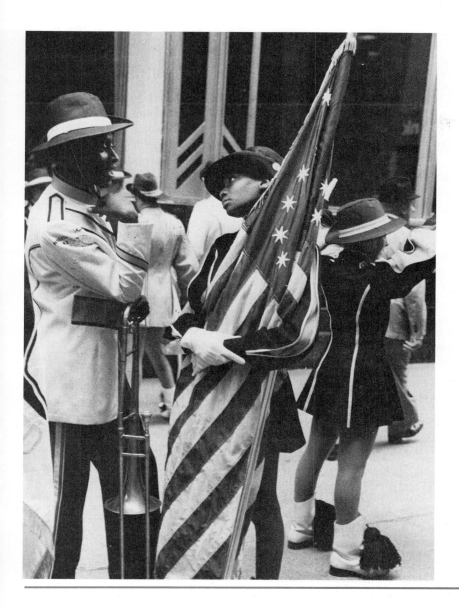

Sex roles and the sexual stereotypes associated with them have become more indefinite in recent years.

tend to agree that masculine characteristics are more desirable (Wesley & Wesley, 1977).

Considerable literature has been devoted to discussing the basic inequities of contemporary sex roles and the extent to which these are culturally determined and hence modifiable. Many of the issues implicit in this discussion are directly relevant to your attitudes toward children as males and females. And it is during childhood and adolescence that sex typing (the adoption of sex-role behavior and attitudes) is profoundly influenced by peers, parents, and other cultural forces.

Determinants of Sex Roles

The development of sex-role differences appears to involve the interaction of three separate forces: biological, family based, and cultural (Lynn, 1974). Biological influences would be manifested in innate (genetic) predispositions for the sexes to think, act, or feel differently; family influences would be most evident in sex-role differences determined by the characteristics and behaviors of parents and siblings; cultural determinants of sex-role differences would be implicit in the models provided for children in schools, in literature, in movies, and on television.

The ways in which each of these factors influences sex typing is still a matter of considerable speculation. Predominant theoretical beliefs maintain that environmental factors (cultural and family based) are influential through processes of imitation and identification. It appears reasonable to suppose that boys learn to behave like "boys" and girls like "girls" through identifying with their parents and with other males and females and through reinforcement that follows their imitation of behaviors that are appropriate for their sex. A more cognitive explanation suggests that once children become aware of their gender identity, they actively participate in organizing their behaviors as well as their environments to conform with sex-appropriate patterns. Thus, having decided that he is male, a boy selects masculine toys and behaviors (Kohlberg, 1966). This process begins in infancy and continues in early childhood.

Evidence supports the notion that genetic influences are also an important factor in determining some sex-role differences. Lynn (1974) presents the following argument: If a difference is genetically based, it would (1) be manifest at a very young age, before environmental forces could have influenced it, (2) be evident in a wide variety of cultures, (3) be evident among subhuman primates, and (4) be related to the effect of hormones on masculinity and femininity. All these criteria appear to be satisfied with respect to the observed greater aggressiveness of males relative to females. Males are more aggressive than females at an early age (Bandura & Walters, 1959); this finding is consistent in most cultures, and nonhuman primates also manifest this sex difference (Mitchell, Arling, & Moller, 1967). The injection of male hormones into pregnant mothers affects the subsequent aggressiveness of female children who are in utero at the time (Money & Ehrhardt, 1968).

However, the greater aggressiveness of males in this culture is not necessarily inevitable, given probable genetic differences related to aggression. The influence of cultural and family-based factors cannot be discounted. Considerable evidence indicates, for example, that parents treat manifestations of aggression in children differently according to their sex. They are more likely to tolerate and even to encourage aggression in boys than in girls (Lewis, 1972). In addition, a large number of occupations requiring physical aggression and strength have traditionally been restricted to males, whereas those requiring nonaggressive, passive, nurturant behavior have been considered more appropriate for women. Are these sociocultural facts a result of innate biological differences? Or do sociocultural expectations simply exaggerate these differences? In other words, do basic, genetic sex differences cause societies to ascribe different roles to the sexes, or do these different roles cause the sex differences? Is this a chicken-and-egg problem?

Sex Differences

The obvious biological differences between the sexes are clearly innate rather than learned. Are there also basic psychological differences between the sexes? The answer is by no means as obvious as many have believed. (See *Cross-Cultural Sex Differences*.) Indeed, there is widespread agreement among parents, teachers, and children themselves with respect to characteristics that are considered primarily feminine and those considered to be more masculine, even as there is widespread agreement concerning which of these characteristics are preferable in society. Rosenkrantz, Vogel, Bee, Broverman, & Broverman (1968) investigated beliefs about masculinity and femininity among college students and found overwhelming agreement concerning which traits were masculine and which feminine (correlations upward of 0.95 between ratings by men and women). There was also marked agreement that many more of the "masculine" traits were socially desirable than "feminine" traits. Lambert, Yackley, and Hine (1971) investigated parents' notions of how boys and girls ought to behave and again found high agreement with respect to sex differences. Boys are expected to be more aggressive, more boisterous, more adventurous; girls are supposedly more passive, more emotional, more tender (Holland, Magoon, & Spokane, 1981).

The nature of sex differences has been the subject of some debate. A number of studies have noted girls' superior verbal development (Maccoby, 1963). Consequently, girls tend to have less difficulty learning how to read, do better on measures of achievement related to reading, and do at least as well as boys do in mathematics in the early years. That they do not continue to do as well in mathematics may be explained in terms of culturally determined interest and motivational factors (Hetherington & McIntyre, 1975).

Achievement orientation also appears to differ *on the average* in men and women. Hoffman (1972) reports that girls score lower on tests of achievement motivation than do boys, a finding that has been corroborated in other studies (for example, Horner, 1969). Hoffman also reports higher affiliative needs among women. Such needs are manifested in girls' greater desire to establish mutually supportive emotional relations with others. Accordingly, boys' and girls' motives for achievement-oriented behavior appear to be different. Whereas boys appear to be motivated largely by a desire to achieve mastery, girls are motivated by a desire to please—hence to affiliate. Consequently, boys tend to attempt more difficult tasks than do girls (Veroff, 1969).

Following their review and summary of research on sex differences, Maccoby and Jacklin (1974) identify four areas with more consistent agreement among research results concerning male-female differences: Females have greater verbal ability than males, particularly at an early age; males excel in **spatial-visual ability;** males excel in mathematical ability; and males are more aggressive (see also Benbow & Stanley, 1982; Boles, 1980; DeFries, 1980).

With respect to achievement orientation, Maccoby and Jacklin point out that apparent sex differences disappear when measures involve noncompetitive situations but that boys do excel in competitive settings. Because achievement in contemporary society frequently involves competition and aggression, it follows that boys would appear to be more achievement oriented. Similarly, because aggression and independence are highly related, a number of researchers have argued that girls are

CROSS-CULTURAL SEX DIFFERENCES

Studies of sex differences in other cultures have not always yielded results comparable to those obtained in our culture, thereby providing additional indirect evidence that these differences are to a great extent culturally based. MacArthur (1973, 1974, 1975) administered a large battery of tests (thirty-five measures) to 177 Central Eskimos (from the Northwest Territories), 176 Greenland Eskimos, 192 Nsenga Africans, and 206 Alberta Caucasians. His findings: almost no sex differences within groups on any of the tests! Specifically, Greenland Eskimo males were very slightly superior to Eskimo females in inductive reasoning tests and on measures of spatial orientation; Central Eskimo and Alberta females showed a slight superiority to males in verbal-educational tasks. One of MacArthur's striking findings is that there were no sex differences among Nsenga Africans. He explains this finding by reference to the absence of any differences between the sexes on measures of need achievement, occupational plans, and parental aspirations for their children. In our culture, these variables typically reflect major sex differences.

less independent and, consequently, more easily influenced than boys. But after a detailed review of research on persuasion and conformity, Eagly (1978) found little evidence of any sex differences in this area.

Note that studies of sex differences reveal *average* differences (more or less accurately); they do not provide data that would be sufficient for making inferences about specific individuals. Nor would it be accurate to conclude that those individuals whose manifested characteristics do not follow the directions observed in these studies are abnormal in any sense. It is important to remember that an average is not a description of the "normal" but is simply a mathematical indication of central tendencies among a group of scores consisting of a wide range of different scores.

Parental attitudes appear to be very important in determining sex-role behavior of children. Parents typically provide daughters with less reinforcement for manifestations of independence and aggression and are more protective of daughters than of sons (Hoffman, 1972). In addition, daughters are less likely than sons to be permitted the kinds of independent explorations that are closely related to the development of spatial-visual abilities (McDaniel, Guay, Ball, & Kolloff, 1978; Russell & Ward, 1982). Studies have shown, for example, that when mothers are asked at what ages they would allow their children to play alone outside, to cut with scissors, and so on, ages are almost always higher for girls than for boys. Sex-role training apparently begins very early in life.

Subsequently, cultural models provided on television, in books, and throughout most of society tend to reinforce children's developing notions of behaviors, attitudes, and interests that are most clearly appropriate for their sex (Biller, 1977). Studies of the role of television in sex typing, for example, have found that children who are exposed to conventional, stereotyped portrayals of male-female roles tend to have stereotyped conceptions of what these roles are and should be (Tan, 1976). By the same token, when researchers have presented children with programs designed to reduce sex-role stereotypes, results have been encouraging (Roberts & Bachan, 1981). In this connection,

tremendous strides have been made in the past several decades in removing sexual biases in books, films, television, and also in our attitudes—which is not to say that we have yet gone as far as we should. But, to quote an original statement by my grandfather, "Times are changing."

■ Sex

This section deals with an area of profound preoccupation for many adolescents—an area that consumes a great deal of their time and energy and to which they sometimes devote themselves with rarely equaled ardor. I speak of Sex—a subject that is capitalized once only, for emphasis.

To begin with, sex is simply a category: male or female. As a category it is rather easily defined by some obvious biological differences between members of the sexes just named. Indeed, the differences are obvious enough that from the moment of birth it is possible for someone to pronounce "It's a girl!" or "It's a boy!"

Sex is more than a category; it is also a psychoanalytic term referring to thumb sucking, defecation, masturbation, fantasies, repressions, and, indeed, to all of living. According to Freud, sex is the source of energy that motivates all of us from birth to death, whether by way of the "normal" psychosexual stages or through the labyrinth of neuroses and psychoses springing from the constant warring between our ids and superegos. Needless to say, not all theorists agree with this Freudian notion.

Sex is also more than a psychoanalytic term. It can mean (as it does in this section) nothing more or less complicated than the physical union between male and female, or variations thereof, or the wish thereto, or the fantasy thereof.

Extensive data have been gathered concerning the sexual beliefs and behavior of the adolescent—data that indicate a marked change in sexual beliefs in recent generations. Some interpret this change as a movement toward promiscuity and shallow, meaningless relationships between casual acquaintances. Others interpret the change as a significant and long overdue recognition of the desirability of what is regarded as the highest form of communication between humans. Fortunately, my role is not to judge, but to report. You may judge if you wish.

Kinsey and his associates (Kinsey, Pomeroy, & Martin, 1948; Kinsey, Pomeroy, Martin, & Gebhard, 1953) provided one of the first major sources of information about sexual behavior in the United States. Among other things, the Kinsey data reveal that although most children have engaged in some form of sexual play prior to adolescence, it is not until puberty that they become capable of an adult sexual response. There is also evidence in the Kinsey data that immediately following puberty boys experience sexual arousal in response to a wider range of stimuli than do girls, a finding that no longer appears to be true (Fisher & Byrne, 1978). This arousal gives rise to a rather urgent desire for orgasm. In the Kinsey surveys, virtually all male adolescents studied reported experiencing orgasm by the time of marriage, while only 30 percent of the females reported doing so. Similarly, far more males than females reported engaging in premarital sexual intercourse.

More recent research contradicts these figures and conclusions. By the middle 1960s, incidence of premarital sexual intercourse among girls was approaching that reported for males (40 and 60 percent, respectively; Packard, 1968); by 1970, the figures were almost identical and higher (78 and 80 percent; Athanasiou, 1973). Other research, employing erotic slides, films, and stories, has generally found that the sexual responsiveness of men and women is not significantly different and that both sexes are aroused by much the same sorts of stimuli (Schmidt & Sigusch, 1973).

The Kinsey finding that fewer women than men engaged in premarital sexual behaviors might have been due in part to women's reluctance to admit having had intercourse—even to as nonthreatening an object as a questionnaire (or as nonthreatening a person as a psychologist). At the same time, it is likely that men might have exaggerated their exploits. It is no secret that male society actively reinforces its members for the frequency and range of their sexual experiences. Female society is much quieter about its reinforcement, although there is evidence of impending change with the emergence of the newly liberated woman. Note, too, that the majority of studies of adolescent sexual behavior involved college or high school students and might therefore not always represent the general population.

The most common form of sexual outlet for adolescent males and females is masturbation. Sorensen (1973) reports that 49 percent of all adolescents age thirteen to nineteen have masturbated at least once. The practice is often accompanied by feelings of guilt and occasionally by totally unfounded fears of impotence, mental retardation, or some other affliction. Males masturbate more frequently than females, reaching their peak sexual activity (*peak* is defined as frequency of orgasm, regardless of its cause) between their sixteenth and seventeenth years. Kinsey et al. (1948) reported that the average frequency for this peak period is 3.4 orgasms per week.

In addition to masturbation, other usual (and unusual) sources of sexual gratification are available to mature humans. A study of unmarried students (Luckey & Nass, 1969) reports that 58 percent of college males and 43 percent of females have had intercourse. The average age for The First Time was 17.9 for boys and 18.7 for girls. In another survey of college students, most of whom were under twenty-five, taken by *Psychology Today* magazine, 80 percent of the males reported having engaged in premarital sexual intercourse. The figure for females was not appreciably lower—78 percent (reported in *Involvement in Developmental Psychology Today*, 1971). Other interesting findings from this survey are that women tended to have fewer one-night (or day) affairs; that first intercourse most often occurred with a steady date, never with a prostitute, and infrequently with a casual acquaintance; that women engage in extramarital sex almost as often as men (36 percent compared to 40 percent for men) and that 20 percent of the females rarely or never reached orgasm. The Sorensen (1973) study reports that by the age of nineteen, only 5 percent of all adolescents remain sexually inexperienced, although not all of the other 95 percent have actually had intercourse.

Although marital sex is not substantially different from premarital sex, its psychological effects might be very different indeed. Despite this generation's professed liberalization and its vociferous espousal of the hang-loose ethic, many of its members are characterized more by *hang-ups* than by loose hanging. Premarital sex frequently results in feelings of guilt, anxiety, remorse, and self-recrimination and may damage the adolescent's all important self-image. These problems do not ordinarily accompany marital sex.

It is sad to note that despite the apparent sophistication of this generation of adolescents, and despite the widespread availability of birth control information and devices, pregnancy or fear of pregnancy is a deciding factor in close to half of all high school marriages; approximately 20 percent of all new brides are pregnant when they marry (Vincent, 1966). Surveys suggest that more than half of all adolescent couples do not use any form of birth control at the time of first intercourse (Apkom, Apkom, & Davies, 1976). Herold and Goodwin (1979) report that of these, 28 percent continue to use no contraception later, and that of those that do, 38 percent attempt withdrawal prior to ejaculation. Others try to use *rhythm* methods, but some, sadly misinformed, believe that the

Despite the effectiveness and availability of birth control, pregnancy (or fear of pregnancy) is a deciding factor in a great many teenage marriages. The breakup rate for these marriages is very high.

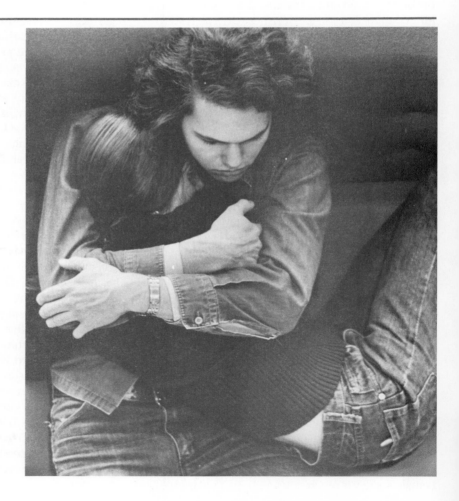

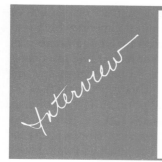
Subject: Male; age sixteen; tenth grade.
(about marriage)

Marriage! Don't rush me. Not for a long time. I suppose I probably will get married and have kids. Doesn't everybody? But I sure won't be in a hurry. I mean, there's so much to do and see, and if you don't when you're young, you probably never will. Like my parents. I know it was different in those days. I mean, harder to travel and such, and everybody got married pretty young. But they got married and they've pretty well been sitting in one place and doing the same thing ever since. I'd like a chance to do something before I settle down.

probability of getting pregnant is greatest during, immediately before, or immediately after menstruation. The break-up rate for adolescent marriages is approximately three times greater than that of the general population (Landis & Landis, 1963; Shearer, 1977).

Adolescent attitudes toward homosexuality were investigated in the Sorensen (1973) study. His primary conclusion was that, despite the visibility of homosexuality in contemporary society, it is not a major adolescent concern or behavior. His findings also contradict the widely held Freudian belief that most young boys engage in relatively innocent homosexual experiences prior to adolescence or in its early stages. Sorensen found that only 9 percent of all adolescents had had one or more homosexual experiences, with more boys than girls reporting such an experience (11 compared with 6 percent). The majority of adolescents, however, are tolerant of homosexuality. Sorensen (1973, p. 294) identifies the following as the main reasons for this tolerance:

The homosexual is playacting a role to satisfy a basic need.

Love is so accidental that no one can predict when and with whom it will occur.

Preassigned sex roles are rejected in favor of "being yourself."

It is the behavior rather than the person that is labeled homosexual; the person underneath is the most important.

Sex—the activity, the category, and its psychoanalytic connotations—is frequently a problem for adolescents but is not their only problem. Nor is it their only source of joy. It has been said that sex gets tiring if it is considered too long, even in an academic textbook. We shall therefore move to the personalities and self-concepts of adolescents before returning to some of their other problems and joys in the final section of this chapter.

■ Personality, Self, and Identity

Of crucial importance to a study of adolescence is a consideration of the self. In one sense, personality is the external manifestation of self; the self is the invisible, unique essence of an individual. Carl Rogers (1951) and other humanistic psychologists maintain strongly that an individual's self can only be understood from that individual's point of view; because a self is necessarily private and alone, it can never be completely known by any outsider. And perhaps it cannot be known very well by that individual either.

What is self? Quite simply, my self is me. It includes what I think of me, what I think I am capable of, what I think others think of me. And my notions of what *I* am—in other words, my *self-concept*—are not the same today as they were when I stole molasses cookies in Aunt Lucy's kitchen.

The self-concept develops, as does the rest of the child. In general, it becomes more abstract and less concrete. When Montemayor and Eisen (1977) had 262 boys and girls from grades four, six, eight, ten, and twelve provide twenty answers for the question "Who am I?" they found a progressive increase in the number of responses relating to basic beliefs, values, personal style, self-determination, and other *abstract* personal qualities. At the same time, there was a dramatic reduction in the number of responses relating to geographical area, citizenship, possessions, and physical attributes. For example, a typical nine-year-old boy's responses included: "I have brown eyes; I have brown hair; I have seven people in my family; I live on 1923 Pinecrest Drive." An eleven-and-one-half-year-old girl provides somewhat less concrete notions of self: "I'm a human being; I'm a girl; I'm a truthful person; I'm a very good pianist." And a seventeen-year-old girl presents a highly abstract self-concept, based largely on interpersonal style and emotional states: "I am a human being; I am an individual; I don't know who I am; I am a loner; I am an indecisive person; I am an atheist" (Montemayor & Eisen, 1977, pp. 317, 318).

Self-Esteem

It has been observed that children spend the first seven years of their lives trying to determine *where* they are, the following seven wondering *who* they are, and the next seven pondering the question of *why* they are. We might add that throughout these twenty-one years and far beyond, an equally important question is not where, who, or why, but simply *whether* or not the self—my me—is worthwhile, lovable, and other goods things that most of us want to believe we are. What I think of me—my self-esteem—is of profound importance to my behavior and to my happiness. If I think I am what I should be, then my self-esteem is high. In other words, there is little discrepancy between my self-concept and my self-ideal. If, however, I am less than I think I can or should be, my self-esteem is low.

That one of the most fundamental aspects of all development is the development of high self-esteem is a notion shared by a large number of psychologists, although they have not all made their beliefs equally explicit or employed the same language. Erikson's (1968) work is probably the best example of a theoretical position devoted to clarifying the importance of self (see Chapter 2). The expression he employs, essentially synonymous with the term *self*, is *identity*. For him, the development of strong feelings of identity—of clear feelings of who one is—is the most important developmental task facing the adolescent. The primary developmental crisis facing the adolescent is accordingly the conflict between accepting, choosing, or discovering an identity and the diffusion of the adolescent's energies resulting from conflict and doubt concerning the choice of identities. Recall that the fifth of Erikson's eight developmental stages is labeled *identity versus role diffusion*.

Resolution of adolescents' identity crises can take a variety of forms, the most common of which is the selection of an identity that conforms to societal norms and to the individuals' expectations of themselves. (See *Adolescent Crisis and Commitment*.) Erikson points out that one of the major social functions of prolonged adolescence is simply to serve as a breathing space (a moratorium in his terms) during which adolescents can experiment with a variety of roles in their quest for identity. He is not particularly alarmed that some of these roles constitute negative identities (delinquency and other forms of rebellion, for example), because in most cases they are temporary, eventually giving way to more acceptable and happier identities.

Psychological research on the development and importance of **self-esteem** reveals some interesting and important findings. The classic study in this area is Coopersmith's (1967) intensive investigation of self-esteem among eighty-five boys between the ages of ten and twelve. These boys were divided into groups according to their self-esteem, a concept defined in terms of the degree to which an individual's attitudes toward the self are favorable. In Coopersmith's words, self-esteem

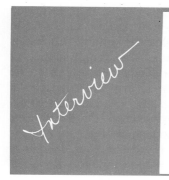

Subject: Male; age nineteen; freshman college student.
(concerning future plans)

Well, no, I guess I really haven't decided what I'm going to be. There are lots of different things I think I'd like for a career. Something social, probably. I've thought off being a social worker or a psychologist even. Like maybe a counselor. But I've thought about going into business too, which is what I think my dad would like. It would probably be a lot easier and I'd maybe make a lot more money. Maybe that's important too, but I want to do something that I'd really like. Something that I'd be proud to say, "I'm a such and such!" I just don't know for sure what that's going to be.

indicates the "extent to which the individual believes himself to be capable, significant, successful, and worthy. In short, self-esteem is a *personal* judgment of worthiness that is expressed in attitudes the individual holds toward himself" (1967, p. 5).

Coopersmith's most important findings with respect to manifestations of self-esteem were that individuals with high self-esteem were more likely than others to be selected as friends, found it easier to make friends, were more likely to assume an active rather than a listening role in group discussions, were less likely to be highly conformist, scored higher on measures of creativity, were more outspoken, were less sensitive to criticism, and were less self-conscious. The major portion of his investigation, however, was concerned with an attempt to identify factors related to the development of high or low self-esteem. In this connection, he found that social class was not a significant factor. Other research (Rosenberg, 1965) has not always supported this finding, a contradiction that may be partially explained by the fact that Coopersmith's sample was relatively homogeneous with respect to social class; that is, none of the extremes were represented. Coopersmith did find, however, that boys whose fathers were least often unemployed tended to have higher self-esteem scores. Similarly, absence of the father was related to self-esteem, with boys whose fathers were most often absent tending to have lower self-esteem. The absence of mothers for work was not related to self-esteem.

Of special interest is Coopersmith's finding of significant relationships between parental characteristics and child-rearing modes and their children's self-esteem. Parents with high self-esteem tended to have children who also thought highly of themselves; mothers with low emotional stability were more likely to have children with low self-esteem. Mothers of boys with high self-esteem tended to have closer rapport with their sons and greater affection for them than did mothers of boys with low self-esteem. Boys with high self-esteem tended to disagree less with their families than those characterized by lower self-esteem and to have more friends who were well known by parents, indicating a generally closer family relationship. Families of these boys were significantly more democratic than others in terms of decision making. Perhaps most striking, families of boys high in self-esteem were significantly less permissive ("stricter"), more demanding, and more consistent in the enforcement of rules but more prone to reinforcing good behavior.

Other findings of interest from this study were that boys high in self-esteem tended to be more intelligent, to appear happier to their mothers, to have developed more rapidly in locomotor areas, and to achieve more in school than other boys.

In summary, the Coopersmith study indicates that self-esteem is closely related to adjustment and behavior, and an individual's chances for success, as it is commonly defined, increase with his or her self-esteem. What is not clear is the extent to which high self-esteem determines success and happiness and the extent to which happiness and success contribute to the development of self-esteem. But perhaps it remains irrelevant to decide between the chicken and the egg. What does appear clear is that parental attitudes and behaviors are closely implicated in the development of self-esteem and that high self-esteem might go a long way toward preventing some of the turmoil sometimes associated with adolescence.

■ The Turmoil Topics

Adolescence is undoubtedly a time of turmoil for many; at the same time, keep in mind that it is quite the opposite for numerous adolescents who pass exuberantly through their teen years. Such individuals discover the joys of their increased powers of mind and body and are successful in overcoming or avoiding the turmoil that besets their less fortunate peers. The average adolescent is considerably more difficult to describe than the younger child. Research may be incapable of determining which quality best characterizes the largest number of adolescents for the longest periods of time: turmoil, ambivalence, or exuberance. Although we may be dealing with the minority, we consider now some of the forms, causes, and manifestations of turmoil; for this minority, if it is one, is significant.

Adolescent Frustration

There are two principal sources of **frustration** for adolescents: their inability to define their role—

ADOLESCENT CRISIS AND COMMITMENT

The central concept in Erikson's description of adolescent development is *identity*. According to him, the key psychological task facing the adolescent is that of selecting and developing a clear identity—of developing a commitment to being a certain kind of person. Given the many choices of *identity* available, many adolescents are frequently in conflict about these choices. In Erikson's terms, many adolescents undergo identity crises.

Considerable clarification of Erikson's description of this developmental stage is provided by Marcia's investigations of the development of identity in adolescence (Marcia, 1966; Marcia and Friedman, 1970). Marcia describes the adolescent in terms of the extent to which a positive, stable identity has been achieved—in other words, by what is called *identity status*. Four distinct types of identity status have been identified. Distinctions among them are based on whether or not the adolescent has undergone (or is currently undergoing) a crisis and on whether or not a commitment has been made to a specific identity.

Identity Diffusion   Adolescents in this state are characterized by a total lack of commitment and the absence of an identity crisis. These are individuals whose political, social, and religious beliefs are ambiguous or perhaps nonexistent and who have no vocational aspirations. Muuss (1975) suggests that while identity diffusion is common and normal in early adolescence, it is less normal in late adolescence. Individuals who have not developed a mature sense of identity by late adolescence are sometimes recognizable as full-time fun seekers (what Marcia, 1966, calls "playboys") or as disturbed individuals characterized by high anxiety, low self-esteem, and lack of self-confidence (Bronson, 1959).

Foreclosure   A second identity status is defined in terms of strong commitment to an identity, although the adolescent has not experienced a crisis. Foreclosure is most clearly illustrated in those instances where political, religious, and vocational decisions have effectively been made for the adolescent and are accepted without question. This is frequently the case, for example, in close-knit religious or political communities where the roles of each individual (as well as their beliefs) are predetermined and are decided upon by individuals other to achieve a sense of identity—and their sense of the depressing distance between the utopia of which they dream and the world as they see it.

Adolescents' difficulty in defining their role is in part a failure of the culture. With the advent of puberty, they suddenly find themselves physically mature. Not only are they capable of being in love, of having intercourse, and of producing offspring, but many actively desire to do so. In many cases, however, they must resort to frequently unsatisfactory means of achieving sexual relief. And when the means are physically more satisfactory, they are perhaps less so psychologically, for the guilt accompanying masturbation is often less severe than that for premarital sexual intercourse.

Economic unemployment is perhaps as frustrating for the adolescent as sexual unemployment. Cultural demands for schooling make it difficult for most children to become economically independent. Thus, at a time when they are struggling to become psychologically independent from parents, they find themselves turning to them with greater frequency and with bigger economic demands. The inherent frustration is obvious: An adolescent cannot afford to ignore parental dictates when desiring the family sedan.

Adolescents may also feel frustrated by ambivalence about where childhood ends and adult status begins. The responsibilities that are occasionally placed on their shoulders—as in time of war, for example—are clearly adult responsibilities. At the same time, however, the privileges granted them are frequently those of children. Until recently, and even now in many places, they could not drink alcohol publicly, could not vote, and could not run for public office, although boys could get maimed or killed for their country. This, at least in their view, is sufficiently unfair to cause frustration.

than the adolescent. Foreclosure also occurs when adolescents simply allow parents or sometimes peers to make important identity-related decisions for them. These adolescents do not go through an identity crisis. Their most striking characteristics appear to be high adherence to authoritarian values (obedience and respect of authority) (Marcia, 1966).

Moratorium Individuals   A large group of adolescents actively explore a variety of roles and experiment with different commitments for periods of varying duration. These periods are termed *moratoria*. According to Erikson, one of the important functions of adolescence is to serve as a period during which it is not essential to be fully committed to one life style, one vocation, one set of beliefs—a period during which the adolescent can explore the tremendous variety of alternatives that might be available. This period is a moratorium—a time when commitment is not required. During the moratorium stage, adolescents have vague, changing commitments. In this sense, they are in crisis. But it is a useful crisis for most adolescents, for in the absence of a moratorium of exploration, there is a danger of premature commitment (as in the case of foreclosure) or of continuing lack of commitment (as in identity diffusion).

Identity Achieved   Adolescents who have experienced the moratorium—having experienced a *crisis* of some degree—and who have arrived at a choice—a commitment—may be described as *identity achieved*. Marcia (1966) reports that these adolescents are more independent, respond better to stress, have more realistic goals, and have higher self-esteem than adolescents in any of the other three categories.

In summary, the development of identity involves making a selection among the various alternatives that present themselves to the adolescent with respect to social, political, religious, and vocational commitments. In short, it involves determining *who* and *what* one is and will be. These four states of adolescence also include those of us who remain adolescent throughout life.

Additional frustration derives from conflicting cultural pressures that surround adolescents. They have been led to believe that kindness, generosity, modesty, and affection are among the highest virtues, and yet they observe cruelty, selfishness, ambition that is quite incompatible with modesty, and the affectionless impersonality of existence in large cities and sometimes in small homes as well. They are taught that people should be individuals, that they should "do their own thing," and yet the advertising media constantly urge them to conform. Indeed, most adult culture urges conformity. These contradictions are powerful sources of conflict and frustration.

All the frustration that stems from adolescents' ambivalence about their role and from conflicting demands that are made of them is frequently less important to the individuals than the distance between the ideals they dream of and the reality they observe. This is the time in their moral development that they question and examine established social and religious rules, in order to arrive at self-chosen moral principles. And implicit in these principles are beliefs about desirable states of affairs—about what *ought* to be—in short, about the *ethical* aspects of human existence. There are people starving, people in pain, people dying needlessly, people fighting, people destroying their environments. There is injustice, greed, anger, rape, murder, dishonesty, and a thousand forms of hypocrisy. There is a callous disregard for the humanity of persons in the depersonalized movements of technology. Adolescents are acutely aware of these realities and of other evils of greater or lesser magnitude; as a result, they often drop out in some way, or they rebel quietly or violently.

Delinquency

Delinquency is a legal rather than a scientific category. Its definition varies from one legal jurisdiction to another, depending on the particular laws of that jurisdiction. Most simply, a *delinquent* is a juvenile who has been apprehended and convicted for transgression of established legal rather than moral laws. Adults in similar situations are criminals rather than delinquents.

When delinquency is defined in this manner, surveys of its prevalence can be based quite accurately on police and legal records. One such survey, involving 25,000 boys and girls aged six to seventeen, found that the incidence of delinquency in Kentucky was 2 percent for boys and 0.5 percent for girls (Ball, Ross, & Simpson, 1964). This same study found that the incidence of delinquency among boys doubled between ages eleven and twelve and tripled between ages twelve and seventeen, with 7 percent of all seventeen-year-old boys being delinquent. Among girls there was little change between the ages of six and seventeen.

It is noteworthy that when delinquency is defined simply in terms of legal transgression, rather than in terms of transgression, apprehension, and conviction, the picture changes dramatically. Short and Nye (1957–1958) studied delinquency through interviews rather than by going to police records. They report that over 80 percent of all subjects in their sample had been guilty of breaking some law at least once. As Vaz and Lodhi (1979) note, the majority of crimes are never reported.

A number of factors appear to be related to delinquency. Given the correlational nature of most of the studies that have investigated delinquency, however, it is impossible to identify its specific causes. Age, for example, is related to delinquency; there is no evidence that it *causes* delinquency. Other related factors include social class, sex, family background, and peers. Note that these are *related* rather than *causal* factors.

Literature pertaining to the relationship between social class and delinquency is ambiguous and inconclusive. Although there is little doubt that the less advantaged social classes, as well as some racial subgroups, are greatly overrepresented among delinquent groups, it is by no means clear that there are, in fact, many more delinquents among these groups. Given the nature of present law-enforcement systems, the often unconscious prejudices of the systems, and their consequently greater likelihood of recognizing and apprehending delinquents among minority and lower-class groups, it is hardly surprising that more of these adolescents are classified as delinquents. At the same time, however, to the extent that delinquency is a form of rebellion sometimes motivated by the desire for material possessions, it is reasonable to expect that more poorer adolescents would be delinquent. Miller (1958) also points out that lower-class delinquents are frequently not rebelling against middle-class values but are simply expressing their adherence to lower-class values—values that sometimes prize the successful law breaker and that emphasize trouble, street smartness, toughness, excitement, and daring. Furthermore, there is a greater tendency for lower-class parents to look to the police for help with their children; middle-class parents turn to therapists (Chambliss, 1974).

The influence of peer groups is also related to delinquent behavior and has been extensively investigated, particularly in the study of gangs (for example, Cartwright, Tomson, & Schwartz, 1975). Like other peer groups, the delinquent gang serves to reinforce its dominant values and serves, as well, as a model for translation of these values into actual behaviors (Buehler, Patterson, & Furniss, 1966). Examples of the importance of peer groups in establishing values and in encouraging certain kinds of behavior are prevalent in television programs. They are also prevalent in various detention centers and other correctional institutions. Because the populations of correctional institutions are primarily delinquent peer groups, it is not particularly surprising that some 60 percent of all admissions are, in fact, readmissions (Stuart, 1969). The same observation could be made with respect to adult correctional institutes. (The term *correction* is a euphemism.)

Research has also indicated that the father is perhaps the most influential parent with respect to delinquency (Schaefer, 1965). Fathers of delinquent boys are, on the average, more severe, more punitive, more prone to alcoholism, more rejecting, and more likely to have engaged in delinquent behavior themselves than are fathers of nondelinquent boys. Herzog and Sudia (1970) report a higher probability of delinquency among boys from fa-

therless homes. They speculate that absence of the father may contribute to delinquency in sons, perhaps by failure to provide adequate male models, perhaps as a function of protest against female domination, or simply because of inadequate supervision. Girls, too, appear to be more prone to delinquency in homes in which the father is absent (see Lynn, 1979). Friedman (1969) suggests that delinquency in such cases may result in part from the girls' sexual "acting out," in retaliation against mothers who deprecate absent fathers.

As was noted earlier, there is also a close relationship between self-esteem and delinquency. Research has shown, for example, that delinquents typically think less well of themselves than do nondelinquent adolescents (Ahlstrom & Havighurst, 1971). And adolescents characterized by negative self-concepts are more likely to be delinquent. Those factors described earlier as being related to the development of high and low self-esteem may also be indirectly implicated in delinquency (Coopersmith, 1967).

As might be expected, the incidence of delinquency is considerably higher among boys than girls. This observation may be partly explained in terms of the male's greater aggressiveness and lesser acquiescence. Traditionally, delinquency among males has involved more aggressive transgressions, with girls being apprehended more often for sexually promiscuous behavior, shoplifting, and related activities. There is evidence that this pattern is now changing, with more girls being involved in aggressive delinquent acts, including breaking and entering, car theft, and even assault (Vaz & Lodhi, 1979). Drug-related offenses also account for an increasing number of detentions.

In summary, a complex of psychological and social forces impinge upon the potential delinquent, although no single factor can reliably predict delinquent behavior. Social class, age, sex, home background, and peer influences are all implicated, but these, alone or in combination, cannot provide a complete picture. Clearly, numerous adolescents from the most deprived of backgrounds are not delinquents, and many from apparently superior environments are.

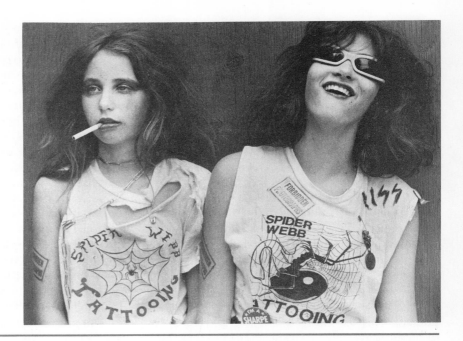

Rebellion can take many different forms, not all of which are necessarily dangerous, undesirable, or even silly.

Rebellion

It would be impossible to provide a complete analysis of the "turmoil topics" selected for this discussion—not only is there insufficient space but there is also insufficient current knowledge. Nevertheless, knowledge has progressed some distance beyond some of our favorite stereotypes and several of these stereotypes can now be discounted.

To begin with, popular belief maintains that the rebel—the adolescent activist—is a malcontent, a social misfit, a disturbed individual, a potential criminal, a lower-class complainer, or some other form of undesirable individual. When adolescent rebellion is defined by student activism, a somewhat different picture of adolescents-as-rebels emerges: They are, in fact, typically well adjusted, middle-class individuals—social malcontents to be sure, but no more potential criminals than you or I.

A second stereotype asserts that most adolescents and college students are radicals—that the

only reason they go to college is to join demonstrations, to sit in hallways of administration buildings, to burn anyone in effigy, to protest their country's attitude toward internal and external problems, to agitate against the stupidity of all people. This belief is only partly correct. Certainly, some students' social consciences demand that they express their dissatisfaction and concern, but the total number of students involved in this demonstrative behavior, even at the height of student activism in the 1960s, was seldom more than 15 percent of the student body and usually much lower than that (Trent & Crais, 1967; Trent & Medsker, 1967). One of the traditional weaknesses of stereotypes is that they are applied to all individuals who have superficially similar appearances.

But not all adolescents who are dissatisfied, disillusioned, or in need of the community of groups join them in protest. A significant number of the severely dissatisfied drop out of society. Lest another stereotype be fostered, one must point out that the methods of dropping out described here are undertaken by the adventurous and by the timid, by the weak and by the strong, by the deluded and by the rational. Frequently, they are not attempts to drop out but merely attempts to intensify the experience of living.

Dropping Out Through Drugs

Drug use is a fact of life. Drugs are with us constantly in the guise of coffee, tea, headache tablets, cocktails, and in thousands of other forms. Humans have been familiar with drugs for centuries, although they have not always known the chemical components of the substances that they ate, drank, chewed, applied to wounds, inhaled, put in ears, or otherwise used on their persons. But the label is much less important than the effect and sometimes the availability.

For adolescents, the discovery of drugs is considerably simpler than it might have been some centuries, or even decades, ago. One need no longer go about testing brews made from plant leaves or chewing on roots and seeds. The communications media have discovered drugs for today's youth. It takes only nominal intelligence for a teenager to be aware of the availability of drugs. Not only do the media serve as a source of information, they also convey an image of adolescents and drugs that often misleads. The frequency of drug use among teenagers has increased dramatically in the past decade, just as alcohol consumption increased drastically several generations ago. At the same time, however, reports of the seriousness of the "problem" and of the extent of drug use are seldom based on more than conjecture and opinion.

Recent surveys of drug use in high schools and colleges have not yielded consistent results, but the majority of the reports have presented a less terrifying picture than might have been predicted on the basis of trends that seemed apparent in the 1960s. Present indications are that the use of at least some drugs, most notably LSD, has leveled off or even dropped slightly. Leon (1977) surveyed 465 people under the age of twenty-six and compared reported drug use in 1974 with previous surveys of drug use in 1970. He found no important patterns of difference for those two

years. In contrast, Kopplin and Greenfield (1977) found significant increases in uses of alcohol, LSD, and marijuana between 1969 and 1973. Similarly, Hollander and Macurdy (1978), following 1970, 1974, and 1978 surveys of approximately 10 percent of a total population of 28,000 secondary school students in Vancouver, British Columbia, reported increases in the use of tobacco, alcohol, and marijuana. Use of LSD and amphetamines had not changed appreciably. In addition, these researchers found no consistent differences between males and females with respect to frequency of drug use or types of drugs used, but they did find considerable evidence of multiple drug use. For example, of those students who said that they used alcohol more than once a week, over 85 percent also reported having used marijuana; in contrast, of those who did not use alcohol, fewer than 4 percent reported using marijuana.

Marijuana is derived from hemp, a tall annual plant appearing in male and female forms. It is from the flowering top of the female hemp plant and from leaves on both male and female plants that the drug *Cannabis sativa* is derived. The specific chemical grouping that apparently accounts for its effects is termed **tetrahydrocannabinols** (THC).

Marijuana is ordinarily smoked, although it can also be eaten or drunk. According to Goode (1969), its primary effect is a pleasant emotional state, although he describes it as having more of an "experience enhancement" effect than as an experience that is highly pleasurable in itself. Thus, it is often taken ("done") prior to listening to music, eating, or engaging in sexual activity. Marijuana has sometimes been reported to enhance the enjoyment of all three, although the majority of the adolescents in Sorensen's (1973) study did not think it increased their sexual pleasure. An additional effect sometimes associated with marijuana is an increased ability to become involved with people, to interact sensitively. It should be pointed out as well that marijuana is occasionally reported to have no discernible effect on the psychological state of the user. If taken in sufficient doses and in sufficiently pure forms (which are extremely rare), it may evoke the same types of hallucinogenic reactions sometimes associated with stronger drugs, such as LSD.

Marijuana does not appear to be physically addictive, although there is a possibility that regular use might be associated with psychological dependence (see *Cannabis Marijuana and Hashish*, 1976). There is evidence, as well, of apathy and loss of motivation following prolonged abuse (Coleman, Butcher, & Carson, 1980).

The widely held fear that marijuana is the first step toward heroin addiction has generally been discounted. There is no evidence that tolerance to marijuana develops, as does tolerance to some of the so-called hard drugs. Hence the marijuana user does not need to go to more powerful drugs to continue to achieve the same "high." Nor is there any evidence that using marijuana leads to a psychological craving for heroin. It is true, however, that procuring marijuana, because it is illegal, frequently exposes the adolescent to underworld figures who would like nothing better than to "hook" someone else. In that sense, marijuana may lead to other drugs. In addition, patterns of multiple drug use indicate that those individuals who try one drug are more likely to try another than are those who do not try a drug to begin with.

LSD-25 (d-lysergic acid diethylamide tartrate) is the most powerful synthetic hallucinogen known. Because it is a synthetic chemical, it can be made by anyone who has the materials, the equipment, and the knowledge. Lysergic acid is derived from *ergot,* a fungus that grows on rye and sometimes on other grasses. Its medical use is relatively widespread. For example, derivatives of ergot are often administered to women directly after childbirth to cause contraction of the uterus, thereby indirectly preventing bleeding. Ergot is also known to cause abortions (Bookmiller & Bowen, 1967). Common street names for LSD-25 are barrels, California sunshine, acid, blotters, cubes, wedges, purple haze, jellybeans, frogs, and microdots.

LSD-25 (ordinarily referred to simply as LSD) is usually taken orally, commonly in the form of a white, odorless, and tasteless powder. Much more is known about its chemical derivation and its production than about its effects. The most objective comment that can be made about its effects is that they vary widely from one person to another, as well as from one occasion to another for the same person. The predominant characteristic of an LSD experience (called an "acid trip") is the augmented intensity of sensory perceptions; color, sound, taste, and vision are particularly susceptible. On occasion, an acid trip is accompanied by hallucinations, some of which may be mild and amusing. At other times, the hallucinations can be sufficiently frightening to lead to serious mental disturbance in the subject, even after the immediate effects of the drug have worn off (Louria, 1966). On occasion, LSD may have effects that can be interpreted by the user as spiritual experiences (Smith & Steinfield, 1970). There is also very tentative evidence, based on studies of rats, that LSD may produce changes in chromosomes that could affect the offspring of the user, if the fetus is not aborted first (Alexander, 1967). More recent research, using psychiatric patients who had been given LSD for therapeutic reasons, found no evidence of chromosomal damage (Robinson, Chitham, Greenwood, & Taylor, 1974).

Other drugs employed by some adolescents include alcohol, other hallucinogens such as STP and MDA (methyl amphetamines), PCP (phencyclidene), cocaine, and various barbiturates and other, milder tranquilizers. Of these, alcohol is still the drug of choice, both among adolescents and adults. (See Table 12.1 and *Adolescents and Alcohol.*)

Dropping Out Through Suicide

Suicide, the deliberate taking of one's life, is final—an end that is sought when individuals can see only two choices: life as it is now or death. Evidently they prefer to die. If he is a male, he will probably shoot himself; a female is more likely to use poisoning or asphyxiation. There are obviously many other methods available, but some of these result in a death that appears accidental (drowning, a car accident) and is difficult to identify as suicide unless the person has left a note, letter, or other message that can be interpreted as a farewell. Because a

Table 12.1 Symptoms of drug use and abuse.

Drug	Signs and Early Symptoms	Long-Term Symptoms
Narcotics	Medicinal breath Traces of white powder around nostrils (heroin is sometimes inhaled) Red or raw nostrils Needle marks or scars on arms Long sleeves (or other clothing) at inappropriate times Physical evidence may include cough syrup bottles, syringes, cotton swabs, and spoon or cap for heating heroin	Loss of appetite Constipation
Sedatives	Symptoms of alcohol consumption with or without odor: poor coordination and speech, drowsiness, loss of interest in activity	Withdrawal symptoms when discontinued Possible convulsions
Stimulants	Excessive activity Irascibility Argumentativeness Nervousness Pupil dilation Dry mouth and nose with bad breath Chapped, dry lips Scratching or rubbing of nose Long periods without sleep Loss of appetite	Loss of appetite Possible hallucinations and psychotic reactions
Hallucinogens, marijuana	Odor on breath and clothing Animated behavior or its opposite	None definite
LSD	Bizarre behavior Panic Disorientation	Possible contribution to psychoses Recurrence of experiences after immediate effects of drug
Inhalants	Odor of glue, solvent, or related substance Redness and watering of eyes Appearance of alcoholic intoxication Physical evidence of plastic bags, rags, aerosol glue, or solvent containers	Disorientation Brain damage

suicide note appears in only 15 percent of all reported suicides, many apparent accidents are probably unidentified suicides.

Suicide is not a pleasant topic—it so violently contradicts our implicit belief in the goodness of life. Consequently, there is a powerful social stigma attached to the act, and the event is often covered over both by the information media and by the attending physician. As a result, people know only of suicides of people whom they have known, or of particularly prominent persons, or of people who commit the act so flagrantly that it compels attention. There are relatively few scientific investigations of suicide, its causes, and the personalities of those who deliberately choose their time and method of departure. Do children commit suicide? How often? How about adolescents, disillusioned idealists that they are, caught up in the stress and turmoil of the transition to adulthood? Here are some facts.

The suicide rate in the United States is slightly less than 15 per 100,000. Although few children under the age of fifteen commit suicide, that number is increasing; however, the most dramatic increase in suicide rates during the past decade involves those aged fourteen to nineteen (Cantor,

ADOLESCENTS AND ALCOHOL

Alcohol, the most commonly used and abused drug in contemporary societies, is a central nervous system depressant. In relatively moderate doses, its primary effect is to suppress inhibition, which is why many individuals who have consumed alcohol behave as though they had taken a stimulant. In less moderate doses, the individual progresses from being "high" or "tipsy" to intoxication. Literally, to be "intoxicated" is to be *poisoned*. Behavioral symptoms of varying degrees of intoxication may include impaired muscular control, delayed reflexive reactions, loss of coordination and balance, impaired vision, uncertain speech, faintness, nausea, amnesia (blackouts), and, in extreme cases, paralysis of heart and lung muscles sometimes leading to death (Harger, 1964).

Alcohol is physiologically addictive, although prolonged or excessive consumption is generally required before symptoms of physical addiction are present. Signs of psychological dependency (a strong desire to continue taking the drug) may appear considerably sooner. One of the major physiological effects of alcohol relates to its contribution to cirrhosis of the liver—a major cause of death in the United States (Jones-Witters & Witters, 1983). In addition, it is implicated in more than half of all motor vehicle deaths, a large number of which involve adolescents.

Alcohol consumption among adolescents is widespread. Most surveys report that extremely few teenagers have not tried alcohol at least once (Torres, 1982). Swift (1975) found that somewhere around 60 percent of high school students claim that they get drunk at least once a month. And in a large-scale survey of Massachusetts teenagers (1,269 subjects), Brown and Finn (1982) found that by age fourteen, 66 percent of teenagers drank with their friends (when they met for "parties, etc.") at least "sometimes"; 29 percent did so "usually" or "always." By the age of seventeen, the percentage of subjects who "sometimes" drank with friends had increased to 88,

and 47 percent now claimed that they "usually" or "always" drank in this situation.

Why do adolescents drink? The numerous reasons include social pressure, experimentation, insecurity and other personal problems, as well as simply for the sensation of being "tipsy," "high," or "drunk." One U.S. government survey reports that as many as one-quarter of seventh-grade students claim to get drunk at least once a year—and an astounding 10 percent of twelfth-grade students get drunk an average of once a week (U.S. Department of Health and Human Services, 1974). Brown and Finn (1982) suggest that deliberately drinking to get drunk (as opposed to getting drunk as a result of foolishly having the proverbial "one too many") underlies a great deal of teenage drinking. In their sample of 1,269 teenagers, 36 percent of the twelve-year-olds thought that getting drunk is the purpose of drinking. As in other studies, this number increases around ages fourteen and fifteen (59 and 64 percent, respectively), but drops subsequently (42 percent at age seventeen).

Why do adolescents want to get drunk? To feel good, have fun, celebrate, let off steam, cheer up, forget worries, feel less shy, and impress friends, they claim (Brown & Finn, 1982). But when they are asked what their actual behaviors and feelings are when they are drunk, while a large number do "feel good" and "laugh a lot," a significant number fall asleep, feel unhappy, cry, damage property, and get into fights. And approximately one-third at all age levels occasionally get sick.

When is alcohol consumption by adolescents deviant or problematic? Is it problematic only when the adolescent gets into trouble? Does it become a problem when alcohol consumption becomes habitual or excessive? When it interferes with normal social or physical functioning? Or is it always a problem, given that the behavior is generally illegal? There are no easy answers.

Students reporting drinking with friends.

Age	"Never" (%)	"Sometimes" (%)	"Usually" (%)	"Always" (%)	At Least "Sometimes" (total %)	Total Number of Students
12	72	24	2	2	28	163
13	62	29	6	3	38	142
14	34	37	23	6	66	242
15	20	42	28	10	80	208
16	13	35	35	17	87	249
17	12	41	33	14	88	219

From Brown and Finn, *Journal of Alcohol and Drug Education*, 1982, p. 15.

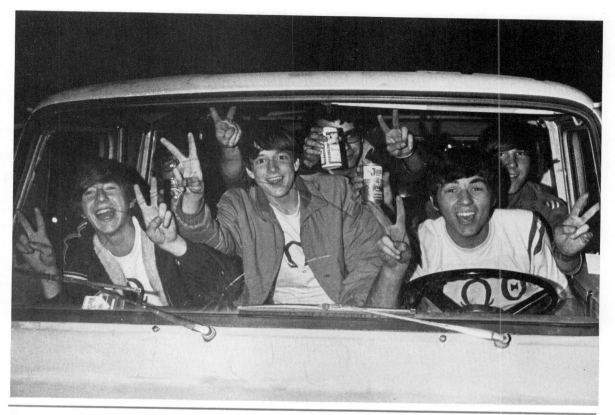

Teenage drinking can be the result of social pressure, insecurity, or personal problems. Even the desire to just have fun can lead to serious alcohol abuse.

1977). In spite of this increase, suicide rates do not peak until the ages between seventy-five and eighty-four (21.5 per 100,000). After the age of eighty-five, the rate declines again (*Monthly Vital Statistics*, 1979). Among adolescents, far more girls than boys attempt suicide, but a much higher percentage of the boys are successful. In the United States, there are approximately 12 percent more male than female suicides (Marks & Haller, 1977). Divorced and widowed men are especially prone to suicide, their rates sometimes exceeding 100 per 100,000. College students are twice as likely to commit suicide as their noncollege peers (Beck & Young, 1978). Foreign students in American colleges are much more likely to kill themselves than native Americans. Older college students are more sui-

cide prone, as are those students who have been referred for psychiatric care (Seiden, 1966). Suicide proneness in college students can be attributed to three major areas of anxiety and conflict: concern over studies, physical complaints, and—probably most important—difficulties with interpersonal relationships. Suicide accounted for at least 34 percent of all student deaths during a ten-year period at the University of California, Berkeley (Seiden, 1966).

Suicide is still the solution of an isolated few. Most of us choose to wait for death and hope that it will be a long time in coming. And for most adolescents, life is only occasionally turbulent and stressful; most of the time, it abounds with joy and excitement.

1 Social development progresses from a stage of relative dependence on the parents to a stage of relative independence. As adolescents become less closely attached to their immediate families, they become more dependent on peer groups.

2 Peer groups begin as small single-sex groups in early adolescence and progress through four additional stages. The first is a period when the single-sex groups interact as groups but remain intact, followed by a stage when the crowd has begun to form but still consists of single-sex groups interacting in a closer fashion. Eventually, a large heterosexual group is formed. In the later stages of adolescence, this crowd breaks into less cohesive groups of couples.

3 The adolescent's acceptance by peers is profoundly important for social and psychological well-being. Friendships tend to be highly age segregated.

4 Sex roles are influenced by siblings and parents as well as by larger environmental forces. Evidence indicates that some sex differences may be partly genetically based.

5 Among the most dramatic examples of culture-linked sex differences are those provided by Margaret Mead's study of three New Guinea tribes in which men and women both showed feminine characteristics (Arapesh), both showed masculine traits (Mundugumor), or had reversed masculine-feminine roles (Tchambuli).

6 Sex roles are defined as the predominant behaviors, interests, attitudes, and characteristics of males and females, respectively. Sex typing refers to the acquisition of sex roles—in other words, to the learning of sex-appropriate behavior.

7 Among the relatively firmly established psychological differences between the sexes are the greater aggressiveness of males, their greater spatial-visual ability, and their greater mathematical ability; females excel in verbal ability.

8 Although some observed sex differences are genetically linked, many are culturally determined and therefore not an inevitable consequence of gender.

9 Sex, the activity and the topic, is highly significant to the adolescent. Masturbation is common among boys but less so among girls. Premarital sexual intercourse is more or less frequent, depending on the interpreter's point of view.

10 There is an intimate relationship between self-esteem and adjustment.

11 Adolescents may be frustrated by their inability to define their role and by the distance that they observe between the ideal world they contemplate and the one in which they live. Not all adolescents are frustrated, and some are less so than others.

12 Delinquency is a legal category that appears to include more lower-class than middle-class adolescents. Factors related to delinquency include sex, social class, self-esteem, home, and peer influences.

13 Only about 15 percent of college students join demonstrations and other similar amusements; many are pacific; very few are drug addicts; and some are sincere, well intentioned, and occasionally justified in their beliefs and demands.

14 The Indian hemp plant produces hashish, bhang, Acapulco gold, Maui wowie, grass, ganja, marijuana, grefa, pot, reefers, stick, and tea.

15 LSD-25 (d-lysergic acid diethylamine tartrate) is the most powerful known synthetic hallucinogenic drug. Both LSD and marijuana are nonaddictive, but both can cause psychoticlike reactions, although these are less common with marijuana.

16 Suicide is an uncommon end, although it accounted for at least 34 percent of all student deaths during a ten-year period at the University of California, Berkeley.

■ FURTHER READINGS

A highly comprehensive discussion of research on sex differences is found in:
Maccoby, E. E., & Jacklin, C. N. *The psychology of sex differences*. Stanford, Calif.: Stanford University Press, 1974.

Two readable books on male-female differences are:
Deaux, K. *The behavior of women and men*. Monterey, Calif.: Brooks/Cole, 1976.
Grambs, J. D., & Waetjen, W. B. *Sex: Does it make a difference?* North Scituate, Mass.: Duxbury Press, 1975.

A careful, contemporary consideration of factors involved in the development of sex roles and an examination of differences between male and female roles is provided by:
Sorensen, R. C. *Adolescent sexuality in contemporary America*. New York: World Publishing Co., 1973.
Wesley, F., & Wesley, C. *Sex-role psychology*. New York: Human Sciences Press, 1977.

There are numerous sources of information about drugs and their effects. Cohen's book is informative about recent trends. Ebin's book presents autobiographical and somewhat literary accounts of the effects of various drugs including marijuana, opium, peyote, and LSD. Among the various well-known authors who describe their drug experiences in this book are Allen Ginsberg, Havelock Ellis, Aldous Huxley, and Charles Baudelaire. Williams and Long present some very practical suggestions for coping with various behavioral problems including those relating to drinking and smoking.
Cohen, S. *The drug dilemma*. New York: McGraw-Hill, 1976.
Ebin, D. (Ed.). *The drug experience: First person accounts of addicts, writers, scientists and others*. New York: Orion Press, 1961.
Williams, R. L., & Long, J. D. *Toward a self-managed life style* (2nd ed.). Boston: Houghton Mifflin, 1978.

Information relating to the frequency and causes of student suicide is given in:
Klagsbrun, F. *Too young to die: Youth and suicide*. Boston: Houghton Mifflin, 1976.
Seiden, R. H. Campus tragedy: A study of students' suicide. *Journal of Abnormal Psychology*, 1966, *71*, 389–399.

For a more comprehensive description of adolescence, see:
Lefrancois, G. R. *Adolescents* (2nd ed.). Belmont, Calif.: Wadsworth, 1981.

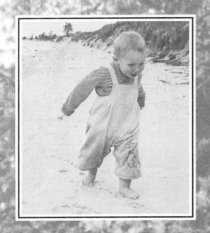

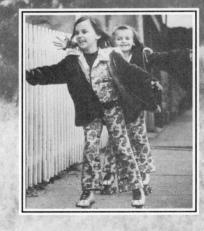

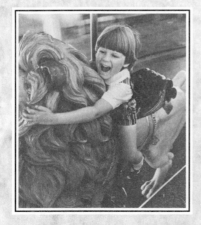

PART FIVE   ADULTHOOD

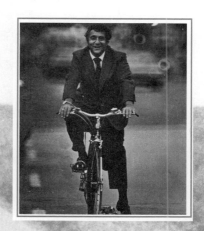

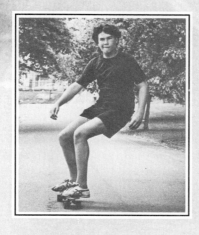

13

THEORIES OF ADULT DEVELOPMENT

What we call the beginning is often the end
And to make an end is to make a beginning
The end is where we start from.

We shall not cease from exploration
And the end of all our exploring
Will be to arrive where we started
And know the place for the first time.

T. S. Eliot
"Little Gidding"

I n Meadow Lake, at a small restaurant with the humble and rather common name "Cafe," I order what the menu calls a "hot hamburger sand." The description is optimistic, but I have little hunger. A "hot hamburger sand" could never come close to filling the void I sense.

The others eat with a gusto that I can scarcely even envy. Grandma, with bright-eyed anticipation, has ordered chicken. She who has killed, plucked, and cooked 10,000 plump, grain-fed chickens in her lifetime—perhaps even 20,000—now relishes the miserly left half of a scrawny, force-fed, six-week-old fryer. For her, eating in a restaurant, even one with a single, unstable kitchen table and a name like *cafe* is always a great treat.

"Eat," Grandma says gently, nodding at my plate. "Would you like a little of my chicken?"

"I've had lots," I answer. We both know it isn't true. I try to sip a little more coffee. It tastes very hot, and not much else. "I'll go gas up. Just come out when you're done." I leave money.

Outside the feeling is of late afternoon. In summer the sun sets reluctantly and briefly in these northern woods. And the afternoons stretch lazily far into that part of day that would be evening or even night elsewhere.

I fill the gas tank, check the oil, and inspect the tires. There is little else to do. I wait.

The waiting seems long. I know it really isn't. And I know, too, that I can usually wait for long periods with almost absolute patience; I have trained myself to do so. But now I have no patience. Instead, I am tormented by a mixture of confused emotions: It seems that the closer we get, the more I want to be there—and the more I am afraid.

Paul drives again. I offered quickly, before he could ask, knowing that he would and knowing that it is easier to offer, magnanimously, than simply to agree or disagree. He drives proudly, attentively, happy to be able to impress his grandmother.

"Stop!" I probably sound more urgent than I need to; Paul hits the brakes too hard, the tires screech, and we all lurch forward, still a long distance from where the man with the orange sock stands waving his arms in the middle of the highway. Next to him, in the ditch, the brown pickup—the same pickup that danced in the mirror behind us this morning and that weaved delicately in front of us in the afternoon. It has now woven its way off the highway and into a great muddy bog next to a poplar grove. Seven or eight Indians have climbed out of it, onto higher ground beyond the ditch. They now squat around a fire, warming their hands, talking, laughing. A great kettle steams on the fire.

"You got room for a wet Indian?" the man with the orange sock asks, grinning widely. Grandma opens her door and moves over at once.

"You guys don't drink all the tea," he shouts as he gets in; his friends laugh uproariously.

"Call me Tommy One Sock," he laughs again, holding up the foot with the sodden, muddy orange sock, "but my name is really Tommy Lachance."

Tommy smells faintly of poplar woodsmoke, black mud, and shaving lotion. He asks everybody's name, laughs gleefully at each, and proceeds to entertain the children and Grandma hugely with the story of how he and his friends all managed to crawl into the truck cab during the hailstorm. Then he launches into a second story, twice as funny he assures us. This one tells of how his friend, who doesn't have a driver's license yet, drove all the way from Ashmont without making a single important mistake, and how, just after they passed Meadow Lake, he stuck his head out the window to say something funny that he had just thought of to the guys in the back of the truck and drove right off the road into the ditch. At this point, Tommy One Sock laughs so hard he would surely fall over except that Grandma's shoulder bounces his head back upright once or twice. She and the children, easily infected by the contagious nature of his laughter, quickly fill the car with great hee haws, har hars, heh heh hehs, and several giggles. I control myself.

"And what's even funnier," Tommy continues when the laughter begins to subside, "was that Pete and Joey, who was sitting in the back, come flying over the top of the cab when we hit that mudhole. Pete, he bounced off the hood once on his head, and then it got buried in the mud, with just his two legs sticking out." Another great, side-aching burst of laughter, my family contributing their full share.

"And Joey, he never touched the cab. He just went sailing right over, about twenty feet in the air, flapping his arms like a big black goose, and hollering like he wanted to get somebody's attention. And he hit them poplars way up high in them little leaves and branches and got all tangled up and ended up perched in a tree about fifteen feet off the ground with one of his arms still flapping. And he was scared to climb down, so we had to coax him with a cup of tea."

In between guffaws, Tommy manages to inform Paul that he needs to get off right here by the corner, because his friend's house is here and he has a truck big enough to go and pick everybody up so they can go dancing at Rosie's house where Frank is playing fiddle tonight. Do we want to come, because we'd sure have a good time and Grandma'd probably sure like to dance to that fiddle? Grandma almost looks tempted as I say no, thank you, but we have a long way to go yet tonight.

"Stay on the road unless you like flying," are his last words, and his laughter follows us down the highway. Miles behind us now, I can still hear it echoing.

Is this unbridled *joie de vivre*, this madness and whimsy, normal in an adult? For Tommy and his friends are not eighteen or twenty, but more like thirty or even forty. Will our continuing tale of the lifespan tell us?

Let us turn to it quickly, before dusk begins to settle on the land, and see what we can discover of what is normal in the long space between adolescence and old age.

■ A Look Backward and Forward

In our travels through the lifespan, we have followed the gradual unfolding of the "average" child from the lucky union of two microscopic cells, through the stages of prenatal growth and birth, into infancy and childhood, and finally through adolescence—a period we labeled "a transition." Throughout the dozen chapters that tell this tale, we have repeatedly emphasized that there are numerous individual exceptions to the "normal" processes and stages of human development; at one point, we devoted almost an entire chapter to looking at the most extreme of these exceptions (in a section appropriately titled "exceptionality").

Very early, we also pointed out that although infants vary considerably one from the other immediately after birth, individual variation becomes far greater with increasing age. Thus, the predictions that psychology can make about the likely behaviors, capabilities, and personality characteristics of one-year-old infants are far more likely to be accurate than the predictions it might care to make about young adolescents. This is so, not only because our behaviors and personalities become more complex and more difficult to understand but also because our individual environments differ—sometimes dramatically—and accordingly affect us in very different ways. Partly for these two reasons, psychology has ventured only timidly and relatively recently into adulthood.

There is at least one other reason why developmental psychology has historically devoted itself mainly to childhood and adolescence. Our prevalent developmental models have historically maintained (implicitly if not explicitly) that development ends with adolescence. These models have viewed human development as a cumulative process of growth and development, beginning in infancy and culminating in adolescence. And adolescence has commonly been seen as a period of transition between the developmental progression of childhood and the stability of adulthood. Following adulthood, those of us who live so long (clearly an increasing number) then enter a final developmental period—one that proceeds, more or less rapidly, in a direction quite opposite to that which characterized our first eighteen or twenty years on this planet. This period, variously referred to as old age, aging, or senescence, has also been of some historical interest to developmental psychologists and is reflected in studies and courses that deal with *aging, geriatrics*, or *gerontology*.

In summary, our traditional, global view of the lifespan has emphasized the positive growth and development characteristic of childhood and adolescence, the stability of adulthood, and the relatively rapid decline of old age. How accurate is this view?

■ Theories of Adult Development

Our more recent models suggest that the traditional view of the lifespan is vastly oversimplified—that adulthood is characterized not only by considerable change but that in this change there is also potential for significant positive growth and development.

In Chapter 2, we looked in some detail at a number of developmental theories that relate primarily to children and adolescents (Freud's and Piaget's, for example) or that are general rather than strictly developmental (learning-theory approaches, for instance). These theories were covered early in the text, because they are important for understanding much of what comes between there and here. A number of other developmental theories that relate primarily to adult development are covered in this chapter where their placement is more useful. Note, however, that much of what was covered in the second chapter is also relevant to an understanding of adult development and behavior. A case in point is Erikson's psychosocial theory, which straddles the entire lifespan.

■ Erikson's Psychosocial Theory

Recall from Chapter 2 that Erikson's theory, based largely on the work of Freud, describes a series of eight stages through which individuals progress as they develop (Erikson, 1959). Each of these stages involves the resolution of an important conflict that arises out of the individual's *social* interaction—hence the label *psychosocial* theory. Progression from one stage to the next requires the resolution of this conflict, an achievement that evolves through the development of a new competence. The first of Erikson's stages, for example, is labeled *trust versus mistrust*. It describes a period in early infancy, in which the infant is beset by fear and mistrust about a strange and foreign world but also senses a need to trust the social environment. The competence that marks a successful transition from this stage to the next is expressed in the development of the ability to trust.

In similar fashion, the individual progresses through each of the remaining stages of childhood and adolescence: autonomy versus shame and doubt, initiative versus guilt, industry versus inferiority, and identity versus identity diffusion. Note, however, that the conflicts specific to each stage are never completely resolved during that stage, but continue, in one form or another, throughout life. But as we develop and grow, our social environments change, and as a result, so too do our most important conflicts.

With the advent of adulthood, the adult is faced with a series of new social demands that require additional adjustments. These too may be expressed in terms of competing tendencies, which give rise to crises of greater or lesser severity and which will be resolved through the development of new competencies. Erikson describes three developmental stages that span adulthood and old age: (1) intimacy and solidarity versus isolation, (2) generativity versus self-absorption, and (3) integrity versus despair.

Intimacy and Solidarity Versus Isolation   The search for identity does not end with puberty but continues through adolescence and beyond. One of the primary functions of adolescence is to serve as a period during which the child need not make a final decision concerning a self. "Negative identities," identities that are not ordinarily conducive to normal adjustment to society, can be experimented with during this period. Essentially, a negative identity simply retains negative aspects of earlier crises: mistrust, guilt, and so on. In a real sense, adolescents must incorporate into their identities the notion that at times they are also guilty and incompetent.

One of the principal ways in which adolescents and young adults arrive at a sense of worth and personal identity is through the development of feelings of intimacy with others, particularly with a person of the opposite sex for the heterosexual majority. The culmination of feelings of intimacy and solidarity (versus isolation) is, according to Erikson, most often found in a marriage.

Generativity Versus Self-Absorption   With increasing maturity, the adult is now faced with the task of establishing the sorts of caring and work relationships that will benefit the world and the community—in other words, of being generative

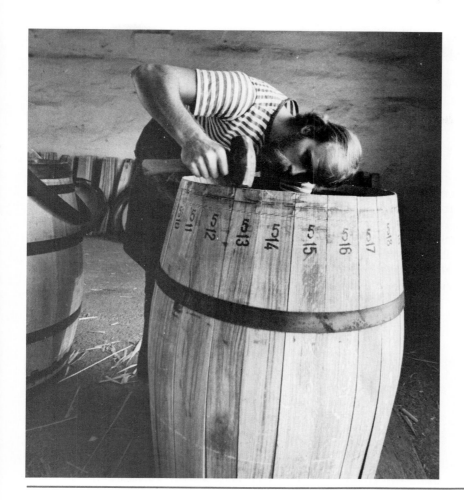

One of the important developmental tasks of adulthood is to assume productive, worthwhile roles—roles that are generative, or productive, rather than self-absorbed. These roles may be assumed at work, as shown here, or in relationships with family and community.

or productive rather than absorbed in self. People can become generative or productive in a number of areas. One is obviously in terms of work. As we note in Chapter 15, for a great many, work is far more than a means of earning a living or of "killing time." It can be a way of *being* someone, a means of self-discovery and self-expression, an essential aspect of feeling worthwhile, as well as a means of contributing to family and to society in significant ways. Another way of expressing generativity is through the establishment of a family, by producing children and acting as a parent. Note, again,

Erikson's continuing emphasis on the individual's relationship to the social-cultural environment.

Integrity Versus Despair   The last of Erikson's eight stages of life presents a conflict that will be resolved when (and if) the individual comes to realize that life has a meaning and integrity of its own. The basic conflict here is one between a sense that life is worthwhile and purposeful and the despair that can easily result as we contemplate the inevitability of our physical ends. Failure to develop this sense of worth may be accompanied by feelings of despair and by loneliness and depression. But for most elderly people, this is not the case; old age is often a time of happiness and contentment—of integrity rather than despair. (See Figure 13.1 for a summary of Erikson's theory.)

Peck's Elaboration of Erikson

A number of theorists have criticized the global and rather vague descriptions of development provided by Erikson, particularly with respect to the adult years. Among them, Peck (1968) suggests that the last two stages, spanning the last forty or fifty years of life, are not detailed enough to take into account some of the critical issues during those years. Accordingly, he suggests a number of additional crises related primarily to the physical and mental changes of adulthood, as well as to some of the more common social changes. These crises describe an additional seven stages, the first four of which are applicable primarily to middle age (around thirty-five to sixty-five); the last three relate to old age (see Figure 13.1).

Valuing Wisdom Versus Valuing Physical Powers   Among the important physical changes of middle age is a gradual decline in stamina, elasticity, muscle tone, and other components of strength, endurance, and athletic prowess. Thus it becomes progressively more difficult for laborers to toil without pain, for professional athletes to continue participating in their sports, or even for fathers to beat their sons at racquet sports or Indian leg wrestling. As these changes occur, it becomes more important for individuals to place greater emphasis on qualities other than those relating solely to the physical. The athlete must develop other competencies, the laborer must work differently or change employment, and the father might consider less physically demanding sports, such as bowling, curling, or billiards, or more cerebral competitions, such as chess or poker—hence the label for this particular psychosocial conflict.

Socializing Versus Sexuality   In the same way as physical powers decline, so too are there often changes in sexual interest, behavior, or capability. And some of the important interpersonal relation-

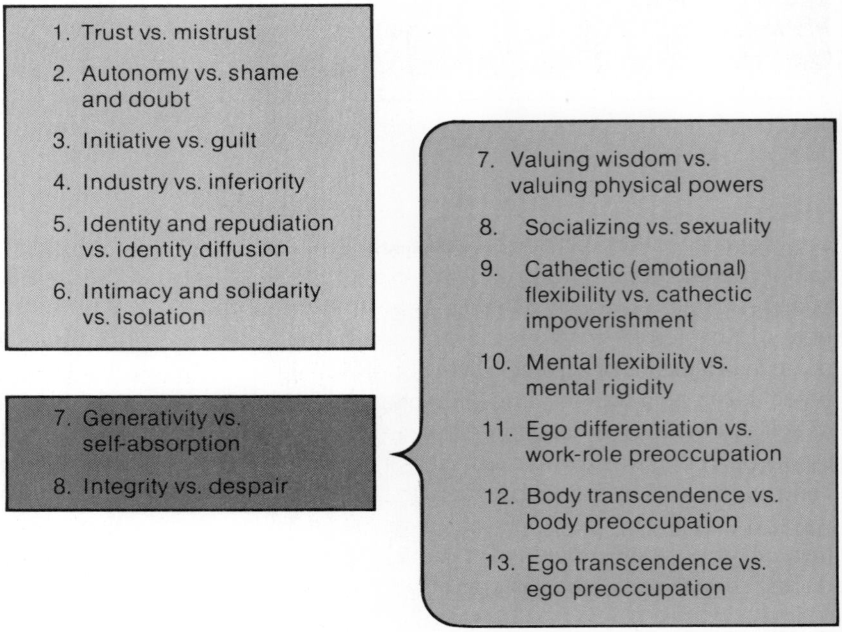

Figure 13.1
Erikson's theory revised. Peck defines seven additional adult development tasks during the last two stages of Erikson's scheme.

1. Trust vs. mistrust
2. Autonomy vs. shame and doubt
3. Initiative vs. guilt
4. Industry vs. inferiority
5. Identity and repudiation vs. identity diffusion
6. Intimacy and solidarity vs. isolation

7. Generativity vs. self-absorption
8. Integrity vs. despair

7. Valuing wisdom vs. valuing physical powers
8. Socializing vs. sexuality
9. Cathectic (emotional) flexibility vs. cathectic impoverishment
10. Mental flexibility vs. mental rigidity
11. Ego differentiation vs. work-role preoccupation
12. Body transcendence vs. body preoccupation
13. Ego transcendence vs. ego preoccupation

ships that characterize early adulthood, and that might initially have had a strong sexual component, change accordingly. Friendship, trust, emotional and moral support, companionship, and other dimensions of social relationships become more important as sexuality loses some importance.

Emotional Flexibility Versus Emotional Impoverishment   The various crises and conflicts described by Erikson and Peck stem, in large part, from social and physical changes in the lives of individuals. These changes, in turn, require adaptation and change in the individual. The third of Peck's stages is a particularly good illustration of this need for adaptability. Through middle age (sometimes much earlier and sometimes much later), many of our emotional ties are strained or ruptured for any of a variety of reasons: People die, children leave home, couples separate and get divorced, careers end, and dogs run away. Adjusting to these emotional changes often requires considerable emotional flexibility.

Mental Flexibility Versus Mental Rigidity   In the same way as changes in our emotional lives require us to be able to form new relationships and sometimes to forget old ones, so too do a variety of social and cultural changes require us to accept new ideas and sometimes to reject old ones. Hence the need for mental flexibility—we cannot always rely on old beliefs and opinions or on old attitudes.

Ego Differentiation Versus Work-Role Preoccupation   According to our current models, development does not end with middle age but continues well into old age. With retirement, for example, it often becomes necessary to develop new interests—to shift one's preoccupations from work and career to other aspects of living. In the same way, as children leave home, preoccupations centered on parenting must be abandoned, but they need to be replaced if the individual is to maintain a sense of integrity and worth.

Body Transcendence Versus Body Preoccupation   One of the common prices we pay for

our longer lives is a longer period during which we are beset by aches, pains, and disabilities of greater or lesser severity. As these become more evident, there is a tendency to become preoccupied with affairs of the body. Resolution of the resulting psychosocial conflict requires that the individual's preoccupation *transcend* the flesh.

Ego Transcendence Versus Ego Preoccupation   In the same way as the aging individual must transcend preoccupation with bodily aches and pains, so too is there a need to transcend a concomitant preoccupation with the inevitability of death. Those who fear death unduly must also fear life, for one is surely the price we pay for the other.

Erikson and Peck: A Summary

Erikson and Peck present a theory that describes human development in terms of progression through a series of stages, each of which is characterized by a basic conflict. Progression through each stage requires resolution of the conflict, a process that generally involves the development of a new set of attitudes, behaviors, or preoccupations—in Erikson's terms, some new social competence. None of the conflicts is ever completely resolved at a given stage, so that each of us, throughout life, carries remnants of old fears, insecurities, and conflicts (Freudian influence).

The first five of Erikson's eight stages deal specifically with development from infancy through adolescence; the last three relate to adulthood and old age. Peck's elaboration of Erikson's theory involves the description of seven separate stages (psychosocial conflicts) to replace the last two of Erikson's eight stages, in an attempt to provide a more detailed and more realistic portrayal of the many important developmental events that fill the long spread of years from the onset of adulthood to death.

Theories such as those of Erikson and Peck do not lend themselves easily to specific age-related predictions for any given individual. Nor can they easily be validated experimentally. Their principal

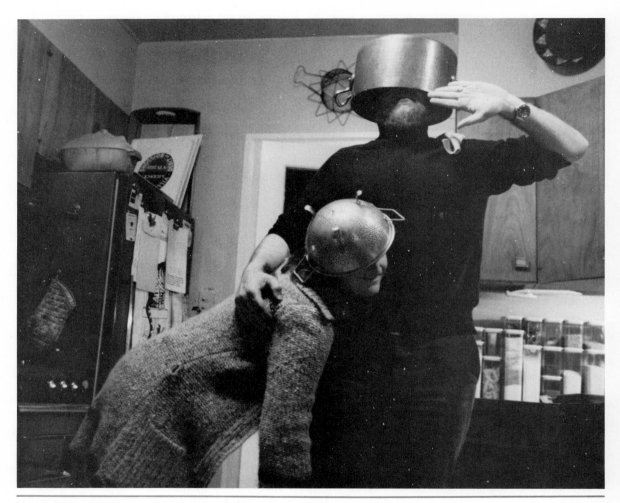

Friendship, trust, companionship, and just plain silliness often become more important as sexual interest and sexual activity decline.

usefulness lies in the insights they provide for understanding the concerns and preoccupations of adults.

■ Levinson's Seasons

In a widely read book, Levinson (1978) attempts to organize the lives of forty men around common, universal themes and changes. These men, aged between thirty-five and forty-five, belong to four occupational groups, with ten subjects in each group: novelists, biologists, business executives, and industrial workers. Each subject was interviewed in depth during a series of between five and ten separate meetings, each lasting an hour or more, and all were interviewed again two years following the initial series of interviews. In Levinson's (1978) term, these were *biographical interviews*, intended to uncover the sequence of each man's life, the major changes in that sequence, and the forces underlying these changes.

Following these interviews, Levinson (1977, 1978, 1981; Levinson, Darrow, Klein, Levinson, & McKee, 1976) advanced a lifespan developmental theory—an account of *the seasons of a man's life*. Like Erikson's and Peck's accounts, this too is a psychosocial theory: It deals primarily with psychological and social change and their relationship to one another. Also like those of Erikson and Peck, it may be described as a theory of *developmental crisis*, although Levinson emphasizes crises somewhat less than does Erikson.

The Five Ages of Man

Levinson (1981) suggests that the human lifespan divides itself roughly into five major *eras* or *ages*, each lasting twenty to twenty-five years, although age boundaries overlap somewhat. These he labels as follows: preadulthood (birth to twenty-two); early adulthood (seventeen to forty-five); middle adulthood (forty to sixty-five); late adulthood (sixty to eighty-five); and late late adulthood (eighty to death). Clearly, not all of our spans will spread so far.

Since the oldest of Levinson's forty subjects was only forty-five at the time of the initial studies, most of his detailed analyses are limited to early adulthood and the first few years of middle adulthood. Within these eras, he identifies a sequence of stages that appear to be common to each of the forty subjects. These are described briefly here and summarized in Figure 13.2.

Early Adult Transition All of Levinson's developmental periods may be described in terms of a major developmental task. The period begins when the task becomes predominant in the person's life, and it ends with its resolution and with the recognition of the next developmental task.

In the first of Levinson's periods, the developmental task that predominates involves separating from the immediate family and beginning to establish an independent, adultlike identity. This period of transition between pre- and early adulthood often begins during the late teen years and may last until the age of twenty-two or so. Labeled "youth" by a number of writers (Coleman, 1974,

for example), this period corresponds closely with the Erikson stage labeled "identity versus role diffusion." For many of Levinson's subjects, attending college was probably the major transitional event (70 percent completed college). However, this was not true of the workers' group; only two of them had any college experience and half had not completed high school.

Entering the Adult World Following the transition between pre- and early adulthood, the person is now faced with two somewhat contradictory tasks. The first is to explore the variety of adult roles that might be suitable for the person's skills, temperament, and inclinations. These roles are not limited to work or career but include, as well, important decisions concerning peer relationships, marriage, and general life style.

The second important developmental task of this period involves the establishment of some degree of stability with respect to adult roles. Thus on the one hand, the period is one of exploration and tentative choice; on the other, it requires commitment and stability. And, as Levinson (1978) notes, finding a workable balance between these two tasks is not always easy. If the young adult explores too long without commitment, the succeeding life may seem rootless and meaningless. But if commitment occurs too strongly and too early, there is a danger that the best choice will not have been explored. Some of the occasional turmoil of adolescence may also be the turmoil of youth and young adulthood.

The period that Levinson labels "entering the adult world" begins in the early twenties and generally ends toward the end of that decade. Its ending is often characterized by the adoption of what Levinson refers to as a "dream." This dream is an idealized sort of fantasy that includes the goals and aspirations of the dreamer. In one sense, the dream is a tentative blueprint for our lives.

Age Thirty Transition The period of entering the adult world is followed by an approximately five-year transition period appropriately labeled "age thirty transition." During these five years of transition (between ages twenty-eight and thirty-

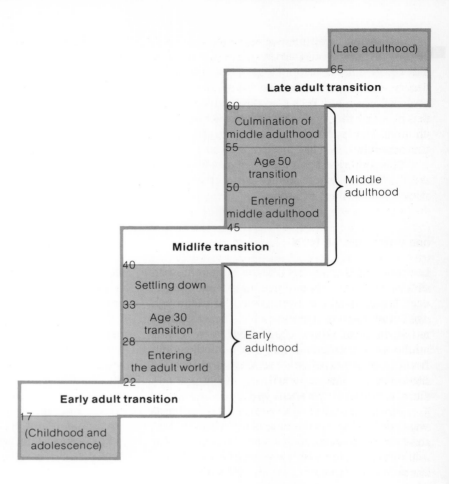

Figure 13.2
Levinson's description of major developmental periods through early and middle adulthood. (From D. J. Levinson et al., *The seasons of a man's life.* Copyright © 1978 by Daniel J. Levinson. Reprinted by permission of Alfred A. Knopf, Inc.)

The figure shows, from bottom to top, with ages marked: (Childhood and adolescence), 17, Early adult transition, 22, Entering the adult world, 28, Age 30 transition, 33, Settling down, 40 — Early adulthood; Midlife transition, 45, Entering middle adulthood, 50, Age 50 transition, 55, Culmination of middle adulthood, 60 — Middle adulthood; Late adult transition, 65, (Late adulthood).

three), individuals are faced with the task of re-evaluating the choices made during the preceding period and are required to make some fundamental decisions concerning these choices. Specifically, it is necessary to commit oneself even more firmly to initial choices regarding work and life style or to change these commitments before too little of the lifespan is left to make the dream come true. Not surprisingly, during this transitory period, Levinson's subjects were most likely to change occupations or to seek divorce.

The three stages described thus far are referred to as "novice" phases of early adulthood; they are primarily a preparation for years yet to come. Hence the age thirty transition is of absolutely critical importance. Levinson (1978) argues that if the "life

structure" (work and life-style) decisions adopted at the termination of this transitory period are consistent with the individual's talents, capabilities, and personality predispositions, as well as with his dreams, the basis will have been laid for a rich and satisfying life. In contrast, if the final choices and commitments are inadequate and inappropriate, the individual may suffer gravely in the next period.

Settling Down   The major developmental task of the *settling down* period is to "make it" in all important areas touched by the dream: social, career related, economic, political, family related, and so on. In describing the tasks of this period, Levinson (1978) repeatedly uses the analogy of the "ladder"—the proverbial ladder that all successful men must climb. Its various rungs may be tied to specific promotion or salary timetables that individuals set for themselves ("I want to be vice-president by the time I'm thirty-five"). The individual's sense of worth and of accomplishment are often tied directly to his own perception of where he is on the ladder, as well as to how he thinks important others evaluate his progress.

The settling down period lasts from around age thirty-three to approximately forty. Levinson also identifies another phase that appears during the last four or five years of this period (ages thirty-five to forty, approximately). Labeled "becoming one's own man," it is characterized by feelings of frustration at not being completely autonomous and independent. At this point, for example, the majority of Levinson's subjects felt that work superiors, family members, and society in general exercised too much control over them. During this phase, the major developmental task continues to be the same as it was earlier during the settling down period: specifically, to achieve success in the chosen career, life style, and community. But now there is added emphasis on reaffirmation as an important, autonomous individual. Job promotions and other external signs of success and acceptance often become very important to the individual. Consequently, their absence can have important consequences for the individual's happiness and satisfaction.

The Midlife Transition   Probably the most highly popularized of all adult develomental stages is the midlife transition—often referred to as the *midlife crisis*. It lasts from about forty to forty-five and is characterized by a number of developmental tasks, all of which are related to evaluating one's life in relation to earlier commitments. The urgency of these tasks is aggravated by a fundamental change that now occurs in the individual's perception of time—and in this change lie the roots of the midlife crisis. Specifically, as Neugarten (1968) put it, our notions of the relationship between our own lives and time change from a perspective that can be described in terms of "time from birth" (age, in other words) to one preoccupied with "time until death." Any of a variety of what Levin-

son calls "marker events" can contribute dramatically to this change in time perspective: death of parents, children leaving home, death of friends and age peers, sickness, and so on. Following these and a variety of less dramatic events (such as being beaten at racquetball or golf by one's son), individuals become progressively more conscious of their own mortality and of the idea that there may not be enough time for the dream. For a great many, it now becomes fundamentally important to modify the dream—to change commitments and life styles and to begin to emphasize those aspects of life that might have been neglected. For some men, the result is a resolution to spend more time with family and friends—and perhaps less with work and career. For others, it might involve a complete abdication of earlier responsibilities and commitments—and new commitments to what are sometimes dramatically different life styles. Some middle-aged individuals do, in fact, "drop out."

Entering Middle Adulthood   Individuals enter middle adulthood at around age forty-five. Some bring with them renewed commitment to family and career; others, following the crises of the preceding period, enter middle adulthood with new commitments and new life styles. All, according to Levinson (1978), experience fundamental change following the midlife transition, even if they continue in the same external roles. Detailed examinations of the lives of his subjects leads him to observe that there are typically changes in relationships with work, family, and others—sometimes for better and sometimes for worse. Thus there is tremendous variation in the extent to which men find their lives satisfactory during this period.

Subsequent Periods   Unfortunately, Levinson's subjects were too young to provide detailed information concerning later periods of the lifespan. Accordingly, Levinson (1978) provides only a quick sketch of developmental phases after the age of forty-five. He suggests that at around age fifty, another period of transition involves tasks very similar to those of the midlife transition: namely, to re-examine accomplishments and relationships in relation to the dream espoused in early adulthood. For those who have accomplished this task inadequately in their early forties, there may be a crisis similar to that of the midlife; for others, the period may be relatively free of turmoil.

Following this period of transition, there is a relatively stable, "settled" period during which the individual's career will begin to end. In a final period of transition, bridging middle and late adulthood, the key tasks will involve reconciling the dream with reality, accepting again the notion of one's own mortality, and preparing for what are sometimes drastic changes brought about by retirement and all that it entails.

A Summary of Levinson's Theory

Levinson's theory of the adult lifespan, applicable to males and limited largely to ages preceding forty-five, is essentially a *crisis* theory. It describes major tasks during developmental phases that last between five and seven years. These tasks typically involve making important choices concerning life style and career.

In an overly simplified sense, the primary preoccupation during early adulthood revolves around work: climbing the "ladder," being recognized, achieving success, being somebody in the community. Between ages forty and forty-five, the individual confronts his dreams and evaluates his life in relation to earlier goals and ambitions. This confrontation often translates itself into a crisis ("Where am I going? What do I want out of life? What is really important?"). Subsequently, work and external marks of success may become less important; the self and the family, more.

It is revealing that a number of other studies of the lifespan present a global picture highly similar to that advanced by Levinson. For example, Vaillant's (1977) study of ninety-five Harvard graduates (classes of 1922–1924) reveals a period of commitment to work and success during early adulthood, a critical period of reappraisal at the midlife, and a tendency to become more concerned with "the world within" following this midlife crisis. Similarly, Sheehy's (1976) journalistic account of the lives of 115 men and women also describes a developmental progression very much like that described by Levinson. We look briefly at Sheehy's descriptions next.

■ Sheehy's Passages

Sheehy (1976), a journalist, suggests that the word *crisis* is often misinterpreted—that we interpret it too seriously. It hints of impending catastrophe, of calamity just a short distance around the corner. For this reason, crisis is not entirely appropriate to describe most of the events that characterize the adult lifespan—hence her use of the term *passages* in its place.

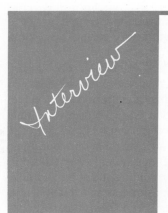

Subject: Male; age forty-six; divorced; no children; involved in film business.

Question: "Do you think you experienced a midlife transition or crisis?"

Do I! I have a couple every week. Seriously, though, sure. Doesn't everybody? I mean, there was a period, there, just about the time I turned forty, when I figured—I guess I just wasn't that certain anymore. Here I was, forty, I'd been divorced for about three years, and I was feeling an awful lot of pressure about deciding if I was ever going to get married again and about whether I was going to have kids. I mean, at forty it didn't seem like I had forever left anymore, and whatever I was going to do I better get on and do it. And then I thought, "What the heck, Bob, you're doing exactly what you want to do, so go with the flow." Maybe that's my philosophy. "Go with the flow."

Sheehy's study of our individual passages through adulthood involved collecting detailed biographical histories of 115 men and women, the majority of whom were couples. They ranged from eighteen to fifty-five years of age and represented a wide variety of social levels and occupations. Among them were high-achieving women and men, as well as those who walk through life more modestly. Accordingly, the biographies provide useful information for examining the lives of women as well as men and provide a more balanced description of the lifespan than is possible with Levinson's all-male sample.

The Stages

Sheehy's stages are essentially identical to Levinson's; only their labels have been changed. Thus the *early adult transition* becomes *pulling up roots*. The expression is descriptive and accurate. Similarly, *entering the adult world* is *the trying twen-*

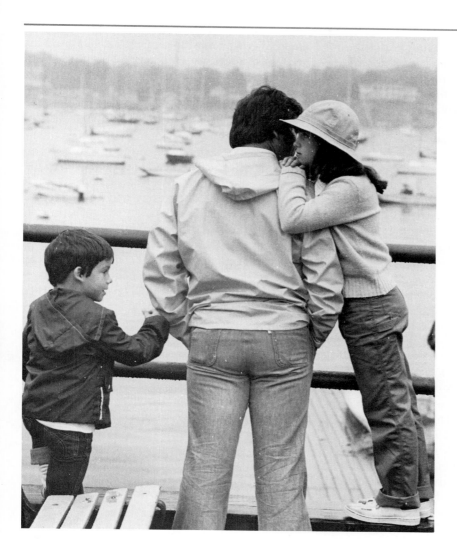

The "midlife crisis," which may occur around age 40 in men, sometimes leads to a de-emphasis on career-oriented goals and a new or renewed emphasis on self, family, and relationships. Among women the "midlife passage" often occurs earlier and frequently leads to renewed interest in achievement-related goals.

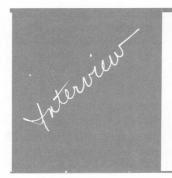

Subject: Female; age forty-eight; widowed; two children, both independent; manager of a cleaning business.

Question: "Do you think you experienced a midlife transition or crisis?"

What the heck is that? My whole life is a bloody crisis! . . .

I get'cha, but the answer is no, I never had no crisis like that. I was too bloody busy bringin' up the kids and tryin' to make ends meet which they never did. If my husband hadn't of died, I might've had enough time. No, I'm afraid I can't help you there at all.

ties; *age thirty transition* becomes *Catch 30; settling down* is *rooting and extending; midlife transition* is *the deadline decade;* and *entering middle adulthood* becomes *renewal or resignation.*

As their labels imply, the major developmental tasks that Sheehy describes for each of these stages are also very similar to those of Levinson's theory. Thus, *the trying twenties* describe a period in which the individual begins attempting to carve a niche in the adult world, when initial choices of career and life style are made. *Catch 30* describes a transition between this first phase of adulthood and the next period, when life style becomes more firmly anchored and where the emphasis is largely on stability and on "making it" (*rooting and extending*). In the next developmental phase, *the deadline decade*, Sheehy departs most significantly from Levinson. This phase, corresponding to the *midlife transition*, is accorded a longer age span by Sheehy (ages thirty-five to forty-five, compared with thirty-eight to forty-three). Other researchers tend to support Sheehy's observation that midlife crises can occur during a much wider age range than Levinson suggests. For example, Vaillant (1977) suggests that critical midlife changes can occur at any time between ages thirty to fifty.

A second important observation made by Sheehy concerns male-female differences. Specifically, Sheehy notes that although the general developmental pattern of men and women is highly similar, the midlife *passage* often occurs considerably earlier for women—frequently at around

age thirty-five (compared to forty or forty-five for men). Perhaps most important, resolution of this crisis sometimes takes a dramatically different form among men and women.

As we saw earlier, both Levinson and Vaillant describe very similar patterns of development among men to and beyond the midlife crisis. To oversimplify somewhat, men spend much of their early twenties deciding on a "life structure," commit themselves to their early decisions during the thirties, subject their lives to profound re-examination around the age of forty, and frequently end up more concerned with family and self than with aggressive, achievement-related goals after the midlife crisis (see *Seasons and Passages for Teachers*).

In contrast to this general male pattern, Sheehy suggests not only that women begin their re-examination of goals and priorities considerably earlier but also that the resolution of any resulting crisis often takes the form of greater assertiveness and more achievement-oriented goals. Thus, whereas many men become more passive, more oriented toward *feeling*—perhaps more "feminine"—many women become more active, more aggressive—perhaps a little more "masculine." As Sheehy notes, one of the ways in which couples can sometimes resolve their midlife dilemmas and find new excitement and meaning in the next decades is to "renegotiate" traditional roles. Perhaps the wife can contribute salary and vacations to the family—and the husband can provide nurturance, clean clothing, and pot roasts.

SEASONS AND PASSAGES FOR TEACHERS

Declining birthrates means fewer babies, fewer school children, and ultimately fewer teaching positions. Fewer teaching positions means fewer young teachers. And, in the end, what all this means is a graying and increasingly stable teaching force. Whereas perhaps 40 percent of all teachers are now over the age of forty, projections are that by the turn of this decade, more than 80 percent will be.

And how do teachers age and develop with respect to their lives and careers? Miller and Taylor (1983) interviewed 56 elementary and secondary school teachers and presented questionnaires to another 383. The questions dealt primarily with job satisfaction and career aspirations. Responses were analyzed in terms of the extent to which they revealed patterns similar to those described by Levinson and Sheehy.

How do teacher aspirations and expressions of satisfaction compare with the general developmental pattern? Remarkably well, according to Miller and Taylor. For example, teachers in their twenties expressed more *dissatisfaction* with their careers than other age groups and spent more time questioning goals and career decisions. But, as Levinson's model would predict, after the age of thirty there is a renewed focus on career for male teachers. This is not yet the case for women; for many, the primary focus is still on family and on goals related to child rearing.

For male teachers, work satisfaction and commitment are both high during their thirties. And a great many have, as part of the *dreams* they have formulated in their thirties, aspirations related to administrative, supervisory, or consulting positions in education. But by the age of forty, an increasing number have become dissatisfied with opportunities for promotion and are being forced to re-examine their goals and priorities. Not surprisingly, most teachers over age forty-five no longer aspire to more advanced positions.

Male-female differences in career aspirations and commitment also appear to correspond closely with what would be predicted on the basis of Levinson and Sheehy's models. Thus, women tend to become career oriented later than men (around age thirty-five rather than thirty) and continue to express strong aspirations longer than men do. Thus, while men are beginning to re-examine careers and, in many instances, to shift some of their emphases from career to self, home, and family, many women are moving in the opposite direction. For

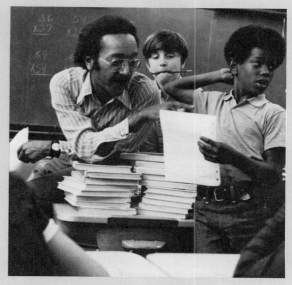

As Levinson's model predicts, there is often a renewed focus on career for male teachers after the age of thirty. For female teachers, families and child-rearing remain the primary focus until after age 35.

them, the shift is from home and family toward career. Miller and Taylor caution, however, that this does not mean that men and women abandon previous commitments during this *crossover* but simply that they begin to accept additional roles and to reallocate priorities.

What are the implications of observations such as these? Are they of value to anyone? Clearly, yes. To begin with, they might contribute in important ways to greater knowledge of self and to a clearer understanding of motives, aspirations, and emotions. And it is not unreasonable to suppose that greater self-knowledge might lead to wiser or happier decisions. At a more practical level, knowledge of likely concerns and preoccupations during the working years of the lifespan might be of tremendous value to managements that are concerned with the development and welfare of their workers; such understanding could lead to some innovative and useful programs in the work place.

■ Gould's Transformations

One final description of the adult phase of the human lifespan is presented in this chapter: that formulated by Gould (1972, 1978). Gould studied a relatively large sample (more than 500 individuals) and included both men and women between the ages of sixteen and sixty. What was most unusual about this sample, however, was that members were outpatients at a psychiatric clinic (at the University of California, Los Angeles), involved in group therapy. Subjects in this sample were divided into different groups according to age and were interviewed by psychiatrists, who attempted to uncover feelings and statements that would be most characteristic of each age group. In this way, Gould hoped to arrive at a sequential description of important changes in the adult lifespan. Following these initial interviews, questionnaires were sent to a sample of 524 individuals who were *not* psychiatric patients. These questionnaires were based primarily on patients' statements that appeared to be characteristic of specific age groups. This aspect of the study was intended simply to corroborate initial findings and to establish that the patient population was not fundamentally different from a nonpatient population.

Gould's description of adult development is summarized in Table 13.1. At first glance, it appears to be very similar to that advanced by Levinson and Sheehy. Thus early preoccupations center on separating from the family and establishing an adult identity (work, family, social responsibility); crises occur at around age thirty and again at forty, the latter being tied to a recognition of mortality and a sense of urgency with respect to goals.

Closer examination reveals that Gould's *transformations* present a different emphasis than do Levinson's *seasons* or Sheehy's *passages*. Gould, a psychiatrist, is concerned less with the individual's relationship to work, career, dreams and family and more with the person's *self-consciousness*— that is, with the individual's understanding of the self and with the gradual transformations that change a child's *consciousness* into adult consciousness. Thus, development is described through developmental tasks that involve getting rid of the false, "childish" assumptions of early years and replacing them with more adult assumptions. For example, between ages sixteen and twenty-two, the principal false (or immature) assumption that dominates the individual's life concerns the rightness of parents: "I'll always want to be with my parents and believe in them—and they can always rescue me if I need help." Accordingly, the major developmental task of this early period is that of leaving home—but not simply in a physical sense. To really "leave" home is to discard these false

Table 13.1 Gould's transformations.

Age	Major False Assumptions	Major Tasks
16–22	"My parents will always be my parents. I'll always believe in them."	Moving away from home; abandon idea that parents are always right.
22–28	"If I want to succeed, I need to do things the way my parents do." "If I make mistakes and need rescuing, they'll rescue me."	Become independent; explore adult roles; abandon idea that things will always turn out if done in the manner of parents.
28–34	"Life is pretty straightforward, especially if you're on the right track. There aren't too many contradictions."	Explore aspects of inner self; become more sensitive to emotions; begin to realize inner contradictions.
34–45	"I have all the time I need. I am doing the right thing."	Recognize and accept idea of one's own mortality; develop strong sense of personal responsibility. Reassess values and priorities.

assumptions concerning the rightness and potency of parents and to accept that parents can be wrong. External manifestations of this process might well include moving from home physically, working or studying independently, and beginning to make decisions concerning one's personal future life style.

In a similar fashion, progress through the lifespan requires shedding a variety of other false assumptions and adopting others that are more realistic (see Table 13.1). The result, according to Gould, is greater self-understanding and greater self-acceptance.

■ A Brief Summary of Lifespan Theories

In this chapter, we have looked at four "stage" theories of adult development. Each is summarized very briefly in this section.

Erikson's *crisis* theory describes a series of eight psychosocial stages that spread across the lifespan. The first five pertain to preadult years; only the last three deal specifically with adulthood. Each of these eight stages is identified in terms of a conflict relating to the individual's need to adjust to social reality—a conflict manifested in two opposing tendencies (for example, tendencies to be isolated and independent versus tendencies toward establishing intimate relationships during the period of transition between home and outside). The resolution of conflicts at each stage results in a new sense of competency and self-worth and prepares the individual for the next developmental stage.

Levinson's description of *the seasons of a man's life* is based on detailed interviews with forty men belonging to four occupational groups (novelists, biologists, business executives, and industrial workers). He describes a series of stages characterized by specific developmental tasks (for example, getting away from home and settling down) and a number of transition periods between major stages, these occurring at around the turn of each decade. Thus there is a transition from adolescence to early adulthood at approximately age twenty; an "age thirty transition," a well-popular-

ized "midlife transition" at around forty, and an "age fifty transition." The emphasis in Levinson's description of the lifespan is on the man's relationship to his career, family, and goals ("dreams").

Sheehy's description of *passages* resembles Levinson's, although it is based on a study of women and men. She too describes a series of developmental phases based largely on the individual's relationship to work, family, and self and punctuated by transition periods that constitute crises (*passages* is her gentler term) of greater or lesser severity. Her notable departures from Levinson include two observations. First, the midlife crisis can occur considerably earlier or later than Levinson's study suggests (at ages thirty to fifty, as opposed to an approximately five-year span around age forty), and it typically occurs earlier for women than for men. Second, resolution of the midlife crisis is often very different among men and women. Whereas men frequently become more tender—more concerned with emotions and family—women often become more assertive and aggressive—more concerned with interrupted dreams and careers.

Gould's account of *transformations* is oriented toward discovering uniformities in how individuals relate to parents and to self through adulthood. It describes how our typical childish consciousness, characterized by false and immature assumptions concerning self and parents, is gradually replaced by more realistic and more mature assumptions.

■ Words of Caution

Early in this chapter, we noted that there is tremendous variation among human beings and that this variation becomes progressively greater with the passing of years. Thus pairs of infants selected at random are likely to resemble each other far more than random pairs of adults. The point is worth repeating again. Although our lifespan developmental theories might give us convenient guidelines within which to interpret the lives of a specific individual, they must also admit uncounted exceptions. And the number of these exceptions will increase with increasing age. Thus our theories are likely to suffer from fewer exceptions in infancy and in adolescence than they will at midlife.

A second important caution, one made by Brim (1976), concerns the danger of overemphasizing those aspects of the life cycle that have been most highly dramatized in popular writings. Chief among these, of course, is the midlife crisis, the inevitability and seriousness of which have sometimes been grossly exaggerated (Rossi, 1980).

Third, our current lifespan theories are sometimes based on quasi-anecdotal research or on observations limited to relatively small groups of individuals who are not always highly representative of the general population. Gould's sample of psychiatric outpatients is one example; Levinson's all-male group of only 40 individuals is another, as is Sheehy's 115 largely middle-class, work-oriented couples. It has not yet been established that the resulting lifespan models are widely applicable to other groups.

Fourth, none of this research has been able to take into account the possibility that observed developmental sequences are particular to the cohorts under investigation and might not apply to different cohorts. As Rossi (1980) notes, almost all subjects used thus far in this type of research were born between 1920 and the early 1930s. Jacobs (1979), in describing this cohort, emphasizes that its relation to the Depression, involvement in the Second World War (though sometimes in very different ways), and its adjustment to rapid changes in the postwar years (including bringing up children during the social unrest of the 1960s) would necessarily have a profound influence on it. Clearly, our lives do not unfold in our personal, individual vacuums—though it might sometimes seem that way. Although understanding the concept of the midlife crisis might be very useful for understanding the lives of the 1920s cohort, it might be of absolutely no value in trying to understand the lives of our children when they are forty. Their crises might occur on the heels of some nuclear catastrophe, the magnitude of which we have yet to imagine, or they might never occur.

■ MAIN POINTS

1 It is worth emphasizing that there are numerous exceptions to the "normal" processes and stages of development.

2 Our prevalent developmental models have been concerned primarily with childhood and adolescence and, to a lesser extent, with old age. More recent models also include the adult years.

3 Erikson has advanced a psychosocial, ego-oriented theory of human development, premised partly on Freud's theories but more culturally based.

4 According to Erikson, the individual progresses through a series of stages characterized by basic conflicts, the resolution of which results in the appearance of new capabilities and attitudes.

5 Erikson's stages are, in order: trust versus mistrust, autonomy versus shame and doubt, initiative versus guilt, industry versus inferiority, indentity versus identity diffusion, intimacy versus isolation, generativity versus stagnation, and integrity versus despair. Only the last three of these relate to adulthood.

6 Peck proposes seven additional psychosocial crises that occur during Erikson's last two major stages and that take into account some additional important adjustments required in middle and old age. The first four of these apply primarily to middle age (approximately to age sixty-five); the last three apply to old age.

7 Peck's stages, with self-explanatory labels, are: valuing wisdom versus valuing physical means, socializing versus sexuality, emotional flexibility versus emotional impoverishment, mental flexibility versus mental rigidity, ego differentiation versus work-role preoccupation, body transcendence versus body preoccupation, and ego transcendence versus ego preoccupation.

8 Following biographical interviews with forty men representing four different work roles (novelists, biologists, business executives, and industrial workers), Levinson describes uniformities that he maintains apply to all of our lives; they are the *seasons* of our lives.

9 Levinson describes five "ages" in our lifespans: preadulthood (birth to twenty-two); early adulthood (seventeen to forty-five); middle adulthood (forty to sixty-five); late adulthood (sixty to eighty-five); and late late adulthood (eighty to death).

10 According to Levinson's investigations, early and middle adulthood are characterized by a number of developmental phases, each of which may be identified in terms of one or more important developmental tasks (for example, leaving home and making life-style decisions). Between these major phases, there are important transition periods, occurring at approximately the turn of each decade (ages twenty, thirty, forty, and so on).

11 The most highly popularized of transition periods in adult life is the midlife transition—also called the midlife crisis. Levinson suggests it occurs at around age forty and that it entails a serious re-examination of the individual's life, particularly in relation to earlier goals and ambitions ("dreams"). One of the significant changes related to the occurrence of the midlife crisis is a recognition of one's mortality.

12 Sheehy describes *passages* through the lifespan, claiming that the term *crisis* is too strong, too suggestive of impending calamity. Her descriptions are based on interviews with 115 couples and are highly similar to Levinson's *seasons,* except with respect to her observations that (1) the midlife crisis spans a wider age range (thirty to fifty rather than four or five years around age forty) and occurs earlier for women than for men, and (2) whereas resolution of the midlife crisis often results in a "turning inward" among men (becoming more concerned with self, family, and emotion), the opposite is often true among women.

13 Gould describes a number of *transformations* whereby a childish consciousness, characterized by false and immature assumptions (particularly concerning the infallibility and power of parents), is gradually replaced by a more adult consciousness.

14 Although lifespan developmental theories are useful in understanding the nature of change through adulthood, they are limited for at least four reasons: the tremendous variability in the lives of adults, a tendency to overemphasize the more dramatic aspects of these theories (the midlife crisis, for example), the nature of their research (sometimes barely removed from anecdotal evidence and often based on groups that may not represent the general population), and difficulties involved in separating universal developmental patterns from sequences that are specific to given cohorts.

■ FURTHER READINGS

Probably the best sources of additional information with respect to models of the lifespan are original books written by Levinson, Sheehy, and Gould. Jacobs' much shorter account is based on the lives of women and provides some interesting insights into female adult development.

Gould, R. L. *Transformations: Growth and change in adult life.* New York: Simon & Schuster, 1978.

Jacobs, R. H. *Life after youth.* Boston: Beacon Press, 1979.

Levinson, D. J. *The seasons of a man's life.* New York: Alfred A. Knopf, 1978.

Sheehy, G. *Passages: Predictable crises of adult life.* New York: E. P. Dutton, 1976.

14 CHARACTERISTICS AND CHANGES OF EARLY AND MIDDLE ADULTHOOD

"You are old, Father William," the young man said,
"And your hair has become very white;
And yet you incessantly stand on your head—
Do you think, at your age, it is right?"

Lewis Carroll
Alice in Wonderland

Lord, how ashamed I should be of not being married
before three and twenty!

Jane Austen
Mansfield Park

T he sign above the door says *Green Lake Service*; for just a few minutes, I'd forgotten where I was. But the sign, *Green Lake Service*, brings me back abruptly. I am in the car, it is still Friday—and I am going home. We are stopped by the pumps at one of Green Lake's two service stations. Here, after we fill up with gasoline and after my children buy the food they need to survive for the next little while, we come to a fork in the road. Not really a fork; more like a dead end. Our highway, eastbound, stops abruptly where it meets the north-south highway. North is Beauval, Lac La Plonge, Patuanak, and other places whose names can be found on maps only because they identify navigable waterways or places where there are many fish; south, only a short distance now, is what is left of home.

I feel vaguely that I should make a choice here in Green Lake, but quickly push the thought aside; the choice has already been made.

"What's that way?" Denise asks, pointing north. We just turned south.

"Fishing." I answer. "Good fishing. The ice should just be going at Lac La Plonge and the lake trout'll be biting."

"Why don't we go?" Paul asks. He's serious. His young roots don't pull as strongly as mine.

"There's still time if you want to go," Grandma says. "No one is expecting us." Our eyes meet briefly in the mirror. We both know what she means. But there is no turning back.

"We're close now. We'll be there not long after dark," I answer.

Darkness is closer now. The shadows, inching eastward since noon, imperceptibly at first, have now turned southeast, stretching more and more rapidly as the day ages. Our car's dark shadow lies across a narrow pale-green ditch and reaches halfway up the spruce forest wall. It streaks raggedly southward. And wherever there is a clearing in the forest, it stretches instantly away until it loses itself in the jumbled muskeg humps in the distance. I point out the shadow and we all watch it for a while.

I am reminded of another time, many years ago, when I watched a similar shadow. Same place, but an older, noisier car with a taller and slightly narrower shadow. My dad and I had driven some Indians up to Green Lake, where they were going to fish; in exchange, when they returned in the fall, they would give us enough gunnysacks of fat frozen whitefish to last through most of the winter.

I remember that my dad was already very old the night we journeyed to Green Lake. In fact, my very first clear recollections of my father are of a rather elderly person. But thinking back on it now, I know that the night he and I drove from Pascal to Green Lake, he was younger than I now am. I find the thought strangely disturbing.

"Do I seem old to you?" I ask abruptly.

The silence hangs, awkward. The question has surprised them. They don't see where it's going and are uncertain how to answer. Nor do they see where it came from. But my grandmother does. She looks up from her green knitting.

"You seem awfully young to me," she says, but her eyes are worried. "Are you having a midlife crisis?"

I force a laugh, trying to shape it into something round, full, humorous. But it is a brittle, empty shell. I suddenly understand what a hollow laugh is. It occurs to me that I have always thought the theories and facts about which we weave the tale of the lifespan describe other people. But maybe it is not so any more; perhaps the tale has finally reached me. And perhaps this journey with my grandmother *is* my crisis. Or does it simply bring the crisis speeding to meet us?

But if we hurry as we hurtle through the darkening spruce shadows and pick up the tale where last we left it, it might again sweep beyond my temporary space in the span. Our personal spaces in the span are always temporary.

■ Organizing Adulthood

The lifespan does not usually divide itself nicely into sections and chapters, organized neatly by age. That happens only in textbooks and theories where we sometimes stretch or squeeze to make things fit. We can only hope that the resulting distortions do not change our subject too drastically—that it will still be recognizable in the end.

There are, of course, different ways of squeezing and stretching. One way is to attempt to organize topics primarily by age. Within each age division, we can then consider the social, cognitive, physical, and emotional aspects of human development. This is, in fact, what we have done in many of the preceding chapters. In childhood and adolescence, change often seems to be tied quite closely to age—hence the usefulness of a chronological approach.

But in these chapters that deal with adulthood, it is more difficult to tie change to age without squeezing and stretching unforgivably. The adult part of the lifespan is, after all, an extremely large part of the entire span—far more than half of it in most cases. And the changes that characterize adulthood are often subtle, usually related to a complex of other changes, and only loosely related to chronological age—hence the value of considering change across a wide spread of ages.

In this chapter, we look specifically at the characteristics and changes of early and middle adulthood—a period that stretches roughly from adolescence to somewhere around age sixty-five. Accordingly, we cover three major aspects: physical, cognitive, and personality. In the next chapter, we look in more detail at individual life styles as they are reflected in careers, marriage, family relationships, and other alternatives, and we examine how life style affects individuals.

■ Youth

As we saw in Chapter 11, adolescence is generally considered to begin with pubescence (changes leading to sexual maturity) and to end with adulthood. Unfortunately for those of us who would like things to be simple, both of these events can occur at very different times for individuals of the same sex and do occur at typically different times for individuals of different sexes. Thus adolescence, as a transition period, has rather fuzzy boundaries.

Youth, also a transition period spanning the adolescent years, has somewhat clearer, though arbitrary, boundaries. Coleman (1974) defines it as the period from the age of fourteen to twenty-four. He selects these boundaries because, as he puts it, nobody can be called an adult prior to the age of fourteen, and nobody can still be classed a child after the age of twenty-four. That, of course, is not to say that all fourteen-year-olds are childish and all twenty-four-year-olds mature. Our definitions are only definitions; they do not alter the exceptions that reality provides.

Developmental Tasks

According to Coleman, a successful transition between childhood and adulthood requires meeting a number of developmental objectives, some of which concern the individual's own capacities and abilities; others have to do with how the individual relates to others. He refers to the first grouping of these objectives as *self-centered* and to the second as *other centered*.

Perhaps most obvious among the self-centered objectives are those that relate to the development of the skills required for achieving eco-nomic independence. Generally these skills have to do with specific occupations or careers. Thus this class of self-centered objectives might be met through postsecondary schooling, through apprenticeship programs, or through the cultivation of some special talent or skill, such as that of a musician or singer, for example.

Adulthood also requires some confidence and skill in the management of one's own affairs. The rapidly increasing complexity of life in contemporary society, coupled with the scant preparation that schools and families offer children for wisely selecting among the thousands of choices with which the adult is constantly faced, makes this a particularly difficult and highly important task. Handling financial affairs and resisting the lure of easy credit are only two of the obvious management tasks that face the young adult. Less obvious, but perhaps no less important, are such tasks as obtaining accommodation, arranging for utilities, looking after a house or an apartment, cooking, making decisions about leisure time, and on, and on. It is small wonder that my cousin Luke keeps moving in with my grandmother.

A third important *self-centered* objective has to do with acquiring the skills that are required to be an intelligent consumer, not so much of goods but of the "cultural riches of civilization" (Coleman, 1974, p. 4). We all consume goods—though not all very intelligently; perhaps the same is true of culture. Presumably, consuming culture intelligently implies learning to enjoy both the more esoteric aspects of culture (plays, concerts, museums, literature) as well as those more mundane (sports, television situation comedies and soap operas). Unfortunately, perhaps, schools and parents don't always do a great deal to prepare their charges to consume culture intelligently. Nor is it completely clear that doing so is highly desirable and beneficial, although we suspect this to be the case.

The final requirement for effective participation in adult society described by Coleman is the ability to engage in concentrated activity. By this, Coleman means that a completely successful transition to adulthood requires individuals to dedicate themselves to certain endeavors. In many cases,

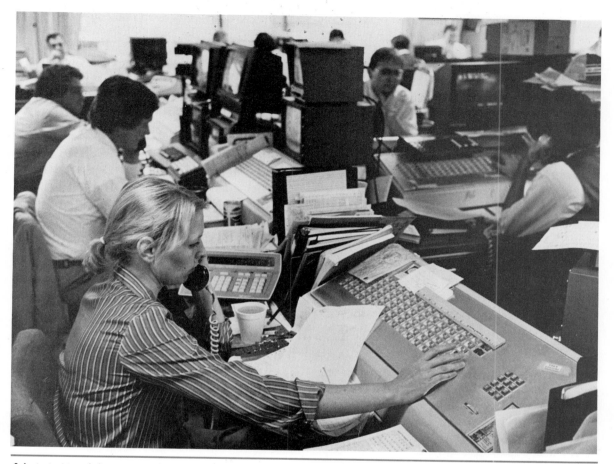

Admission to adult society requires the ability to engage in concentrated activity. For many, these activities center on work and are tied to the necessity of earning a living.

these endeavors will be job related; in other cases, they might relate to community activities, specific hobbies, religious beliefs, or political interests. He suggests that the greatest of human achievements in all areas are usually the result of such concentrated activity.

Among *other-centered* objectives, Coleman lists three types of experiences that contribute significantly to the adoption of mature social roles. These include the opportunity to interact with a variety of individuals from many different social classes, races, age groups, religions, and occupations;

experience in situations where the individual is *responsible* for others; and experience in activities where the outcomes depend on the cooperation of a number of individuals.

To the extent that meeting these objectives will facilitate the transition between youth and adulthood and will result in better-adjusted and happier adults, anything that existing social and cultural institutions can do to bring them about should be strongly encouraged. Chief among these institutions are home, school, and church; their responsibilities have always been clear. What has not always been clear is precisely what can be done. Coleman's description of objectives that must be met during youth provides a useful source of ideas. (These objectives are summarized in Table 14.1.)

The Transition

How do we know when the transition is complete? When does youth become adulthood? There is no simple, widely accepted answer. In general, however, the beginning of adulthood coincides roughly with attaining of economic and emotional independence from the family. The most common manifestations of independence are, accordingly, finding some means of financial support (obtaining a job, for example) and establishing a new home, sometimes alone, but very often with a mate.

Note that in the same way as adolescence is partially a cultural phenomenon, so too is youth. Thus, although we might argue that adolescence *as a biological event* is common to people everywhere, in many cultures (sometimes described as "primitive") where rites and ceremonies are employed to mark the passage between childhood and adulthood, the period of adolescence as we know it apparently does not exist (see Chapter 11).

Youth, as defined in this section, is essentially a prolongation of adolescence that has been created by complex, technological societies, where simply achieving puberty does not provide the child with the skills required for optimal participation in adult life. In the days of our grandparents, being able to work on the land or in the house and being able to make babies might have been sufficient qualification for admission to the rank of adulthood. Today, however, a great many of us are required to spend an increasing amount of time learning the skills that we are likely to need later. And during this time, whether we are in college, in the military, or elsewhere, we are likely to be neither child nor adult but somewhere in between—still financially dependent on our parents in many cases but progressively less dependent on them emotionally.

We should note again, however, that this swiftly brushed picture of youth paints only one of several

Table 14.1   Skills required for effective transition to adulthood.

Self-Centered Skills	Useful for
Work and occupational skills	Attaining economic independence
Self-management skills	Making reasonable decisions in the face of wide choice
Consumer skills	Learning how to use and enjoy culture as well as goods
Concentrated involvement skills	Succeeding in undertakings; making significant contributions in many areas

Other-Centered Skills	Useful for
Social interaction skills	Effective commerce in a variety of situations with different people
Skills relating to management of others	Assuming responsibility for those who are dependent
Cooperative skills	Engaging in joint endeavors

Based on J. S. Coleman, *Youth: Transition to adulthood.* Chicago: University of Chicago Press, 1974.

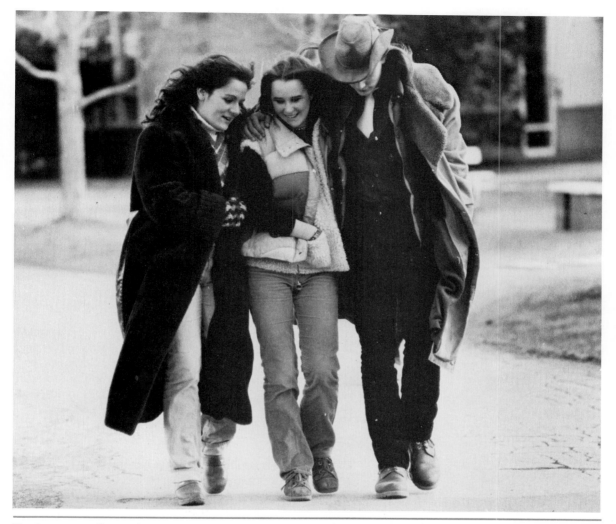

Youth is essentially a prolongation of adolescence—a stretching of the period during which the individual is clearly no longer a child, but is nevertheless not clearly an adult either.

possible scenes. Growing up in today's technological world does not always entail a prolongation of adolescence—a period of youth. There are many who still enter the work force during adolescence, and among these, many become adult in all significant ways far before others of identical age. Similarly, even in the time of our great grandparents and beyond, during a period when we imagine life to have consisted largely of idyllic meanderings through pastoral scenes, many people prolonged their adolescence for long periods, unable or perhaps simply unwilling to become adult. Then, as today, there were some people who knew very clearly that we do not all have to become adults (in terms of work roles, responsibilities, and attitudes toward self, others, and life in general). There are those who can dream and play—like children—through the entire span.

The important point of the preceding paragraph is simply that whether we become adults when puberty first makes that possible, whether we struggle through a lengthy and sometimes fitful transition period, or whether we continue to frolic through life like children may be a function of two different sets of forces: our personality characteristics, on the one hand, and the social and economic conditions that affect our particular cohort, on the other. In most cases, the function is likely to be a complex interaction between the two.

Table 14.2 Age ranges: peak creativity, leadership, and achievement.

Discipline or Area	Age Range
Physial Sciences, Mathematics, and Inventions	
Chemistry	26–30
Mathematics	30–34
Physics	30–34
Electronics	30–34
Practical inventions	30–34
Astronomy	35–39
Biological Sciences	
Psychology	30–39
Medical discoveries	35–39
Music	
Instrumental selections	25–29
Vocal solos	30–34
Symphonies	30–34
Grand opera	35–39
Writing	
Poetry	25–29
Short stories	30–34
Novels	40–44
"Best books"	40–44
Best sellers	40–44
Art	
Oil paintings	32–36
American sculpture	35–39
Modern architecture	40–44
Income	
Movie actors who are "best money-makers"	30–34
Movie actresses who are "best money-makers"	23–27
Outstanding commercial and industrial leaders	65–69
Athletics	
Professional football players	22–26
Professional prizefighters	25–26
Professional hockey players	26
Professional tennis players	25–29

From *Age and achievement* by Harvey C. Lehman. Copyright 1953 by the American Philosophical Society; reprinted by permission of Princeton University Press.

Physical Development

One of the reasons why developmental psychology has traditionally been concerned with children and not with adults is simply that children appear to change a great deal—sometimes very rapidly and dramatically; changes among adults are usually less dramatic and less uniform. Hence the temptation is to think of adulthood as a *plateau*—a resting state following development and preceding decline. It is worth emphasizing again that contemporary models of development depart significantly from this conception.

In the area of physical development, it is clear that adulthood is not a plateau. Although change might not be as predictable or as dramatic as it was in earlier years, there are still some small mountains to climb and a few slopes to descend.

Strength

Early adulthood sees the very peak of our physical development in terms of speed, strength, coordination, and endurance, as well as in terms of general health (Bromley, 1974). Thus during our twenties and early thirties, we can lift more, run faster, throw farther, work longer, climb higher, and crawl lower than at any other time in our lives. It is not surprising that Lehman's (1953) studies of the ages at which people were most likely to achieve in a variety of fields found that the twenties and sometimes early thirties were periods of highest achievement for sports requiring strength, stamina, and coordination. As Table 14.2 indicates, highest achievement in other areas tends to occur somewhat later, though not often after the age of forty-four. Only popes, presidents, and other important leaders typically *peak* later. Note, however, that Lehman's survey was conducted more than three decades ago and therefore deals with cohorts exposed to social conditions quite different from those that now prevail. Although strength and stamina are still likely to peak in early adulthood, peak achievement in areas more susceptible to social influence might now occur at slightly different ages.

The normal developmental pattern with respect to physical strength sees a very gradual decline following the peak years. This decline is often not particularly noticeable until the forties and is most apparent with respect to back and leg strength. Clement (1974) reports that loss of upper body strength (particularly arm strength) is often no more than 10 percent by the age of sixty (see *Exercise*).

In addition to a gradual loss of strength following the peak in early adulthood, there is a more noticeable loss of stamina, usually related to poorer aerobic functioning (heart-lung efficiency) (Tanner, 1978). Few forty-year-olds can still compete with younger individuals in athletic events re-

quiring strength and endurance (marathon races, for example).

Appearance

This gradual decline in physical functioning through the adult years is accompanied by a number of other important physical changes. Our cultural standards of beauty and attractiveness, closely tied to physical appearance, dictate that peak attractiveness will generally occur during early adulthood. This is particularly true for females and is quite evident in the physical appearance of the models that the advertising industry employs to sell its clients' wares. It is also evident in the enormous salaries that many of these models command between ages sixteen and twenty-five.

Physical changes that account for our progressively changing appearance are highly varied and initially very subtle. The most obvious are changes in height and weight. After the late teens or early twenties, height does not generally increase.

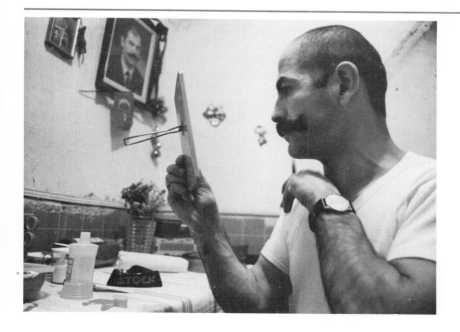

As we age, some of us will lose our hair; some will watch it turn gray or white, and others will retain their hair's thickness and color well into old age.

However, after the age of forty-five (sometimes earlier and sometimes later), there are frequently decrements in height. On the average, these decrements are greater for women than for men. Rossman (1977) reports average lifetime losses of 4.9 centimeters (almost 2 inches) for women and 2.0 centimeters (about 3/4 inch) for men.

Although changes in height occur late in adulthood and are usually so gradual that they are not often detected, changes in weight are often far less subtle. As Bischof (1976) notes, after we stop growing at the ends, we begin to grow in the middle. Thus, adulthood is often accompanied by the accumulation of fatty tissue, which tends to be distributed differently in men and women. Typically, excess fat first finds its way around the middles of men; it is more likely to be deposited on the hips among women. In general, percentage of body weight that is fat is higher for women than for men throughout the adult years, whether or not they are overweight. Figure 14.1 presents the results of a study that looked at relative distributions of fat among 520 adults (215 males, 305 females) between the ages of eighteen and eighty-five.

Other physical changes that contribute to the adult's changing appearance include loss of skin elasticity, thinning of hair, loss of muscle tone, loss of flexibility in joints, gradual recession of gums (hence the expression "long in the tooth"), and the appearance of longer, stiffer hair in the eye-brows, ears, and nose. In addition, even among those adults who remain trim, there is a gradual thickening of the torso but an eventual thinning of the legs and arms. It is partly for this reason that, as Troll (1982) notes, a skinny old person does not look like a skinny young person.

The majority of these physical changes are very gradual and seldom dramatic while they are occurring. In addition, there are extremely wide individual variations, not only in the speed with which we age physically but also in the ways we age. Some of us will lose all our hair; the hair of others will turn snowy white. And some, like my paternal great-grandfather, will retain a head of raven-black hair right into their tenth decade of life.

The Senses

Like most of our physical systems, our senses too are subject to the influences of time. Vision, for example, appears to be best at around the age of twenty and typically remains relatively constant until the age of forty. After that age, most individuals become more farsighted, so that those who were initially nearsighted sometimes experience better vision (Timiras, 1972). In one longitudinal study of aging, it was found that by the age of fifty, 88 percent of the women and all of the men had at

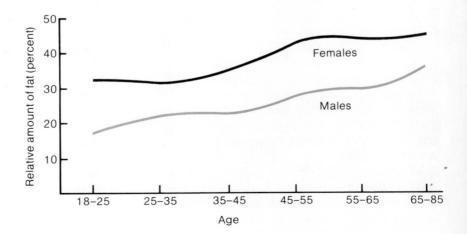

Figure 14.1
Relative amounts of body fat by age and sex. (From L. P. Novak, Aging, total body potassium, fat-free mass, and cell mass in males and females between ages 18 and 85 years. *Journal of Gerontology*, 1972, *27*, 438–443. Data on p. 440. Reprinted by permission of the Gerontological Society of America.)

least one pair of eyeglasses (Bayer, Whissell-Bue-chy, & Honzik, 1981).

Hearing losses are also very gradual during the early years of adulthood but are typically more severe for men than for women. Bayer et al. (1981) report that hearing complaints at the age of thirty are very few (2 percent of the men and none of women in the sample). By the age of forty-two, however, while very few women had experienced noticeable hearing loss, 14 percent of the men had— a figure that had risen to 32 percent by the age of fifty.

Changes in the ability to taste appear to be very slight until later adulthood, although by the age of fifty, some individuals are less sensitive to spices, salts, and sugars—a fact that most are not likely to have noticed. Loss of taste sensitivity is common during adulthood—a condition that might be linked to heavy drinking and smoking as well as to the excessive use of salt. Loss of taste sensitivity often leads elderly individuals to flavor their foods with quantities of salt and pepper that children would find almost unpalatable.

Health

In the same way as early adulthood is characterized by the peak of physical strength and endurance, as well as of sensory capacity, so is it characterized by the peak of physical health. In particular, many of the infections of childhood become far less common in early adulthood and remain so throughout life. With increasing age, however, there is increased susceptibility to chronic (recurring) medical complaints, such as back and spine problems, heart ailments, and so on. Whereas the leading causes of death among young adults are accidents, heart disease is the leading cause of death among older adults, particularly after the age of thirty-five for men and forty-five for women (Dingle, 1973). In this connection, there have been some dramatic changes in the most common causes of death during the last several decades. In 1940, the leading cause of death was pneumonia and influenza, followed closely by tuberculosis. Thirty years later, influenza and pneumonia were a distant fifth

and tuberculosis had become almost inconsequential as a cause of death. Heart disease, cancer, and cerebrovascular disease now lead the list (Dingle, 1973).

Bayer et al. (1981) have looked at health during early and middle adulthood by summarizing data from three major longitudinal studies. These include the Oakland Growth Study (ages eleven to fifty), the Berkeley Growth Study (birth to thirty-six), and the Berkeley Guidance Study (birth to age forty-two). Among other things, they found that although the majority of adults (more than 80 percent) consider themselves to be in "good-to-excellent" health during their middle years, an increasing number suffer from a variety of complaints. As noted earlier, these tend to be chronic rather than instances of acute infections such as colds and influenza. Among women, the most common complaints relate to the reproductive system. These may involve attempts to become pregnant, pregnancy itself, problems relating to menstruation, ovarian cysts and tumors, and infections. Among men, the most common complaints relate to the digestive system; men have three times the incidence of stomach ulcers that women do.

Another sex difference with respect to adult health is that women generally report more illnesses than do men. Ironically, their life expectancies continue to be significantly higher, which is sometimes explained by the possibility that women are more sensitive to their bodies and perhaps less likely to dismiss symptoms as inconsequential. Accordingly, they are more likely to seek medical help and thus to report more illnesses. Also, they are more likely to receive assistance when it is most likely to be effective.

"Change of Life"

One final area of physical change is particularly important for understanding the adult years. It involves changes in the sex glands and is popularly referred to as the *change of life* or, more properly, the **climacteric**. Among women, the climacteric involves menopause, a dramatic change in physical functioning. Among men, the climacteric is more subtle, which has led to some debate concerning whether it is fruitful or even appropriate to speak of a male climacteric or change of life.

The secretion of the sex hormones by the ovaries (primarily estrogen) and the testes (primarily testosterone) is among the most important changes of pubescence (see Chapter 11). These hormones are closely involved in the development of secondary sexual characteristics (breasts, facial hair, voice changes, and so on), as well as in sexual interest and behavior. Their production continues, relatively unabated, from puberty through early adulthood. But by the late thirties or early forties among women, and perhaps by the early fifties for men, the production of sex hormones begins to decrease. Among men, this decrease is often very gradual and not easily noticed. Among women, it is considerably less gradual, leading eventually to the cessation of menses (**menopause**). The average age of menopause is approximately fifty (Talbert, 1977).

The hormonal changes that cause menopause are sometimes also responsible for a number of other symptoms and complaints, including flushes of perspiration or "hot flashes," dizziness, headaches, mood fluctuations, and so on. These are serious enough to lead women to consult a doctor in as many as one-third of all cases (Weideger, 1976). Although similar symptoms have sometimes been reported by men, there is little evidence that they might be tied to hormonal changes that are common to most men. In fact, hormonal changes among men are seldom sufficient to lead to infertility, although they often do lead to a reduction in the number of viable sperm that are produced.

EXERCISE

Participate! Play tennis! Racquetball! Squash! Dance! Join a spa! An exercise class! Skate! Ski! Swim! Run! Jog! At least walk.

Literally millions of adults, many of whom had engaged in virtually no unnecessary physical activity since high school or college—and perhaps not even then—have now embarked on exercise programs. And many undertake these programs with the same dedication and serious determination that they bring to their careers—and perhaps to other aspects of their lives. Why? Simply, to be happy and healthy. That is, after all, what most of us want. Exercise, we are told, will make us healthier, may enable us to live longer, and should make us trimmer, more fit, and perhaps even more attractive, given our contemporary cultural standards of physical attractiveness.

How valid are these claims? Research leaves little doubt that exercise contributes significantly to good health. Numerous studies of cardiovascular fitness have repeatedly found higher levels of fitness and lower incidence of coronary heart disease among those who exercise regularly than among those whose lives are more sedentary (for example, Blumenthal, Sanders, Williams, Needels, & Wallace, 1982; Fox & Haskell, 1978). In addition, it has been clearly established that exercise is importantly involved in reducing the percentage of body fat and in increasing muscle and bone density.

But does exercise make us happier? Does it affect us psychologically? Blumenthal et al. (1982) provide some answers, following an investigation of the effects of exercise on a group of sixteen subjects who had registered for a ten-week adult fitness program. The average age of this group was forty-five years; the youngest subject was twenty-five and the oldest sixty-one. At the very beginning of the program, all subjects were administered a battery of three psychological tests. The Profile of Mood States assesses six emotional states: depression, tension or anxiety, anger, vigor, fatigue, and confusion. The State-Trait Anxiety Inventory provides two measures of anxiety or tension: present level of tension (state) and habitual level of tension (trait). Finally, a retrospective change questionnaire was designed to uncover subjects' perceptions of how they might have changed with respect to health, sleep habits, social life, sense of personal achievement, and so on. A control group, consisting of healthy but sedentary individuals of similar age, was also administered these same tests.

The exercise program that the sixteen experimental subjects then undertook consisted of a ten-minute routine of stretching exercises, followed by forty-five min-

Where complaints accompanying menopause are sufficiently serious, they can easily and effectively be treated with estrogen—a form of therapy appropriately labeled *estrogen replacement therapy*. Unfortunately, there is some possibility that estrogen therapy might increase risk of cancer (Rosenwaks, 1981).

Sexual functioning among men and women does not necessarily change with the climacteric. Most women continue to be interested in sex and to be capable of orgasm, although there might be some reduction in vaginal lubrication following arousal. Among men, changes in sexual interest and functioning vary a great deal. For example, it may now take longer for the man to achieve an erection, both before and after intercourse, and this erection might not always be as firm as it was some decades ago. In addition, ejaculation itself will typically be less forceful. Unfortunately, these highly common changes are seldom discussed openly and are often interpreted as evidence of rapidly declining sexual prowess—an event that can lead to considerable anxiety concerning sexual performance and that is often implicated in the man's resulting impotence. In fact, among men, the process of aging does not entail the loss of ability to perform sexually.

■ Cognitive Changes

Many of the physical changes of aging are obvious. We can *see* the wrinkles and sags, the stiffenings and tightenings, the slackings, the graying and the drooping. Cognitive changes do not flaunt themselves so flagrantly. Do they even occur? We have

utes of walking or running, three times a week over a period of ten weeks. All exercise periods were under medical supervision. The intensity of the activities for each individual was determined by the maximum heart rate attained by each subject on a treadmill, prior to the program. Exercises were designed to allow the individual to attain 70 to 85 percent of this maximum. Control-group members continued as before, without any regular exercise program.

At the end of the ten-week period, individuals in both the experimental and the control group were again administered the three psychological instruments. The results are clear and striking. Whereas the groups had initially been identical on each of these instruments, the experimental group now felt less tension, fatigue, depression, and confusion and experienced significant reductions in immediate and general anxiety. And, as expected, physiological measures indicated significant improvements in the experimental groups.

It appears that middle-aged individuals who are inactive but basically healthy can increase their well-being, as well as their *sense* of well-being, through exercise. There is little reason to suppose that this might not also be the case for many who are less healthy and for people of different ages.

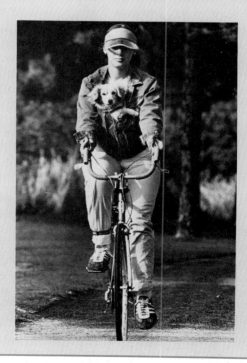

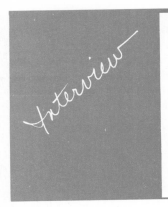

Subject: Female; age thirty-one; never married; university education; successful career in a helping profession.

Question: "When do you think the 'prime of life' is?"

I'm not sure. Some people say around forty. I think maybe it's earlier. Like around . . . in the twenties. That's when you're the strongest and everything, and all your goals and your life is still ahead of you. But maybe men are in their prime later than women, because after the age of forty or maybe even thirty women are getting old but men don't seem that old even when they're forty or even fifty. Men can get married and have children when they're pretty old; when a women is past thirty-five, she's pretty well finished. If she hasn't had any yet, too bad. Her prime, at least for having kids, is finished.

had little difficulty in answering this question with respect to childhood and adolescence when, at every succeeding age, we could detect increases in comprehension and reasoning and in the ability to analyze, synthesize, and solve problems. The task is not so simple with respect to adults and has led to considerable controversy. Does cognitive ability, like strength, vision, and the elasticity of our skins, reach a peak in early adulthood and begin a downhill slide from there—slow and imperceptible at first, but gradually more rapid until, in the words of Shakespeare, we reach again our "second childishness"? Or does it continue to grow so that, when we are finally old, we might also be truly wise?

Learning, Remembering, and Solving Problems

In practice it is very difficult to separate learning from memory, although the ways in which each is studied are often different. Thus, although evidence that something has been learned is identical to evidence that it is remembered, studies of memory often look at the effects of experience after a time lapse, whereas studies of learning are generally more concerned with the immediate effects of experience. What is often unclear in memory research, however, is whether the inability to remember something is due to faulty memory or

whether it might be due to the fact that it was never learned.

There are a number of different ways of assessing memory. If I want to know whether you remember the people in your first-grade class, I might ask you to name them for me. This illustrates a *recall* procedure; you simply retrieve material from memory as best you can. Alternately, I might show you a great number of photographs of different individuals, among whom are the members of your first-grade class, and ask you to point these out to me. This method relies on *recognition* rather than recall. A third method for assessing memory is to have individuals *relearn* material that was previously learned. To the extent that it takes less time to relearn than to learn initially, there is evidence of memory of the initial learning.

Of these three methods—recall, recognition, and relearning—the last is the most sensitive. That is, it is most likely to provide evidence of memory. In the same way, the first, recall, is the least sensitive (the most difficult); it is most likely to provide no evidence of memory.

These distinctions between methods of measuring memory are particularly important when comparing the memories of older and younger people, because it appears that they change in different ways with age. Following a review of relevant research, Troll (1982) concludes that our abilities to *recognize* do not suffer from the ravages of time in the same way as our ability to *recall*

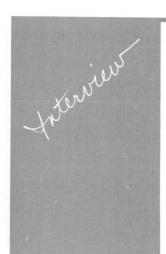
Subject: Male; age thirty-three; first marriage; two children; university education; professional career.

Question: "When do you think the 'prime of life' is?"

The prime of life. It depends exactly what you mean.

. . .

Okay. Well, generally, the prime of life is right at the peak. I'd say it probably goes from the time you're grown up and finished with education—twenty or twenty-five maybe—right up until you're "over the hill," and I suppose for most people that wouldn't happen for quite a long time. Retirement, maybe. Sixty or sixty-five.

. . .

Well, if I had to narrow it down to just five years, I'd say maybe around . . . well it depends. My physical prime is different. Probably from twenty-five to thirty. But intellectually and in my work, I haven't reached my prime yet. Maybe around forty-five years.

does. For example, Bahrick, Bahrick, and Wittlinger (1975) found virtually no changes in the ability of individuals to recognize the names and photographs of those with whom they went to high school, whether they were tested three months or almost fifty years after leaving school. During the entire span, recognition hovered around 90 percent. This figure is very close to that reported by Standing (1973), who presented subjects with more than 10,000 photographs and who later paired a number of these photographs with others that the subjects had not seen. Under these conditions, subjects were able to recognize more than 90 percent of the pictures they had already seen.

Unfortunately, our ability to recall does not appear to fare quite as well as does our ability to recognize. In the Bahrick et al. (1975) study, recall of high school colleagues was less than 80 percent accurate after only three months, had dropped to around 60 percent after four years, and was below 50 percent twenty years later (see Figure 14.2).

A gradual decline in problem-solving ability is also evident during adulthood. For example, with respect to Piagetian tasks that are typically used to investigate formal operations, older subjects *on the average* do less well than young adults (Denney, 1979). It must be emphasized, however, that

differences in favor of younger subjects are very small and far from completely general. A great many older adults continue to do at least as well as most of those who are younger.

Intelligence

Does intelligence, like problem-solving ability, ability to recall, and physical strength, also decline with the passing of years? Much of the relevant research seems to provide a clear answer: When the intelligence test scores of older subjects are compared with those of adolescents or young adults, they do significantly less well (for example, Schaie, 1979). In fact, with respect to general intelligence tests such as the Stanford-Binet and the WAIS, the highest scores are almost always obtained by adolescents (or young adults), with progressively lower scores for older age groups. Does this mean that most of us become less intelligent as we age?

Perhaps not—numerous reasons, other than lowered intelligence, may explain why older subjects might perform less well than younger subjects. Perhaps most important among these might be a large number of *cohort* variables that cross-sectional studies cannot take into account. Recall

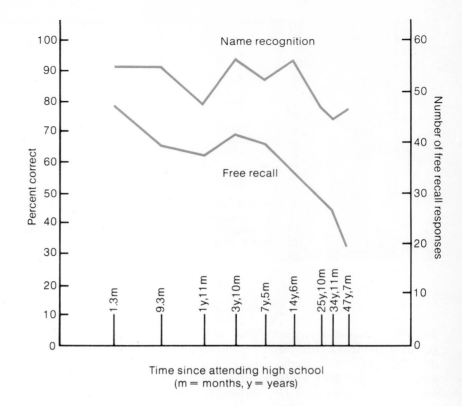

Figure 14.2
Free recall and name recognition as a function of age. Between 1.3 months and almost 50 years after leaving school, subjects were asked either to recall the names of their former classmates or to recognize their names from a list. (From H. P. Bahrick, P. O. Bahrick, and R. P. Wittlinger, Fifty years of memory for names and faces: A cross-sectional approach. *Journal of Experimental Psychology: General,* 1975, *104,* 54–75. Data on p. 62, figure on p. 66. Reprinted by permission of the publisher and the author.)

that a cross-sectional study compares different age groups at one point in time. For example, a cross-sectional study might present intelligence tests to groups of seventy-year-olds and twenty-year-olds in 1984 and then compare results obtained by these two groups. The major weakness of this type of study, with respect to questions concerning changes as a function of age, is their comparison of individuals who are born at different times (different cohorts) and who have sometimes been exposed to dramatically different environmental influences. With respect to the example just given, the study actually compares people born in 1914 with those born in 1964. Thus it compares people whose educational experiences, motivations, and values are vastly different. Specifically, individuals born in 1914 have spent considerably less time in school than those born in 1964, are often totally unfamiliar with the types of items in most intelligence tests, may never have been exposed to electroni-

cally scored answer sheets with their fine print and their demand for careful eye-hand coordination, and might be quite intimidated by the entire testing procedure.

Longitudinal studies do not bring with them the same problems that cross-sectional research does. Recall that a longitudinal study compares the performance of the same individuals at different points in time. For example, a study that presents intelligence tests to a group of twenty-year-olds in 1944 and presents the same test to the same individuals in 1964 and again in 1984 is longitudinal. It compares the performance of a single cohort with itself at different points in time and provides far better data for reaching conclusions with respect to changes that are age related rather than specific to cohort variables.

An impressive number of longitudinal studies have *not* found decrements in measured intelligence of the type typically reported with cross-

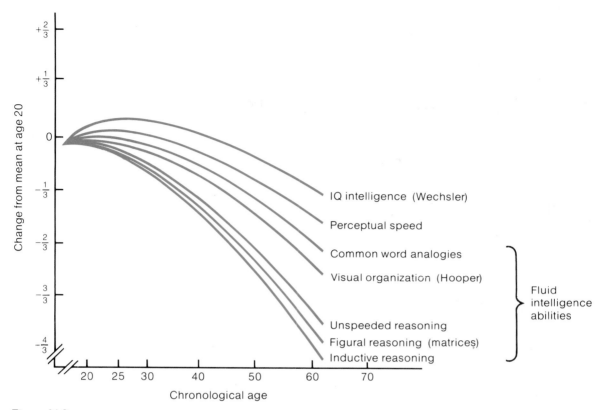

Figure 14.3
Smoothed curves summarizing several studies on aging and fluid intelligence.
(From Horn and Donaldson in Brim and Kagan, 1980, p. 469.)

sectional studies (for example, Baltes & Willis, 1979). In fact, a number of these studies report actual increases in intellectual performances into the fifties and even beyond, particularly for those individuals with professions that require the daily practicing of problem-solving and related skills. More detailed investigations reveal, however, that while increases in some intellectual abilities may continue well into middle age, decrements in others are common (Horn, 1975, 1976). Specifically, those abilities that are highly influenced by experience and education (verbal and mathematical skills, for example) tend to increase with age. Cattell (1971) labels these abilities *crystallized*, in contrast with abilities that seem to be basic to intellectual functioning but that are not affected by experience—

labeled *fluid*. Fluid abilities are reflected in general reasoning, memory and attention span, ability to understand analogies, and so on. Figures 14.3 and 14.4 summarize the results of a number of studies that have looked at age changes in measured intelligence. Note that decrement in fluid abilities contrasts with the increase in crystallized abilities.

What should we now conclude? Does intelligence, in fact, decrease with age? Horn and Donaldson (1980) and others say yes, although the decline is not usually very significant until well into old age. Schaie and others (Baltes & Schaie, 1976; Schaie, 1974, 1979; Schaie & Gribbin, 1975) are more cautious. Although they do not deny that decline is frequently observed, they maintain that

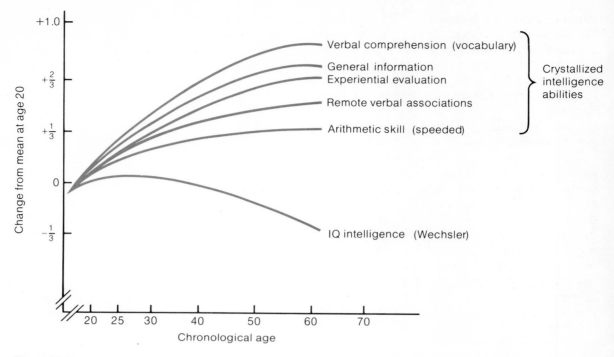

Figure 14.4
Smoothed curves summarizing several studies on aging and crystallized intelligence. (From Horn and Donaldson in Brim and Kagan, 1980, p. 471.)

belief in its inevitability and irreversibility is largely a myth. Furthermore, decline in important areas such as verbal ability, reasoning, and numerical skills is usually inconsequential until well into the sixties and appears to be occurring later for succeeding generations (Schaie & Labouvie-Vief, 1974). These authors argue that, given appropriate environmental stimulation, not only will many cognitive abilities not decrease with age, but a number may also actually continue to increase well into old age. Wisdom, which we discuss in Chapter 16, may be a case in point.

■ Personality

We are *persons; personalities* are what make us what we are. Do our personalities, like our bodies, change with age? The answer is simple: yes. Our personalities are made up of all the stable char-

acteristics of a person, including abilities, talents, habits, preferences, weaknesses, moral attributes, and other important qualities that vary from one person to another. As we have seen, many of these characteristics do change (abilities, for example); hence our *personalities* change with age. However, precisely what characteristics change, how they change, and why are more difficult questions.

Traits Versus Situations

Personality theorists have been particularly interested in the extent to which knowledge of personality characteristics can be useful for understanding, predicting, and explaining people's behaviors. Thus, a person whose personality is *aggressive* would be expected to behave aggressively in different situations. Indeed, the decision that a person is aggressive is generally based on the observation of aggressive behavior at different times. The personality trait (characteristic) simply labels a predictable consistency in behavior. If behavior is inconsistent—that is, if it varies in unpredictable ways from one time to the next—then the concept of personality characteristics becomes largely meaningless.

Most personality theorists have assumed without question that behavior is indeed highly consistent with underlying personality characteristics, even though some of these characteristics might change with age and experience (for example, Cattell, 1974). Accordingly, their efforts have been directed primarily toward identifying the most useful ways of classifying personality and the best ways of assessing the presence and importance of personality characteristics in individuals. Thus it is that theorists such as Jung (1923) and Eysenck (1967) describe *introverts* and *extroverts* and develop elaborate theories designed to help us understand the differences between these two major *types* of personality. Other theories have been more concerned with identifying a variety of specific personality *traits* (characteristics) and relating these to behavior.

And others have recently challenged the assumption that behavior is sufficiently consistent that it reveals the existence of underlying personality characteristics. Mischel (1968, 1977) and others argue that behavior is far more influenced by the immediate situation in which it occurs than by any underlying personality characteristic. Indeed, these theorists suggest that personality traits are more often in the observer than in the person behaving—that is, the situation predicts the behavior far more accurately than does any notion we might have about personality characteristics that determine consistency in human behavior. Because of their emphasis on the immediate situation, these theorists are often described as *situation* theorists in contrast with *trait* theorists. Accordingly, the resulting controversy is labeled the situation-trait controversy.

Who is right? Probably both, although in different ways and for different reasons. Although it is true that knowledge of specific traits has not proven very valuable in attempts to predict specific behaviors in isolated instances, there nevertheless appears to be a general consistency to a given individual's behavior. Thus, when Block (1971) readministered personality tests to the same individuals as much as ten years later, he found a high similarity between results on the two tests.

Age-Related Personality Changes

Although some aspects of personality do not appear to change dramatically, careful investigations reveal that others change a great deal (for example, Moss & Susman, 1980; Nesselroade & Baltes, 1974). These studies suggest that intellectual characteristics (measured IQ, self-concept, typical approach to problems) change the least (Mischel, 1979); in contrast, characteristics having to do with interpersonal behavior and attitudes are most susceptible to change.

In one longitudinal study, Kelly (1955) administered a long battery of personality tests to a sample of 300 students. Between sixteen and nineteen years later, 86 percent of the original sample was retested. Of thirty-eight different personality characteristics that were assessed, twenty had not changed, the remaining eighteen had changed but usually only moderately. Attitudes (toward religion, for example) appeared to be most unstable; values had changed the least.

In a widely reported study of aging, Neugarten (1964) has identified some important general patterns of changes in personality. The study involved a group of more than 700 subjects between forty and seventy and a second group of over 300 individuals between fifty and ninety. Among the important findings of this study was the tendency of men and women to alter their dominant approaches to life following the period of the mid life crisis (ages forty-five to fifty-five). As we saw in Chapter 13, Neugarten observed a tendency for males to become less aggressive, more passive, more concerned with emotions and with internal states, and, in short, somewhat more "feminine." In contrast, women frequently become more aggressive, more active, and more concerned with achieving personal goals.

A similar study, also conducted by Neugarten (1968), looked at the *self-concepts* of one hundred middle-aged men and women. All of these individuals were highly articulate, well educated, successful business and professional leaders. Interviews revealed that most felt that middle age is, in fact, "the prime of life." As one of the subjects put it, "There is a difference between wanting to *feel* young and wanting to *be* young" (Neugarten & Datan, 1981, p. 281). That is, although subjects would have liked to retain the appearance and the vigor of youth, most would have been reluctant to exchange the competence, confidence, power, and other rewards that had come with maturity.

Middle age, Neugarten informs us, is characterized by a tremendous increase in self-awareness and introspection and by greatly heightened self-understanding. Accordingly, the prevalent theme of these middle years is the reassessment of self. And, as we saw, the result of this reassessment often takes the form of greater femininity for males and greater masculinity for females. In short, the dramatic differentiation between the sexes that our culture encourages throughout the more plastic years of childhood is often softened in our middle ages, when we become more **androgynous**—more a combination of masculine and feminine characteristics.

How valid are Neugarten's observations with respect to male-female personality changes in midlife? Other evidence provides corroboration. Gutmann (1977) studied personality changes in a number of different cultures (American, Israeli, Navajo, and Mayan, among others) and found patterns very similar to those described by Neugarten. In brief, he found that by the age of fifty-five, women had become noticeably more aggressive and men more passive in all of these cultures. His tentative explanation is that the roles that men and women must play with respect to child rearing during their early adulthood require that women be unaggressive and nuturant if they are to be good mothers and that men be aggressive and active if they are to be successful breadwinners. Following midlife, when men and women are finally freed of parenting roles, they are now able to concentrate on those aspects of their personalities that had previously been repressed. Thus men now compensate by becoming more feminine as women become more masculine.

Two important points must be noted here. First, these patterns of personality change are far from universal, nor are they usually dramatic. In other words, most men do not become highly (or even noticeably) feminine after the age of fifty-five, nor do most women become dramatically more aggressive. Second, if Gutmann's explanation for this slight reversal of sex roles following the midlife is accurate, it follows that changing male-female roles with respect to parenting, economic support of families, and decision making may do a great deal to lessen personality differences that now exist between younger males and females. In the end, it may no longer be possible for males to become less aggressive—or females more active and aggressive. Put another way, male-female personality differences in adulthood, and the changes described by Neugarten and Gutmann, might well be cohort specific rather than age related. This, of course, makes them no less real or important, but it might significantly alter our explanations and understanding. (See *Types A and B.*)

■ Happiness and Satisfaction

"Taking all things together, how would you say things are these days—would you say you are very happy, pretty happy, or not too happy?" (Campbell, 1981, p. 27). When this question was first asked in a psychological survey in 1957, more than one person in three described himself as being "very happy"; only one in ten was "not too happy." The remaining 54 percent thought they were "pretty happy." But by 1972, only one in four was willing to describe himself as being "very happy," a finding that seems strangely curious in view of the tremendous growth in prosperity between 1957 and 1972 and the concomitant rise in the standard of living. Is happiness inversely related to owning two cars and having quail and other exotic meats in many pots? Does it increase or decrease with age? Who is most likely to be happy?

TYPES A AND B

Our personalities are complex and often perplexing. We are not easily reduced to a handful of traits. And the *types* of which novels and grandmothers speak—as in "he's the aggressive type," or "she's the manipulating type"—are highly misleading at best. We are too unpredictable and too complicated to be nothing more than one of several consistent types. In spite of this, psychology has sometimes found it useful to categorize individuals into broad categories such as extroverted, authoritarian, independent, or introverted, and A and B. Of these, A and B are particularly intriguing.

Type A individuals may be described as hard driving, loud, aggressive, achievement oriented, and impatient. These are individuals who drive themselves mercilessly, who sense most keenly the unrelenting pressures of time and the urgency of their lives. In contrast, Type B individuals are slow, relaxed, easygoing. They speak more softly, tend to impose few deadlines on themselves, and do not, in general, respond to life with the same sense of urgency that drives Type A's.

Type A and B individuals can easily be recognized in the work place. Psychology also provides a number of instruments that can be employed to distinguish between them (for example, Jenkins, Zyzanski, & Rosenman, 1971). These questionnaires ask questions such as: "Do people sometimes tell you that you eat too fast?" Or "Do the people with whom you work see you as being aggressive and achievement oriented?" Using such questions, researchers have found that perhaps 40 percent of the population is Type A; the remainder are Type B. Clearly, however, the types are less a dichotomy than a continuum. That is, some Type A individuals would manifest extremes of Type A behavior and others would be only slightly different from Type B individuals.

The medical profession has found this typology particularly useful because of the close relationship that exists between Type A behavior and coronary problems (Corse, Manuck, Cantwell, Giordani, & Matthews, 1982).

Indeed, some studies indicate that Type A individuals are approximately twice as likely as Type B individuals to suffer fatal heart attacks. And if they survive the first attack, they are more likely to have a second (Rosenman et al., 1975). In addition, approximately three-fourths of all men suffering from hypertension (high blood pressure) are Type A's ("Down with Type A," 1983). Small wonder that being a Type A individual is sometimes accorded the same weight as a contributor to coronary problems as high blood pressure, high cholesterol level, smoking, and obesity. Miller (1983) notes that the prevalence of most of these factors (obesity, smoking, and hypertension) had been increasing until the mid-1960s and that incidence of coronary heart disease had also been increasing. Since then, however, widespread public campaigns drawing attention to their role in heart disease seem to have been somewhat successful in reversing the trend, and incidence of death from strokes and coronary heart disease has also been decreasing. Although this observed correlation does not constitute proof that factors such as smoking and obesity *cause* hypertension and coronary heart problems, it does provide evidence in that direction.

Several words of caution are appropriate at this point. To begin with, not all Type A's are doomed to coronary problems or hypertension, nor will all Type B's escape. Second, these are crude categories that do not recognize the possibility that some individuals may be Type A's in a variety of ways (aggressive, hard driving, and so on), but may nevertheless be able to relax very effectively, thereby lessening the risk of coronary problems. And finally, although there appears to be some inherited predisposition to be Type A or Type B (Ovcharchyn, Johnson, & Petzel, 1981), we can do a great deal to control our behavior. Type A's can, with proper motivation and training, become Type B's. Perhaps the opposite is also true.

In a very personal way, these are fundamentally important questions to each of us, for it is happiness, in any of its many disguises, for which we all strive (even though some strive for happiness *after* rather than *during* the lifespan). But happiness, like so many other qualities of the human experience, is not easily investigated. As Yensen

(1975) notes, there are no physiological ways of measuring happiness. Nor, indeed, are there any other *objective* means. We are left with having to resort to *subjective* questions such as the one that opens this section. We either ask directly, "Are you happy?" or we must ask, less directly, "Is life boring, exciting, miserable, or worthwhile?" "Are you

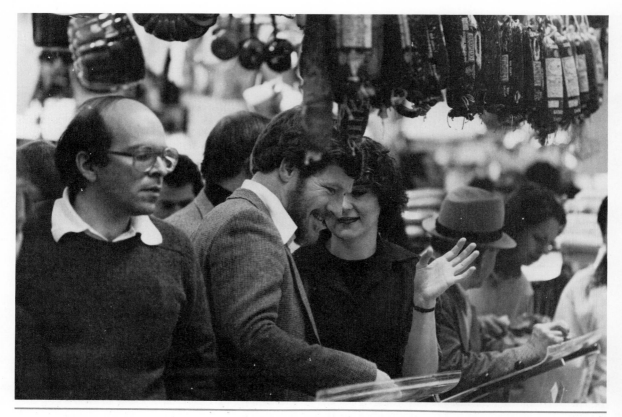

We are *satisfied* to the extent that our goals and aspirations have been met; we are *happy* to the extent that we feel content and joyful. Satisfaction is relatively stable; it doesn't change much from one day to the next, while happiness is more subject to fluctuations of mood. As we age, we often become more satisfied. Do we also become happier?

satisfied with your work, your husband or wife, your children, and your income?" And if we ask these questions, as Campbell and his associates have since 1957 (Campbell, 1976, 1981; Campbell, Converse, & Rodgers, 1976), we soon find that, contrary to what we might have expected, satisfaction and happiness are different. Nor do they always go hand in hand.

Satisfaction is, in effect, a relatively stable dimension. If I am satisfied with my job, my wife, or my life in general today, I am still likely to be satisfied tomorrow, next month, and perhaps even next year. In this context, to be satisfied is to confess either to the fulfillment of one's goals and

aspirations or to a resignation to the way things are. Thus, if I am satisfied with my job, it may be because this is the job I wanted; it has lived up to my expectations and given me what I desired and anticipated. Alternately, it might be because I realize that I am incapable of succeeding in the job I really wanted or that it is impossible or unlikely that I will obtain that job or any other more satisfying; therefore I have resigned myself to this one.

Happiness, on the other hand, is more subject to the fluctuations of mood. It is a personal, highly subjective *feeling*, easily sensed and interpreted by each of us but not always easily communicated to others. Nor can it readily be tied to satisfaction.

Campbell et al. (1976) found that although "completely satisfied" individuals most often saw themselves as being "very happy," a number were only "pretty happy." And a large number of individuals were dissatisfied with the major domains of life, such as job, health, housing, and marriage, but nevertheless felt "pretty happy" or even "very happy" (see Figure 14.5).

Who are the happiest people? The rich or poor? The married or single? The young or the old? Some tentative answers are available, following massive interview studies reported by Campbell and his associates. These studies involved randomly selected samples representative of the entire population of the United States. The samples ranged in size from 2,164 to 3,692 individuals and totaled more than 12,000 subjects. Interviews were conducted on five separate samples between 1957 and 1978. They provided information concerning satisfaction with various important dimensions of life, self-esti-

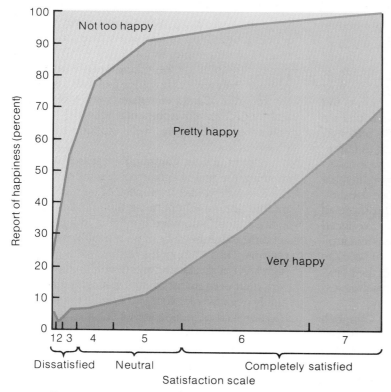

Figure 14.5

Reports of happiness by degree of overall satisfaction with life. The figure shows the distribution of responses to the happiness item for respondents at each level on the overall satisfaction item; for example, of those who said they were "completely satisfied," 59 percent were "very happy," 40 percent were "pretty happy," and 1 percent were "not too happy." Of those who were completely dissatisfied (at 1 on the satisfaction scale), very few were "very happy," approximately 20 percent were "pretty happy," and around 75 percent were "not too happy." The length of the space devoted to each of the seven points on the scale corresponds to the number of people who described themselves as "dissatisfied" or more satisfied. Thus, the majority see themselves as quite highly satisfied (scores of 6 or 7); only a few admit to high dissatisfaction (scores of 1, 2, or 3). (From *The quality of American life* by Angus Campbell, Phillip E. Converse, and Willard G. Rogers. © 1976 by Russell Sage Foundation. Reprinted by permission of Basic Books, Inc., Publishers.)

mates of happiness, and detailed information concerning sex, age, marital status, and so on.

A word of caution is appropriate at the outset. The results of studies such as these have to be interpreted tentatively, primarily because of the highly subjective nature of some of the central questions involved. Not only might there be systematic differences in the ways in which different groups interpret the questions, but there might also be systematic biases in the ways in which people choose to respond.

Not surprisingly, health is among the most important of all variables in predicting whether people will describe themselves as being happy—a finding that has been corroborated by a number of other researchers (for example, Clemente & Sauer, 1976; Flanagan, 1978). And among the most surprising findings, at least on the surface, is the observation that adolescents and young adults are typically less satisfied than older people, although they are not necessarily less happy. But, as Campbell (1981) explains, this finding is perhaps not so surprising when one considers the possibility that younger adults may be dissatisfied not because their lives are objectively less satisfying than those of older adults but because they have not yet resigned themselves to not having all their dreams and aspirations fulfilled. In contrast, adults past middle age might well have resigned themselves to the objective realities of their lives, feeling themselves less able to make significant changes in them.

Other intriguing findings from the Campbell studies are that women generally report less happiness than men, single women are happier than single men, married people are typically happier than the unmarried (single, widowed, or divorced), divorced women are less happy than divorced men, childless couples are as happy as couples with children, and couples whose children have left home continue to report high levels of satisfaction and happiness (the empty nest does not always lead to unhappiness).

Age-related changes in satisfaction and happiness are somewhat difficult to separate from those

associated with major personal events, particularly since many of these events (marriage, child bearing and rearing, career advancement and retirement) are closely tied to chronological age. Thus it is difficult to determine whether our popular notions of youth as a time of carefree abandonment and happiness and of old age as a period of contentment and serenity are accurate portrayals of age-related changes. Campbell's (1981) research, as well as a number of other studies reviewed by him, indicates that there has been a systematic change in professed happiness of young people since the early 1970s. Specifically, fewer of them report a high level of happiness. The same is not true of older people. As Campbell (1981, p. 176) put it, "In 1978 ... the young people were less positive than any of the older generations except the very old." Campbell suggests that social, political, and other environmental variables that are cohort specific might well account for these observations.

Unfortunately, Campbell's research does not shed a great deal of light on questions concerning the satisfaction and happiness of people beyond middle age, largely because the samples did not include those who were not living independently at home, either because of poor health or for other reasons. Thus Campbell's findings of a generally high level of satisfaction and of contentment (little very high excitement or anticipation but also few highly negative reactions) apply only to those who had survived as independents in older age.

A Recipe

If psychology were to be so bold as to attempt to provide us with a recipe for happiness, it might urge, among other things, that we all remain healthy, that we marry (we need not have children), and that we try to die at least as early as our spouses. But psychology would not yet dare be so bold or so flippant. To each his or her own. What is sauce for the goose is *not* necessarily sauce for the gander.

1 Many of the important developmental changes that occur during childhood and adolescence appear to be closely tied to chronological age. This is less true of changes that occur during adulthood.

2 Youth describes a developmental period that includes both adolescence and early adulthood (ages fourteen to twenty-four, according to Coleman) and that serves as a transition between childhood and adulthood.

3 According to Coleman, a successful transition from youth to adulthood requires the development of a number of important "self-centered" competencies (relating to economic independence, management of one's affairs, intelligent consumption of culture as well as of goods, and the ability to engage in concentrated activity). It also requires some related "other-centered" capabilities (relating to social interaction, cooperation with others, and assuming responsibility for those who are dependent).

4 Although we have sometimes been tempted to view adulthood as a *plateau* between childhood and old age—a period characterized by *no* change, following the rapid growth of childhood and preceding the rapid declines of very old age—our current models suggest that this view is misleading. Adulthood too is characterized by change, although this change is not always as dramatic or as predictable as it sometimes appears to be at the more extreme ends of the lifespan.

5 For most individuals, the twenties are characterized by a peak in many areas of human functioning, including strength and stamina. Noticeable declines in strength and stamina often become apparent by the forties and occur for the back and legs before the upper body.

6 Physical changes that eventually contribute significantly to the changing appearance of adults include cessation of growth in height and frequently a slight decrement in height in later years, the accumulation of a greater proportion of fatty tissue (often on the hips for females and around the midsection for males), loss of skin elasticity, thinning of hair, stiffening of joints, loss of muscle tone, and an eventual reduction in muscle tissue.

7 Changes in sensory capabilities with age include a gradual reduction in visual acuity, tending toward greater farsightedness, so that most fifty-year-olds require glasses; gradual loss of hearing ability, particularly for higher tones, and more serious for men than for women; and a gradual reduction in taste sensitivity to salt, sugar, and spices.

8 Changes in health and sickness that accompany adulthood include a reduction in the number of *acute* conditions (infections such as colds and flus) but an increase in chronic conditions (back and spine problems, heart disease, and so on). Women report more illnesses than men (but live longer). The most common medical complaints among women relate to the reproductive system; the most common among men concern the digestive system.

9 The most common causes of death among adolescents and youth are accidents; among older adults, heart disease is the number-one killer, followed by cancer.

10 By the late thirties or early forties for women, and perhaps by the fifties for men, the sex glands' production of hormones decreases (primarily estrogen from the ovaries and testosterone from the testes). This reduction leads to what is termed the *climacteric* or "change of life," an event that is not dramatic among men but that takes the form of menopause among women.

11 Menopause has generally occurred for most women by the age of fifty. It is sometimes accompanied by physical symptoms such as "hot flashes," trembling, dizziness, and headaches, which, in approximately one-third of all cases, are serious enough for women to seek medical advice. These symptoms can often be prevented through *estrogen replacement therapy*.

12 On the average, cognitive functioning declines with age. Among memory functions, the ability to *recall* declines more rapidly than does the ability to *recognize*. Problem-solving ability also appears to decline very slightly. In old age, these decrements are sometimes clearer, although they are not inevitable and universal.

13 There has been considerable controversy concerning whether or not measured intelligence changes with age. Numerous cross-sectional studies indicate that it does. However, these studies cannot take into account the possibility that important cohort-specific variables might account for the poorer performance of older people (their early experiences, educational level, familiarity with tests, and so on might place them at a disadvantage that is not related to lower intelligence).

14 Longitudinal studies indicate that those cognitive abilities that are highly dependent on experience do not decline with age, but may continue to increase into old age (verbal and numerical abilities, for example, labeled *fluid* abilities by Cattell). In contrast, abilities that are less dependent on experience do not fare as well (reasoning, attention span, and analogies, for example, labeled *crystallized* abilities by Cattell).

15 To the extent that personality includes all our capabilities, habits, predispositions, and so on, it changes with age. Research indicates that personality characteristics related to cognitive functioning (IQ, for example) are less susceptible to change than are the more interpersonal characteristics such as attitudes toward others.

16 There is considerable controversy concerning whether behavior is consistent with underlying personality characteristics (traits) or whether it is more influenced by the situation in which it occurs (the situation-trait controversy). Evidence suggests that both are importantly involved in behavior.

17 Among the important age-related personality changes that have been observed is a tendency for men to become more passive, more introspective, and more concerned with feelings following midlife and a corresponding tendency for women to become more outgoing and more aggressive during this period.

18 Satisfaction relates to the extent to which various objective aspects of our lives correspond with our goals and aspirations. Satisfaction is therefore a state of affairs that does not fluctuate greatly from day to day. Happiness, on the other hand, is an emotional state, susceptible to fluctuations of mood; it is not necessarily closely tied to satisfaction.

19 The past several years have seen an apparent decline in the number of individuals willing to describe themselves as "very happy"—a finding that is most noticeable among adolescents and young adults.

20 Isolated findings from happiness surveys include the following: Married individuals report more happiness than those who are alone (single, widowed, or divorced); women report less happiness than men; childless couples report as much happiness as those with children; couples whose children have left home (the "empty nest") do not, as a result, report lower levels of happiness, and perceived health is closely related to happiness.

21 Psychology does not yet have a good recipe for happiness.

■ FURTHER READINGS

The following are two very short, easily read books that discuss the transition between childhood and adulthood. Bocknek describes the experience of young adulthood from a psychological point of view. Coleman looks at the competencies that adulthood requires and the changes that might be made in social and educational institutions to facilitate the development of these competencies.

Bocknek, G. *The young adult: Development after adolescence*. Monterey, Calif.: Brooks/Cole, 1980.

Coleman, J. S. *Youth: Transition to adulthood*. Chicago: University of Chicago Press, 1974.

Davitz and Davitz present some useful insights into the lives of the middle aged in the following book. It is based primarily on interviews with over 200 individuals.

Davitz, J., & Davitz, L. *Making it from forty to fifty*. New York: Random House, 1976.

The following is an excellent, although frequently technical, collection of articles dealing with a variety of topics relevant to middle age. Among them are articles on physical health, mental health, and drinking, as well as on marriage, parenting, and careers—topics that we examine in the next chapter.

Eichorn, D. H., Clausen, J. A., Haan, N., Honzik, M. P., & Mussen, P. H. (Eds.). *Present and past in middle life*. New York: Academic Press, 1981.

The classic studies of satisfaction and happiness in the United States, conducted by Campbell and his associates beginning in 1957, are summarized in:

Campbell, A. *The sense of well-being in America: Recent patterns and trends*. New York: McGraw-Hill, 1981.

15 LIFE STYLES: CAREERS, MARRIAGE, AND FAMILY

To youth I have but three words of counsel—
work, work, work.

Otto Von Bismarck

Times are changed with him who marries; there are no more
by-path meadows, where you may innocently linger, but the road
lies long and straight and dusty to the grave.

Robert Louis Stevenson
Virginibus Puerisque

Darkness lies lightly upon the land as we approach Big River. On our right is Cowan Lake, a long, thin stretch of water reaching far into the north toward Green Lake. The lake's flat surface shimmers with the dark gold and orange reflections of a faded sunset.

Can the others sense the peace on this land—the tranquility? Does my grandmother, whose knitting disappeared with the sun and who now smiles out the western window, sense it in the marrow of her old bones as I do in mine? Can Paul and his brother and sister feel it too, this restfulness that comes upon the land with the end of the day? Or are they too young to have learned it?

I am about to ask them, but something stops me. Perhaps a fear that if I ask, it will go away. Or a fear that the feelings of the land aren't really feelings of the land at all—that they are just my own feelings.

I turn left onto the main street, and we suddenly lose the last glow of sunset among street lights and garish pink and blue neon. I pull up in front of the largest building on the street. Its name flames brightly in moving pink: "Hotel." The establishment immediately to the right announces itself in a more subdued blue: "Billiards."

"Where are you going?" Paul's voice is tight, high pitched, and for a second he looks small and frightened.

"I'll just get a case of beer for Uncle Raoul. Be right back." The relief is almost palpable. I meet grandmother's eyes in the mirror. She looks preoccupied, her smile small and unfocused. "I'll be right back," I repeat, as though the echo will bring more relief, as though they might trust me more if I urge them to trust me. But will I ever trust myself?

Inside, the air is abruptly heavy with smoke and drink. It reeks of old memories. I feel them tug, urgently it seems, but I ignore them as I walk through the noise toward the bar.

"Hey! Hey you! Is that you?" I am the only newcomer. I face the voice.

"Is that Guy Lefrancois?" The tone is neutral. Probably not a long-lost bosom buddy of my childhood, nor, if I am lucky, one of those who might have been around in those later years.

I hold out my hand, squinting through the smoke. A dark, burly, bearded individual, dressed in workshirt and coveralls, hat low over his ears.

"Maurice Frenette. You forgot me, hey?" Is the tone less friendly?

"Just for a minute there, Maurice. You've changed." When I shake his hand, huge and heavily calloused, I feel small. "What are you doing now?" Even as I ask the question, I know what the answer will be. The Frenettes have always lived here, halfway between Big River and Debden, and they have always farmed.

"Same," he says, "You?" I hesitate. "Hear you're a big-shot writer up there. Hear you made it big there." The question is no longer a question, more an accusation. I shrug, preparing a noncommittal, inoffensive answer, grinning harmlessly all the while. "Is it true," he continues, sounding more belligerent with every word, "that nobody up there knows about . . ."

"What are you drinking?" I interrupt him quickly. "Let me buy you a drink. Molson's, hey? Here, I'll get one."

I turn quickly toward the bar, order a case of Molson's Canadian for Uncle Raoul, and consider briefly whether or not I want to placate Maurice Frenette with a bottle of same. I decide that I don't want to, but buy him one just the same. He has now turned and is busily talking to someone at the table next to his.

"Tell him I had to leave," I say to the bartender. "And tell him I'll be back sometime," I add as an afterthought. Even as I say it, I wonder whether or not I ever will be back.

Everyone seems happy to see me so soon. Chatter fills the car as we drive through the last of Big River's streets and turn once more onto the highway. It is now a black highway, snaking stealthily through a moonless night. For the first few miles it courses through heavy spruce forests. Later the woods become less dense, there are more poplar groves, and scattered farms have eaten small clearings into the forest.

This is almost home. I can feel its closeness and smell it in the black night air. Where would I be now—what would I be, I muse, if I had never left this place? Would I, like Maurice Frenette, answer "same" if someone were to ask me? When did I make the decisions that are most responsible for the life style that is now mine? And did *I* actually make those decisions, or were they determined by circumstances over which I had no personal control?

We must turn immediately to these and related questions. Now, while we speed darkly over these last miles. Quickly, before we arrive. For if we reach my past too soon, I may find it impossible to continue the tale of the lifespan.

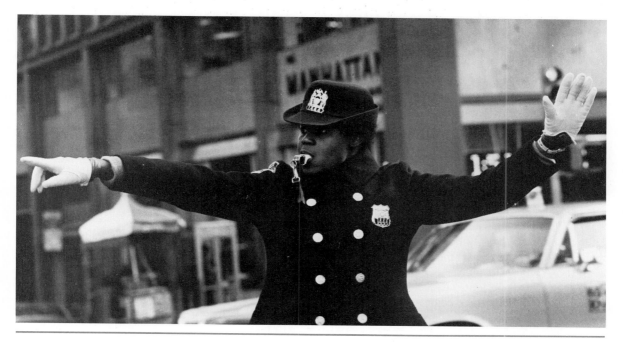

Although most people work to earn a living, the majority claim that they would continue to work even if they didn't have to. Clearly, we get far more from working than simply "a living."

■ Work

The telling of tales is now my work. It is a large part of the "dream" I had in distant years—a "dream" of which Levinson speaks in his description of the *seasons* of our lives. Most of us work. Indeed, work is an absolutely fundamental part of the lives of most adult men and women and is also, accordingly, a fundamental part of the dreams that fill our young lives and against which we later measure the happiness and satisfaction of our lives. Given that most of us will spend somewhere between twenty-five and forty years of our lives in work, its selection, the satisfaction it brings, and the ease with which we make the transitions between work and nonwork are all fundamentally important. These transitions include going from school (or adolescence) to work at the one end and going from work to retirement at the other. We look at these topics in the first major section of this chapter, as

well as at some important recent changes in the work of women outside the home. (See *Employment: Some Definitions,* on p. 413, for clarification of work terms.)

Why Work?

At the most basic and most obvious level, most of us work to earn a living. However, it would be highly misleading to suggest that that is the only, or even the most important, reason for working. Clearly, some individuals have little need of the income associated with their work, but they continue to work in any case. And even for those for whom work-related income is essential for "earning a living," work may also provide other rewards and satisfactions. Thus, a majority of men and women claim that they would continue to work even if they did not have to (Crowley, Levitin, &

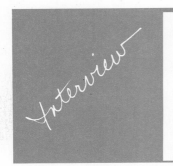

Interview

Subject: Male; age twenty-four; single; high school dropout; varied history of short-term employment, primarily as laborer for construction firms.

Question: "What do you want out of life? What do you dream of being or doing? Say when you're forty or so."

Well, I sure wouldn't want to be doing what I'm doing now. And I won't be. No way, Jose! Maybe I'll win the lottery.
. . .
What would I do then? Heck, nothing. Drink beer and party. Have a good time.

Quinn, 1973). When Sobol (1963) interviewed working women and asked them why they worked, even those who said they needed the money (48 percent of all respondents) also claimed they were committed to working for reasons *other* than the money. Most important was a need for "accomplishment." Also important was the desire to meet people and to occupy time that might otherwise be boring.

The reasons why men work are similar. Although a large majority of those working need to do so to provide a living for their families or for themselves, most obtain far more than just income from their work. Perhaps most important, it is through working and earning that people achieve a sense of self-worth and satisfaction. More than this, it is from our work that many of us derive important aspects of our identities. It is no accident—no careless slip of the tongue—that leads many of us to answer the question "What do you do for a living?" with "I am a(n) . . ." In a sense, we *are* what we do.

■ Changes in Work Opportunities

Unfortunately, the choice of what we will do and consequently be is perhaps far more difficult today than it might have been for my grandfather and grandmother. For her, there was almost no choice. Although she might have worked outside the home for a very short period of time between school and marriage, unless she was black or very poor, this would have been the exception rather than the rule. Her sex had already determined that she would spend most if not all of her working years occupied as a parent and homemaker.

My grandfather, on the other hand, had somewhat more choice since his sex had determined that he would be working outside the home. However, he and the majority of his cohorts were already working by the age of twenty, many having begun permanent work by the time they were sixteen (Havighurst & Gottlieb, 1975). And the great majority of them would be employed in blue-collar occupations, often identical to those of their fathers and even of their grandfathers. Career selection frequently presented no choice whatsoever.

Today's highly industrialized, "high-tech" society presents an incredible array of jobs, an increasing number of which have replaced blue-collar occupations. Furthermore, the nature of these jobs is in a constant state of flux, as are the markets that provide employment. Thus, the 1965 edition of *The Dictionary of Occupational Titles* (the third edition; U.S. Department of Labor, 1965) listed more than 22,000 separate occupations. The fourth edition of this publication lists approximately 1,800 *fewer* occupations. However, there are slightly more than 2,100 *new* occupations in the fourth edition, but more than 3,500 distinct jobs have now been deleted (U.S. Department of Labor, 1978).

Another important change in current employment concerns vastly increased mobility among different occupations within a single career and also among different careers. As Toffler (1970)

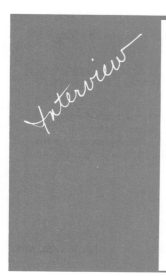

Subject: Male; age twenty-six; single; recent university graduate; permanent employment with government department.

Question: "What do you want out of life? What do you dream of being or doing? Say when you're forty or so."

You're sure this is going to be anonymous?

. . .

Okay. What I'd really like, I guess, is a good administrative position in this department or in another one. It doesn't really matter. As long as I'm in charge. Of people and decisions. I know I've got the right background, and if I play my cards right I should be assistant director by the time I'm thirty-five. I'll be in line for a supervisor's job by next summer. But there's lots of politics, and if it doesn't work out—like if I don't go as fast as I think I should—then I'd move. Transfer to another department, or maybe even run for politics. If the situation looks right. I don't want to waste my time and run if it doesn't look like I can win. Here you have to be in the right party. But mostly I think I can make a heck of a good career here if I play my cards right.

suggests, present conditions dictate that many of us should be looking not at a single career but at *serial* careers. Not only is there time, within a single life, to engage successfully in more than one career, but doing so may also be required by the rate at which old jobs disappear and new ones take their place. But through it all, we must be prepared for adjustments and adaptations that were not likely to be demanded of our grandparents, lest we too be overcome by *future shock*.

Theories of Career Choice

But how is the adolescent to choose from among so many careers? Or the adult, for that matter? Do we *naturally* drift toward a career? Do our personal talents and interests urge us gently down the right paths? Or should we be guided? And if we are to be guided, how should it be done?

There are two general groups of theories that influence much of our thinking in career guidance. One is based on the notion that individuals should be matched with respect to their interests and talents and is referred to as *trait-interest job matching*. The other emphasizes the development of career-related abilities rather than simple job-

interest matching and includes what are termed *developmental models of guidance*.

Among the very earliest systematic attempts to provide guidance for those who need to make career decisions were theories based on the notion that jobs and individuals should be matched on the basis of talents or interests. According to this approach, guidance takes the form of identifying which talents are most essential for specific occupations, administering batteries of tests to those who require guidance in order to discover their particular combinations of talents, and matching the two. The matching itself generally takes into account the individual's interests as well as talents. A well-known example of this trait-interest, job-matching approach is that of Holland (1964, 1966). His instrument, the Holland Vocational Preference Inventory (Holland, 1975), identifies six specific combinations of traits and interests that he labels *coping styles*, as well as five personality traits. The coping styles are called *realistic, intellectual, social, conventional, enterprising,* and *artistic*. Each of these, in combination with specific personality characteristics, is thought to be appropriate for different careers. In effect, then, this inventory is both an interest and a personality measure (Herr & Cramer, 1979).

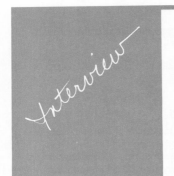
A second measure widely employed to provide information for matching occupations and individuals on the basis of talents and abilities is the Differential Aptitude Tests (Bennett, Seashore, & Wesman, 1981). They provide a profile of eight separate classifications of abilities as well as a general summary of abilities in the form of an average. These eight classifications include verbal reasoning, numerical ability, abstract reasoning, mechanical reasoning, space relations, spelling, language usage, and clerical, speech, and accounting. An analysis of the individual's profile with respect to each of these groupings of abilities can sometimes provide useful suggestions concerning career choices.

Although the trait-interest matching approaches to career guidance have proven highly useful and continue to be widely used both in schools and in placement and employment offices, the *developmental models* are also important and useful. These are based on the notion that the *development* of careers is at least as important as any attempt we might make to match individual interests and abilities with specific occupations.

Among the best known of developmental guidance models are those advanced by Ginzberg (1951, 1972) and Super (1957, 1974; Super & Hall, 1978). Ginzberg's model describes three sequential preadult stages in career development. The *fantasy* period lasts until approximately age eleven and is often characterized by highly unrealistic notions of career choice. There is no distinction between what is possible (or probable) and what is not. This is the stage during which children want to be astronauts, baseball players, physicians, poets, and popes.

During a second stage, termed the *tentative* period (ages twelve to sixteen), adolescents gradually become aware of the requirements of different careers, as well as of their own personal interests and capabilities. The third stage, the *realistic* period, begins at around age seventeen and generally involves the beginnings of career decisions. However, final decisions might be some distance in the future, particularly in view of the extent to which postsecondary education extends adolescence and often postpones the need to enter the work world. And even after a career choice has been made, it will remain *tentative* for some time. Career evaluation continues to occur not only in early adulthood but also sometimes throughout much of the remainder of the lifespan.

Work Selection

It would be naive and misleading to suggest that most of us make our career choices on the basis of well-reasoned decisions based on what we know of our interests and abilities—that each of us undertakes a careful examination of available careers and a thoughtful analysis of their requirements as well as of their potential contributions to our eventual growth and satisfaction. In fact, a great

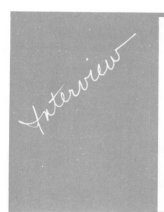

Subject: Male; age forty-six; divorced; no children; involved in film business.

Question: "How or why did you become a _____? And is this the type of work (career) that you think you would have chosen when you were in high school?"

Sure. When I was in high school we had a communications course and everybody made little 8-millimeter films. I guess I had some talent which the teacher recognized. I'll never forget that teacher. It's probably because of him that I went into this business. I mean, it wasn't just an accident. I *decided* this is what I wanted, and I've been working at it ever since. I haven't done everything I want to yet, but it's shaping up. It's a lot of work and learning and contacts. This is a tough business, but I wouldn't want to be anything else.

many of us select our careers (or are selected for them) in very different ways. Thus fortune, the occupations of our parents, and our sex may each contribute significantly to what we eventually become. For its part, fortune may provide a variety of chance happenings that mold great chunks of our lives. A father dies and leaves his child a business, a farm, or a family to look after; a teenage girl becomes pregnant; a dedicated young doctor marries into great wealth. Events such as these can profoundly influence the course of an individual's career, as can the simple availability of jobs. For those who attempt to enter the labor market directly from high school, or even before completing high school, the first job obtained is likely to be the one that is first available. And in many cases, the individual's eventual career may be related to this first accidental job.

Our sex, socioeconomic backgrounds, and the occupations of our parents may also have important effects on our career choices. Despite rapidly changing social conditions (discussed later in this chapter), stereotypes concerning appropriate male-female career divisions are still prevalent. Thus, almost two-thirds of young girls still claim they would like to be teachers or nurses (Tibbetts, 1975). The sciences, the medical and legal professions, and other high-status occupations such as those related to engineering, architecture, and finance are seen largely as male employment.

Socioeconomic background, too, influences choice of careers, with people from higher levels being the most likely to obtain postsecondary education or training and consequently being most likely to select professional, white-collar, and high-technology occupations. People from lower levels are more likely to be found in blue-collar occupations. Similarly, parental occupation often has a strong bearing on the child's selection of careers. This is true not only when parents are in a position to bring children into a family business but in many other cases as well. When Werts (1968) looked at the occupations of sons and their fathers among more than 76,000 high school graduates, he found an overwhelming tendency for sons to choose the *same* career as their fathers or a career that would be highly similar in terms of status, often in a related field.

Following a review of literature on careers and career guidance, particularly as it relates to women, Tittle (1982) suggests four things that schools should do to foster intelligent career decisions. First, and perhaps most important among these, is her suggestion that schools have a responsibility to attempt to counter a subtle "hidden" curriculum that often continues to foster sexual stereotypes concerning occupations that are most likely and most appropriate for males and females. Second, she urges schools to help students look at the various work-related roles that are implicit

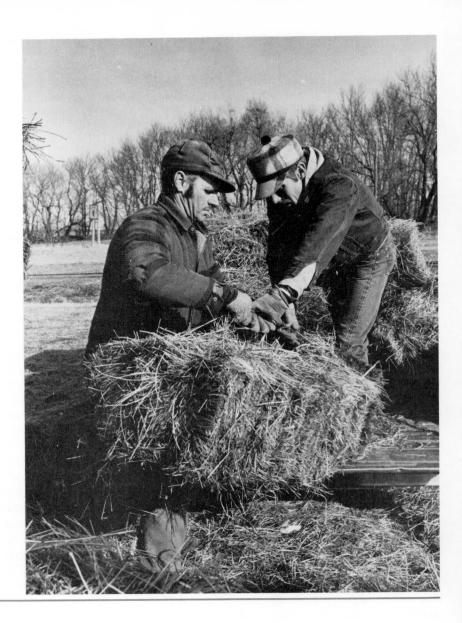

Few of us select our careers on the basis of careful analysis of our interests and talents. Our socioeconomic backgrounds, parents' occupations, and various fortunes and misfortunes have important effects on our career choices.

not only in specific careers but that are also part of being a homemaker or parent. Third, schools should stress the economic importance of education. This is especially critical for women because earning disparities between males and females are such that even with a college degree, a woman earns no more than the average male blue-collar worker with no college experience whatsoever (see Troll, 1982). Finally, Tittle suggests that students need to understand the tremendous social implications of being male or female with respect to occupations, particularly as these are reflected in occupational segregation and differences in earnings.

EMPLOYMENT: SOME DEFINITIONS

Although terms such as *career, vocation, job,* and *occupation* are often used interchangeably, their precise meanings are somewhat different. The narrowest of these terms is *job,* which refers to the specific tasks or duties that the worker performs. Thus, one of the jobs undertaken by a caretaker might be to empty wastebaskets. In much the same way, there are jobs associated with being a lawyer or a dentist—specific tasks that are part of the individual's work.

Occupation is a somewhat more general term than job and refers to a broad employment classification such as accounting, clerking, selling, being a mechanic, and so on. Occupations are categories of work that cover a variety of related jobs.

The term *career* is far broader than either occupation or job. It does not refer to any specific occupation or employment but to an entire range of related occupations (Super & Hall, 1978). Thus, a career will often span an entire lifetime of work and may include a host of related occupations (each with their own jobs). A career in food services, for example, might include occupations as busboy, waiter, bartender, food manager, convention manager, and chain food–services supervisor. Similarly, a career in law might include a variety of employments (occupations) for different legal firms or government agencies, private practice, and so on. It is possible, of course, to have more than one career in a single lifetime (Reardon & Burck, 1975).

In its strictest sense, the term *vocation* refers to a "calling" and has traditionally been restricted to the clergy and to certain white-collar professions. Thus one can have a vocation for the ministry, a vocation for medicine, or a legal vocation; it is less appropriate to refer to a laborer's or a secretary's vocation.

In this text, as in many other contexts, *work* is often employed as a general term to include all manner of occupations, careers, professions, jobs, and vocations.

Job Satisfaction

Not many decades ago, the primary purpose of a job was to provide a living. Not only did every man (and some women) have a *duty* to work, but each also had a duty to support himself and his dependents. Thus, the primary motivations for work were money, perhaps security, and often duty. And the emphasis was on being a successful, productive worker (Getzels, 1972). But when Yankelovich (1972) interviewed youth about their attitudes toward work, he found overwhelming agreement that the financial aspects of an occupation are far less important than its nature, its purpose, its social significance, and the extent to which growth and happiness are likely to be associated with it. As Kuder (1977) notes, it is no longer sufficient just to have a job; we also want to be *happy* in our work and to feel that our contributions are worthwhile. In Terkel's (1972) words, work is "a search for daily meaning as well as daily bread, for recognition as well as cash, for astonishment rather than torpor; in short, for a sort of life rather than a Monday through Friday sort of dying. Perhaps immortality, too, is part of the quest" (p. xiii).

How satisfied and happy are most of us with what we do? Here, as in the more general areas of satisfaction with their lives, few adults are willing to describe themselves as very dissatisfied or very unhappy (see Chapter 14). Indeed, in a wide-scale study of workers, Quinn, Staines, and McCullough (1974) found that at least three-quarters of all workers at any age level describe themselves as being satisfied with their jobs and happy. And the percentage of those who so describe themselves increases with age. Thus, 75 percent of those under the age of twenty-one describe themselves as happy; 84 percent of those between twenty and thirty, and an amazing 90 percent of those above thirty, also describe themselves as happy.

Why do we become progressively more happy with our jobs? In addition to the fact that work gives meaning to a great many lives and that we therefore *want* to be satisfied, perhaps finding it difficult to admit even to ourselves that we might not be (Yankelovich, 1978), there are at least three reasons why people seem to become happier with their work as they age. The first and most obvious is that those who are truly unhappy with their careers will often change them early in their lives. The second is that it is possible to grow to love (or at least accept) a career that at first seems unpleasant. And third, as we age, many of us might modify our original *dream*, dropping our aspirations, lowering our estimates of what our contributions and rewards should be; perhaps we become satisfied with less as it becomes clearer that we are unlikely to be given more.

Not all of us are bound to succeed, to climb the high ladders of corporate achievement, to accumulate great power and status, to become, as Kanter (1977) puts it, "fast trackers." Many more will simply be "dead enders"—those who never reach the high ceilings toward which the "fast trackers" climb so rapidly. "Dead enders," Kanter tells us, include those who initially enter occupations that have low ceilings, those who are in high-ceiling employment but who fail somewhere along the line, and those who simply take the wrong paths. Low-ceiling jobs are those that do not ordinarily lead to advancement and include many labor and clerical jobs. High-ceiling occupations include opportunities for advancement. Dead enders in low-ceiling employment are relatively satisfied; those in high-ceiling employment but who fail to climb upward are most unsatisfied. And those who simply climb the wrong ladders in the beginning find themselves at an intermediate level of satisfaction.

Clausen (1981) identifies three factors that appear to be closely related to the satisfaction workers experience with their occupations. Most important is the extent to which the job reflects personal interests. Also crucial is the extent to which it requires full use of the worker's capabilities and provides an opportunity to develop ideas. Finally, income also contributes to job satisfaction. It is revealing that although each of these factors was important both for white- and blue-collar workers in Clausen's sample, more than half of the blue-collar workers also indicated that job security was also extremely important. In contrast, fewer than 20 percent of those in white-collar occupations thought job security was critical. Clausen specu-

lates that this might be because white-collar occupations are frequently such that job permanence or security is seldom an issue. Such is not the case for blue-collar occupations, particularly during economic recessions.

Women at Work

Between 1900 and 1970, the number of adult women working for a salary in North America more than doubled (from 20 to 45 percent; Sheppard, 1976). Age groups most likely to work outside the home include young adults prior to marriage and those whose children have left home (ages forty-five to sixty-four). In addition, black women and those from poorer groups have always been more likely to work than the more affluent, white, middle-class woman. Figure 15.1 shows the relative distribution of the U.S. work force in 1981 by age and sex. Note that the curve for females is bimodal. That is, there are two age periods of peak employment for females rather than a single period as for males—one occurring shortly after twenty (prior to marriage or children) and the other shortly after the age of forty-five (after children have left home).

The percentage of the labor force that is female has changed dramatically in recent decades. In 1960, 13 percent of adult women worked outside the home, a figure that had increased to 33 percent by 1970 and to 37 percent in 1974 (Turner & McCaffrey, 1974). By 1978, 42 percent of adult women now worked outside the home, a number that apparently continues to increase (Hoffman, 1979). Among other important recent changes is a greater tendency for mothers of preschool children to work.

A number of male-female differences in the work place should also be noted, in addition to the fact that far fewer women work for a salary than men. As mentioned earlier, typical female occupations are not yet on a par with male occupations in terms of status, prestige, or income (Tittle, 1982). Average income for females is perhaps 60 percent that of males (England, 1979). And in 1977, women with four years of college earned less than men who had quit school after eighth grade (Tittle, 1982). Unemployment rates are typ-

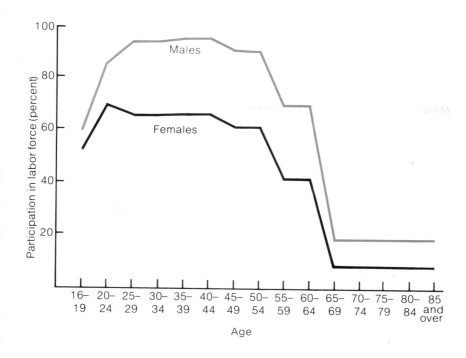

Figure 15.1
Labor force participation rates by age and sex in the United States, 1981. (From U.S. Bureau of the Census, *Statistical Abstract of the United States, 1983*, p. 377.)

ically higher for women than for men. They are lowest for white adult males above the age of twenty and highest for black teenage females (Tittle, 1982).

The reasons why women work are often not very different from those for which men work, although the majority are not as career oriented as men (Crowley et al., 1973), a fact that may well be due to the greater number of low-status, dead-end jobs that many women occupy. Where women enter careers with higher ceilings, their work attitudes and achievement orientations are very similar to those of men in similar positions (Stroud, 1981, cited in Skolnick, 1981).

Research on job satisfaction reveals that working women are, on the average, happier than those who do not work outside the home. In addition, middle-aged career women tend to have higher self-esteem than other women, whether they are single or married. Also, work satisfaction appears to increase with age, even for those women who are responsible for the dual roles: career, on the one hand, and homemaking and child rearing, on the other (Huston-Stein & Higgins-Trenk, 1978).

There appears to be relatively little conflict between being a mother and working at the same time, although there is a possibility of work overload (Stroud, 1981, cited in Skolnick, 1981).

Changing Social Conditions

In the relatively recent past, women who continued their education after twelfth grade or who took one of various job-training courses often claimed that they were doing so in order "to have something to fall back on later." The implicit, and sometimes explicit, assumption that these women made was that they would find Mr. Right, marry him, and have and raise their children while he earned their bread and other good things. Having "to fall back" was something that would happen only in the wake of some great misfortune that would make it impossible for the husband to provide for his wife and children any longer. Death was clearly one such misfortune, but as those who sell death insurance (usually misnamed *life* insurance) had surely informed the husband, if enough of this insurance were purchased, even in the event of so unlikely a catastrophe, she might not have to leave her rightful place in the home and enter the world of work.

Not so any longer. There are fewer and fewer who still believe that the home is woman's only rightful place. And an increasing number of women continue their education, not to have something to fall back on but so that they can pursue their own careers. However, since more than 40 percent of all young adult marriages eventually end in divorce (Corcoran, 1979), there is sometimes a real need to have something to fall back on.

Changing social conditions are reflected not only in the increasing numbers of women who have entered the work force but are reflected as well in the fact that the *expected* family pattern, where the man works outside the home and the woman inside, describes fewer than 20 percent of all contemporary American families (Eisenstein, 1982). Approximately 57 percent of two-parent families also have two wage earners. Furthermore, single-parent families headed by a woman are now as common as the more traditional two-parent family, where the male is the sole wage earner (Eisenstein, 1982). Clearly, there have been some profound changes in the American family. There have also been some important changes in the alternatives that now confront new adults.

■ Life-Style Choices

At some point, usually in early adulthood or even before (though sometimes much later), many of us make a very basic life-style choice: to marry or not to marry. And although we might be tempted to believe that the choice was far simpler in the misty days of our grandparents, assuming that in those years almost all who could did marry, the situation is still very much the case today. More than 95 percent of all adults marry at least once (Rawlings, 1978).

The choice, to marry or not to marry, is certainly not as simple as it might at first appear, since there are a number of different nonmarried life styles, as well as a number of different types of marriages. Nor is it always a rational choice, made only by the individuals most directly affected. In many cases, parents or other circumstances (such as total physical repulsiveness) might make our choices for us.

Cohabitation, homosexuality, singlehood (with or without children), and a variety of communal living arrangements are among the other life styles adults follow. We look briefly at each of these before turning to the most common adult life style: marriage.

Cohabitation

When my Uncle Raoul moved in with Elizabeth Proulx, all my other uncles and aunts told my grandparents that he had moved to a boardinghouse in Debden. All of my relatives objected. We objected on social and moral principles, on religious grounds, and for countless other reasons. And the ensuing scandal was at least as large and as overwhelming as our objections were numerous. The eventual resolution was not a happy one and cannot be disclosed here, hidden as it is among other things in that closet.

My Uncle Raoul should have attended Cornell University many years later, where one-third of a large sample of senior and sophomore students admittedly shared accommodation with a member of the opposite sex (Macklin, 1972) and where more than 95 percent of the sample, whether or not they lived alone, considered cohabitation of unmarried couples totally acceptable. Or he should have lived anywhere in the United States some years later, where one out of twenty-three couples is unmarried (Glick & Norton, 1978). Or, better yet, he should have gone to Sweden, where more than one out of every eight couples is not married (Trost, 1975).

There are a number of reasons why couples might live together without marrying. Among college students, for example, it has become increasingly common to share accommodation for financial reasons. Sexual relations might, or might not, also be part of the arrangement. Among couples where relations are intimate, cohabitation is some-

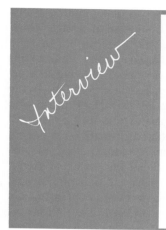

Subject: Female; age thirty-one; never married; university education; successful career in a helping profession.
(concerning a recently ended relationship with a man with whom she had been living)

I read an article which described a couple making love. They both liked different music, so she would listen to one thing on headphones and he would listen to something else. Sometimes making . . . well, not even making love with him reminded me of that article. It was like we both wanted to be listening to something else. We were so different we never heard or saw the same things even when we were together.

. . .

I don't think I will get married now. At least not for a while. I'm not saying no, period. I might like to have a child someday. But I guess it wouldn't really matter if I was married or not.

times preferred over marriage because the legal obligations are different, because partners want intimacy and friendship without a long-term commitment, or because marriage is simply being delayed. In many cases, cohabitation serves as a sort of "trial marriage," during which couples explore their compatibility and assess the rewards that each is likely to obtain from a permanent relationship.

Cohabitation does have legal status in a number of jurisdictions and can, therefore, entail the same sorts of legal responsibilities that are more explicit in conventional marriage. Where cohabitation defines a legally recognized union of partners, it is termed a *common-law marriage*. Common-law marriages apparently originated on the frontier, where ministers, priests, rabbis, and ships' captains were scarce and where couples were often forced to exchange "marriage" vows, sometimes in the presence of witnesses but often in private as well. Subsequently, these common-law marriages were upheld as being valid in the courts (Leslie, 1979). The end result is that, to this day, if it can be established that a couple intend to live together with the same commitments as a married couple, theirs may be a legal, common-law marriage. It was on these grounds that Lee Marvin's companion of many years, Michelle Triola Marvin, sued him for half the wealth he had accumulated during the years they lived together. In the end, the judge awarded her considerably less than half of the several million dollars in question.

Homosexuality

A number of life styles are available to those whose sexual preferences are directed toward members of their own sex (*homo*sexual) rather than to members of the opposite sex (*hetero*sexual). Here, as elsewhere, however, things are seldom simply black or white. The research of Kinsey et al. (1948) revealed that sexual preference is, in many respects, a continuum, with the vast majority of individuals being primarily attracted to members of the opposite sex, a small minority being attracted primarily to members of the same sex, and others falling in between. Estimates of actual numbers that can be considered to be homosexual vary a great deal and tend to be highly unreliable. Many still view homosexuality as deviant and unnatural, although it has now been deleted from the American Psychiatric Association's manual of mental disorders (American Psychiatric Association, 1980). Accordingly, given that many homosexuals have preferred to remain incognito, some surveys have probably provided underestimates. In contrast, the 1960s and 1970s witnessed a dramatic increase in a sense of community among homosexual groups and a some-times militant tendency to agitate for rights and recognition. And estimates of homosexuality that have been provided by outspoken members of this community have perhaps sometimes been overestimates.

Gebhard (1972) suggests that between 4 and 5 percent of the male population and between 1 and 2 percent of the female population can be considered to be overtly homosexual. Choice of life style for these individuals does not include marriage, since same-sex marriages have not been legalized in the United States, despite several test cases in the courts. There are, however, a number of possible living arrangements. Bell and Weinberg (1978) describe five of these. The *closed couples* consist of single homosexual pairs who live together with the same sorts of commitments that are characteristic of traditional marriage. *Open couples* include those who live together in close pairs, but who are also open to other relationships in addition to the primary one. This living arrangement parallels the open marriage described by the O'Neills (1972). *Functionals* include those who live alone or in groups and who seek a variety of relationships rather than a primary commitment (homosexual "swingers"). A fourth group, the *dysfunctionals*, includes those whose sexual preference is a source of conflict and unhappiness and who frequently vacillate between expressing and hiding this preference. *Asexuals*, the fifth group, effectively suppress their sexual preferences. They typically function without intimate homosexual or heterosexual relationships.

Many who might have been far more secretive some decades ago have now become very outspoken about their sexual preferences.

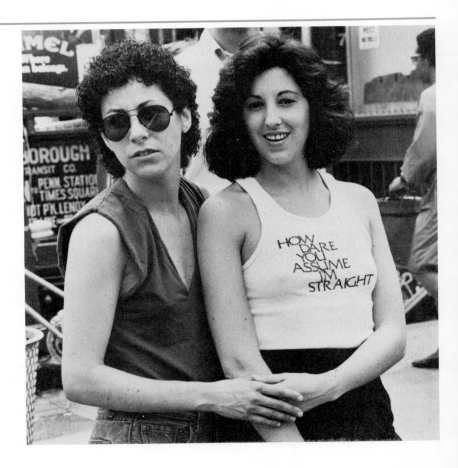

Singlehood

Single adults include not only those who have consciously decided not to marry (or, as noted earlier, for whom the decision has been made by other circumstances) but also those who are divorced, widowed, or separated.

Current indications are that somewhere close to 5 percent of the adult population never marries (95 percent do at least once). And there is evidence, still tentative, that this number may be rising (Schulz & Rodgers, 1980). In addition, many are now getting married later, a fact that increases the number of young single people in the population. This trend is reflected in a growing number of clubs, bars, housing associations, and other organizations that cater specifically to single individuals.

Contrary to the popular images we might have of the lives of bachelors, the happiness research we looked at in Chapter 14 indicates that married people are *on the average* happier than those who are single. In addition, single women report more satisfaction with their lives than single men. In the main, however, our society continues to be oriented toward marriage, an attitude that might at least partly account for these findings.

Communes

Communes are, by definition, *communities*—joint, cooperative attempts to carve a happy or useful life style. Although they present a life style that is different from, and hence an alternative to, the more or less conventional life styles we have looked at thus far, they are compatible with any of them. Thus, there are communes for conventionally married couples as well as for people involved in group marriages; there are homosexual and heterosexual communes, religious and political communes, utopian communes, and all manner of other possible communal arrangements. As Ramey (1972) notes, so many communes are possible that "being a commune is almost a state of mind" (p. 477). Some communes are established so that members can do their own, presumably unconventional,

"thing"; others function primarily to pool individual resources as a means of coping more effectively with society. And still others result from fundamental religious beliefs that can more easily be encouraged and practiced in relative isolation from society.

■ Marriage

Although we have a choice of many life styles, marriage is the choice of the vast majority. It is perhaps notable, however, that we choose it somewhat later than did our parents—and they later than theirs. Skolnick (1981) reports the average age of first marriage for men as twenty-four and for women as twenty-one and one-half, in a sample of 232 members.

For most of us, there is only one officially approved form of marriage: that where each partner is entitled to only one other partner—*monogamy*. Having more than one wife or husband is, in fact, illegal in North America and is termed *bigamy* by the courts. **Polygamy** is a more general expression for the same state of affairs. It includes *polygyny*, where the man is permitted to have more than one wife, and *polyandry*, where a wife is permitted more than one husband. Murdock (1957) looked at 554 of the world's societies and found that only 24 percent sanctioned only monogamy. The vast majority (75 percent) permit polygyny; only 1 percent permit polyandry (Table 15.1). Note, however, that even in those societies that permit

Table 15.1 Common forms of marriage among 554 of the world's societies.

Type of Marriage	Number of Societies	Percentage
Monogamy	135	24
Polygamy	419	76
Polyandry	4	1
Polygyny	415	75

Based on data reported by G. P. Murdock. World ethnographic sample. *American Anthropologist*, 1957, *59*, 664–688. Reprinted by permission of the American Anthropological Association.

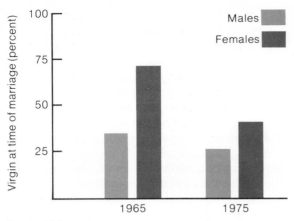

Figure 15.2
One example of the sexual revolution: the decrease in the percentage of people who are virgins when they marry.

of men and that they would no longer be denied. In 1965, 65 percent of all males were no longer virgins at the time of their marriage; only 29 percent of all women were in the same state. But by 1975, when the percentage of nonvirgin males had risen by 9 percent to 74, the corresponding percentage for females had increased a whopping 28 percent to 57 (King, Balswick, and Robinson, 1977). These figures are even more staggering when we note that the percentage increase for males was approximately 14, but that it was almost 100 percent for females. In short, *twice* as many females were no longer virgins at the time of marriage in 1975. The sexual revolution had happened, but it affected females far more than males (Figure 15.2).

Contrary to some popular reports, however, this sexual revolution did not translate itself into widespread, indiscriminate, totally recreational sex, although there is clearly more of this type of sexual activity now—as the current herpes epidemic indicates—than there was when my grandfather cut mustard and sowed his particular species of oats. True, the sexual revolution of these past decades does manifest itself in greater sexual permissiveness. But it is a permissiveness that, with some notable exceptions, insists on *affection*. As Scanzoni and Scanzoni (1981) explain, there are four categories of premarital sexual behavior. The first, abstinence, belongs largely to another age. The second, the double standard, was recently common and still lingers, although it is a battered and torn standard, ravaged by the forces of women's liberation. The third, permissiveness with affection, appears to be increasingly common. And the last, permissiveness without affection, has its place too in the contemporary world, although sexual activity is a long distance from having become as indiscriminate, as matter of fact, and as casual as many had feared—or hoped.

one or more forms of polygamy, these are typically the exception rather than the rule. Often only the old and the wealthy can afford more than one wife (or husband). Often, too, only the very highly placed in the social hierarchy are permitted polygamy.

Although contemporary Western societies do not permit polygamy, they do permit what Mead (1970) calls *serial monogamy*. We are free to marry, divorce, and remarry an unlimited number of times. In addition, various group-sex arrangements, mate swapping, open marriages, and other forms of sexual and emotional permissiveness, while not a dominant part of the current social mainstream, are nevertheless not altogether uncommon.

Premarital Sex

Indications are clear, then, that monogamy is not what it used to be. This is particularly true for those many women whose roles were determined largely by the well-known double standard that was rampant until recently and that still rears itself on occasion in various male bastions: "Boys will be boys, you know." It went without saying that "girls will not be girls; if they must be anything, they will be angels."

Later, we discovered that women, too, have sexual feelings that are at least as intense as those

Extramarital Sex

Although extramarital sex, *adultery* if a spade is to be called a shovel, is apparently not uncommon, most societies discourage its practice, often on the grounds that it threatens the family unit. There is ample evidence, however, of a powerful double standard here, as there is with respect to premarital sex. In Japan as well as in many European countries, it is quite acceptable for a man to have a mistress, providing he is reasonably discreet about the affair and continues to discharge his familial obligations. The same behavior is far less easily tolerated among married women and, indeed, is often grounds for punishment or divorce; such is seldom the case when the man is the adulterer.

In North American societies, the mistress and the male lover are less clearly condoned or condemned, but the *affair* is common. An affair is a sexual-emotional episode of varying duration and intensity involving two people, one or both of whom is married but not to each other. It implies an element of deception, such that if the other partner were to "find out," there would follow some consequences of greater or lesser severity. How common are affairs?

Thirty years ago, Kinsey and his associates (Kinsey et al., 1953) reported that by the age of forty, 26 percent of all married females and almost half of all males had engaged in at least one extramarital affair. More than twenty years later, Maykovich (1976) reported an increase to 32 percent for females. Major surveys conducted by Hunt (1974) and Athanasiou (1973) report that the incidence of adultery is now almost as common among women as it is among men (somewhere between 33 and 50 percent by middle age). It is somewhat more common among women who have also experienced premarital sex (Krishna Singh, Walton, & Williams, 1976). And although affairs might be implicated in the breakup of some marriages, Strean (1980) suggests that it is relatively rare that a husband or wife will disrupt a marriage specifically to live with the lover.

Affairs, by definition, are clandestine and secretive. They are seldom openly tolerated by the other marriage partner. And where they are, they are no longer labeled affairs. One type of marriage that openly tolerates extramarital encounters is labeled "open" and is described by the O'Neills (1972) as providing both freedom and the "relatedness" that we all crave. But the freedom of the successful open marriage is not the freedom of the unmarried "swinger"—a freedom without responsibility. "Freedom in open marriage does not mean freedom to 'do your thing' without responsibility. It is the freedom to grow to the capacity of your individual potential through love—and one aspect of that love is caring for your partner's growth and welfare as much as your own" (1972, p. 258). We have little evidence that truly "open" marriages are common. On the other hand, marriages where partners engage in group sex or in mate swapping (also termed consensual adultery) are not altogether uncommon.

Bartell (1971), who employed a participant-observer approach for studying 280 "swingers," provides some insights into the causes and effects of these sexual practices. He reports that the most common reasons for mate swapping include boredom, feelings of alienation and loneliness, and, particularly for men, the desire to explore sexual fantasies. And although ages of participants in Bartell's study ranged from eighteen to seventy, very few were still "swinging" after eighteen to twenty-four months. Reasons for stopping included feelings of jealousy and guilt, occasional boredom, and frequently a renewed strengthening of the marriage. Denfeld and Gordon (1970), in a separate study, found that it was not uncommon for swinging couples to develop a stronger and closer relationship with each other, a finding also reported by Bartell. At the same time, in both these studies, a number of marriages did not outlast the mate-swapping experience.

Good and Bad Marriages

We know that some 40 percent of all new marriages now end in divorce. We know, too, that between one-third and one-half of all married people, even if they remain married all their lives, will not always be sexually faithful. But we also know that married people describe their lives in more satisfactory terms and see themselves as being happier than those who remain single (or who are separated, divorced, or widowed).

To describe marriages as being either good or bad would be overly simplistic. There can be much that is good and much that is bad in any marriage. But it might be important to know what a "good" marriage can be like. Cuber and Harroff (1965) provide us with the beginnings of some answers. They studied 211 men and women—all upper-middle-class and highly successful professionals. Each had been married for at least ten years and *none* had ever seriously contemplated separation or divorce. The marriages were *good* at least to that extent.

Among the most notable findings of this study was the tremendous variation in the nature of the marriage relationships among these individuals. In the end, Cuber and Harroff identified five different types of relationships among these couples. The *conflict-habituated* couple lives in the continuously stormy atmosphere of domestic disagreement and conflict, as though each of the partners wants and perhaps even needs constant disagreement so that, in spite of the quarrels, the marriage endures.

The *devitalized* marriage is a lifeless affair; it has no fire, no passion, and little intimacy. Couples in this type of marriage typically remember that they were quite madly in love when younger, that their relationship was intense and fiery, that they were deeply intimate. Now habit and memory bind them in an apathetic but enduring relationship.

Those in a *passive-congenial* marriage are, in essence, trapped in the same dull, lifeless relationship that characterizes the devitalized marriage. Sadly, however, a passive-congenial marriage is one that was devoid of any of the sweet excesses of romantic love from its beginning. Such marriages are often simply convenient arrangements for both parties, socially expected, proper, and sometimes useful in the advancement of careers or for clinging to the proper rungs in the social ladder, but they are emotionally barren.

A *vital* marriage is one where the marriage relationship is fundamentally important to both partners and where there is a genuine sharing of important experiences and values. While both husband and wife devote much of their time to the marriage relationship and are genuinely happy with it, the partners retain their individuality.

A *total* marriage describes a relationship that is very similar to that characteristic of the *vital* marriage, except that it involves a greater commitment to the relationship, much closer and more intense agreement on most issues, and a total, unreserved, and intimate sharing of all aspects of life. For those in a total relationship, the marriage and the marriage partner are the absolutely dominant facts of life.

These five types of marriages describe the nature of the relationships that are possible between husband and wife, but they do not describe whether a marriage is good or bad. However, because the sample studied by Cuber and Harroff did not include any obvious instances of serious marital discord, we can conclude that each of these relationships can be characteristic of an enduring marriage.

Marital Satisfaction

There is, of course, a great deal more to marital satisfaction than might be evident in the simple longevity of a marriage. Indeed, a great many abjectly miserable marriages, for one reason or another, endure magnificently. And, as my grandmother recently observed, a number of perfectly contented marriages may end too abruptly.

We ask a great deal of our marriages and careers. As we saw earlier, we used to ask only that our jobs fill our time and our bellies. Now we ask not only that they continue to fill our bellies but also that they bring us joy, feelings of worth, and perhaps a small measure of growth and development. In the same way, our foreparents asked mostly that marriage bring them a workable, child-rearing arrangement with a clear division of duties and responsibility. Now we expect marriage to make us *happy*; we think happiness is our right. And if it does not come sooner, we seldom wait for it to come later. We simply try again.

But the married are happier, though perhaps not vastly so (Freedman, 1978). And happiness, of course, is relative and highly individualistic. Skolnick (1981) provides some insights into who might be happier and why. Her findings are based on

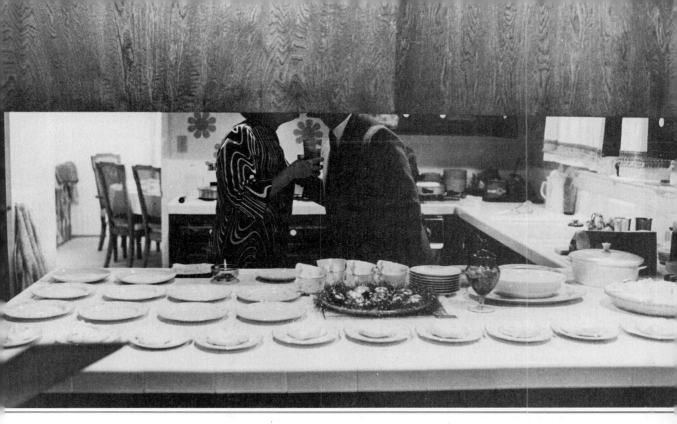

In general, the married are happier than the never-married or no-longer-married.
Women who marry when older and men in high-status occupations tend to be happiest.

intensive interviews with 232 members of the Oakland Guidance Study and the Berkeley Guidance Study, conducted in 1958 and in 1979. Members of these longitudinal samples were born in 1920 or 1921 and in 1928 or 1929 and were therefore between twenty-nine and thirty-eight in 1958 and fifty and fifty-nine in 1979. Seventy-five percent of the group were still in their first marriage; 19 percent had divorced, and more than half of these had remarried. Only 6 women and 5 men of the original 232 had not married. Data concerning marital satisfaction and happiness were based on self-reports as well as on more objective assessments by teams of experienced raters.

A number of social factors appeared to be closely related to marital satisfaction. For women, the most important of these was age at first mar-riage. In general, the older the woman, the more likely she is to be happily married later. That teen-age marriages break up twice as frequently as older marriages is additional corroboration of this find-ing. For men, the social variable most highly related to marital satisfaction is occupation, with socio-economic status, a closely related variable, being almost equally important. In general, executives and professionals tend to be more happily married than other men.

For both men and women, amount of education is positively related to marital satisfaction, as is socioeconomic status. The number of marriages relates positively to satisfaction for men (second marriages are happier) but is negatively related to satisfaction for women (second mar-riages are less happy) (Skolnick, 1981).

In addition to these social variables, Skolnick also looked at personality variables. Like most other researchers, she found that opposites do not attract, complement each other, and live happy lives because the strengths of one make up for the weaknesses of the other. Quite the contrary, similar people are attracted to each other. Indeed, the more similar members of a pair were, the more likely they were to report high marital satisfaction. This was particularly true of cognitive variables such as intelligence and whether or not the person is impulsive or reflective. It is also true of social characteristics. Couples in which both members share some major social characteristic (for example, both are highly aggressive or highly sociable) tend to live in greater harmony than those in which each is the opposite of the other.

In Skolnick's study, as in a number of others, marital satisfaction did not appear to decline with age *on the average*, although it sometimes changed a great deal over time for any given couple. In a study of eighty middle-aged couples, Abrioux and Zingle (1979) found, for example, that a majority of these couples considered their present marriages to be better than they had ever been. Among these couples, those whose last child had been gone from home for more than one complete year reported somewhat more satisfaction than those whose last child had left home within the year immediately preceding.

In Skolnick's (1981) investigation, a number of observations seemed to consistently be *most characteristic* of those marriages that were rated satisfactory. These included:

1. Person likes spouse
2. Person admires and respects spouse
3. Person and spouse enjoy each other's company
4. Person would marry spouse again
5. Marriage has improved over time. (p. 289)

Conditions that were *least characteristic* of satisfactory marriages were:

1. Marriage is a utilitarian living arrangement (as opposed to a close personal relationship)
2. Person has seriously considered leaving spouse
3. Serious conflicts and disagreements occur between the spouses

4. Person and spouse have discordant personality traits
5. Sexual adjustment is or has been a source of tension. (p. 289)

Skolnick also describes some of the conditions that are most and least common in unsatisfactory marriages. Among the *most common* characteristics are the following:

1. Person is critical of spouse
2. Serious conflicts and disagreements exist between the spouses
3. Spouses have discordant personalities
4. Person tries to avoid conflict with the spouse
5. Marriage is a utilitarian living arrangement (rather than a close personal relationship). (p. 289)

Items *least* descriptive of unsatisfactory marriages are:

1. Marital relationship has improved over time
2. Person sees spouse very much like self in temperament
3. Spouses basically agree on child rearing
4. Person is pleased with spouse's performance of daily tasks
5. Person feels loved by spouse. (p. 290)

There is perhaps a great deal in these simple descriptors that might be of value for those who are now married, for those who would give them advice, and for those who are contemplating either step.

■ Marriage and the Family

A marriage is simply the legal union of two individuals. Its social function, however, goes considerably beyond these two individuals; it makes possible the *family*.

As we saw in Chapter 8, there have historically been two types of families. The one most common in Western societies consists of parents and their immediate children and is termed the *nuclear* family. That which is most prevalent throughout the world includes grandparents and assorted other relatives in addition to children and their parents and is labeled *extended*.

Among recent changes in the family in North America are a reduction in its longevity, a decrease in the absolute number of *intact* nuclear families, and a corresponding increase in one-parent families. These changes are due largely to divorce rates that have increased dramatically in the past several decades (Bronfenbrenner, 1977).

In spite of these changes, the nuclear family continues to be the most prevalent child-rearing unit in North America; more than 85 percent of all children live with their mothers and fathers and perhaps with one or more siblings as well. Much of Chapter 8 is devoted to examining the importance of the family from the child's point of view, as well as to a discussion of the impact of divorce and of one-parent families—again primarily from the child's point of view. In the remaining pages of this chapter, we look at the family as a sociological unit and at the impact of children *on parents*.

The Family Life Cycle

One of the most useful ways of approaching a study of the family is to look at it in terms of the series of relatively predictable changes that occur from its beginning to its end. This, the **family life cycle**, is perhaps best described by Duvall (1977), who identifies eight sequential stages in the evolution of the family. These stages often overlap and can

The family is a dynamic social organism. It changes dramatically with the advent of children and changes again as children age and begin to leave home. Duvall describes eight stages in the family life cycle, defined by age and status of children.

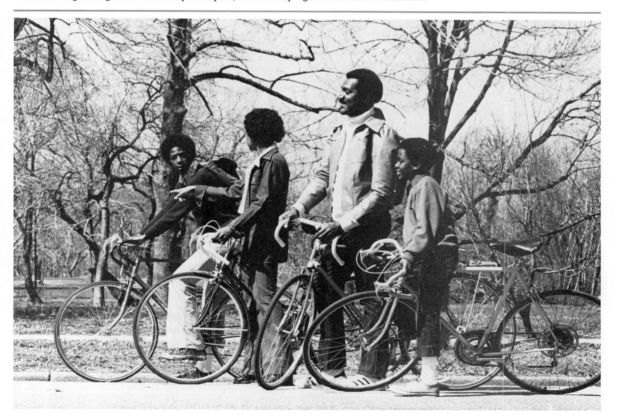

also be very different for different families. In the main, however, they describe a relatively common progression premised, at least in part, on Duvall's belief that families, like individuals, are exposed to a series of important developmental tasks. But whereas individual developmental tasks, described by theorists such as Erikson, center on the resolution of personal conflicts and the development of individual competencies, those tasks that relate to the family center on child rearing. Thus all but the last of Duvall's stages of the family life cycle deal specifically with the family in relation to its

children. These stages, together with the amount of time the *average* couple spends in each, is summarized in Figure 15.3 and discussed briefly here.

Most families begin as a childless couple, a period that lasts approximately two years and that brings with it a series of developmental tasks relating to the adoption of responsible marital roles. These tasks may include finding and keeping a job for the man and sometimes for the woman as well. In addition, both are faced with important tasks relating to sexual fulfillment and the development of a reasonably harmonious marriage.

Figure 15.3
The family life cycle by length of time in each of eight stages. (From Duvall, 1977, p. 148. Based upon data from the U.S. Bureau of the Census and from the National Center for Health Statistics, Washington, D.C.)

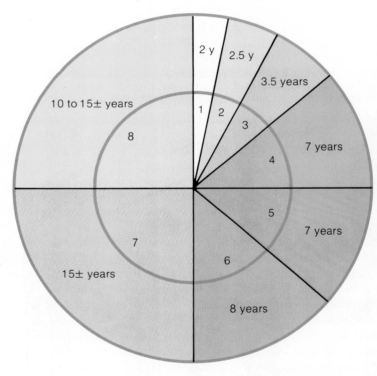

1. Married couples without children

2. Childbearing families
(oldest child birth–30 months)

3. Families with preschool children
(oldest child 30 months–6 years)

4. Families with schoolchildren
(oldest child 6–13 years)

5. Families with teenagers
(oldest child 13–20 years)

6. Families launching young adults
(first child gone to last child leaving home)

7. Middle-aged parents
(empty nest to retirement)

8. Aging family members
(retirement to death of both spouses)

The second stage in Duvall's life cycle begins with the birth of the first child and lasts approximately two and one-half years. This time of very rapid changes and adjustments in the family brings with it a variety of demands for both mother and father. Among other things, the mother is called upon to develop and clarify her roles as mother, wife, and person; needs to learn how to care for and cope with infants and young preschoolers; continues to maintain a satisfying relationship with her husband; and must, through all this, nevertheless maintain some sense of personal autonomy (Duvall, 1977). And the father too is required to make numerous adjustments, including reconciling conflicting conceptions of his role as father, accepting new responsibilities for parenting, conforming to changes in schedules, coping with the reduced time and attention that the wife can now devote to him, maintaining a satisfying marital relationship and a sense of autonomy and of self-worth.

As the first child reaches the preschool age, the family enters the third stage of Duvall's family life cycle. It begins when the first child is two and one-half, ends with school age (six), and brings with it a continuation of most of the developmental tasks that were first introduced in the preceding stage. Few of these tasks are ever completely resolved during any one phase of the cycle. Indeed, such important tasks as maintaining a sense of autonomy and worth while striving for the development of a mutually satisfying and happy marriage continue from the beginning to the very end of the family life cycle. In addition, the presence of preschoolers in the family brings additional demands for income, space, equipment, time, and attention, as well as a new set of child-rearing responsibilities and problems. And to complicate matters, only those families with a single child can be described as being in only one developmental phase at one time. For many families, there is considerable overlap among stages as additional children are born.

The fourth stage, much longer than any of the first three, spans the preteen school years of the first child (ages six to thirteen). It brings three important developmental tasks, none of which is exclusive to this developmental phase, but all of which are fundamentally important to the happy and effective functioning of the family. These include providing for children's special as well as ordinary needs, enjoying life with children, and encouraging children's growth. And although these tasks are difficult and demanding, most parents raise their children without a great deal of deliberation or guidance, relying primarily on intuition, folk wisdom, and their recollection of the child-rearing techniques of their parents (Lunde & Lunde, 1980).

The fifth phase in the family life cycle spans the teen years of the oldest child (thirteen to twenty) and brings with it the occasional parenting problems of adolescence. These present a number of family developmental tasks, including working out changing financial problems, reallocating the sharing of responsibilities, bridging the communication gap between generations, and, all the while, continuing to maintain the marriage relationship (Duvall, 1977).

As a social unit, the family functions mainly to produce and socialize children. Its primary social functions therefore end with the *launching* of children into the world. This *launching* phase, the sixth in Duvall's cycle of the family, begins with the first child's leaving home and ends when the youngest child is launched. The launching phase lasts as long as the space between the oldest and youngest child, which averages approximately eight years. It too brings new demands on the family, including those relating to the rearrangement of physical facilities and resources, additional expenses relating to the launching (college or wedding expenses, for example), and reassigning responsibilities among grown and growing children. Clearly, the launching phase will be longer, more expensive, and perhaps more difficult in those families where there are many children and where the space between oldest and youngest child is greatest. By the same token, it will be far shorter for those families in which there is a single child.

The "empty nest" phase, seventh in the family life cycle, begins with the launching of the last child and lasts perhaps fifteen or more years. The average age of the contemporary mother at the beginning of this stage is around fifty-two (fifty-four for the average father). Although the family

VIOLENCE IN THE FAMILY

Prophets and others who specialize in gloom and related states have been warning us for some time that violence is rapidly becoming a way of life in contemporary societies. And perhaps they are correct. Certainly, police reports indicate that incidence of violent crimes in Western industrialized nations has increased sharply during recent decades.

Although it might be tempting to assume that violence typically involves strangers and that surrounding ourselves with friends and family will therefore protect us, that, sadly, does not appear to be the case. Indeed, more than 25 percent of all assaults and homicides that are reported to police involve members of the same *family* (Gelles, 1972). And a large percentage of the remainder involve friends or at least acquaintances. More than half of all rapes, crimes that most of us attribute to disturbed strangers in dark parking lots, are committed by acquaintances or relatives (Gelles, 1979). As Gelles (1978a) puts it: "We have discovered that violence between family members, rather than being a minor pattern of behavior, or a behavior that is rare and dysfunctional, is a patterned and normal aspect of interaction between family members" (p.169).

Violence in the family takes a variety of forms. It is perhaps most evident in the observation that more than nine out of ten parents admit to using physical force to punish children (Martin, 1978). It is even more dramatically apparent in instances of child abuse (discussed in Chapter 8). And it is present as well in countless episodes of violence among siblings. Indeed, violence among siblings seems to be highly prevalent among young children, although it diminishes rapidly with increasing age. In a sample of 2,143 families, Straus (1980a) found that 74 percent of all three- to four-year-old children who had siblings occasionally resorted to some form of physical aggression in their interactions. Only 36 percent of those aged fifteen to seventeen behaved in similar fashion.

Violence in the family is also apparent in instances of wife and husband beating. And surprisingly, the latter is almost as common as the former, although generally less serious (Straus, 1980a). In Straus's investigation of 2,143 nationally representative American families, 3.8 percent of all husbands admitted to activities that the authors define as wife beating. These activities include kicking, biting, hitting with the fist or some other object, threatening with a knife or a gun, or actually using a knife or a gun. And an amazing 4.6 percent of all wives admitted to similar activities with respect to their husbands (see the figure opposite). However, Straus cautions that wife beating tends to be hidden and secretive more often than is husband beating and that wives are, in fact, far more often *victims* than are husbands.

The picture presented by surveys such as these is probably only a partial sketch, given the privacy of the family. Its affairs are not easily accessible to social science or to law-enforcement agencies. In addition, our prevailing attitudes concerning the *right* of parents to punish their children physically, the normalcy of siblings fighting, and, yes, even the right of a husband to beat his wife, tend to obscure the prevalence and seriousness of violence in the family. Thus when Shotland and Straw (1976) staged a series of events where one individual attacked another, bystanders almost invariably tried to assist the victim unless the attack involved a man and a woman. When a man attacked a woman, bystanders usually assumed that the couple was married and that they should therefore not interfere. It is perhaps the same sort of reasoning that generally makes it legally impossible for a husband to rape his wife. In most jurisdictions, rape is defined as forcible sexual intercourse with someone *other* than a spouse (Gelles, 1979). This same implicit acceptance of a husband's right to use physical force on his wife accounts for the reluctance of many law-enforcement agencies to charge husbands with assault when wives are the victims—unless the results of the assault are obvious and serious (Straus, 1980b). English common law maintains that a man is still king in his castle—however humble that castle might be.

But winds of change have begun to blow more strongly over our kingdoms. In the jurisdiction in which I write, for example, the Attorney General's office has just issued new guidelines governing procedures to be followed by police officers investigating domestic disputes ("Crackdown on Wife Beaters," 1983). According to these guidelines, assault charges will now be laid—"where warranted." In practice, this apparently means that assault charges may be made when there is obvious *physical* evidence that a beating has occurred. The important change that this implies is that, since police officers are the ones laying charges, wives can then be subpoenaed to testify against their husbands. Previously, if wives refused to lay charges (often because of fear of reprisals) and to testify, police could take no action.

Why do some husbands beat their wives? There is no simple answer. Some, probably a minority, might be classified as suffering from a psychological disorder. In one study involving one hundred battered wives, 25 percent of the husbands had received psychiatric help in the past. And, according to the wives, many more were in need of such help (Gayford, 1978). A great many of these husbands came to their marriages with a history of violence. Many had been physically abused and beaten as children. And compared with the general population, more of them were chronically unemployed and poorly educated.

Other factors that contribute to violence in the family include the high incidence of violence in society, cultural attitudes that accept violence as a legitimate reaction in certain situations, and our predominantly sexist attitudes toward the role of husband and wife in contemporary marriage. These and other contributing factors are summarized in the flow chart on p. 430.

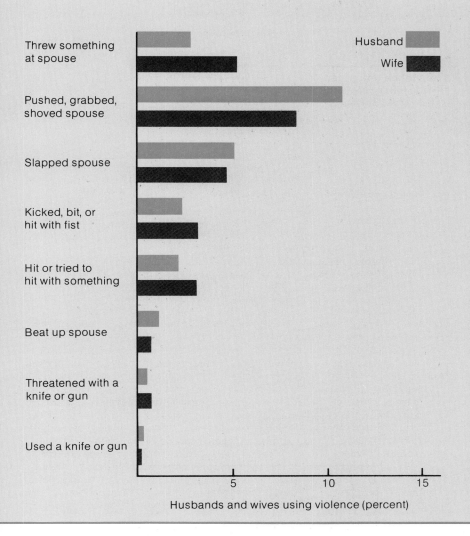

Percentage of spouses admitting to an act of violence during the last 12 months. (Adapted from Straus, 1980a, and Gelles, 1972. Reprinted by permission of University of Minnesota Press, and Sage Publications, Inc.)

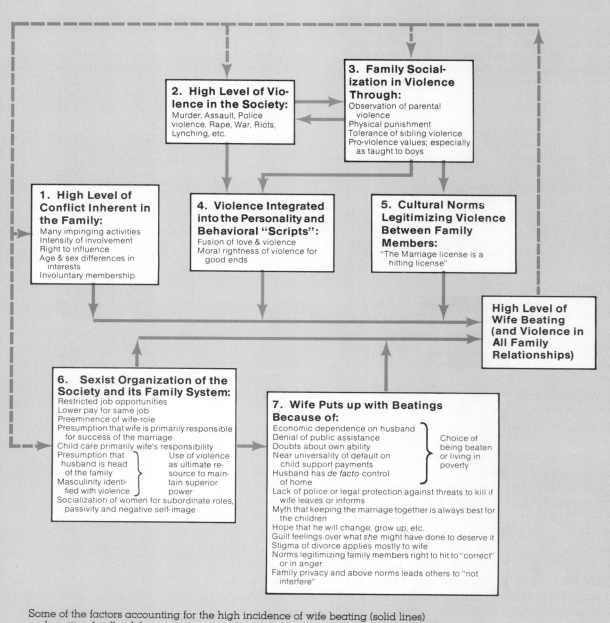

2. High Level of Vio-lence in the Society:
Murder, Assault, Police violence, Rape, War, Riots, Lynching, etc.

3. Family Social-ization in Violence Through:
Observation of parental violence
Physical punishment
Tolerance of sibling violence
Pro-violence values; especially as taught to boys

1. High Level of Conflict Inherent in the Family:
Many impinging activities
Intensity of involvement
Right to influence
Age & sex differences in interests
Involuntary membership

4. Violence Integrated into the Personality and Behavioral "Scripts":
Fusion of love & violence
Moral rightness of violence for good ends

5. Cultural Norms Legitimizing Violence Between Family Members:
"The Marriage license is a hitting license"

High Level of Wife Beating (and Violence in All Family Relationships)

6. Sexist Organization of the Society and its Family System:
Restricted job opportunities
Lower pay for same job
Preeminence of wife-role
Presumption that wife is primarily responsible for success of the marriage
Child care primarily wife's responsibility
Presumption that husband is head of the family
Masculinity identi-fied with violence
Use of violence as ultimate re-source to main-tain superior power
Socialization of women for subordinate roles, passivity and negative self-image

7. Wife Puts up with Beatings Because of:
Economic dependence on husband
Denial of public assistance
Doubts about own ability
Near universality of default on child support payments
Husband has *de facto* control of home
Choice of being beaten or living in poverty
Lack of police or legal protection against threats to kill if wife leaves or informs
Myth that keeping the marriage together is always best for the children
Hope that he will change, grow up, etc.
Guilt feelings over what *she* might have done to deserve it
Stigma of divorce applies mostly to wife
Norms legitimizing family members right to hit to "correct" or in anger
Family privacy and above norms leads others to "not interfere"

Some of the factors accounting for the high incidence of wife beating (solid lines) and positive feedback loops maintaining the system (dashed lines). (From Straus, 1980a. Used by permission of University of Minnesota Press.)

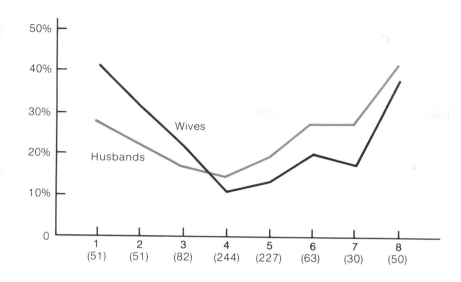

Figure 15.4
Percentage of individuals at each stage of the family life cycle (from Stage 1, "beginning families," to Stage 8, "retirement") reporting their marriage was going well "all the time." (Figures in parentheses indicate the number of husbands and wives in each stage. There was a total of 1,598 cases.) (From Rollins and Feldman, 1981, p. 308. Used by permission of Columbia University Press.)

continues to function as an important social unit and continues to encourage the development of autonomy among its sons and daughters, its primary developmental tasks shift away from children and refocus on the husband and wife. Among these tasks are those that relate to maintaining a sense of well-being, developing and enjoying career responsibilities, relating to aging parents, and establishing and maintaining a useful or enjoyable position in the community.

Although folklore has often associated the leaving of children with unhappiness and even depression among parents—and especially among mothers—remarkably consistent research findings contradict this belief. As an example, Rollins and Feldman (1981) looked at marital satisfaction through Duvall's stages among 850 couples. Like other researchers, they found that the majority (around 80 percent) of husbands and wives thought their marriages were "going well" either all or most of the time. But they also found that happiness and satisfaction tend to be highest in the first stage of the cycle (prior to the advent of children) and begin to decline with the first child, reaching a low at about the time that the oldest child is entering adolescence. By the time of the "empty nest" stage, happiness and satisfaction again begin

to increase and continue to do so until the retirement years (see Figure 15.4).

The final stage in Duvall's family cycle begins with retirement and ends with the death of both spouses. Since in most instances one will die before the other, one of the important tasks of this phase is to adjust to life as a widow or widower. Other important tasks relate to adjusting to retirement, coping with changing physical, cognitive, and sexual interests and abilities, and facing dying. Each of these topics is covered in the next chapter.

An Evaluation of the Life-Cycle Approach

One of the principal advantages of the life-cycle approach to studying the family is that it greatly simplifies an incredible complex of dynamic relationships. Too, it provides some structure on which to hang our facts and to examine and understand them. But it does have a number of disadvantages—some of which relate to its simplicity. Among these are its assumption that families with more than one child progress through the same general phases as one-child families, its failure to take into account the impact of family crises such as death and divorce, and its inability to take into account the vast number of families that do not fit the traditional mold of working father and homemaking mother. Divorce, one-parent families, career mothers, and a variety of other family situations that have become increasingly common in recent decades present different sets of problems and tasks. In spite of this, however, we should not forget that no matter the nature of their families, children still progress in similar ways through their infancies and childhoods, into their adolescence, and finally into the world. And it is children who, after all, define the very existence and nature of the family.

Following a massive study of 1,746 couples at all stages of Duvall's family life cycle, Nock (1979) concludes that two family variables are most important for predicting such factors as satisfaction with the marriage, as well as satisfaction with self, occupation, living standard, and so on. The first of these is simply the presence or absence of children; the second is length of marriage. Specifically, the most happily married couples are those *without* children, whether they be couples who have not yet had children, who will never have children, or couples whose children have already left home. In addition, childless couples are least likely to contemplate divorce. And the longer couples have been married, the more likely they are to express satisfaction with their lives, their spouses, and their marriages and the less likely they are to think of divorce, to disagree over finances or over child-rearing practices, or to be unhappy with their standard of living.

■ MAIN POINTS

1 Most of us spend between twenty-five and forty years of our adult lives working—inside or outside the home. We do so to earn our livings as well as to achieve a sense of identity and of worth. We work to *be* somebody.

2 Recent changes in the work place include an increasing number of different jobs, the majority of these being white-collar and high-technology jobs, a concomitant decrease in the number of blue-collar jobs available, and a significant increase in job mobility and in the percentage of women in the work force.

3 The trait-interest matching theory of vocational choice argues that we should select occupations on the basis of a "match" between our interests and abilities and the requirements of specific occupations. Career development theories are more concerned with the progressive development of career choice and with *preparation* for careers. Several tests provide information concerning interests and abilities that is sometimes valuable in making career choices.

4 Actual selection of careers is often less a matter of conscious and rational deliberation than a matter of luck (which job is available when we need it). Sex, socioeconomic status, and parental occupations are also important factors in determining career choice.

5 We ask not only that our jobs fill our bellies but also that they make us happy. And approximately three-fourths of all workers claim happiness and appear to become happier the longer they are at one occupation. Job satisfaction is related to personal interest in the work, the extent to which it requires use of the individual's capabilities, and income. Job security is also important for blue-collar workers.

6   The percentage of adult women who work has more than doubled in this century. Women's occupations are still not at a par with those of men with respect to status and income. In addition, some occupations are still stereotypically female (secretarial and nursing), while others are stereotypically male (engineering and airline piloting).

7   Our one fundamental choice of life style is to marry or not to marry. If we opt not to marry, we might select from among singlehood, cohabitation, homosexuality, or one of a variety of communes. About 5 percent of the adult population is single by choice.

8   Cohabitation now appears to be far more socially accepted than it was several decades ago. Approximately 1 out of 23 couples in the United States lives together unmarried. Reasons for unmarried cohabitation include economic and sexual advantages, the elimination of the legal responsibilities of marriage, and the possibility of using cohabitation as a "trial" marriage. In many legal jurisdictions, cohabitation may be interpreted by the courts as constituting "common-law marriage," a situation that is in some ways identical to a more conventional, legal marriage.

9   Under 5 percent of the male population and less than half that number among females is overtly homosexual. Homosexual life styles include couples who live together in a marriagelike bond, those who live together but also seek outside relationships, homosexual "swingers," those for whom sexual preference is a source of conflict and in whom sexual expression varies, and those who do not actively seek or engage in intimate relationships.

10 Communes include a vast array of communities whose members have in common a desire to remove themselves from the social, economic, political, or religious mainstream. Some are utopian (devoted to developing a better society), some are purely economic, and others are primarily religious.

11 Marriage is our most commonly selected adult life style (95 percent). Monogamy is the only legal form of marriage in North America, although our customs and laws make *serial* monogamy possible—even easy. Some form of polygamy is permitted in most of the world's societies, with polygyny commonly being allowed and polyandry (the wife having more than one husband) rarely being allowed.

12 Historical progression in social standards governing premarital sex has moved from a period that encouraged and even demanded total abstinence, through a period characterized by a double standard that condoned sexual activity among males but not among females (vestiges of this standard linger still), and finally to a period where premarital sexual activity is seen as being permissible for women as well as men, providing there is affection between partners. Sex without affection, a fourth period, does not appear to be generally descriptive of the majority of today's premarital sex.

13 A double standard governs the attitudes of many societies toward extramarital sex (adultery). In North America, extramarital affairs are engaged in by between one-third and one-half of men and women at least once. Marriages that tolerate extramarital sexual encounters may be *open* or may deliberately engage in group sex or mate swapping.

14 Reasons for "swinging" include attempts to relieve boredom and reduce alienation and loneliness, as well as a desire to explore sexual fantasies. Most couples who "swing" stop doing so within two years, sometimes because of boredom, jealousy, or guilt and sometimes because the marriage has either broken up or has actually improved.

15 It is possible to classify "successful" marriages in five groups: *conflict habituated*, where partners live in continual disagreement and conflict; *devitalized*, where couples remember being very much in love, but where no passion remains; *passive-congenial* marriages, where there never was any fire; *vital* marriages, where couples share intimately and the relationship is important, but each remains an individual; and *total* marriages, where the single most important thing for each member is the relationship and the other person.

16 We ask not only that our marriages provide a social institution for raising our children but that they also make us happy. And, in general, they do. Important factors contributing to marital satisfaction among women include age at first marriage (later is better), education, and socioeconomic status. Among men, occupation, socioeconomic status, and education contribute to marital satisfaction.

17 Opposites do not attract, but similars do. The more alike two people are, the more likely they are to describe their marriage as a happy one. The statement most often selected as characteristic of a happy marriage was that spouses like each other; the characteristic *least* descriptive of a happy marriage was that spouses view the marriage as a utilitarian living arrangement.

18 The nuclear family (consisting of parents and immediate children) is a common Western family arrangement, although the extended family (parents, children, and assorted relatives) is most common throughout the world. The contemporary North American family can be described in terms of a life cycle with a number of stages. Each stage reflects different developmental tasks that occur as children are born, grow up, and leave home.

19 Duvall's eight stages in the family life cycle include the initial childless years, the first child, the phase of the preschool child, a seven-year period during which the oldest child is school aged but preteen, another phase of approximately seven years during which the oldest child is a teenager, a "launching" phase lasting approximately eight years, the empty nest to retirement period lasting around fifteen years, and a final period spanning retirement until the death of both partners.

20 Although this life-cycle approach to understanding the family is highly useful, it cannot easily take into account the increasingly common families that result from unwed parenthood, divorce, and death. Nor is it sensitive to differences among families that might relate to the parents' occupations, to the family's socioeconomic status, to parents' attitudes toward each other and their children, or to the number of children in the family.

21 Two variables relating to the family life cycle are the most important predictors of marital and life satisfaction: presence of children and length of marriage. In general, childless couples report more satisfactory marriages than those with children, and the longer a couple has been married, the more likely that members will report high satisfaction with life as well as with marriage.

■ FURTHER READINGS

A detailed and comprehensive look at career education and vocational guid-ance is provided by the following text, which should be of particular value for those who are concerned with career education at different stages in the lifespan:
Herr, E. L., & Cramer, S. H. *Career guidance through the life span: Systematic approaches.* Boston: Little, Brown, 1979.

Terkel's interviews with workers and his analysis of work form the basis of his classic book on this topic:
Terkel, S. *Working.* New York: Random House, 1972.

The following are two excellent texts on marriage and the family. The first is somewhat more comprehensive and detailed than the second, a highly readable text, which relies less on research.
Eshleman, J. R. *The family: An introduction* (3rd ed.). Boston: Allyn & Bacon, 1981.
Schulz, D. A., & Rodgers, S. F. *Marriage, the family, and personal fulfillment* (2nd ed.). Englewood Cliffs, N.J.: Prentice-Hall, 1980.

An excellent account of recent changes in the family is contained in:
Schulz, D. A. *The changing family: Its function and future.* Englewood Cliffs, N.J.: Prentice-Hall, 1982.

Those with a psychoanalytical orientation might be interested in the following Freudian analysis of the extramarital affair:
Strean, H. S. *The extramarital affair.* New York: Free Press, 1980.

A well-known textbook that presents an Eriksonian, developmental task analy-sis of the family through its various cycles is:
Duvall, E. M. *Marriage and family development* (5th ed.). New York: Harper & Row, 1977.

16

AGING AND DYING

All would live long; but none would be old.

Benjamin Franklin
Poor Richard's Almanac

Old women sit, stiffly, mosaics of pain . . .
Their memories: a heap of tumbling stones,
Once builded stronger than a city wall.

Babette Deutsch
Old Women

An aged man is but a paltry thing,
A tattered coat upon a stick, unless
Soul clap its hands and sing.

William Butler Yeats
"Sailing to Byzantium"

I would like to stop here, in Debden. Just for a minute. Just long enough to run in and see whether any of my old friends are, by chance, in Debden's only tavern—Bad Bernie's Bar. And perhaps to rest for just a minute before continuing the last few miles of our journey. But my grandmother, looking fragile and tired after this long day, will not hear of it.

"It's getting late," she insists, "and they don't even know we're coming."

So we drive quickly down the main street, past Courchene's Grocery, Brunet's Hardware, Boutin's Insurance and Liquors, and the church. There is little else; darkness joins us at the west end of town almost as quickly as it left us on the east. I turn left on the gravel road just out of town.

"This is it," I inform my children. "Home. We lived just fifteen miles from here. Uncle Robert's is right there, at the corner where the road turns. And Uncle Raoul, where we're going, is only about five miles down the road. By the lake."

"Why don't we stop here?" Marcel asks. There have been far more than enough miles for him this one day.

"We should stop and let them know we're here. Nobody knows we're coming," Grandma suggests, although it is perhaps more a command than a suggestion.

I pull into the yard. It has been a long time; almost two decades. Little seems to have changed. The house is still narrow, too tall for its width. And it is still faintly pink, even in the half-gloom of a single yardlight. The same weather-beaten shed crouches next to the tractor; the same four wooden granaries are backed against the corral. But there is a new dog, a dirty-yellow dog who growls low in his throat, ears laid flat, hair bristling. I am about to send Paul to the door, but there is no need. My Aunt Lucille has come out on the porch. There are large pink curlers in her hair; great wrinkles course sadly through her drooped cheeks.

"They're waiting for you at Raoul's," she says. Her voice is older, tighter. She doesn't smile.

"How did they know I was coming?" I ask, surprised.

"They heard." She sees Grandma and approaches the rear window, smiling now. They embrace and she meets my children, who have gotten out of the car. There are tears in her eyes, and the dog wags his tail. I start to open my door, the beginnings of a tear in my eye as well. But the dog growls again. No one else seems to hear him, but I do. Very clearly.

"We should get going." My door is closed again.

There is an urgency upon me now. They know I am coming. Why? How?

If this tale is not soon completed, there may be no time left for the telling. Fortunately, we no longer need great reaches of space and time, for the vast stretches of childhood and adulthood now lie behind us, and all that is left of the lifespan are its graying years and its final ending. We turn to these now as we crunch noisily through this day's last few graveled miles.

■ Ageism

"How old are you?" Few questions are more important to any of us when we first meet someone. Of course, it is not always proper to ask; there are many for whom age is very private.

But if we do ask and find out how old someone is, what have we actually discovered? A great deal, most of us think, for we all have definite opinions about what people of different ages are like—and perhaps even stronger opinions about what they *should* be like (Troll & Nowak, 1976). We know, for example, that children should be immature and impulsive; that adolescents should be moody and sometimes rebellious; that young adults should be adventurous, bold, and energetic; that middle-aged adults should be responsible, controlled, and strong; and that older adults should be cautious, rigid, and narrow minded. Armed with these bright tidbits of folk knowledge, we glibly judge people to be "old" or "young" for their age. And, in fact, our judgments are probably often accurate and useful. At other times, however, our age-based expectations are inaccurate and highly prejudiced. **Ageism** is the term employed to describe *negative* attitudes toward a group that are based solely on age (Butler, 1969).

Ageism is most common with respect to old age, which is often described by the young in terms such as "used up," "ready to die," "narrow mind-

ed," "prejudiced," and "worn." Negative attitudes such as these are sometimes manifested in age discrimination, in which older and younger people are treated differently simply on the basis of age. Kalish (1982) notes, for example, that the medical treatment of the elderly often reflects ageism. Not only do the medical professions assign a much lower priority to geriatrics and to research dealing with diseases of aging, but the actual care that medical facilities provide for the aged is also often inferior to that which would be provided for a younger person in the same circumstances. Another example of ageism may be found in immigration policies, which have traditionally favored the young and which, earlier in America's history, allowed parents to bring their children from foreign countries but often did not permit them to bring their parents (Gruman, 1978). Similarly, ageism is illustrated in those customs and rulings that have made retirement mandatory at a specific age. Finally, it is evident in the negative media portrayals of the old as doddering, feebleminded, wrinkled, and laughable men and women, standing weakly and foolishly on the last of their worn legs.

Is ours the only society that sometimes views its elderly in these terms? Was it always this way? Although it might be tempting to suggest that we honored our old ones more in days past, when the family was strong and our roots stretched lovingly among our kinfolk, Ward (1979) cautions against

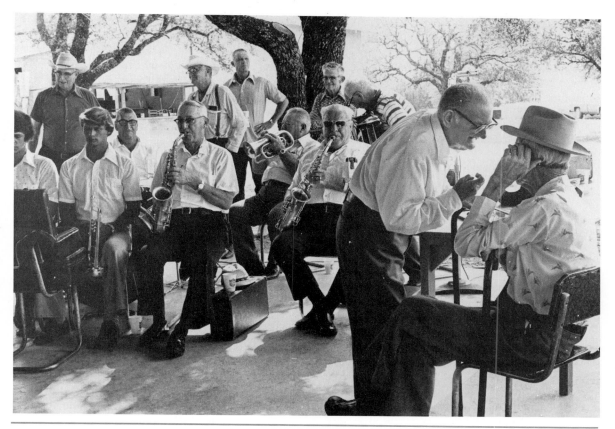

Ageism describes negative, prejudicial attitudes toward a group, based on age alone. Most common with respect to the elderly, ageism is highly evident in media caricatures of doddering, foolish old people. Ageism is not evident in this photograph.

doing so. In the first place, only recently have the old become numerous. Only a century ago, less than 1 percent of the population was over sixty-five. Being old in such unlikely circumstances might have been somewhat more prestigious than being old now. Thus our social attitudes toward the old might well have something to do with their numbers. In addition, Ward (1979) suggests that these attitudes often reflect environmental, economic, political, and social conditions. For example, in harsh and demanding environments, where survival is at a premium, the old quickly become a burden. And, in the same way that children who were an economic burden were sometimes killed during the Middle Ages, there are societies where

the elderly were also killed or customarily committed suicide (Mowat, 1952; Simmons, 1960).

Lest this paint too cynical a picture, let me hasten to point out that perhaps no more than one-quarter of us are actually guilty of ageism with respect to the old (McTavish, 1971). Furthermore, the rapidly increasing number of old people in contemporary society is having a profound effect on public opinion as well as on social policy. And the middle aged and the elderly are increasingly breaking traditional age barriers. Many go back to school, begin new careers, marry for the first time, and otherwise devote themselves to dramatically new life styles, at ages that many would have considered far too advanced only a few decades ago.

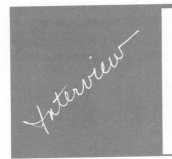

In one study of attitudes toward the aged, involving 456 subjects aged fourteen to forty, the five major dimensions that emerged as being most descriptive of the elderly were: integrity, fortitude, social appeal, dependableness, and open-mindedness (Signori, Butt, & Kozak, 1980). In general, this sample did not exhibit ageism, although a number of individuals in the sample did hold negative attitudes toward the aged. The authors suggest that our attitudes toward the aged are, in fact, generally very positive but that a number of studies of ageism have sampled gerontologists and other professionals who often worked with biased samples of the elderly—that is, with those suffering from mental or physical impairment—and have consequently obtained misleading impressions of ageism.

Ageism describes negative attitudes that are prejudicial because they are based on age alone. Attitudes that are based on fact, even though they might be negative, do not illustrate ageism. Thus the sometimes gloomy pictures that we have of social, physical, and psychological changes in old age might, to some extent, be fact—negative and uncomfortable fact, to be sure, but fact nevertheless. And social policies that sometimes appear to favor the young might often be based not on a stereotyped and prejudiced ageism but on the sometimes painful recognition that the elderly present much greater risk in terms of decline in all areas. Indeed, they are at much greater risk of death, and it would be a pointless exercise in wish-ful thinking to behave as though this were not the case. But, as is made clear in this chapter, all is not sudden gloom with the advent of old age.

■ Definitions and Demography of Old Age

When does old age actually begin? Most of us think of age sixty-five as the boundary between middle and old age, perhaps because age sixty-five has been a common retirement age. In addition, Social Security programs for the aged, "old age" pension plans, and the various concessions that some public and private entities grant the "elderly" are typically for those aged sixty-five and above. In fact, however, variability among individuals is at least as great at age sixty-five as it is at any other time in the lifespan. It is important to keep in mind that there are sixty-five-year-olds whose interests, activities, and vitality are comparable to those of an average fifty-year-old. Too, there are some who are "old before their time."

Although it is convenient and simple to group all those above age sixty-five in a single category, we should also bear in mind that there is a tremendous spread of years between a sixty-five-year-old and an eighty-five- or ninety-year-old. With this in mind, a number of researchers have proposed different divisions within this part of the lifespan. For example, Neugarten (1978) suggests that it might be fruitful to consider two major periods during old age. The "young-old" are those who are still highly active physically, mentally, and socially, although they might already have retired from their main careers. The young-old are found between the ages of fifty-five and seventy-five. Beyond this age are the "old-old"—those for whom physical activity is far more limited and among whom the effects of decline have become more apparent and more rapid. These unimaginative and somewhat clumsy labels reflect our lack of more common terms with which to discuss the elderly and are another indication of how we have historically had little interest in aging. Unfortunately, being called "old-old" or even "young-old" may not be looked on with great favor by those who are now often labeled "seniors" or "senior citizens."

As noted earlier, numbers of older people have increased dramatically both in absolute numbers and in relation to the remainder of the population. For example, while the population of the United States increased almost two and one-half times during the first six decades of this century, the number of people over the age of sixty-five increased by a factor of five (Blau, 1973). This tremendous increase is due in part to a high birthrate early in the century and in part to immigration policies that increased the number of young people in North America. Initially, therefore, there were relatively few old people. Later there were more, not only because the children of the high-birthrate group had grown up but also because medical advances, as well as changes in nutrition, have contributed to our increased life expectancies. The net result was that, by 1981, more than 11 percent of the population of the United States was aged sixty-five or older—more than twenty-five million individuals. And the percentage continues to increase.

■ Lifespan and Life Expectancy

In North America, life expectancy has increased by almost one-quarter of a century in little more than three-quarters of a century. At the turn of the century, the average individual did not live fifty years;

now we can reasonably expect to live to around age seventy-three—less if we are male, more if we are female. Table 16.1 presents life-expectancy data for nineteen countries. Note the tremendous variation for different countries, as well as the consistent differences between males and females in all countries. In Canada and the United States, for example, women live an average of between seven and eight years longer than men, a fact that is partly explained in terms of the greater susceptibility of men to stress-related disease (heart disease, for example) and to their traditionally less restrained life styles (more smoking, for example). But part of the explanation must also lie elsewhere, since male infants and children are also more likely to die than are female infants and children. Thus, although approximately 105 males are born for every 100 females, the numbers of each still alive are equal by early adulthood. And by age sixty-five, only sixty-nine males are still alive for every one hundred females. Social and cultural sex biases may have favored males; nature has been less kind.

Although improved nutrition and medical care have given us 25 more years than our late-nineteenth-century predecessors, our lifespans still remain virtually identical to what they have always been. If we live until age seventy, our life *expectancy* is another twelve years—only a few years more than it was almost a century ago. In other words, while it is now far more likely that we will reach old age (approximately two-thirds of us can expect to reach age seventy), the very oldest among us will, in the end, live no longer than the very oldest who lived a long time ago. If disease, accident, or boredom do not claim us, old age surely will.

■ Theories of Biological Aging

Contrary to what we might like to believe, age is probably fatal. We all suffer from the same terminal condition: life. Although **life expectancy** (the average anticipated years of life) might continue to increase for some time, it is not likely to go

Table 16.1 Life expectancies of men and women in selected countries.

Country	Date	Men	Women
Algeria	1970–1975	52.9	55.0
Belgium	1968–1972	67.8	74.2
Canada	1970–1972	69.3	76.4
Chile	1969–1970	60.5	66.0
China	1970–1975	60.7	64.4
Costa Rica	1972–1974	66.3	70.5
Egypt	1960	51.6	53.8
France	1976	69.2	77.2
Gambia	1970–1975	39.4	42.5
Kuwait	1970	66.4	71.5
Mexico	1975	62.8	66.7
Morocco	1970–1975	51.4	54.5
Netherlands	1977	72.0	78.4
Pakistan	1962	53.7	58.8
Peru	1960–1965	52.6	55.5
Poland	1976	66.9	74.8
Senegal	1970–1975	39.4	42.5
Switzerland	1968–1973	70.3	76.2
United States	1975	68.7	76.5

From *Demographic Yearbook, 1978,* by the Statistical Office of the United Nations. Department of Economic and Social Affairs. New York: United Nations, 1979.

beyond **lifespan** (the maximum length of life in the absence of disease or accident). The span of human life is not likely to be increased until (and unless) we achieve control over the biological processes of aging (Hayflick, 1975). And even if we could control the biology of aging, whether we *should* do so remains a highly debatable point.

Strong evidence indicates that the limits of the lifespan are biological and are inherent in the cells of which we are composed (Hayflick, 1975). When tissue cultures are raised in the laboratory, these cultures initially regenerate and multiply at a high rate. But they do not do so indefinitely; eventually they begin to atrophy and finally die. What is perhaps most striking about this observation is that while cultures based on human embryonic lung tissue regenerate perhaps fifteen times before dying, cultures from animals with shorter lives regenerate correspondingly fewer times. And when cultured cells are taken from an adult organism rather than from an embryo, they too multiply fewer times before dying. In fact, there is an almost per-

fect relationship between the normal lifespan of the organisms and the number of times cultures derived from their tissue will regenerate (Hayflick, 1975). Only certain defective, usually cancerous, cells regenerate indefinitely.

Although we do not yet know exactly why we age, these and related observations have led to a number of theories of biological aging. A *genetic* theory holds, for example, that cells are programmed to die—that, in other words, the limits to life implicit in the fact that cells eventually cease reproducing and die are an intrinsic part of the DNA material of all body cells.

Several other theories of aging also relate directly to body cells. *Error* theory suggests that, with the passage of time, certain changes occur in DNA material so that the cell eventually ceases to function. These changes are seen as *errors* rather than as genetically preprogrammed occurrences.

The *toxin* theory of cell malfunction maintains that there is a gradual buildup of foreign material in the cell. Although much of this material is poisonous, it is initially present in insufficient quantities to affect cell function. With the passage of time, however, it continues to accumulate until the cell dies.

The *free-radical* theory argues that portions of cells sometimes become detached during normal metabolic processes. Many of these "free radicals" are highly unstable chemical compounds that may interact with various enzymes and proteins in the body and significantly affect the cell's ability to function normally.

A last cell-related theory refers to *cross linking*, a process whereby bonds ("cross links") form between molecules or parts thereof, changing the properties of the component cells and altering their functioning.

In addition to these genetic and cell-based theories of biological aging, other theories speculate that various body systems undergo age-related changes that eventually lead to their breakdown or malfunction. Such theories sometimes argue that aging results from reductions in the efficiency of those body systems that control temperature, blood-sugar level, and so on. Perhaps best known among these theories is that involving our immune systems. These are the systems in our bodies designed to guard against foreign invaders. They protect us from cancer, for example, as well as from a variety of infections. With advancing age, however, not only do our immune systems weaken so that they can less effectively protect us from infection and disease, they also sometimes make errors and interpret some of our own cells as invaders. This process, known as **autoimmunity**, leads to the production of antibodies that may attack the body itself. Autoimmunity is thought to be involved in some diseases of aging, such as rheumatoid arthritis (Waring, 1978).

As Shock (1977) notes, aging is an extremely complex process that probably cannot be well understood within the context of any single theory. It is likely that various processes are involved and that genetic factors, cellular changes, and failing or weakening bodily systems are all implicated. Furthermore, these explanations are probably largely interdependent. That is, genetic factors may well account for many of the cellular changes that occur with age; cellular changes may, in turn, be responsible for functional changes in body systems.

■ Longevity

As of this writing, and as far as science knows, our life*spans* are the upper biological limits of our lives. But our life *expectancies* will seldom reach the limit of our spans. Some of us will die sooner, others later. Why these differences in longevity?

A number of factors contribute to longevity. As we saw in Table 16.1, sex and race are two such factors. Women live longer than men, whites live longer than blacks, and Americans live longer than people from Senegal. Some of the reasons for this are clearly environmental and relate to nutrition, medical care, health habits, and various vices and virtues having to do with life style—exercising, drinking, smoking, and so on (see *Ripening Without Rotting*). Other reasons for longevity are genetic and relate to inherited susceptibility to various diseases, as well as to other genetically linked strengths and weaknesses.

When present life expectancy is calculated on the basis of sex, race, and present age, a number of other variables can then be employed to predict the likelihood that the person will live longer than expected. Information based on longitudinal samples in North Carolina indicates that four factors are good predictors of longevity. In order of importance, these are physical mobility, education, occupation, and employment (Palmore, 1969). At all ages, those who are physically mobile (active) lived longer, as did those with higher levels of college education, those whose careers were professional or white collar, and those who were employed rather than retired. Notwithstanding these factors, however, heredity is still the best overall predictor of longevity.

A variety of other factors have also been found to be linked to longevity. These include physical condition (overweight individuals have shorter life expectancies; those who exercise are more likely to live longer), nature of occupation (people whose jobs require little physical activity live less long on the average), locale (rural people live longer than those in urban environments), wars (life expectancies of those actively engaged in such contests are understandably less), and religious calling (nuns live longer than monks; other things being equal, both live longer than you and I) (see Table 16.2).

So, should we all become athletic monks and nuns and move to the country? Perhaps not. Birren and Renner (1977) caution that the most important factors in determining a long life are those over which we do not have any control—namely, genetic factors, the environments of our grandmothers and

RIPENING WITHOUT ROTTING

In most parts of the world, only 2 or 3 people out of every 100,000 live to be 100; 1 in 1 million reach 105; and only 1 in 40 million live to be 110 (Hayflick, 1975). Occasionally, however, the popular press tantalizes us with visions of healthy old people, sometimes 120 or more years of age, living happily clustered in some remote, exotic, dreamlike, and certainly very faraway place. Three such groups of people have received the

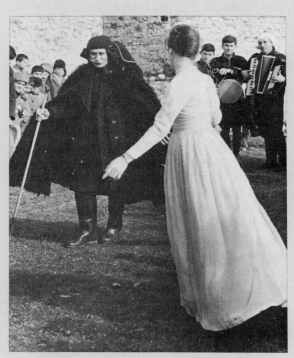

The gentleman shown in this photograph is an octogenarian and a bridegroom.

greatest amount of attention: the Vilcabambans in Ecuador, the Hunzukuts in the Karakoram Range of Kashmir, and the Soviets in parts of the Caucasus of the Georgian Republic, U.S.S.R. Scientists have visited each of these parts of the world, interviewed the inhabitants, and attempted to determine what they might have in common (Leaf, 1973).

The Vilcabambans live in primitive circumstances, far removed from the sanitary conditions of our own lives. Their average caloric intake per day is 1,200 for each adult, with very little animal fat or protein. Pigs and chickens share their modest mud huts, situated along the banks of a river in which they only rarely bathe (some had not had a bath for ten years). Infant mortality is high, but so is longevity. Indeed, had there been 100,000 villagers, 1,100 of them would have been over 100 (compared with 2 or 3 in the United States).

Among their more interesting and potentially significant habits are those of smoking between forty and sixty cigarettes per day and imbibing an unspecified amount of a potent local rum. Is that why they live so long? Why else might they live so long?

More pertinent, do they live so long? Leaf (1973) reports that ages were verified by reference to birth certificates. Hayflick (1975) reports that birth certificates were not always in existence, and those that were found proved highly unreliable. In addition, a gerontologist (aging specialist) who revisited the Vilcabambans five years later interviewed a number of villagers who now claimed to be seven to ten years older than they had been when interviewed five years previously.

The Hunzukuts and the Georgians provide data that are no less unreliable. Identity cards came into use in the Soviet Union in 1932 and were, at that time, based solely on verbal reports, totally unsubstantiated by any documentation. The Hunzukuts are illiterate and have no written language. As Hayflick (1975) says, "They cannot even point to falsified birth records" (p. 37). Rum and cigarettes may not be the answer after all.

Table 16.2 Secrets of longevity.

You may live longer if:
1. You are female
2. Your ancestors lived long lives
3. You are a large tortoise and not a housefly
4. You remain physically active well into old age
5. You are highly educated
6. Your employment is high status
7. You continue to be employed well into old age
8. You are a monk or a nun
9. You are married or cohabit full-time
10. You exercise moderately on a regular basis
11. You drink moderately and do not smoke
12. You avoid wars, accidents, and homicidal maniacs
13. Your job requires physical activity
14. You are not overweight
15. You sleep less than nine hours per night
16. There is no incidence of cardiovascular diseases, cancer, chronic bronchitis, or thyroid disorders among your close relatives
17. You live in the country rather than in the city
18. You obtain regular medical examinations

of our mothers before and during pregnancy, and our own experiences in early childhood. Sadly, we can far more easily shorten our lives than lengthen them. That is, the good that we might do by not smoking or drinking is not likely to be equal, in terms of years, to the bad that we might do were we to smoke and drink. And perhaps living a long time is not all that important. We have to be concerned with the quality of our lives as well as with their length.

■ Physical Changes in Old Age

Those who study aging sometimes speak of three great stages in human development. The first, from conception to early adulthood, is ordinarily described as a stage of growth and development. The second, from early adulthood to somewhere in upper middle age, is sometimes seen as a plateau—a period during which relatively few dramatic changes occur. And the final stage is marked by physical, social, and cognitive deterioration. The technical term for this period of decline is *senescence*. Senescence can begin at very different ages

for different individuals, and the losses it entails are not always dramatic or rapid. In addition, manifestations of aging are not always identical for all individuals. Those results of aging that are universal are referred to as *primary aging*. One example of a primary aging process is arteriosclerosis—a gradual hardening of the arteries—which begins very early in life and becomes progressively more serious, although its severity varies greatly among different individuals.

Numerous physical changes of old age are not inevitable and therefore not universal, but the probability of undergoing them increases greatly with age. They are referred to as *secondary aging* and are illustrated by such diseases as cancer, arthritis, Parkinson's disease, and acute brain syndrome.

Appearance

Most of the physical changes characteristic of old age begin well back in middle age and progress, more or less rapidly, through the remainder of the lifespan. For example, as we saw in Chapter 14, strength and endurance both peak in early adulthood (through the twenties and sometimes early thirties) and begin to decline very slowly from that point. In the same way, height usually reaches its maximum in early adulthood and begins to decline very slowly after age forty-five, partly because of tendons that shrink and harden, feet that become flatter, a spinal cord that shortens, and muscles that have begun to atrophy. And the combined result of these changes can often be seen in the characteristically stooped posture of the very old.

Among the many changes that contribute to the appearance of age, perhaps none are more apparent than those that occur in the skin, on the face, and on the head. Our skins are truly marvelous things. Indeed, it is difficult to imagine a better wrapping for our bodies—totally flexible, self-regenerating and self-repairing, sensitive to heat and cold as well as to pain, highly elastic, porous yet impervious to wind and rain, and totally washable. But with age, these wrappings become thinner, far less elastic, and are often flecked with little

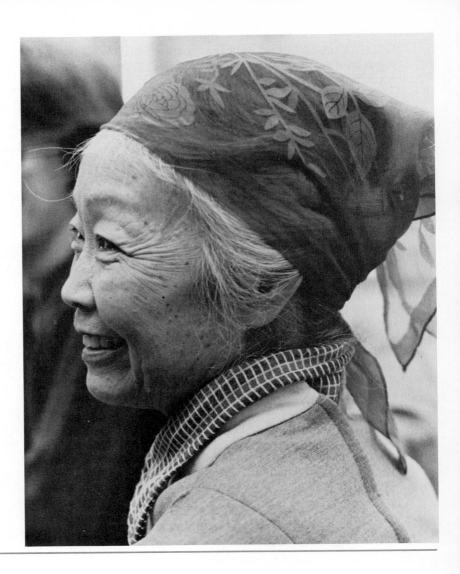

Among the physical changes of aging are wrinkling and loss of hair and hair color. As this photograph shows, the predominant wrinkles follow definite patterns near the eyes and mouth and on the forehead. Only among the very old do wrinkles become more random.

splotches of brown pigment (popularly called "liver spots") as well as with warts, bristly hairs, and the blackish bruises of tiny leaks in blood vessels. And as fatty cells die, old skin is no longer sufficiently elastic to cover the loss; it sags and droops under our arms and chins, and it creases and wrinkles. And the wrinkles of the very old are quite different from those of the middle aged. No longer do they follow the contours of muscles that have repeatedly stretched the skin in the same way—the laugh lines on the cheek as well as the "crow's feet" at the corners of the eyes and the frown lines on the forehead. The wrinkles of the very old are an almost random arrangement of tiny little creases running in all directions between larger crevices. But these are the wrinkles of the very old; there is a long space of time between the appearance of our first wrinkles and the wizening of very old age. Some people have a mechanical retightening of the skin in the interim—a "facelift."

Other physical changes that have begun in middle age (or earlier) also continue. Hair becomes thinner or loses pigment; wear on remaining teeth (if any still remain) becomes more apparent, and gums continue to recede. Thus the caricature of an "old codger" might be either "toothless" or "long in the tooth."

The timing and the exact manifestations of these changes are sometimes very different in different individuals. Not only can nutrition and physical activity affect their appearance but so can different genetic backgrounds.

Health and Strength

As we noted in Chapter 14, muscular strength may begin to decline very slowly in the thirties or forties, particularly for the back and lower body; the upper body (arms and torso) retains its strength for a longer time. But with the advent of old age, there is a progressive decline in strength. This relates not only to the gradual deterioration of muscles but has to do as well with the shortening and stiffening of tendons and ligaments and with the weakening of bones. The bones of the old are far more brittle than those of the young, consequently break more easily, and mend more slowly and with more difficulty—a condition whose medical label is *osteoporosis*.

We have noted earlier that susceptibility to diseases changes from childhood through middle adulthood. Whereas the young are more susceptible to acute infections (colds, for example), those who are older suffer more from chronic complaints (back problems, heart disease). This pattern continues into old age. But note that whereas the old are perhaps less susceptible to acute infections, they also experience greater difficulty in coping with them. Upper respiratory infections are not often fatal among children, but they more often are among the old.

With age, the entire cardiovascular system becomes less efficient, slower, and less able to cope with strenuous demands. In the same way, lungs typically do not function as well, kidneys and the liver are less efficient, and there may be changes in glandular functioning as well as in nervous system activity.

The most common chronic conditions in people above the age of sixty-five include arthritis (44 percent of the population), hypertension (39 percent), hearing impairment (28 percent), heart conditions (27 percent), visual impairments (12 percent), and arteriosclerosis (12 percent) (Brotman, 1981, cited in Kalish, 1982). Other diseases to which the elderly are susceptible include Parkinson's disease, which is linked to a deficiency in the neurotransmitter dopamine and which is often characterized by coarse tremors, generalized weakness, slow movement, sleep disturbances, and sometimes depression; cancer; kidney and urinary problems; osteoporosis, which involves loss of bone calcium, resulting in greater brittleness of bones, and which is more common among women than among men; Alzheimer's disease, also called senile dementia, characterized by confusion, loss of memory, disorientation, and other symptoms associated with degeneration of the brain; and acute brain syndrome, which may be characterized by confusion, speech disturbances, hysteria, paranoia, or other symptoms of mental disturbance, but which, to the extent that it is acute (as opposed to *chronic* or recurring), will generally respond to treatment. Acute brain syndrome often results from drug overdoses, from taking toxic drug combinations, or from excessive ingestion of alcohol. The elderly are particularly susceptible to acute brain syndrome, not only because of age-related changes in the brain and nervous system but also because a great many of them take an alarming number and variety of prescription drugs.

Lest this brief examination of the health consequences of aging paint too grim a picture, let me hasten to point out that although some 86 percent of the elderly suffer from one or more of these conditions, the majority do not consider their health to be a very serious problem (Butler & Lewis, 1977). Remarkably few are bedridden, dependent, or hospitalized. In fact, only 5 percent of those over sixty-five and 17 percent of those over eighty-five are in any kind of institution (Troll, Miller, & Atchley, 1979).

Sensory Changes

As we saw in Chapter 14, virtually all individuals require at least one pair of prescription eyeglasses by the end of middle age, with men generally requiring them at younger ages than women. The most common problem seems to be one of increasing farsightedness, which is thought to be related to decreasing elasticity of the lens and its consequent inability to focus clearly on material that is near. In addition, peripheral vision, depth perception, color vision, and adaptation to the dark generally suffer with age (Corso, 1971).

Hearing losses also often begin in midlife and become more serious after the age of sixty. They are again more common for men than for women and are most evident in decreased sensitivity to higher tones and in difficulty in discriminating among different sounds. It is partly for this reason that older people sometimes find it very difficult to follow conversations when there is background noise (other conversations, radio or television, or children playing, for example). The desire that many older people have for quiet environments may well be related not to an aversion to noise so much as to a desire to follow normal conversation without strain.

Evidence concerning changes in other senses is less clear, perhaps because these senses are so subjective that it is difficult to measure them. For example, we cannot easily determine whether things smell, taste, or feel different to different people, except in those cases where sensory processes are grossly deficient. When a blindfolded individual insists that an onion tastes like an apple or that ammonia smells like roses, we might suspect that something is wrong. There is, nevertheless, some evidence that taste sensitivity decreases in old age (older people use more salt and spices).

Sexuality

One of the myths that we have long entertained with respect to the old is that they are essentially sexless—affectionate and emotional, perhaps, but generally devoid of either the desire or the ability for sexual expression. It bears repeating that this view *is* a myth.

Although human sexual activity, defined in terms of frequency of orgasm, often peaks in late adolescence or early adulthood among males and somewhere between the ages of thirty and forty among females (Kinsey et al., 1948, 1953) and begins to decline thereafter, it does not end with old age.

The climacteric (discussed in Chapter 14) does bring with it some important changes in sexual functioning. Most notably, it brings a cessation of reproductive capacity for women—an event that has generally occurred by age fifty. Total loss of reproductive capacity for males may not occur until very old age, if at all. But in both sexes, the climacteric involves a significant reduction in the production of the sex hormones that are most closely associated with sexual interest and behavior in early years. Does that mean that the old must therefore lose their sexual interest?

Our best evidence indicates that this is not the case. Although sexual activity *does* decline with age, most people with partners remain sexually active into their seventh and eighth decades—and perhaps even later (Rubin, 1968). But there are some differences in sexual responsiveness between the young and the old. In the female, for example, following the climacteric there is a gradual shrinking and loss of elasticity in the uterus, a thinning of the walls of the vagina, and a loss of fatty tissue and elasticity surrounding the vagina. In addition, lubrication may be slower to occur and less plentiful. As a result of these changes, some women may experience pain and irritation during foreplay or intercourse (Masters & Johnson, 1970). However, these changes are much less noticeable in some women than in others. Furthermore, in most women, the clitoris remains sensitive to stimulation, so that the vast majority of women who were capable of orgasm when younger will not lose this capability.

Among men, there is a higher incidence of impotence with advancing age (Kinsey et al., 1948).

However, only a small number of cases of impotence in old age are related directly to physiological changes. In other words, aging does not appear to cause impotence, in spite of its greater frequency in old age. But, as noted in Chapter 14, a number of changes occur in sexual functioning of males as they become older. For example, it may now take longer to achieve an erection and to reach orgasm, the intensity of the orgasm is generally reduced, and more time is required between erections or ejaculations.

In summary, what we know of biology and what little we have discovered of the private behaviors of the elderly indicates that most individuals continue to be capable of sexual activity well into old age, this being more the case for women than for men, given differences in their sexual roles. And we do have some indication that sexuality continues to play an important role in the lives of many people, particularly if they have been sexually active throughout life (Ludeman, 1981). But sexual behavior is a highly private matter for a great many and may be even more so for the cohorts that have thus far reached old age. In addition, sexual behavior has not been widely accepted among these cohorts except within the context of marriage. Since the majority of very old women are *not* married but the majority of very old men are, opportunities for sexuality in old age may be highly limited for a great many women, though less so for men. Succeeding cohorts may tell a different story.

■ Cognitive Changes

When I was quite young and he was already very old, my maternal grandfather gave each of his many grandchildren three peppermint candies every Sunday morning when we gathered in his house before church. "Three of a kind beat two pair," he would always say, that being the reason why we took three rather than four or two. And that was almost the full extent of his knowledge of English—that along with a few other indispensable expressions, such as "check," "pass," "raise," "fold," "flush," "full house," and "straight."

We would sit, then, sucking our peppermints and listening to the old ones talk. Our uncles and aunts were the old ones, and our grandparents were very, very old. And in the end, it was almost always our grandfather who did most of the talking. And the subject was almost always the same: "les guerres des Philippines." He had been an infantryman in the Philippines during the Spanish-American War. Now, some five or six decades later, he told the same war stories over and over, occasionally forgetting or confusing some of his details and sometimes, though rarely, adding a few.

Why did my grandfather learn only enough fragments of English to be able to play poker with those who did not know enough fragments of French? Why did he tell such old stories when so many other things had occurred between the happening of the old stories and now? Are these the inevitable, even the likely, consequences of aging?

Learning and Memory

Let us look briefly at the research before we try to answer these questions. Recall, first, that memory and learning are very difficult to separate. That is, it is often unclear whether failure to remember is a problem of memory or whether it results from incomplete or improper learning in the first place. Evidence that one has learned depends on being able to remember; but then, remembering depends on having learned in the first place.

In Chapter 14, we looked at various ways of assessing memory and at age-related changes in remembering. We noted that free recall (bringing back from memory) is considerably more difficult than recognition (tasks that do not require that something be recalled from memory but that simply require a decision concerning whether or not something is familiar, simply a re-cognition). We saw, as well, that recall appears to become more difficult with increasing age, but that recognition is not affected in the same way. Similarly, we noted that a very gradual decline in problem-solving ability may begin some time late in middle adulthood.

Research that has investigated learning and memory in old age has generally found the same patterns of gradual decline continuing past the age of sixty-five. However, in most instances changes are minimal before age seventy-five. And the most obvious changes after that age are often related to *secondary* aging processes (specific, nonuniversal diseases, for example) rather than to *primary* processes (inevitable consequences of aging). Studies that have looked at sensory memory (immediate recall of visual or auditory material) have found only slight differences between older and younger subjects (Crowder, 1980). However, those that have looked at *speed* of recall have found greater differences, particularly when the material is initially unfamiliar. These differences are not nearly so apparent when the materials are more familiar. Indeed, as Birren, Cunningham, and Yamamoto (1983) note, when the materials employed for assessing learning and memory are meaningful to the individuals concerned and relevant to their lives, age differences are almost always smaller than those typically found with less famil-iar laboratory material. Consequently, an increasing number of researchers in this area have begun to emphasize problems and tasks that are immediately relevant to their subjects. This approach, sometimes labeled *contextual*, looks at such things as the ability to understand sentences, to recall meaningful instructions, and to employ available information in the solution of realistic problems.

In summary, while there do appear to be some age-related changes in memory, these vary greatly from one individual to another. In addition, when the materials employed are meaningful and familiar, observed differences are often negligible. What is not clear from this research, however, is whether observed declines in memory are due to memory deficits, learning problems, or differences in motivation, attentiveness, background, and so on.

Intelligence

The picture with respect to measured intelligence is similar to that with respect to memory and learning. Research reviewed in Chapter 14 indicates that intelligence test scores tend to decline with age and that this decline is more apparent with cross-sectional than with longitudinal research. We cautioned that at least some of the observed declines in measured intelligence probably reflect generational (cohort) differences rather than age-related differences.

Another important finding from this research is that some intellectual abilities, such as those relating to attention span or ability to memorize, seem to decline after midlife (termed *fluid* abilities) but that other abilities, such as those having to do with verbal or numerical skills, do not decline and might even increase well into old age (termed *crystallized* abilities) (see Figures 14.3 and 14.4 in Chapter 14). These patterns of change, which often begin somewhere in midlife but which are initially very minor, continue into old age (Baltes, Reese, & Lipsitt, 1980). Thus, older subjects, *on the average*, do less well than younger subjects on *some* measures of intellect. Most notably, they do progressively less well on the *performance* scales of the Wechsler tests. Among other things, these scales

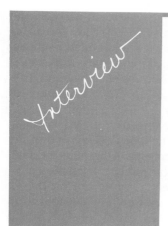

Subject: Male; age seventy-five; retired school teacher.

Question: "Do you notice any difference in how well you remember things now compared to, say, twenty or thirty years ago?"

No. To be quite honest, I don't really. Maybe little things once in a while, but nothing really important. Everybody forgets some things no matter how old they are. I think if I've forgotten more than, say, somebody your age, it's just because I've had that much more time to forget. What I mean is the saying that your memory goes when you get older isn't right. Your memory doesn't get poorer—except maybe if you're really old. What happens is that you forget a lot of things that happened twenty or thirty years ago. And when you're fifty or sixty, the same thing happens. Everybody forgets what happened a long time ago no matter what their age unless it's something important. Then you remember it no matter how old you are. That's what I think.

require motor coordination, speed, dexterity, and spatial-visual abilities. In contrast, however, they continue to do as well on the *verbal* scales of the Wechsler tests. These scales emphasize verbal reasoning, general information, vocabulary, and general comprehension. They deal with familiar rather than unfamiliar items and do not reward speed (or punish slowness), as do the performance scales.

Numerous studies have corroborated that many older people do less well on items where speed is important and where the emphasis is on immediate memory and attention span but that they continue to do as well on items that stress verbal and numerical abilities as well as general information (Botwinick, 1977).

One curious observation based on studies of intellectual change in old age concerns the phenomenon labeled **terminal drop**. Several decades ago, Kleemeier (1962) noticed that among those subjects who died during the course of his longitudinal study, there were a significant number whose measured intelligence dropped noticeably before death. Subsequently, other researchers noticed much the same thing: A great many people experience a sudden drop in intellectual performance one or two years prior to dying (Riegel & Riegel, 1972). This finding has sometimes been explained in terms of a general decline in functioning that might be associated with poorer

health preceding death (Palmore & Cleveland, 1975). It has also been suggested that many older people deliberately *disengage* themselves from life and that one manifestation of this disengagement might be a drastic reduction in motivation to do well on measures of intelligence.

Some Cautious Conclusions

The research leaves little doubt that there are some age-related decrements in cognitive functioning with advancing age. But whether most (or any) of these changes are the inevitable consequences of aging (due to *primary* aging processes) or whether they are due to other factors is not entirely clear. And whether the changes are as great as research sometimes indicates or whether they are as significant in the lives of the elderly as we might think is not entirely clear either.

At least four important considerations must be taken into account when trying to interpret this research. First, we need to keep in mind that *performance* and *competence* are not identical (Baltes & Willis, 1979). That is, a number of reasons other than incompetence might lead an individual to perform poorly on some measure. These include fatigue, to which the elderly are susceptible (Furry & Baltes, 1973); the low education of many older samples; physical and sensory problems such as poor hearing, vision, or motor control; differences in motivation; unfamiliarity with laboratories or testing instruments; and timidity.

Second, cognitive abilities are so complex that we cannot justifiably arrive at single, all-encompassing generalizations that will still be accurate. As we saw, for example, research indicates that some cognitive abilities do *not* decline but that others do. In the same way, sensory memory (immediate recognition of auditory or visual stimuli) does not appear to change with age, but longer-term memory does (Cerella, Poon, & Fozard, 1982).

Third, it is important to note that there are vast differences among individuals with respect to cognitive abilities at *all* ages and that, in addition, there are some fundamentally important cohort differences. That is, not only is there a tremendous variability within a single age group (one cohort), but there may also be great variability between two different cohorts. These observations should make it clear that many observed differences in cognitive competence and performance are related to factors other than age.

Finally, an increasing number of studies demonstrate that intellectual performance can be improved, sometimes dramatically, through various training programs (Denney, 1979). To the extent that this is the case, intellectual decline is not a primary aging process.

In spite of these cautions, however, the reality of decline in performance of intellectual tasks cannot be denied. Many older people learn and remember less effectively and less efficiently, and they perform less well on measures of intelligence. But perhaps they are wiser.

Wisdom

Wisdom is a particular quality of human behavior and understanding that has long been associated with old age. This quality appears to combine the types of intuition, emotion, and knowledge that are not easily available to those whose experiences span only a few years. Thus it is that we believe the ancients—the old ones—to be wise.

Wisdom is not a highly obvious and easily measured human characteristic, which might account for its relative absence in psychological literature. Peck (1968), in his elaboration of Erikson's theory, is one of the few developmental theorists to specifically mention wisdom as an age-related characteristic. According to Peck, as physical strength and endurance decline, one of the important developmental tasks that faces the adult is that of valuing wisdom rather than physical powers. But what, precisely, is wisdom? How does it develop? And does it truly belong only to the old ones?

Psychology suggests a few tentative answers for these questions, but in the main, biblical history and ancient philosophy deal most thoroughly with wisdom. Clayton and Birren (1980) present a review of some of the important literature. Among other things, they note that although wisdom is universally acknowledged as a quality most commonly found in older persons, Eastern and Western beliefs concerning how it is most likely to be acquired are somewhat different.

In the West, it has historically been accepted that there are three paths to wisdom—and that in many cases, all three need to be followed if the individual is to be truly wise. The first of these paths is that of formal education, which historically trained individuals (particularly young men rather than women) to be statesmen or businessmen, emphasizing the ability to make intelligent judgments and thoroughly reasoned decisions. The second path involved listening to and learning from parents or other important and influential mentors. Presumably, then, wisdom is more likely to come to those who are fortunate enough to have wise parents (or perhaps uncles or aunts). The final path that we have traditionally believed capable of leading to wisdom is that of faith—in some ways a far easier path than the first two, since it requires little deliberate learning on the part of the individual. In this case, wisdom does not result from listening, studying, and learning, but from God; some individuals are simply chosen to be wise. These people are given wisdom in the same way that others are given long noses or curly hair.

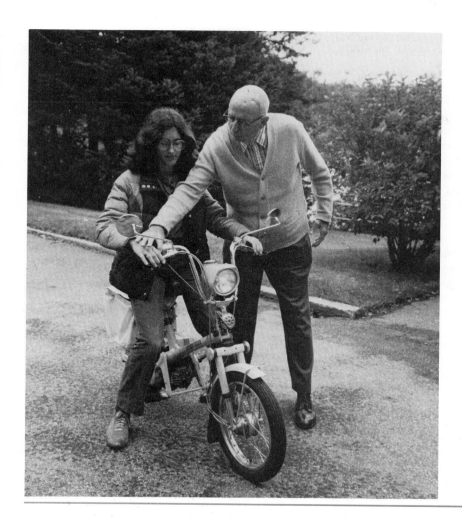

Wisdom is a particular combination of knowledge, gentleness, patience, and intelligence that is associated with age rather than youth. But sometimes, just knowing where the brakes are is sufficient.

Eastern conceptions concerning paths to wisdom are somewhat different. In the main, these are tied to religion, but unlike the Western belief that having faith might be sufficient to be granted wisdom, most Oriental religions require great sacrifice and dedication on the part of those who would be wise. Furthermore, these religions often prescribe specific behaviors and regimens that must be followed by those who are disciples of wisdom. Most have in common the belief that wisdom (often referred to as enlightenment) will be greatly facilitated by meditation and by spending long periods in the presence of a *master* teacher.

Both Western and Eastern conceptions of wisdom view it as a type of knowledge that leads to a greater understanding of reality (of life, its meaning and purpose, and so on). And if the descriptions of its development provided by East and West are accurate, it is unlikely that the young will be very wise.

Psychological investigations of wisdom are scarce, to say the least. Clayton and Birren (1980) conducted a study designed to determine how wisdom is seen by individuals of different ages and whether it is typically associated with the elderly. Their sample consisted of twenty-one-year-olds, forty-nine-year-olds, and seventy-year-olds. Subjects were presented with fifteen terms that might be considered to be related to wisdom (for example, *intuitive, pragmatic, understanding, gentle, sense of humor,* and so on). These were presented in 105 pairs, and subjects were asked to judge how similar each pair was. (For example, are *wise* and *aged* highly similar? Are *experienced* and *knowledgeable* alike?)

In general, this study revealed that most subjects tend to associate wisdom with age. Strikingly, however, older subjects are less likely to see themselves as being wise, although younger subjects view them in that way. Thus, older subjects were less likely to associate *experience* and *aged* with *wise*; they were more likely to judge emotional qualities such as *empathetic* and *understanding* as being more closely related to wisdom. In contrast, younger subjects consistently believed that there is a high similarity between such terms as *aged, experienced,* and *wise.* Does this mean that the wise do not recognize their own wisdom? Or does it mean that the wisdom that the young attribute to the old is merely an illusion? Perhaps research will eventually tell us—or old age.

■ The Implications of Decline

Although it might be somewhat distressing to contemplate the increasing probability of decline with age, most of us will in the end cope successfully and even happily with aging—should we be so lucky as to live that long. We are, after all, human, and part of being human is being resilient, remembering the good things, and always having hope. There is little evidence that age robs us of any of these qualities.

There are other reasons, too, why the aged might cope successfully with the declines and losses they experience. To begin with, changes often occur so slowly that it is often possible to adapt to them without making any major adjustments. In addition, other people of the same age also experience similar changes—and that too presumably makes life easier. And even more dramatic and perhaps more personal changes (knowledge of a serious health problem or death of a spouse, for example), which might initially appear to be totally devastating, can usually be adapted to. (See box for information about those unable to cope independently.) It is important to keep in mind that physical and cognitive decline is only one feature of the lives of the very old. Happiness and joy can continue to come from many sources.

■ Successful Aging

In its clearest sense, to age successfully is to age in relative contentment and happiness. And that must surely be an almost universal goal. And to age unsuccessfully might be to age in misery and despair—and perhaps alone and in poverty as well. As our sensationalist media often remind us, some of the elderly struggle desperately for survival on meager income. And a few do eat foods that the more affluent feed their pets, and do sometimes freeze in unheated dwellings. Fortunately, however, poverty afflicts only a minority. But that this minority even exists is a sad reflection on our humanity.

Attempts to understand and explain the lives and the activities of those who appear to age successfully have led to two essentially opposing points of view concerning the most advisable course for the aged: disengagement theory and activity theory.

Disengagement Theory

Disengagement theory, which originated with Cumming and Henry (1961), is based on the notion that as people age, they progressively withdraw from social, physical, and emotional interaction with the world. Put simply, they gradually *disengage* themselves. And while this process is largely voluntary, it is also two-sided. Not only does the aging person gradually give up active social roles and narrow the sphere of emotional commitment, but society also begins to withdraw its engagement with the aging person. This happens in a number

ALTERNATIVES TO INSTITUTIONS
FOR THE ELDERLY

The term *institution* is not particularly appealing. An authoritarian term, it brings to mind visions of steel bars, cold and comfortless rooms, antiseptic environments, and decisions and procedures that are always made by other people. It also connotes some degree of coercion—some loss of independence and decision-making capacity.

The elderly can be found in a variety of institutions, the most common being hospitals and nursing homes. In general, only the *very* old live permanently in these facilities. And as Tobin and Kulys (1981) note, institutional care is typically sought only after the burden of caring for an elderly person in a private home becomes overwhelming. Hence the great majority of individuals in these institutions are there because of physical or mental impairments. In spite of this, in most cases the institutionalized person feels abandoned and alone and the family suffers from feelings of guilt (Tobin & Kulys, 1981).

There is some evidence of what is termed "excess institutionalization," where individuals are inappropriately given over to the permanent care of an institution. Large-scale surveys, based on the functional capabilities of the institutionalized elderly, suggest that this might occur in 10 to 18 percent of cases (Lawton, 1976). Not surprisingly, individuals are far less likely to be inappropriately institutionalized if they have a spouse than if they are alone. In addition, the more children they have had, the less likely they are to be institutionalized. Thus, the proportion of those *never-married* who are eventually institutionalized is considerably greater than the proportion of those who have been married (Lawton, 1981).

In recent years, the provision of alternatives to institutional care for the elderly has been emphasized. These alternatives include providing community-based assistance for families who care for the elderly in private homes. Such assistance might take the form of home visitations by various personnel with expertise relating to the care of the old; it also includes community-based programs whereby the elderly who live independently in their own homes have hot meals brought to them on a regular basis, are visited by nursing and medical personnel, and might also be visited by community volunteers, who sometimes simply visit with them but who might also assist them with chores such as shopping and might occasionally take them outside the home to various athletic and cultural happenings.

The great variety of other alternatives to institutionalization include the many housing projects that are designed specifically for the elderly. Some of these are government assisted; others are private. They include apartment- or motel-type projects, as well as single-unit, detached dwellings. Some are designed to provide a wide range of services, including residential medical care, much as a nursing home might; others do little more than bring a number of elderly people together, where they can live independently but in close community.

Numerous studies have been designed to assess whether these alternatives to institutions are as satisfactory for the elderly as is simply living in a "normal" community, which is where more than 90 percent of those over age sixty-five live. These studies have typically presented a relatively positive picture in terms of the degree to which residents feel satisfied with their housing, with the social interaction available to them, and with their participation in various activities (Lawton, 1981).

Although most of the elderly would prefer to remain independent or to move in with relatives if they cannot remain independent, the need for other alternatives is increasing rapidly. This demand is occurring not only because the absolute number of elderly people is increasing dramatically but also because of medical advances that now make it possible for individuals to live longer following the onset of a variety of chronic disorders (Gurland, Bennett, & Wilder, 1981). As Lawton (1981) points out, alternatives to institutions are also alternatives to living independently in ordinary communities. And many of these alternatives can perhaps fill the gap between independence and institutionalization and, in the process, make the lives of the very old far happier.

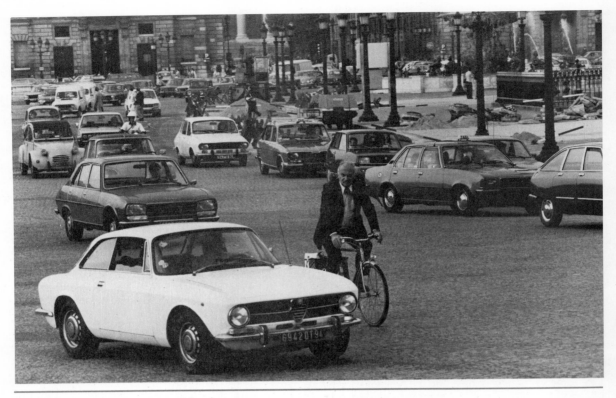

For some, aging successfully and happily means continuing social, emotional, and physical involvement (Activity Theory). For others, it means gradual withdrawal from emotional involvement with life (Disengagement Theory).

of ways, the most obvious relating to the ways in which society often encourages retirement from work and sometimes from other commitments as well.

One of the basic premises of disengagement theory is that withdrawal is not only natural but desirable. The predominant argument is that with declining physical and mental powers, the elderly find it increasingly difficult to continue to engage successfully in work-related activities, as well as in social, emotional, or political involvements. Consequently, they look forward to withdrawing and experience greater satisfaction and happiness if they are permitted to do so.

Although much of the research that has looked at disengagement theory has found that disen-gagement is often an accurate *description* of what happens in old age, this research has been hard pressed to establish that this is what *should* happen. Furthermore, disengagement is not often descriptive of the entire period of old age but occurs later in life. And it often involves less disengagement than strict interpretation of the theory might indicate. That is, although most individuals will have withdrawn from work and from many other involvements by the time they are seventy-five or eighty, few will have completely withdrawn from important emotional commitments. A great many will continue to fulfill crucial social roles as wives and husbands; some will be actively engaged in productive activities, such as looking after grandchildren or raising geraniums and chickens;

and a great many will be active in religious, political, and community organizations (Mindel & Vaughan, 1978).

Activity Theory

Activity theory, attributed to Havighurst, Neugarten, and Tobin (1968), is in some important ways the opposite of disengagement theory. Although it recognizes that a great deal of social and psychological disengagement does occur among older people, activity theory stresses that life satisfaction is highly dependent upon continued active involvement. According to this theory, those who age "best" are those who maintain the highest level of social, emotional, and physical involvement.

Among the variety of studies that have attempted to evaluate these opposing points of view, the majority indicate that continued involvement is often associated with satisfaction in later life. Indeed, some studies provide strong evidence that involvement and continued responsibility may be important for survival itself. In one such study, for example, Langer and Rodin (1976) told one group of nursing home residents that the staff was anxious to care for them and that they would therefore have to do very little for themselves. Each resident was given a small plant but was told that the nursing staff would see to its watering and care. A second group of residents was told that they should be making important decisions on their own behalf and that they would be responsible for many aspects of their own care. They were also given plants but were told that they would be responsible for their watering and care. In short, the first group was encouraged to *disengage*; the second was encouraged to remain *active*.

Some three weeks later, both groups were assessed in terms of physical and psychological health. And although measures for each group obtained prior to the study had been very similar, the *activity* group now showed significant improvement in terms of happiness, alertness, and sense of well-being. Follow-up measures, obtained 18 months later, still showed the same pattern of superiority for the activity group. What is perhaps even more striking, however, is that twice as many people in the disengagement group had died in the interim (thirteen out of forty-four as opposed to seven out of forty-seven).

Note that this study was designed not to investigate the importance of activity relative to disengagement but to explore the role of "perceived control" and of feelings of powerlessness in the lives of the aged. Other research has demonstrated that feelings of powerlessness are closely associated with mental disorder and might also be implicated in physical health; conversely, feelings of control are associated with psychological and physical health (see, for example, Seligman, 1975). Clearly, however, a close relationship exists among continued involvement, responsibility, and activity.

In conclusion, disengagement is usually characteristic of aging. But this does not necessarily mean that it should be required or even encouraged. By the same token, there is considerable evidence that continued involvement might contribute significantly to satisfaction, happiness, and health in many cases. But this too does not mean that continued activity should be required of all people. There are some who crave involvement, responsibility, and activity, and there are others who prefer the contentment of solitary rocking chairs.

■ Satisfaction and Happiness

And who will be the happiest? The old person in the solitary rocking chair or the one writing biographies or catching fish?

Buhler (1961) informs us that both might be happy; too, both might be unhappy. It may be a platitude but is no less true to say that it depends a great deal on the individuals. Some people seek rocking chairs in old age, because they are satisfied that they have done their life's work, and they wish to rest; other people wish to remain active and do so. Both might be very content. But there are also those who find themselves in their rocking chairs not by choice but because the ravages of age have

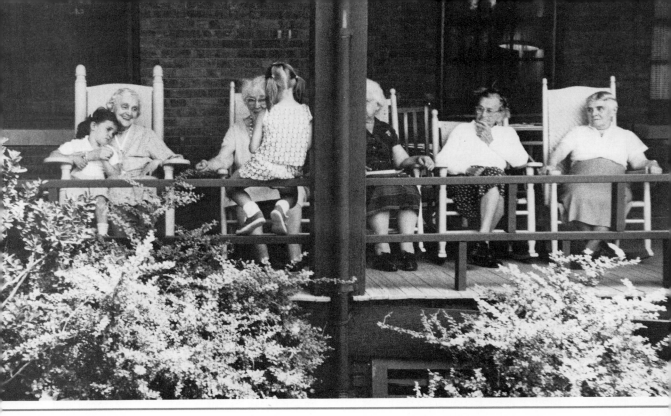

Close friendships, both among the very old and among the young and old, are important for maintaining high morale—a sense of well-being and worth.

put them there, and they now lack the abilities or the strength required to continue their activities. And there are those who remain active but who labor with a sense of frustration, not only because of the insufficient time they have left but also because they recognize the meaninglessness of their lives. And both of these groups might be unhappy.

In general, the research we looked at in Chapter 14 showed a pattern of increasing satisfaction with life, beginning in adolescence (Campbell, Converse, & Rodgers, 1976). Indeed, the highest ratings of satisfaction with life occur between the ages of sixty-five and seventy-four and the second highest, above age seventy-five. This finding is not particularly surprising, however, given that satisfaction is defined primarily in terms of the extent to which family and career goals have been met. The old have had an opportunity to reach their

goals and are therefore satisfied that they have done so—or, alternately, are resigned to never reaching them. And the young, whose dreams are still in the future, still sense some dissatisfaction.

Measures of happiness do not reveal quite the same pattern as measures of satisfaction. In many studies, the young have fared better than the old, with the highest measures of happiness occurring between the ages of twenty-five and thirty-four (second highest between fifty-five and sixty-four) and the lowest being reported for ages seventy-five and above (Campbell et al., 1976). This has not always been the case in more recent studies, however. In a 1978 study, percentages of individuals claiming they were "very happy" were almost identical at *all* age levels (around 30 percent), as was the percentage claiming to be "not too happy" (around 8 percent) (Campbell, 1981, p. 245).

At all stages of the life cycle, health is closely associated with happiness. It becomes an even more critical factor with the physical decline and increased susceptibility to disease of old age (Markides & Martin, 1979). Similarly, income is importantly related to a sense of well-being in old age, perhaps partly because of the sense of security that comes with having enough money and partly because those who are healthy and who have sufficient money are more easily able to remain actively involved.

Close friendships are also extremely important to maintaining what Lowenthal and Haven (1981) refer to as *high morale*—a quality closely related to what we have been calling happiness. In a study of morale, these researchers looked at the importance of intimate friends (confidants) in the lives of 280 individuals above the age of sixty. All resided in the community rather than in institutions, and a number were divorced, married, or widowed. Some had intimate friends in whom they could confide; others did not. For those who were married, the confidant was often, though not always, the spouse.

Results of the study indicate rather strongly that the presence of a confidant can be of tremendous importance in maintaining morale, even in the face of serious and tragic events such as the death of a spouse or serious illness. Perhaps equally important, in the absence of a confidant, progressive social disengagement (withdrawal from old social roles—for example, retirement) was often associated with depression. This was far less likely to be the case for those individuals who had access to an intimate friend. Indeed, even those who *increased* their social roles but had no confidants were more likely to become depressed than those who decreased their roles but did have confidants.

Friendships among the elderly are perhaps especially important for women, since they are far more likely than men to lose their spouses. Whereas more than 80 percent of all men are still married between the ages of sixty-five and seventy-four, only 49 percent of the women are—because of the much shorter life expectancies of men (Brotman, 1981, reported in Kalish, 1982). Thus there are always far more widows than widowers—far more women who need confidants.

Lopata (1981) examined friendship patterns among more than 1,000 widows. She found that surprisingly few of these women had established new friendships after the deaths of their husbands, even when they had lacked close friends previously. More than one-third of them simply kept their old friends, another third had both old and new friends, and almost one-sixth had neither new nor old friends. In fairness, however, it should be pointed out that some of these women still had relatives with whom they might occasionally socialize but who were not considered to be close friends.

Following her investigations, Lopata (1981) identified two types of "friendless" widows: those who do not see friends as an important part of life, who do not miss having them, and who are not dissatisfied as a result; and those who would like to have friends and who are consequently lonely and dissatisfied. She suggests, as well, that our cultural restraints concerning self-disclosure and intimacy make it difficult for women to develop the types of close, confiding relationships that might be fundamentally important to the happiness of their later years. Presumably the same is true for men.

In conclusion, we cannot easily say that old age is a happier or sadder time than any other in the lifespan. For some, it may indeed be happier, or at least as happy; for others, it might be a lot sadder. But whether it brings sorrow, joy, or simple resignation, it will also bring new roles and new problems, and it requires a whole new set of adjustments. Perhaps none of these adjustments is more difficult or painful than the need to face the certainty of death.

■ Death and Dying

As we have all known for some time, although most of us contemplate it reluctantly, death comes to each of us. We are allotted only one span. The only uncertainty concerns precisely when that span will end.

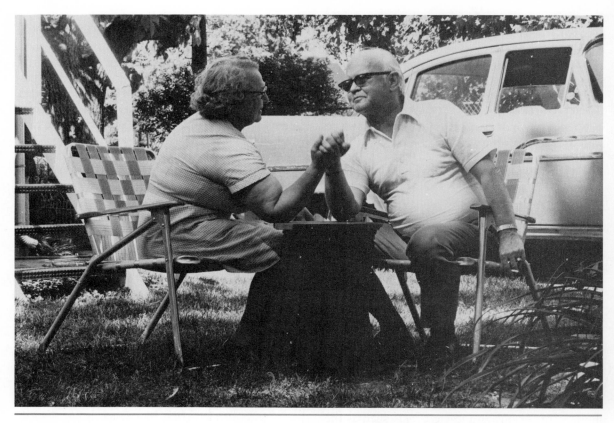

Health and friendship are closely associated with happiness at all stages of the life cycle.

Notions of Death Through the Lifespan

What do children know of death? Early research and theorizing indicated that they typically knew very little. Nagy (1948) interviewed children and identified three stages in their understanding of death. The first, spanning ages three and four, is marked by the first glimmerings of an understanding, although at this stage, children do not understand the finality of death. They believe, for example, that those who are dead are simply "not here"— that they continue to breathe and eat—that they are, in other words, something and somewhere. During the next stage (ages five to nine), children begin to *personify* death. It becomes a "bogeyman," a "witch," or some other wicked something

that is capable of taking people away. And the child now understands the irreversibility of this process of dying. In the third stage (from age nine onward), children begin to understand that the end of life is a biological process, that its cause lies within the body rather than with some outside force.

Although subsequent research has often found evidence corroborating the unfolding of stages like these, it appears that children can develop an understanding of death at considerably earlier ages. Bluebond-Langner (1977) suggests that the reason why children do not understand the nature of death is not that they are not capable of understanding but simply that they have not had experiences with death. This interpretation seems particularly appropriate, since more recent research indicates that children are not nearly as naive as was once thought (Tallmer, Formanek, & Tallmer, 1974). Television has now done a great deal to provide children with vicarious experiences that contribute to their earlier understanding of death and dying. And it is perhaps partly for the same reason that so many adolescents and young adults *expect* to die within a few years, most from violent causes (Teahan & Kastenbaum, 1970).

As children age and become more sophisticated intellectually, their understanding of death becomes progressively more adultlike. But for most of them, thoughts of death are remote and abstract. There is little reason to be concerned with dying when the future stretches almost forever. Yet evidence indicates that by adolescence, thoughts of dying and accompanying fears are not at all uncommon (Zeligs, 1974).

By early adulthood, many events have generally conspired to emphasize the transitory nature of living. These include the sometimes painful observation that with every passing decade, more and more of our friends, acquaintances, and relatives die. In addition, many young adults experience the loss of their own parents or observe signs of aging and of impending loss. And, as Kalish (1981) notes, since we all know that parents are supposed to die before children, we perhaps fear death less while our parents still live—and more after they die. Research does indicate that young adults are more concerned about death and more afraid to die than the middle aged (Kalish & Reynolds, 1976). Kalish suggests that this might be because having lived less, they sense that they have more time coming and have more to lose if they die.

With passing years, the inevitability of death becomes clearer. As Neugarten (1968) notes, sometime in middle age we experience a fundamental shift in time orientation: We cease to think in terms of the number of years we have lived and begin to think in terms of the time that is yet to be lived. This realization is frequently one aspect of the midlife crisis described in Chapter 13.

How do old people feel about dying? Reassuringly, they report less fear of death, although they spend considerably more time thinking about it. Kalish (1981) suggests several reasons why this

might be so. In the first place, the elderly have usually had far more experience with death than younger people, and many of these experiences have involved close friends, relatives, perhaps even a spouse. They have therefore been repeatedly compelled to think about death. In addition, progressive changes in their own bodies, often accompanied by one or more diseases, continue to emphasize that their own end is imminent. Kalish (1981) also suggests that our knowledge of what normal life expectancy is has led us to accept a lifespan of seventy or so years as one over which we have few legitimate complaints.

Stages of Dying

Psychologists have divided much of our lifespans into stages. There is nothing magical about these stages, nor is there anything intrinsically correct about them. They are simply inventions. They simplify our understanding, they make it easier to organize and to remember important observations, and sometimes they lead to important theoretical and practical insights.

Must we also die in stages? Some theorists suggest that this might sometimes be the case. Clearly, we need not resort to stages to understand the immediate and senseless finality of a gun, a bomb, or a plane crash. But perhaps a stage approach might be useful for understanding the process of dying when the patient *knows* that death is near. (See *Euthanasia* for an issue facing dying patients and their families.)

Kübler-Ross (1969, 1974), one of the foremost researchers in this field, describes five stages through which a terminally ill patient progresses after learning of the illness. In the first, *denial*, the patient often rejects the diagnosis and its implications: "This can't happen to me. There must be some mistake." Denial is sometimes followed by *anger*: "Why me? It shouldn't be me." The third stage, labeled *bargaining*, is characterized by the patient's attempts to look after unfinished business (with God, for example), promising to do well in exchange for a longer life or less suffering. The

EUTHANASIA

Popularly referred to as *mercy killing*, euthanasia presents a complicated and controversial collection of issues. These are presented here starkly, with little evaluative comment; our consciences make their own comments.

The term *euthanasia* is of Greek origin and means, literally, *good death*. A distinction is often made between *passive* and *active* euthanasia. *Active* euthanasia involves deliberately doing certain things to shorten life, such as administering a lethal injection or removing a patient from life-supporting systems. *Passive* euthanasia involves *not* doing certain things that might have prolonged life and is illustrated in those instances where heart surgery is *not* performed or blood transfusions are *not* given.

Active euthanasia is dramatically illustrated in the case of twenty-two-year-old Karen Ann Quinlan, whose brain no longer functioned but whose body was being kept alive artificially. Her parents were successful in obtaining a U.S. Supreme Court ruling, permitting them to remove her from life-sustaining equipment. In effect, the Court ruled that the state should not interfere in such decisions but that they should be made by the family in consultation with their physicians. The Quinlan lawyer, Paul Armstrong, has handled more than one hundred similar cases since Karen Ann's case and has won them all. Ironically, however, Karen Ann Quinlan has defied all medical predictions and is still alive, though comatose, more than seven years after being removed from artificial life-support systems ("Quinlans Have No Regret," 1983).

Passive euthanasia is illustrated in another poignant case, recently decided by the British Columbia Supreme Court, that of Stephen Dawson. Stephen, age six, suffered massive and irreversible brain damage following a bout of spinal meningitis as an infant. The disease left him blind, deaf, severely retarded, and apparently in pain. His parents petitioned the courts for the right *not* to perform brain surgery designed to remove cerebrospinal fluid. Without the operation, the boy was expected to die painlessly within a few weeks. On March 12, 1983, the family court judge granted the petition ("Loving Parents Given," 1983). The B.C. Association for the Mentally Retarded and provincial officials immediately appealed the family court decision. Following a week of testimony, Supreme Court Judge Lloyd McKenzie overturned the lower court decision, granted temporary custody of the boy to the province, and ordered that the life-saving operation be performed ("B.C. Judge Orders Operation for Boy," 1983).

Do we have a moral or legal right to decide when we shall die? (Suicide has historically been illegal.) Do we have a right to decide when others shall die? Do conditions such as severe and irreversible pain, coupled with inevitable and imminent death, justify euthanasia? Is passive euthanasia less objectionable than active euthanasia? Are there significant ethical or biological issues that clearly separate suicide, euthanasia, and perhaps even abortion?

These questions are far easier to ask than to answer. But for those whose answers are clear and who believe they would want to chose death under certain circumstances, the Euthanasia Education Council provides a document that can be used to formalize these wishes. It is called a *living will* and is reproduced on the opposite page.

LIVING WILL DECLARATION

To My Family, Physician and Medical Facility

I, _____, being of sound mind, voluntarily make known my desire that my dying shall not be artificially prolonged under the following circumstances:

If I should have an injury, disease or illness regarded by my physician as incurable and terminal, and if my physician determines that the application of life-sustaining procedures would serve only to prolong artificially the dying process, I direct that such procedures be withheld or withdrawn and that I be permitted to die. I want treatment limited to those measures that will provide me with maximum comfort and freedom from pain. Should I become unable to participate in decisions with respect to my medical treatment, it is my intention that these directions be honored by my family and physician(s) as a final expression of my legal right to refuse medical treatment, and I accept the consequences of this refusal.

Signed_____ Date_____

Witness _____ Witness _____

DESIGNATION CLAUSE (optional*)

Should I become comatose, incompetent or otherwise mentally or physically incapable of communication, I authorize _____,

presently residing at _____
to make treatment decisions on my behalf in accordance with my Living Will Declaration. I have discussed my wishes concerning terminal care with this person, and I trust his/her judgment on my behalf.

Signed_____ Date_____

Witness_____ Witness _____

*If I have not designated a proxy as provided above, I understand that my Living Will Declaration shall nevertheless be given effect should the appropriate circumstances arise.

A living will. (Reprinted with permission from Concern for Dying, 250 West 57th St., New York, N.Y. 10017.

fourth stage, *depression,* frequently follows. Finally, the patient may arrive at an *acceptance* of death.

Kübler-Ross's main concerns have been with the needs of the dying and with those who are left to mourn. Accordingly, much of her work deals less with a description of stages of dying than with advice concerning practical questions related to dying: "When should a patient be told?" "Who should do the telling?" "How can we reduce fear of death?" Nevertheless, her description of the stages of dying has had tremendous impact on the various professions that deal with death, as well as on the lay public. However, these stages have been extensively criticized. Not only are they a highly subjective interpretation of the process of dying, but there is also little empirical evidence to support the claim that people typically pass through these five stages and in the order prescribed. As I note elsewhere (Lefrancois, 1983): "The stages leave little room for individual differences and lead to the disturbing possibility that friends and family might react in what would otherwise be regarded as a callous and indifferent manner, rationalizing their behavior by claiming that the patient is simply going through the 'anger' or 'grief' stage. Not all go through these stages and in this order; dying is a highly individualistic process" (p. 377). So too is living.

■ MAIN POINTS

1 Most of us have *expectations* based primarily on age (we *know* what four-year-olds and forty-year-olds should be like). Many are also guilty of *ageism*—negative prejudices that are based solely on age. The elderly are frequently the object of ageism, reflected in the media's portrayal of weak, doddering, and foolish old people who, in their dotage, eat only porridge and other mushy foods.

2 Old age is socially defined as beginning at age sixty-five, but, given the wide spread of interests and abilities that separates age sixty-five from age eighty-five, some researchers make additional divisions. The proportion of people over sixty-five in the United States has increased fivefold in this century, while the entire population has slightly more than doubled. Approximately 11 percent of the population is now over sixty-five (twenty-five million individuals).

3 In many industrialized countries, life expectancies have increased nearly 50 percent since the turn of this century. In the United States, women can expect to live an average of eight years longer than men. But the biological limit of the human life—our lifespan—has remained constant at around one hundred twenty.

4 Theories of aging include genetic theories (lifespan limits are programmed in cells), error theories (with age certain errors occur in cells, hampering their normal functioning), toxin theories (poisons gradually accumulate in cells until they can no longer function), the free-radical theory (portions of cells become detached, interact with enzymes and proteins, and impede cellular activity), and the cross-linking theory (over the years, cells combine in different ways, some of which are detrimental to normal functioning). Some theorists suggest that aging is due to a gradual breakdown of body systems, and particularly of our immunity system (referred to as autoimmunity, a process whereby our immune systems become defective and attack the wrong cells).

5 Longevity is related to sex, race, mobility, education, occupation, employment, locale, heredity, and other factors.

6 *Senescence* describes biological decline as a function of age. Primary aging processes are universal and irreversible (arteriosclerosis, for example); secondary aging processes are not universal but include changes that become more probable with increasing age (cancer or heart disease, for example).

7 Age-related changes that have the greatest effect on appearance include changes in posture, loss of skin elasticity and consequent wrinkling, loss of hair or hair pigmentation, and loss of teeth or recession of gums.

8 With increasing age, people become less susceptible to acute infections (but recover from them more slowly) and more susceptible to chronic conditions. The most common chronic complaints include arthritis, hearing losses, heart disease, visual impairment, and arteriosclerosis. Parkinson's disease, osteoporosis (brittle bones), and acute brain syndrome are also diseases of old age. In spite of these greater health problems in old age, the majority of old people do not consider health to be a very serious problem for them.

9 Changes in sensory functioning that accompany aging include increasing far-sightedness, hearing impairment, and some loss of taste sensitivity.

10 Age-related changes in sexual functioning among women include diminished lubrication and loss of vaginal elasticity; in males, age-related changes include greater time for achieving an erection and orgasm and decline in the violence of ejaculation and the intensity of orgasm. Old age does bring with it some decline in sexual interest and activity. However, in most cases, sexual activity can usually continue well into old age.

11 Learning, memory, and measured intelligence decrease with age. In particular, scores on *performance* tests (attention span, spatial-visual ability) decline, while scores on tests that are more *verbal* often do not decline.

12 Measured IQ appears to drop, sometimes dramatically, in a great many individuals within one or two years before their deaths; labeled *terminal drop*, this phenomenon is sometimes explained in terms of health problems.

13 Declines on measures of intelligence might reflect problems of *performance* rather than lack of *competence* and can perhaps be partly explained in terms of the greater susceptibility of the old to fatigue, differences in motivation and education, physical and sensory problems, and their unfamiliarity with contemporary tests and testing procedures. Intelligence, a complex phenomenon, is difficult to measure for any age group.

14 Wisdom is one of the few positive qualities we typically associate with old age. In the West, it has been thought to be attainable through education, through affiliation with a wise mentor, or through faith. Eastern religions often recommend meditation as well as a master teacher as a path to wisdom (enlightenment).

15 Because decline is gradual and affects everybody, most of the elderly cope with the processes of aging and continue to find contentment and joy in their lives. With respect to successful aging, *disengagement* theory suggests that, with failing physical and mental capabilities, the elderly seek to withdraw from active social roles and that they should be allowed and perhaps even encouraged to do so. *Activity* theory argues that continued involvement socially, physically, and emotionally is important to the physical and emotional well-being of the aged.

16 Although satisfaction with life appears to increase with age (we either achieve our goals or become resigned to not doing so), happiness may decrease somewhat for some individuals. Health, income, and friendships appear to be important for later happiness and high morale.

17 Very young children often do not understand the finality of death, slightly older children may understand its finality but may personalize it in the form of some "bogeyman," and older children understand it as an irreversible biological phenomenon. Fear of death appears to be more common among adolescents and young adults than it is later in life. Although the very old think more about death than others, they do not, on the whole, express as much fear.

18 Kubler-Ross describes dying (when the person knows that death is imminent) in terms of five stages: denial (not me), anger (why me?), bargaining (let me suffer less and I will . . .), depression, and acceptance. Not all people go through these stages and in this order. Dying, like living, is highly individualistic.

■ FURTHER READINGS

The following book presents some useful insights about the impact of rapid cultural and technological change on the old and should serve to emphasize that our understanding of old age is limited to the understanding of a small handful of cohorts. Succeeding generations may tell different tales.
Fischer, D. *Growing old in America*. New York: Oxford University Press, 1977.

A moving look at creativity and learning among the old is presented in:
Koch, K. *I never told anybody*. New York: Random House, 1977.

Far more complete accounts of aging than can be contained in a single chapter may be found in the following two books. The first looks primarily at the social and personal aspects of aging; the second is a comprehensive textbook of aging.
Atchley, R. C. *The social forces in later life* (3rd ed.). Belmont, Calif.: Wadsworth, 1980.
Huyck, M. H., & Hoyer, W. J. *Adult development and aging*. Belmont, Calif.: Wadsworth, 1982.

The following is a candid, short, and highly readable book that deals specifically with many of the problems of aging, including loneliness, illness, spirituality, relationships with aging parents, and so on.
Weininger, B., & Menkin, E. L. *Aging is a lifelong affair*. Los Angeles: Guild of Tutors Press, 1977.

Kalish's book presents a comprehensive look at our understanding of death throughout the lifespan and at the process of dying and of grieving. A classic layperson's book on death and dying is the following one by Kübler-Ross.
Kalish, R. A. *Death, grief, and caring relationships*. Monterey, Calif.: Brooks/ Cole, 1981.
Kübler-Ross, E. *On death and dying*. New York: Macmillan, 1969.

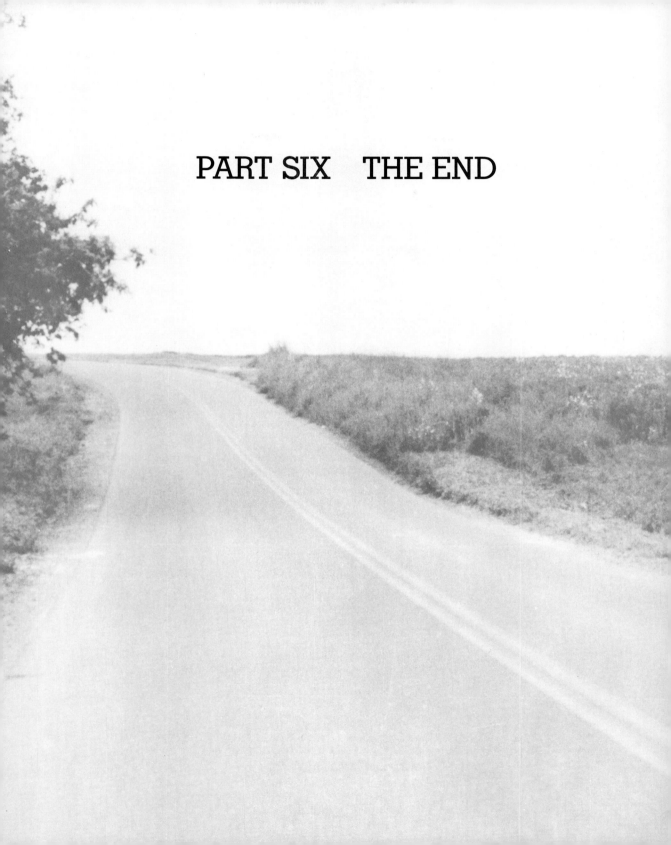

PART SIX   THE END

THE END

Do not go gentle into that good night,
Old age should burn and rave at close of day;
Rage, rage against the dying of the light.

Dylan Thomas
"Do Not Go Gentle"

Old age is no such uncomfortable thing if one gives
oneself up to it with a good grace, and don't drag it
about "To midnight dances and the public show."

Horace Walpole
Letter

In Victoire a sliver of newly risen moon shines dully on Pelletier's store. But even before I see the green lettering, I remember that it is no longer Pelletier's store—that it is now Lalonde's store. And I know that I should have come back sooner—that none of my reasons for not coming were really good enough.

Victoire is only a store, a church, and a small handful of houses not bordering a street, but scattered along a dirt road. From Victoire to Uncle Raoul's is one short mile.

We turn left in front of the store and drive slowly past the graveyard. I remember that I always drove slowly past this graveyard and that I would often think that some day I would never drive past it again—that I would stop and stay there forever. In those days that possibility seemed so remote that I could entertain it almost gleefully. Now the thought is much closer, sadder, and I wonder whether my grandmother's thoughts are also here. But when I look at her in the mirror, I see that she looks not toward the graveyard but toward Uncle Raoul's. His farm lies in an open meadow up against the southern end of Devil's Lake. We should see the lights from the top of this rise.

"There it is," Grandma says, proud that her old eyes have seen it first.

"Where? There. I see it. See it?" The children are excited and happy. We turn down the black dirt driveway. The house lies just ahead, lights shining happily from every window.

"Well, hello!" Uncle Raoul's smile is enormous. Aunt Lucy's too. And we all stand and embrace and laugh and embrace some more. And then I see it, a lone police car pulled up against the side of the house.

"What . . ." I begin to ask, nodding toward the car, but Uncle Raoul answers before I can finish.

"It's the RCMP from Debden. You know Mrs. Watts. The midwife. He brought her down. Cecile just had a baby. A boy!"

"I'm a great-grandmother again," my grandmother says, and everyone can see she's almost as proud as if she had done it all by herself. And in a way, she did. And now, a new life begins and overlaps her old span, as have so many others—so many lives whose roots reach back to this gentle old lady. Everyone connected.

They all hurry into the house, now, anxious to see the new infant, and I am left alone in the warm outside. But only for a moment. The police officer approaches. He smiles, but there is no humor in his smile; it is simply a polite smile.

"You are Guy Lefrancois?" It is only half question. Mostly, it's flat statement. "We want to talk to you. In the station tomorrow would be fine."

"What about?"

We both know, but he answers anyway—carefully and briefly. "The phone calls. The betting. Everything. Your uncles. You. We've known for a long time. Just waiting for you to come back. Knew you would."

Suddenly I understand.

"My phone. You tapped. . . ."

He shrugs noncommittally.

I begin to protest, but realize there is no point. I nod in agreement so that he will again leave me alone. I have no time to think of these things now, for the tale of the lifespan cannot be left unfinished. Quickly now, while everyone hastens to see the new infant, I will put a tail onto this tale.

■ A Global Summary

The tale that is told in this book concerns human development through the entire span of our lives. The book begins at the beginning with a consideration of the scope and methods of lifespan developmental psychology, looks next at some of the theories that have been used to organize what we know and suspect, and then turns to the two great forces that determine the course of development. Heredity certainly determines much of the eventual outcome of development, although we do not know precisely how much. Among other things, it determines most of our physical characteristics— our body type, our general pattern of physical growth, the color of our eyes, skin, and hair, and the shape of other parts of our anatomy. Evidence strongly suggests that heredity is also profoundly involved in determining intelligence and that personality predispositions are also somewhat subject to genetic influences. In short, a great deal about each of us is predetermined when we are born— characteristics that were determined largely by chance and certainly not influenced by anything over which we had any personal control. Indeed, the very fact that such a person as you or I exist is largely a matter of fortune—it could have been another ovum; it could have been any one of several million other sperm cells. And in each case the result would have been someone else. Or would it?

But what you and I are becoming is not solely a function of the intricate arrangements of DNA molecules that our parents passed on to us, and which they in turn received from their parents, and they from their parents, and so on, so that in a remote sense a common pool of genes exists for all of us. What we are is also a matter of where we were at different times in our lives and of what people and things were like around us. Witness the dramatic differences among the Arapesh, the Tchambuli, and Mundugumor. Or closer to home, look at the ideals and aspirations, the typical behavior, the sources of reinforcement, the language, the self-concepts, and the *selves* of the people around you. And if the point is not yet striking enough, look at the painful differences among the inhabitants of your city. What we become is a process of constant interaction between our native endowment and the environment in which we find ourselves. Environment is a complex thing, including everything around us—family, friends, inanimate objects, the media, the air—everything. Really understanding the influence of the environment on an individual means perceiving it from that person's point of view—from what is termed a *phenomenological* standpoint. We will speak of this again shortly.

The bulk of the remainder of the book then followed the usually gradual but sometimes dramatic development of a human life. We began with the very beginning: a microscopic speck in one of the mother's fallopian tubes. Through the next 266 days, this indistinct cellular mass changes into the form and functions that define the newborn infant; although these changes are ordered, systematic, and highly predictable, they are nevertheless subject to external influences. Some of these influences on the child in utero were examined, followed by a description of the process of birth, both from the physician's and from the mother's points of view.

We followed the child through the sequential stages of human unfolding: infancy, preschool, middle childhood, and finally the period of transition between childhood and adulthood—adolescence. At each of these steps, something was said of the physical, social, and cognitive development of the average child. And at each stage, you were urged to keep in mind that we spoke of the nonexistent average child and, further, that we were dividing this child into different layers to simplify the process of communication between us while robbing the child of individuality and robbing the developmental process of its dynamism.

In the end we left the child—somewhere in adolescence or early adulthood; the point is never exact. But development does not end with childhood; it continues to the very end of our spans. So in later sections of the book, we looked at the physical and cognitive changes that aging entails and at the adjustments that are required. We also looked at various life styles and at the unfolding of human personality through the adult years. And we looked at some of the theories that might clarify our understanding of these years. Finally, we came to the biological end of the span.

That part of the story has now been told. There remains only the attempt to bring the various layers and pieces into a cohesive whole, to provide a richer, more accurate, more complete, and more *human* picture of humans in the process of becoming.

■ A Humanistic View of Developing Humans

Who am I? Is the I who is sitting here thinking about who he is different from the I who questioned my grandmother's fertile theories? Was I the same me when, as an adolescent, I wondered about life, its purposes and goals, the reaches beyond its obvious limits, society and the predicaments that it had created for itself, and a thousand other questions of grave and immediate consequence? Was the I who went to school as a freshly scrubbed six-year-old the same person who graduated from college many years later? Who is my self and what is it? How does it become what it is?

Perhaps there is no correct answer to the question of personal identity—a question that has plagued philosophers, psychologists, theologians, and all manner of thinkers since thinking began. But two useful answers are frequently given, both intuitive and highly subjective but still meaningful. The first asserts that there is an unidentifiable something about the self that continues from the dawning awareness of a personal identity until the oblivion of psychotic disorder, acute senility, or death destroys all sense of existence. The other answer does not contradict the first, but simply extends it. The self is continually developing, despite the individual's feeling of a single and unique personal identity throughout life.

Discussions of the self and its development have been a primary concern of humanistic psychology and existential philosophy, both of which might contribute much to our understanding and appreciation of the phenomena of human development. A rigorous discussion of their contributions is beyond the scope of this text. Nevertheless, an introduction of the two points of view is presented here, partly to serve as an alternative to the somewhat unreal picture that inevitably results from attempting to examine people in objective psychological detail and partly as a finishing touch for the painting that has been attempted in this text.

Humanism

Humanism is a concern for humans, for humanity, for the development of *humanness*, and for its expression. It exalts the individual and glorifies the *self*. Thus, the concepts of paramount concern to the humanistic psychologist include such notions as self-structure, self-concept, self-image, self-

understanding, self-acceptance, self-enhancement, and self-actualization. Humanism is concerned with what is most clearly human; accordingly, the development of self (self-actualization) is the goal toward which humans should strive.

The process of *self-actualization* is the act of becoming whatever one has the potential to become through one's own efforts; it is the process of making that potential real or actual. But it is not a static goal toward which individuals consciously or unconsciously strive; it is a process, an ongoing activity. Self-actualization is the process of development. Different terms could have been substituted in this text to make this relationship more apparent. For example, instead of speaking of development, we might have spoken of self-actual-

To self-actualize is to become whatever one can—should be—through one's own efforts. Although self-actualization is more obvious in the lives of great historic figures, it can also be found in humbler, more private lives.

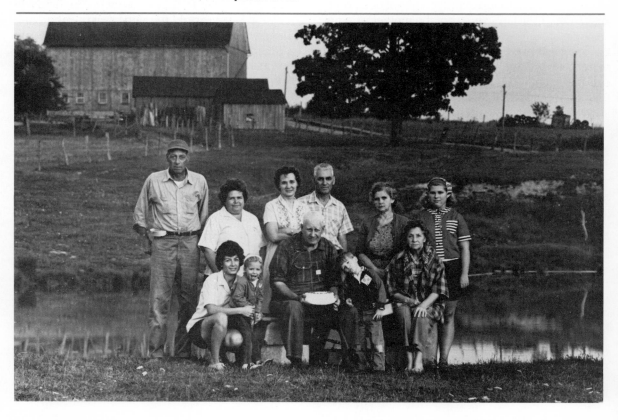

ization or of the development of self; instead of referring to the frustrations of adolescents, who cannot easily determine whether they are child or adult, we could have spoken only of the difficulty of establishing the *identity* of the self during the transition from childhood to adulthood; and instead of discussing forces that impede or accelerate development, we could have discussed self-enhancement or changing self-structure. And the picture that would have emerged might have been a more integrated one, for we would constantly have been speaking of the self. It would also have been a more realistic picture that dealt more with the real person than with the average, normal person—for the self belongs solely to the individual; there is no "average" self. To speak of the average self is to distort the concept unforgivably. At the same time, the portrait would probably have been a more global, less precise, and less informative study of humans.

Existentialism

To complete the description of human life presented here, we might consider the concepts of **existential psychology**, because in some ways they are similar to those of humanistic psychology.

From Jean-Paul Sartre we borrow a description of the human condition—cynical and pessimistic, but one that enables us to understand better the direction of development, particularly in its nearly adult stages. From Martin Buber we borrow ideas from a philosophy of what he calls personalism, which is but a short distance from humanism.

The existential picture of people and of the forces that move them, as presented by Jean-Paul Sartre, can be described by three words: *anguish, abandonment*, and *despair*. These words summarize the human condition—they are both the facts of existence and its consequences. People are forever in *anguish,* because they are constantly forced to make decisions and yet have no guides for these decisions. There is no guarantee that anything one does is correct, for there is no God, Sartre informs us, and without a God all action must be justified in terms of its effects on others. Such resolution is a tremendous and terrible responsibility—an insoluble dilemma—and its consequence is deep and undying anguish. People have also been abandoned, and **abandonment** is an indescribably lonely feeling. They have not been abandoned simply by others but abandoned in a general sense, without a purpose and with no a priori values, abandoned to be free—free to make choices but also required to make them. And so

Subject: Female; age sixty-two; married; three children; four grandchildren; not working outside home; husband recently retired.

Question: "When did you decide that you had finally grown up?"

I can't say that there was ever one special time when I felt—well, grown up. I remember thinking that when I left home I'd be all grown up and maybe I was anxious for that to happen. Then I got married, left, but I'm sure I didn't feel very grown up. Especially at the beginning. I still felt . . . Frank . . . my husband seemed to me like he was grown up. Even when we first got married. He's a bit older. He always seemed to know. . . . Me, I was not sure—confused lots of times. He knew what to do but I often wondered. It's not always easy. . . . I guess I'm not sure I actually *feel* grown up right now. Why do you think I'm taking this university course? (laughter)

Interview

we despair, because we are free but without hope, because to will something is not necessarily to achieve it, and because when we die all our efforts may have been in vain.

Sartre's atheistic existentialism is described here to give a perspective through contrast to the more optimistic reflections of Martin Buber. Buber (1958, 1965) tells us that there are four main evils in the modern world and that the effect of these evils is to highlight the importance of the human self. The first of these evils is our terrible loneliness, and loneliness has long been recognized by existentialists as a concept of extreme importance. Existence as a self is essentially a lonely experience, because the self always belongs only to the individual—it can never be shared completely. Therefore we are always alone. Buber's second evil is the never-ending drive for technological progress, the individual's worth lessening with the increasing importance of machines and sciences. The third evil stems from human duality: the good-versus-evil dichotomy—the id warring with the superego. Finally, Buber contends that the individual is being degraded by the state; the conglomerate, impersonal, and faceless entities that define states are incompatible with the uniqueness and personal worth of the individual.

The result of these evils is summarized in a single existentialist (and humanistic) term: *alienation*. To be alienated is to be separated from, to be a stranger to. In a very real sense, we are alienated from ourselves, from others, and from our environment. In short, we have been uprooted from the relationships that we should have with all three: our private self, those who surround us, and the world we live in. Accordingly, the greatest evil that besets us, social animals that we are, is alienation, and the greatest good is *love*—love of self and love of others. Buber's philosophy is seldom pessimistic, for it asserts strongly that our salvation, our happiness, and our consequent self-actualization can be achieved through love. And love is simply a question of relationships, what Buber terms an I-Thou relationship, one in which the object or person being related to is not being used selfishly, the relationship is mutual, there is dialogue as opposed to monologue, and people say and do what they honestly mean rather than what is merely convenient or socially appropriate.

If the process of human development has a goal—that is, if it ever ceases to be a process of becoming—then its goal must surely be a capacity to feel great love, and the reward for having reached that state must surely be great happiness. Does self-actualization ever become self-realization? Does the old person ever know that the child has grown up?

■ Editor's Note

As this magnificent book goes to press, we still have no definite news about Guy Lefrancois, although we have been in touch with Anne, as well as with his grandmother and with various other people up there. There has not been a trial or even a hearing, as far as we know. Some say the police continue to look for evidence, although we suspect that the whole thing was a complete misunderstanding, brought about by his association, many many years earlier, with people whom we have reason to believe were engaged in illegal gambling. It has never been proven that he was associated with them in any way other than socially. And the few chickens he might have stolen, purely as a prank, have surely been forgotten by now. In spite of what some have said, a handful of scrawny chickens and the occasional harmless wager do not a kleptomaniac and a compulsive gambler make.

Others say that what the police are looking for is not evidence, but Guy Lefrancois himself. We doubt that very much. We tend to believe Anne, who claims that he is writing poetry in a romantic cabin hidden in a black and green forest. Maurice Frenette says he saw him in the bush last winter.

"He was wearing a homemade knitted toque," he told us. "Green, it was, and so big it covered most of his face. But I know it was him!"

We really do not know for sure. But apparently not many chickens have been reported missing up there recently.

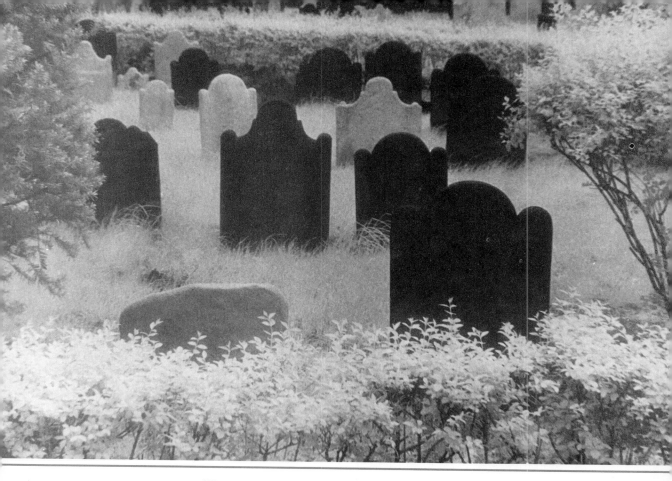

When all is said and done. Or even before . . .

■ Anne's Note

Please allow me to set the record straight, once and for all. It was not the gambling or even the chickens. Both were red herrings. Sure he gambled, and he did steal a few chickens now and again. But I have little doubt that he did so mostly to confuse his detractors. He has always been abnormally fond of doing things simply to confound those he calls "my enemies." And he did succeed in confusing various law-enforcement agencies—maybe too well.

Now Guy says he's writing poetry up there. In that dilapidated shack he calls a cabin. But he probably isn't. He's probably continuing his deception. You see, he really isn't Guy Lefrancois at all! He has never been to any college or university in his life! And he is anything but a psychologist! His real name is . . .

■ Author's Note

There is now too little space left for the whole truth. Besides, chickens and red herrings are close enough. And the adventure is still too young for the entire truth to have yet occurred. Perhaps when the next edition. . . .

BIBLIOGRAPHY

Abrioux, M. L., & Zingle, H. W. An exploration of the marital and life-satisfactions of middle-aged husbands and wives. *Canadian Counsellor*, 1979, *13*, 85–92.

Abroms, I. F., & Panagakos, P. G. The child with significant developmental motor disability (cerebral palsy). In A. P. Scheiner & I. F. Abroms (Eds.), *The practical management of the developmentally disabled child*. St. Louis: C. V. Mosby, 1980.

Acredolo, L. P. Development of spatial orientation in infancy. *Developmental Psychology*, 1978, *14*, 224–234.

Ahammer, I. M., & Murray, J. P. Kindness in the kindergarten: The relative influence of role playing and prosocial television in facilitating altruism. *International Journal of Behavior Development*, 1979, *2*, 133–157.

Ahlstrom, W. M., & Havighurst, R. J. *400 losers*. San Francisco: Jossey-Bass, 1971.

Ainsworth, M. D. S. Attachment and dependency: A comparison. In J. L. Gewirtz (Ed.), *Attachment and dependency*. Washington, D.C.: Winston, 1972.

Ainsworth, M. D. S. Infant-mother attachment. *American Psychologist*, 1979, *34*, 932–937.

Ainsworth, M. D. S., & Bell, S. M. Some contemporary patterns of mother-infant interaction in the feeding situation. In A. Ambrose (Ed.), *Stimulation in early infancy*. New York: Academic Press, 1969.

Ainsworth, M. D. S., Blehar, M. C., Waters, E., & Wall, S. *Patterns of attachment*. Hillsdale, N.J.: Lawrence Erlbaum, 1978.

Aldis, O. *Play fighting*. New York: Academic Press, 1975.

Alexander, G. LSD: Injection early in pregnancy produces abnormalities in offspring of rats. *Science*, 1967, *157*, 459–460.

Als, H., Tronick, E., Lester, B. M., & Brazelton, T. B. Specific neonatal measures: The Brazelton neonatal behavior assessment scale. In J. D. Osofsky (Ed.), *Handbook of infant development*. New York: John Wiley, 1979.

Altus, W. D. Birth order and academic primogeniture. *Journal of Personality and Social Psychology*, 1965, *2*, 872–876.

Altus, W. D. Birth order and its sequelae. *International Journal of Psychiatry*, 1967, *3*, 23–42.

American Psychiatric Association. *Diagnostic and statistical manual of mental disorders*. Washington, D.C.: American Psychiatric Association, 1980.

Ames, L. B. The sequential patterning of prone progression in the human infant. *Genetic Psychology Monographs*, 1937, *19*, 409–460.

Anderson, D. R. Active and passive processes in children's television viewing. Paper presented at the annual meeting of the American Psychological Association, New York, August 1979.

Angelino, H., Dollins, J., & Mech, E. V. Trends in the "fears and worries" of school children as related to socioeconomic status and age. *Journal of Genetic Psychology*, 1956, *89*, 263–276.

Anthony, E. J. (Ed.). *Exploration in child psychiatry*. New York: Plenum Press, 1975.

Anthony, E. J., & Koupernik, C. (Eds.). *The child in his family: Children at psychiatric risk* (Vol. 3). New York: John Wiley, 1974.

Apkom, A., Apkom, K., & Davies, M. Prior sexual behavior of teenagers attending rap sessions for the first time. *Family Planning Perspectives*, 1976, *8*, 203–206.

Arbuthnot, J. Modification of moral judgment through role playing. *Developmental Psychology*, 1975, *11*, 319–324.

Aries, P. *Centuries of childhood: A social history of family life* (R. Baldick, trans.). New York: Alfred A. Knopf, 1962. (Originally published, 1960.)

Arlin, P. K. Cognitive development in adulthood: A fifth stage? *Developmental Psychology*, 1975, *11*, 602–606.

Arnold, A. *Violence and your child*. Chicago: Henry Regnery, 1969.

Asch, S. E. Opinions and social pressure. *Scientific American*, November 1955, 194.

Asimov, I. *The intelligent man's guide to science*. New York: Basic Books, 1963.

Atchley, R. C. *The social forces in later life* (3rd ed.). Belmont, Calif.: Wadsworth, 1980.

Athanasiou, R. A review of public attitudes on sexual issues. In J. Zubin & J. Money (Eds.), *Contemporary sexual behavior: Critical issues in the 1970's*. Baltimore: Johns Hopkins University Press, 1973.

Ault, R. L. *Children's cognitive development: Piaget's theory and the process approach*. New York: Oxford University Press, 1977.

Baer, D. M., & Wright, J. C. Developmental psychology. In M. R. Rosenzweig & L. W. Porter (Eds.), *Annual review of psychology* (Vol. 25). Palo Alto, Calif.: Annual Reviews, 1974.

Bahrick, H. P., Bahrick, P. O., & Wittlinger, R. P. Fifty years of memory for names and faces: A cross-sectional approach. *Journal of Experimental Psychology: General*, 1975, *104*, 54–75.

Bakan, D. *Slaughter of the innocents*. Toronto: CBC Learning Systems, 1971.

Baker, J. B. E. The effects of drugs on the fetus. *Pharmacological Review*, 1960, *12*, 37–90.

Bakwin, H. Psychologic aspects of pediatrics. *Journal of Pediatrics*, 1949, *35*, 512–521.

Baldwin, A. L. *Theories of child development*. New York: John Wiley, 1967.

Ball, J. C., Ross, A., & Simpson, A. Incidents and estimated prevalence of recorded delinquency in a metropolitan area. *American Sociological Review*, 1964, *29*, 90–93.

Baltes, P. B. Prototypical paradigms and questions in life-span research on development and aging. *Gerontologist*, 1973, *13*, 457–512.

Baltes, P. B., Reese, H. W., & Lipsitt, L. P. Life span developmental psychology. In M. R. Rosenzweig & L. W. Porter (Eds.), *Annual review of psychology* (Vol. 31). Palo Alto, Calif.: Annual Reviews, 1980.

Baltes, P. B., & Schaie, K. W. On the plasticity of intelligence in adulthood and old age: Where Horn and Donaldson fail. *American Psychologist*, 1976, *31*, 720–725.

Baltes, P. B., & Willis, S. L. The critical importance of appropriate methodology in the study of aging: The sample case of psychometric intelligence. In F. Hoffmeister & C. Muller (Eds.), *Brain functions in old age*. Heidelberg: Springer-Verlag, 1979.

Bancroft, R. Special education: Legal aspects. In P. A. O'Donnell & R. H. Bradfield (Eds.), *Mainstreaming: Controversy and consensus*. San Rafael, Calif.: Academic Therapy Publications, 1976.

Bandura, A. *Principles of behavior modification*. New York: Holt, Rinehart & Winston, 1969.

Bandura, A. *Psychological modeling: Conflicting theories*. Chicago: Aldine, 1971.

Bandura, A. *Social learning theory*. Englewood Cliffs, N.J.: Prentice-Hall, 1977.

Bandura, A., Ross, D., & Ross, S. A. Vicarious reinforcement and imitative learning. *Journal of Abnormal and Social Psychology*, 1963, *67*, 601–607.

Bandura, A., & Walters, R. *Adolescent aggression*. New York: Ronald Press, 1959.

Bandura, A., & Walters, R. *Social learning and personality development*. New York: Holt, Rinehart & Winston, 1963.

Bane, M. J. Marital disruption and the lives of children. *Journal of Social Issues*, 1976, *32*, 103–117.

Baran, S. I., Chase, L. I., & Courtright, J. A. Television drama as a facilitator of prosocial behavior: "The Waltons." *Journal of Broadcasting*, 1979, *23*, 277–285.

Barber, T. X., & Silver, M. J. Fact, fiction, and the experimenter bias effect. *Psychological Bulletin Monographs Supplement*, 1969, *70*, 1–29. (a)

Barber, T. X., & Silver, M. J. Pitfalls in data analysis and interpretation: A reply to Rosenthal. *Psychological Bulletin Monographs Supplement*, 1969, *70*, 48–62. (b)

Barnett, S. A. *Instinct and intelligence: Behavior of animals and man*. Englewood Cliffs, N.J.: Prentice-Hall, 1967.

Barron, F., & Harrington, D. M. Creativity, intelligence, and personality. In M. R. Rosenzweig & L. W. Porter (Eds.), *Annual review of psychology* (Vol. 32). Palo Alto, Calif.: Annual Reviews, 1981.

Bartell, G. D. *Group sex: An eyewitness report on the American way of swinging*. New York: New American Library, 1971.

Baskin, Y. Spare genes: Tampering with human embryos? *Omni*, March 1982, pp. 52–54; 109–114.

Bates, J. E. The concept of difficult temperament. *Merrill-Palmer Quarterly*, 1980, *26*, 299–319.

Baumrind, D. Child care practices anteceding three patterns of pre-school behavior. *Genetic Psychology Monographs*, 1967, *75*, 43–88.

Baumrind, D. Some thoughts about childrearing. In S. Cohen & T. J. Comiskey (Eds.), *Child development: Contemporary perspectives*. Itasca, Ill.: F. E. Peacock, 1977.

Bayer, A. E. Birth order and college attendance. *Journal of Marriage and the Family*, 1966, *28*, 480–484.

Bayer, L. M., Whissell-Buechy, D., & Honzik, M. P. Health in the middle years. In D. H. Eichorn, J. A. Clausen, N. Haan, M. P. Honzik, & P. H. Mussen (Eds.), *Present and past in middle life*. New York: Academic Press, 1981.

Bayley, N. *Bayley scales of infant development*. New York: Psychological Corp., 1969.

B.C. judge orders operation for boy. *Edmonton Journal*, March 18, 1983, p. A-1.

Beck, A. T., & Young, J. E. College blues. *Psychology Today*, September 1978, pp. 80–92.

Bell, A., & Weinberg, M. *Homosexuality: A study of diversity among men and women*. New York: Simon & Schuster, 1978.

Bell, R. Q. A reinterpretation of the direction of effects in studies of socialization. *Psychological Review*, 1968, *75*, 81–95.

Bell, R. Q. Stimulus control of parent or caretaker behavior by offspring. *Development Psychology*, 1971, *4*, 63–72.

Belsky, J. Early human experience: A family perspective. *Developmental Psychology*, 1981, *17*, 3–23.

Belsky, J., & Steinberg, L. D. What does research teach us about day care: A follow-up report. *Children Today*, July/August 1979, pp. 21–26.

Benbow, C. P., & Stanley, J. C. Consequences in high school and college of sex differences in mathematical reasoning ability: A longitudinal perspective. *American Educational Research Journal*, 1982, *19*, 598–622.

Benda, C. E. Mongolism: A comprehensive review. *Archives of Paediatrics*, 1956, *73*, 391–407.

Bennett, G. K., Seashore, H. G., & Wesman, A. G. *The differential aptitude tests* (6th ed.). New York: Psychological Corp., 1981.

Berg, W. K., & Berg, W. K. Psychophysiological development in infancy: State, sensory function, and attention. In J. D. Osofsky (Ed.), *Handbook of infant development*. New York: John Wiley, 1979.

Berkowitz, L. The concept of aggressive drive: Some additional considerations. In L. Berkowitz (Ed.), *Advances* *in experimental social psychology* (Vol. 2). New York: Academic Press, 1965.

Berkowitz, L. *A survey of social psychology.* Hinsdale, Ill.: Dryden Press, 1975.

Bernard, J., & Sontag, L. W. Fetal reactivity to sound. *Journal of Genetic Psychology*, 1947, *70*, 205–210.

Berndt, T. J. *Prosocial behavior between friends and the development of social interaction patterns.* Paper presented at the annual meeting of the Society for Research in Child Development, New Orleans, 1981.

Bernstein, B. Social class and linguistic development: A theory of social learning. *British Journal of Sociology*, 1958, *9*, 159–174.

Bernstein, B. Language and social class. *British Journal of Sociology*, 1961, *11*, 271–276.

Bettelheim, B. *The uses of enchantment: Meaning and importance of fairy tales.* London: Peregrine Books, 1978.

Bigelow, B. J., & LaGaipa, J. J. The development of friendship values and choice. In H. D. Foot, A. J. Chapman, & J. R. Smith (Eds.), *Friendship and social relations in children.* New York: John Wiley, 1980.

Bijou, S. W., & Baer, D. M. *Child development II.* New York: Appleton-Century-Crofts, 1965.

Biller, H. B. Sex-role learning: Some comments and complexities from a multidimensional perspective. In S. Cohen & T. J. Comiskey (Eds.), *Child development: A contemporary perspective.* Itasca, Ill.: F. E. Peacock, 1977.

Binet, A., & Simon, T. Méthodes nouvelles pour le diagnostic du niveau intellectuel des anormaux. *Année Psychologique*, 1905, *11*, 191–244.

Birch, H. G., & Gussow, J. D. *Disadvantaged children: Health, nutrition and school failure.* New York: Grune & Stratton, 1970.

Birren, J. E., Cunningham, W. R., & Yamamoto, K. Psychology of adult development and aging. In M. R. Rosenzweig & L. W. Porter (Eds.), *Annual review of psychology* (Vol. 34). Palo Alto, Calif.: Annual Reviews, 1983.

Birren, J. E., & Renner, V. Research on the psychology of aging: Principles and experimentation. In J. E. Birren & K. W. Schaie (Eds.), *Handbook of the psychology of aging.* New York: Van Nostrand Reinhold, 1977.

Bischof, L. J. *Adult Psychology* (2nd ed.). New York: Harper & Row, 1976.

Blatz, W. E. *Collected studies on the Dionne quintuplets.* Toronto: University of Toronto Press, 1937.

Blau, Z. S. *Old age in a changing society.* New York: New Viewpoints, 1973.

Blehar, M. C. Anxious attachment and defensive reactions associated with day care. *Child Development*, 1974, *45*, 683–692.

Block, J. *Lives through time.* Berkeley, Calif.: Bancroft Books, 1971.

Bloodstein, O. The development of stuttering. *Journal of Speech and Hearing Disorders*, 1960, *25*, 219–236.

Bloom, B. S. *Stability and change in human characteristics.* New York: John Wiley, 1964.

Bloom, L. *Language development: Form and function in emerging grammars.* New York: Academic Press, 1970.

Bloom, L. *One word at a time: The use of single word utterances before syntax.* The Hague: Mouton, 1973.

Bluebond-Langner. Meanings of death to children. In H. Fecfel (Ed.), *New meanings of death.* New York: McGraw-Hill, 1977.

Blumberg, M. L. Psychopathology of the abusing parent. *American Journal of Psychotherapy*, 1974, *28*, 21–29.

Blumenthal, J. A., Sanders Williams, R., Needels, T. L., & Wallace, A. G. Psychological changes accompany aerobic exercise in healthy middle-aged adults. *Psychosomatic Medicine*, 1982, *44*, 529–536.

Bocknek, G. *The young adult: Development after adolescence.* Monterey, Calif.: Brooks/Cole, 1980.

Bogopolsky, Y., & Cormier, B. M. Économie relationnelle de chacun des membres dans une famille incestueuse. *Canadian Journal of Psychiatry*, 1979, *24*, 65–70.

Boisvert, M. J. The battered child syndrome. *Social Casework*, 1972, pp. 475–480.

Boles, D. B. X-linkage of spatial ability: A critical review. *Child Development*, 1980, *51*, 625–635.

Bookmiller, M. M., & Bowen, G. L. *Textbook of obstetrics and obstetric nursing* (5th ed.). Philadelphia: W. B. Saunders, 1967.

Boring, E. G. Intelligence as the tests test it. *New Republic*, 1923, *35*, 35–37.

Borke, H. Piaget's mountains revisited: Changes in the egocentric landscape. *Developmental Psychology*, 1975, *11*, 240–243.

Bornstein, M. H., Kessen, W., & Weiskopf, S. Color vision and hue categorization in young human infants. *Science*, 1975, *191*, 201–202.

Bornstein, M. H., & Marks, L. E. Color revisionism. *Psychology Today*, January 1982, *16*, 64–72.

Bossard, J. H., & Boll, E. S. *The large family system.* Philadelphia: University of Pennsylvania Press, 1956.

Bossard, J. H., & Sanger, W. P. The large family system—a research report. *American Sociological Review*, 1951, *17*, 3–9.

Botwinick, J. Intellectual abilities. In J. E. Birren & K. W. Schaie (Eds.), *Handbook of the Psychology of Aging.* New York: Van Nostrand Reinhold, 1977.

Bouchard, T. J., Jr., & McGue, M. Familial studies of intelligence: A review. *Science*, 1981, *212*, 1055–1059.

Bower, T. G. R. The object in the world of the infant. *Scientific American*, 1971, *225*, 30–38.

Bower, T. G. R. *Development in infancy.* New York: W. H. Freeman, 1974.

Bower, T. G. R. *The perceptual world of the child.* Cambridge, Mass.: Harvard University Press, 1977.

Bowes, W. A., Jr., Brackbill, Y., Conway, E., & Steinschneider, A. The effects of obstetrical medication on fetus and infant. *Monographs of the Society for Research in Child Development*, 1970, *35*(4).

Bowlby, J. The influence of early environment. *International Journal of Psychoanalysis*, 1940, *21*, 154–178.

Bowlby, J. Some pathological processes set in train by early mother-child separation. *Journal of Mental Science*, 1953, *99*, 265–272.

Bowlby, J. The nature of the child's tie to his mother. *International Journal of Psychoanalysis*, 1958, *39*, 350–373.

Bowlby, J. *Attachment and loss*. New York: Basic Books, 1973.

Boyd, G. A. *Developmental processes in the child's acquisition of syntax: Linguistics in the elementary school*. Itasca, Ill.: F. E. Peacock, 1976.

Brackbill, Y. Acoustic variation and arousal level in infants. *Psychophysiology*, 1970, *6*, 517–526.

Brackbill, Y. Obstetrical medication and infant behavior. In J. D. Osofsky (Ed.), *Handbook of infant development*. New York: John Wiley, 1979.

Brady, K. *Father's days: A true story of incest*. New York: Seaview Books, 1979.

Brandwein, R. A., Brown, C. A., & Fox, E. M. Women and children last: The social situation of divorced mothers and their families. *Journal of Marriage and the Family*, August 1974, pp. 498–514.

Braun, S. J., & Caldwell, B. Emotional adjustment of children in daycare who enrolled prior to or after the age of three. *Early Child Development and Care*, 1973, *2*, 13–21.

Brazelton, T. D. *Neonatal Behavior Assessment Scale*. Philadelphia: J. B. Lippincott, 1973.

Brazziel, W. F. A letter from the south. *Harvard Educational Review* (Reprint Series No. 2), 1969, 200–208.

Brill, A. A. (Ed.). *The basic writings of Sigmund Freud*. New York: Random House, 1938.

Brim, O. G. Theories of the male mid-life crisis. *Counseling Psychologist*, 1976, *6*, 2–9.

Brim, O. G., Jr., & Kagan, J. (Eds.). *Constancy and change in human development*. Cambridge, Mass.: Harvard University Press, 1980.

Bromley, D. B. *The psychology of human ageing* (2nd ed.). Middlesex, England: Penguin, 1974.

Bronfenbrenner, U. *Two worlds of childhood: U.S. and U.S.S.R.* New York: Russell Sage Foundation, 1970.

Bronfenbrenner, U. Nobody home: The erosion of the American family. *Psychology Today*, May 1977, pp. 41–47. (a)

Bronfenbrenner, U. Is early intervention effective? In S. Cohen & T. J. Comiskey (Eds.), *Child development: Contemporary perspectives*. Itasca, Ill.: F. E. Peacock, 1977. (b)

Bronfenbrenner, U. Contexts of child rearing: Problems and prospects. *American Psychologist,* 1979, *34*, 844–850.

Bronfenbrenner, U., Belsky, J., & Steinberg, L. Daycare in context: An ecological perspective on research and public policy. In *Policy issues in daycare*. Washington, D.C.: U.S. Department of Health & Human Services, 1977.

Bronson, G. W. Identity diffusion in late adolescence. *Journal of Abnormal and Social Psychology*, 1959, *59*, 414–417.

Bronson, G. W. Fear of the unfamiliar in human infants. In H. R. Schaffer (Ed.), *The origins of human social relations*. London: Academic Press, 1971.

Bronson, G. W. Infants' reactions to unfamiliar persons and novel objects. *Monographs of the Society for Research in Child Development*, 1972, *37*(3).

Brown, J., & Finn, P. Drinking to get drunk: Findings of a survey of junior and senior high school students. *Journal of Alcohol and Drug Education*, 1982, *27*, 13–25.

Brown, J. L. States in newborn infants. *Merrill-Palmer Quarterly*, 1964, *10*, 313–327.

Brown, R. *A first language: The early stages*. Cambridge, Mass.: Harvard University Press, 1973.

Bruch, H. *Eating disorders*. New York: Basic Books, 1973.

Bruininks, R. H. *Manual for the Bruininks-Oseretsky Test of Motor Proficiency*. Circle Pines, Minn.: American Guidance Service, 1977.

Bruininks, R. H., & Warfield, G. The mentally retarded. In E. L. Meyen (Ed.), *Exceptional children and youth: An introduction*. Denver, Colo.: Love Publishing, 1978.

Bruner, J. S. Early social interaction and language acquisition. In H. R. Schaffer (Ed.), *Studies in mother-infant interaction*. London: Academic Press, 1977.

Bruner, J. S. Learning the mother tongue. *Human Nature*, September 1978, pp. 43–49.

Bruner, J. S., & Kenney, H. J. On multiple ordering. In J. S. Bruner, R. R. Olver, & P. N. Greenfield (Eds.), *Studies in cognitive growth*. New York: John Wiley, 1966.

Bruner, J. S., Olver, R. R., & Greenfield, P. N. *Studies in cognitive growth*. New York: John Wiley, 1966.

Buber, M. *I and thou*. New York: Charles Scribner's, 1958.

Buber, M. *The knowledge of man* (M. Friedman, Ed.). New York: Harper & Row, 1965.

Budoff, M., & Gottlieb, J. Special-class EMR children mainstreamed: A study of an aptitude (learning potential) × treatment interaction. *American Journal of Mental Deficiency*, 1976, *81*, 1–11.

Buehler, R. E., Patterson, G. R., & Furniss, J. The reinforcement of behavior in institutional settings. *Behavior Research and Therapy*, 1966, *4*, 157–167.

Buhler, C. *The first year of life* (Greenberg & Ripin, trans.). New York: Day, 1930.

Buhler, C. Old age and fulfillment of life with considerations of the use of time in old age. *Acta Psychologica*, 1961, *19*, 126–148.

Burt, C. The genetic determination of differences in intelligence: A study of monozygotic twins reared together and apart. *British Journal of Psychology*, 1966, *57*, 137–153.

Butler, R. N. Age-ism: Another form of bigotry. *Gerontologist*, 1969, *9*, 243.

Butler, R. N., & Lewis, M. I. *Aging and mental health* (2nd ed.). St. Louis: C. V. Mosby, 1977.

Campbell, A. Subjective measures of well-being. *American Psychologist*, 1976, *31*, 117–124.

Campbell, A. *The sense of well-being in America: Recent patterns and trends*. New York: McGraw-Hill, 1981.

Campbell, A., Converse, P. E., & Rodgers, W. L. *The quality of American life: Perceptions, evaluations, and satisfactions*. New York: Russell Sage Foundation, 1976.

Campbell, D. T., & Stanley, J. C. *Experimental and quasi-experimental designs for research*. Chicago: Rand McNally, 1963.

Campbell, J. D., & Yarrow, M. R. Personal and situational variables in adaptation to change. *Journal of Social Issues*, 1958, *14*, 29–46.

Campos, J. J., Langer, A., & Krowitz, A. Cardiac response on the visual cliff in prelocomotor human infants. *Science*, 1970, *170*, 196–197.

Cannabis (Marijuana and Hashish). Edmonton: Alberta Alcoholism & Drug Abuse Commission, Public Information Series, 1976.

Cantor, P. Suicide and attempted suicide among students: Problems, prediction and prevention. In P. Cantor (Ed.), *Understanding a child's world*. New York: McGraw-Hill, 1977.

Caputo, D. V., & Mandell, W. Consequences of low birth weight. *Developmental Psychology*, 1970, *3*, 363–383.

Carlson, P., & Anisfeld, M. Some observations on the linguistic competence of a two year old child. *Child Development*, 1969, *40*, 572–574.

Carmichael, L. Onset and early development of behavior. In P. H. Mussen (Ed.), *Carmichael's manual of child psychology* (Vol. 1) (3rd ed.). New York: John Wiley, 1970.

Cartwright, D. S., Tomson, B., & Schwartz, H. *Gang delinquency*. Monterey, Calif.: Brooks/Cole, 1975.

Casler, L. Maternal deprivation: A critical review of the literature. *Monograph of the Society for Research in Child Development*, 1961, *26*(2).

Cattell, R. B. *Abilities: Their structure, growth, and action*. Boston: Houghton Mifflin, 1971.

Cattell, R. B. Travels in psychological hyperspace. In T. S. Krawiec (Ed.), *The Psychologists* (Vol. 2). New York: Oxford University Press, 1974.

Cerella, J., Poon, L. W., & Fozard, J. C. Age and the iconic read-out. *Journal of Gerontology*, 1982, *37*, 197–202.

Chambliss, W. J. The state, the law, and the definition of behavior as criminal or delinquent. In D. Glaser (Ed.), *Handbook of criminology*. Chicago: Rand McNally, 1974.

China fears sexual imbalance. *Edmonton Journal*, March 14, 1983, p. D-4.

Chomsky, N. *Syntactic structures*. The Hague: Mouton, 1957.

Chomsky, N. *Aspects of the theory of syntax*. Cambridge, Mass.: M.I.T. Press, 1965.

Chomsky, N. *Language and mind* (Enl. ed.). New York: Harcourt Brace Jovanovich, 1972.

Churchill, J. A. The relationship between intelligence and birth weight in twins. *Neurology*, 1965, *15*, 341–347.

Clark, H. H., & Clark, E. V. *Psychology and language: An introduction to psycholinguistics*. New York: Harcourt Brace Jovanovich, 1977.

Clark, R. W. *Freud: The man and the cause*. New York: Random House, 1980.

Clarke, A. M., & Clarke, A. D. B. (Eds.). *Early experience: Myth and evidence*. London: Open Books, 1976.

Clarke-Stewart, K. A. The father's contribution to children's cognitive and social development in early childhood. In F. A. Pedersen (Ed.), *The father-infant relationship: Observational studies in the family setting*. New York: Praeger, 1980.

Clausen, J. A. The social meaning of differential physical and sexual maturation. In S. E. Ragastin & G. H. Elder (Eds.), *Adolescence in the life cycle: Psychological change and social context*. New York: John Wiley, 1975.

Clausen, J. A. Men's occupational careers in the middle years. In D. H. Eichorn, J. A. Clausen, N. Haan, M. P. Honzik, & P. H. Mussen (Eds.), *Present and past in middle life*. New York: Academic Press, 1981.

Clayton, V. P., & Birren, J. E. The development of wisdom across the life span: A reexamination of an ancient topic. In P. B. Baltes & O. G. Brim, Jr. (Eds.), *Life-span development and behavior* (Vol. 3). New York: Academic Press, 1980.

Clement, F. J. Longitudinal and cross-sectional assessments of age changes in physical strength as related to sex, social class, and mental ability. *Journal of Gerontology*, 1974, *29*, 423–429.

Clemente, F., & Sauer, W. J. Life satisfaction in the United States. *Social Forces*, 1976, *54*, 621–631.

Clements, S. D. *Minimal brain dysfunction in children: Terminology and identification* (NINDB Monograph No. 3). Washington, D.C.: U.S. Department of Health & Human Services, 1966.

Cobb, E. *The ecology of imagination in childhood*. New York: Columbia University Press, 1977.

Cohen, D. K. Does IQ matter? *Current*, 1972, *141*, 19–30.

Cohen, L. B. Our developing knowledge of infant perception and cognition. *American Psychologist*, 1979, *34*, 894–899.

Cohen, L. B., DeLoache, J. S., & Strauss, M. S. Infant visual perception. In J. D. Osofsky (Ed.), *Handbook of infant development*. New York: John Wiley, 1979.

Cohen, S. *The drug dilemma*. New York: McGraw-Hill, 1976.

Cohn, F. *Understanding human sexuality*. Englewood Cliffs, N.J.: Prentice-Hall, 1974.

Cole, L., & Hall, I. N. *Psychology of adolescence* (7th ed.). New York: Holt, Rinehart & Winston, 1970.

Coleman, J. C., Butcher, J. N., & Carson, R. C. *Abnormal psychology and modern life* (6th ed.). Glenview, Ill.: Scott Foresman, 1980.

Coleman, J. S. The adolescent sub-culture and academic achievement. *American Journal of Sociology*, 1960, *65*, 337–347.

Coleman, J. S. *The adolescent society*. New York: Free Press, 1961.

Coleman, J. S. *Youth: Transition to adulthood*. Chicago: University of Chicago Press, 1974.

Collins, W. A., & Getz, S. K. Children's social responses following modeled reactions to provocation: Prosocial effects of a television drama. *Journal of Personality*, 1976, *44*, 488–500.

Comstock, G. The impact of television on American institutions. *Journal of Communication*, 1978, *28*, 12–28.

Comstock, G., Chaffee, S., Katzman, N., McCombs, M., & Roberts, D. *Television and human behavior*. New York: Columbia University Press, 1978.

Comstock, G., & Lindsey, G. *Television and human behavior: The research horizon, future and present*. Santa Monica, Calif.: Rand Corporation, 1975.

Contat, M. *The writings of Jean-Paul Sartre*. Evanston, Ill.: Northwestern University Press, 1974.

Cook, H., & Stingle, S. Cooperative behavior in children. *Psychological Bulletin*, 1974, *81*, 918–933.

Coopersmith, S. *The antecedents of self-esteem*. New York: W. H. Freeman, 1967.

Corcoran, M. The economic consequences of marital dissolution for women in the middle years. *Sex Roles*, 1979, *5*, 343–353.

Corse, C. D., Manuck, S. B., Cantwell, J. D., Giordani, B., & Matthews, K. A. Coronary-prone behavior pattern and cardiovascular response in persons with and without coronary heart disease. *Psychosomatic Medicine*, 1982, *44*, 449–459.

Corso, J. F. Sensory processes and age effects in normal adults. *Journal of Gerontology*, 1971, *26*, 90–105.

Cottle, T. J. *Barred from school: Two million children*. Washington, D.C.: New Republic Book Co., 1976.

Cowan, E., & Pratt, B. The hurdle jump as a developmental and diagnostic test. *Child Development*, 1934, *5*, 107–121.

Crackdown on wife beaters. *Sherwood Park News*, March 9, 1983, p. A-3.

Cramer, P., & Hogan, K. A. Sex differences in verbal and play fantasy. *Developmental Psychology*, 1975, *11*, 145–154.

Cratty, B. J. *Perceptual and motor development in infants and children*. New York: Macmillan, 1970.

Crick, F. H. The genetic code. *Scientific American*, 1962, *207*, 66–74.

Crick, F. H. On the genetic code. *Science*, 1963, *139*, 461–464.

Crisp, A. H., Hsu, L. K. G., Harding, B., & Hartshorn, J. Clinical features of anorexia nervosa. *Journal of Psychosomatic Research*, 1980, *24*, 179–191.

Crossland, F. E. *Minority access to college: A Ford Foundation report*. New York: Schocken Books, 1971.

Crow, J. F. Genetic theories and influences: Comments on the value of diversity. *Harvard Educational Review* (Reprint Series No. 2), 1969, 153–161.

Crowder, R. G. Echoic memory and the study of aging memory systems. In L. W. Poon, J. L. Fozard, L. S. Cermak, D. Arenberg, & L. W. Thompson (Eds.), *New directions in memory and aging*. Hillsdale, N.J.: Lawrence Erlbaum, 1980.

Crowley, J. E., Levitin, T. E., & Quinn, R. P. Seven deadly half-truths about women. *Psychology Today*, September 1973, *6*, 94–96.

Cruickshank, W. M. (Ed.). *Cerebral palsy: A developmental disability* (3rd rev. ed.). Syracuse, N.Y.: Syracuse University Press, 1976.

Cruickshank, W. M., Morse, W. C., & Johns, J. S. *Learning disabilities: The struggle from adolescence toward adulthood*. Syracuse, N.Y: Syracuse University Press, 1980.

Cuber, J. F., & Harroff, P. B. *The significant Americans*. New York: Appleton-Century-Crofts, 1965.

Cumming, E., & Henry, W. H. *Growing old*. New York: Basic Books, 1961.

Dalby, J. T. Environmental effects on prenatal development. *Journal of Pediatric Psychology*, 1978, *3*, 105–110.

Darley, J. M., & Latané, B. Bystander intervention in emergencies: Diffusion of responsibility. *Journal of Personality and Social Psychology*, 1968, *8*, 377–383.

Darwin, C. A biographical sketch of an infant. *Mind*, 1877, *2*, 285–294.

Dasen, P. R. (Ed.). *Piagetian psychology: Cross-cultural contributions*. New York: Gardner Press, 1977.

Davidson, D. M. Anorexia nervosa in a serviceman: A case report. *Military Medicine*, 1976, *141*, 617–619.

Davies, J. M., Latto, I. P., Jones, J. G., Veale, A., & Wardrop, C. A. Effects of stopping smoking for 48 hours on oxygen availability from the blood: A study of pregnant women. *British Medical Journal*, 1979, *2*, 355–356.

Davis, E. A. *The development of linguistic skills in twins, single twins with siblings, and only children from age 5 to 10 years*. Institute of Child Welfare Series, No. 14. Minneapolis: University of Minnesota Press, 1937.

Davitz, J., & Davitz, L. *Making it from forty to fifty*. New York: Random House, 1976.

Deaux, K. *The behavior of women and men*. Monterey, Calif.: Brooks/Cole, 1976.

de Bono, E. *Lateral thinking: A textbook of creativity*. London: Ward Lock Educational, 1970.

de Bono, E. *Teaching thinking*. London: Temple Smith, 1976.

DeFries, J. C. Mental abilities: A family study. In J. H. Mielke & M. H. Crawford (Eds.), *Current developments in anthropological genetics* (Vol. 1.). New York: Plenum, 1980.

DeFries, J. C., & Plomin, R. Behavioral genetics. In M. R. Rosenzweig and L. W. Porter (Eds.). *Annual review of* *psychology* (Vol. 29). Palo Alto, Calif.: Annual Reviews, 1978.

DeMause, L. Our forebears made childhood a nightmare. *Psychology Today*, April 1975, pp. 85–88.

DeMyer, M. K., Barton, S., DeMyer, W. E., Norton, J., Allen, J., & Steele, R. Prognosis in autism: A follow-up study. *Journal of Autism and Childhood Schizophrenia*, 1973, *3*, 199–246.

Denfeld, D., & Gordon, M. The sociology of mate swapping: Or the family that swings together clings together. *Journal of Sex Research*, 1970, *6*, 85–100.

Denhoff, E. Medical aspects. In W. M. Cruickshank (Ed.), *Cerebral palsy: A developmental disability* (3rd rev. ed.). Syracuse, N.Y.: Syracuse University Press, 1976.

Denney, N. W. Problem solving in later adulthood: Intervention research. In P. B. Baltes & O. G. Brim, Jr. (Eds.), *Life-span development and behavior* (Vol. 2). New York: Academic Press, 1979.

Dennis, W. A description and classification of the response of the newborn infant. *Psychological Bulletin*, 1934, *31*, 5–22.

Dennis, W. Infant development under conditions of restricted practice and of minimum social stimulation. *Genetic Psychology Monographs*, 1941, *23*, 143–191. (a)

Dennis, W. The significance of feral man. *American Journal of Psychology*, 1941, *54*, 425–432. (b)

Dennis, W. Historical beginnings of child psychology. *Psychological Bulletin*, 1949, *46*, 224–235.

Dennis, W. A further analysis of reports of wild children. *Child Development*, 1951, *22*, 153–158.

Dennis, W. Causes of retardation among institutional children: Iran. *Journal of Genetic Psychology*, 1960, *96*, 47–59.

Dennis, W. *Children of the creche.* New York: Appleton-Century-Crofts, 1973.

de Villiers, J. G., & de Villiers, P. A. *Language acquisition.* Cambridge, Mass.: Harvard University Press, 1978.

Dick Read, G. *Childbirth without fear: The original approach to natural childbirth* (4th ed.) (H. Wessel & H. F. Ellis, Eds.). New York: Harper, & Row, 1972.

Diener, C. I., & Dweck, C. S. An analysis of learned helplessness: II. The processing of success. *Journal of Personality and Social Psychology*, 1980, *39*, 940–952.

Dingle, J. *The ills of man: Life and death and medicine.* New York: W. H. Freeman, 1973.

Dobbing, J. The early development of the brain and its vulnerability. In T. A. Davis and J. Dobbin (Eds.), *Scientific foundations of paediatrics.* Philadelphia: Saunders, 1974, 565–577.

Dollard, J., Doob, L. W., Miller, N. E., Mowrer, O. H., & Sears, R. *Frustration and aggression.* New Haven, Conn.: Yale University Press, 1939.

Donaldson, M. *Children's minds.* London: Fontana/Croom Helm, 1978.

Donovan, C. M. Program planning for the visually impaired child. In A. P. Scheiner, & I. F. Abroms (Eds.), *The practical management of the developmentally disabled child.* St. Louis: C. V. Mosby, 1980.

Douglas, J. W. B., & Ross, J. N. Age of puberty related to educational ability, attainment, and school leaving age. *Journal of Child Psychology and Psychiatry*, 1964, *5*, 185–196.

Down with Type A! *Health*, January 1983, pp. 14–15.

Drugs and the human fetus (Pt. I). *PharmChem Newsletter*, 1978, 7 (Whole No. 5).

Duffty, P., & Bryan, M. H. Home apnea monitoring in 'near-miss' Sudden Infant Death Syndrome (SIDS) and in siblings of SIDS victims. *Pediatrics*, 1982, *70*, 69–74.

Dunn, L. M. Special education for the mildly retarded—Is much of it justifiable? *Exceptional Children*, 1968, *35*, 5–22.

Dunphy, D. C. The social structure of urban adolescent peer groups. *Sociometry*, 1963, *26*, 230–246.

Duvall, E. M. *Marriage and family development* (5th ed.). New York: Harper & Row, 1977.

Dweck, C. S. The role of expectations and attributions in the alleviation of learned helplessness. *Journal of Personality and Social Psychology*, 1975, *31*, 674–685.

Eagly, A. H. Sex differences in influenceability. *Psychological Bulletin*, 1978, *85*, 86–116.

Ebin, D. (Ed.). *The drug experience: First person accounts of addicts, writers, scientists and others.* New York: Orion Press, 1961.

Eckerman, C. O., & Rheingold, H. Infants' exploratory responses to toys and people. *Developmental Psychology*, 1974, *10*, 255–259.

Eckerman, C. O., & Whatley, J. L. Infants' reactions to unfamiliar adults varying in novelty. *Developmental Psychology*, 1975, *11*, 562–566.

Edmonton (Alberta) Public School Board. *Learning Disability*, Fall 1978, No. 7.

Egeland, B., & Vaughn, B. Failure of "bond formation" as a cause of abuse, neglect, and maltreatment. *American Journal of Orthopsychiatry*, 1981, *51*, 78–84.

Ehrman, L., & Parsons, P. A. *Behavior genetics and evolution.* New York: McGraw-Hill, 1981.

Eibl-Eibesfeldt, I. *Love and hate: The natural history of behavior patterns.* New York: Schocken Books, 1974.

Eichorn, D. H., Clausen, J. A., Haan, N., Honzik, M. P., & Mussen, P. H. (Eds.). *Present and past in middle life.* New York: Academic Press, 1981.

Eisenberg, R. B. *Auditory competence in early life.* Baltimore: University Park, 1976.

Eisenberg, R. B., Griffin, E. J., Coursin, D. B., & Hunter, M. A. Auditory behavior in the neonate. *Journal of Speech and Hearing Research*, 1964, 7, 245–269.

Eisenberg-Berg, N. Development of children's prosocial moral judgment. *Developmental Psychology*, 1979, *15*, 38–44.

Eisenman, R. Birth order and sex differences in aesthetic preference of complexity-simplicity. *Journal of General Psychology*, 1967, 77, 121–126.

Eisenstein, Z. R. The sexual politics of the new right: Understanding the "crisis of liberalism" for the 1980's. *Signs*, 1982, *7*, 567–588.

Elkind, D. Egocentrism in adolescence. *Child Development*, 1967, *38*, 1025–1034.

Elkind, D. Understanding the young adolescent. In L. D. Steinberg (Ed.), *The life cycle: Readings in human development*. New York: Columbia University Press, 1981.

Elkind, D., & Bowen, R. Imaginary audience behavior in children and adolescents. *Developmental Psychology*, 1979, *15*(1), 38–44.

Elliot, R., & Vasta, R. The modeling of sharing: Effects associated with vicarious reinforcement, symbolization, age and generalization. *Journal of Experimental Child Psychology*, 1970, *10*, 8–15.

Endsley, R. C., & Bradbard, M. R. *Quality day care: A handbook of choices for parents and caregivers*. Englewood Cliffs, N.J.: Prentice-Hall, 1981.

Engels, F. *The origin of the family, private property and the state*. Chicago: Kerr, 1902.

Engen, T., Lipsitt, I., & Peck, M. B. Ability of newborn infants to discriminate sapid substances. *Developmental Psychology*, 1974, *10*, 741–744.

England, P. Women and occupational prestige: A case of vacuous sex equality. *Signs*, 1979, *5*, 252–265.

Erikson, E. H. The problems of ego identity. *Journal of the American Psychoanalytic Association*, 1956, *4*, 56–121.

Erikson, E. H. Identity and the life cycle: Selected papers. *Psychological Issues Monograph Series, I* (No. I). New York: International Universities Press, 1959.

Erikson, E. H. The roots of virtue. In J. Huxley (Ed.), *The humanist frame*. New York: Harper & Row, 1961.

Erikson, E. H. *Identity, youth and crisis*. New York: W. W. Norton, 1968.

Erlenmeyer-Kimling, L., & Jarvik, L. F. Genetics and intelligence: A review. *Science*, 1963, *142*, 1477–1478.

Eshleman, J. R. *The family: An introduction* (3rd ed.). Boston: Allyn & Bacon, 1981.

Ethical standards for research with children. *SRCD Newsletter*, Winter 1973, pp. 3–4.

Eyesenck, H. J. *The biological basis of personality*. Springfield, Ill.: Charles C. Thomas, 1967.

Fagan, J. F., III. Infant color perception. *Science*, 1974, *183*, 973–975.

Falek, A. Ethical issues in human behavior genetics: Civil rights, informed consent, and ethics of intervention. In K. W. Schaie, V. F. Anderson, G. E. McClearn, & J. Money (Eds.), *Developmental human behavior genetics*. Lexington, Mass.: D. C. Heath, 1975.

Fantz, R. L. The origin of form-perception. *Scientific American*, 1961, *204*, 66–72.

Fantz, R. L. Pattern vision in newborn infants. *Science*, 1963, *140*, 296–297.

Fantz, R. L. Visual experience in infants: Decreased attention to familiar patterns relative to novel ones. *Science*, 1964, *146*, 668–670.

Fantz, R. L. Visual perception from birth as shown by pattern selectivity. *Annals of the New York Academy of Science*, 1965, *118*, 793–814.

Faris, R. E. Sociological causes of genius. *American Sociological Review*, 1940, *5*, 689–699.

Farleger, D. The battle over children's rights. *Psychology Today*, July 1977, pp. 89–91.

Faust, M. S. Developmental maturity as a determinant in prestige of adolescent girls. *Child Development*, 1960, *31*, 173–184.

Fein, G., Johnson, D., Kosson, N., Stork, L., & Wasserman, L. Sex stereotypes and preferences in the toy choices of 20-month-old boys and girls. *Developmental Psychology*, 1975, *11*, 527–528.

Feingold, B. F. Hyperkinesis and learning disabilities linked to artificial food flavors and colors. *American Journal of Nursing*, 1975, *75*, 797–803. (a)

Feingold, B. F. *Why your child is hyperactive*. New York: Random House, 1975. (b)

Felsenthal, N. *Orientations to mass communication*. Chicago: Science Research Associates, 1976.

Field, T., & Greenberg, R. Temperament ratings by parents and teachers of infants, toddlers, and preschool children. *Child Development*, 1982, *53*, 160–163.

Fischer, D. *Growing old in America*. New York: Oxford University Press, 1977.

Fishbein, H. D. *Evolution, development, and children's learning*. Pacific Palisades, Calif.: Goodyear, 1976.

Fisher, S., & Greenberg, R. P. *The scientific credibility of Freud's theories and therapy*. New York: Basic Books, 1977.

Fisher, W. A., & Byrne, D. Sex differences in response to erotica? Love versus lust. *Journal of Personality and Social Psychology*, 1978, *36*, 117–126.

Fishkin, J., Keniston, K., & MacKinnon, C. Moral reasoning and political ideology. *Journal of Personality and Social Psychology*, 1973, *27*, 109–119.

Flanagan, J. C. A research approach to improving our quality of life. *American Psychologist*, 1978, *33*, 138–147.

Flavell, J. H. *The developmental psychology of Jean Piaget*. New York: Van Nostrand, 1963.

Fodor, F. N. Delinquency and susceptibility to social influence among adolescents as a function of level of moral development. *Journal of Social Psychology*, 1972, *86*, 257–260.

Fouts, R. S. Acquisition and testing of gestural signs in four young chimpanzees. *Science*, 1973, *180*, 978–980.

Fox, S. M., & Haskell, W. L. Physical activity and the prevention of coronary heart disease. *New York Academy Medical Bulletin*, 1978, *44*, 950–965.

Fraiberg, S. *The magic years*. New York: Charles Scribner's, 1968.

Fraiberg, S. Blind infants and their mothers: An examination of the sign system. In M. Lewis & L. A. Rosenblum (Eds.), *The effect of the infant on its caregiver*. New York: John Wiley, 1974.

Fraiberg, S. The development of human attachments in infants blind from birth. *Merrill-Palmer Quarterly*, 1975, *21*, 315–334.

Frazier, A., & Lisonbee, L. K. Adolescent concerns with physique. *School Review*, 1950, *58*, 397–405.

Freedman, J. *Happy people.* New York: Harcourt, Brace Jovanovich, 1978.

Freeman, D. *Margaret Mead and Samoa.* Cambridge, Mass.: Harvard University Press, 1983.

Freud, A. *The ego and the mechanisms of defense* (C. Baines, trans.). New York: International Universities Press, 1946.

Freyberg, J. T. Increasing the imaginative play of urban disadvantaged kindergarten children through systematic training. In J. L. Singer (Ed.), *The child's world of make-believe.* New York: Academic Press, 1973.

Friedan, B. *The second stage.* New York: Simon & Schuster, 1983.

Friedman, A. S. The family and the female delinquent: An overview. In O. Pollak & A. S. Friedman (Eds.), *Family dynamics and female sexual delinquency.* Palo Alto, Calif.: Science and Behavior Books, 1969.

Frisch, R. E., & Revelle, R. Height and weight at menarche and a hypothesis of critical body weights and adolescent events. *Science*, 1970, *169*, 397–398.

Furry, C. A., & Baltes, P. B. The effect of age differences in ability-extraneous performance variables on the assessment of intelligence in children, adults, and the elderly. *Journal of Gerontology*, 1973, *28*, 73–80.

Furth, H. G. *Deafness and learning: A psychosocial approach.* Belmont, Calif.: Wadsworth, 1973.

Furth, H. G. Piagetian perspectives. In J. Sants (Ed.), *Developmental psychology and society.* London: Macmillan, 1980.

Gale, R. F. *Developmental behavior: A humanistic approach.* New York: Macmillan, 1969.

Gallagher, J. J. *Analysis of research on the education of gifted children.* Springfield, Ill.: Office of the Superintendent of Public Instruction, 1960.

Galton, F. *Hereditary genius: An enquiry into its laws and consequences.* London: Macmillan, 1896.

Garbarino, J., & Crouter, A. The human ecology of child maltreatment: A conceptual model for research. *Journal of Marriage and the Family*, 1977, *39*, 721–735.

Gardner, H. The making of a storyteller. *Psychology Today*, March 1982, pp. 48–53; 61–63.

Gardner, R. A., & Gardner, B. T. Teaching sign language to a chimpanzee. *Science*, 1969, *165*, 664–672.

Garmezy, N. Vulnerable and invulnerable children: Theory, research, and intervention. Master lecture on developmental psychology, American Psychological Association, 1976.

Garretson, M. D. Total communication. *Volta Review*, 1976, *78*, 88–95.

Gayford, J. J. Battered wives. In J. P. Martin (Ed.), *Violence and the family.* New York: John Wiley, 1978.

Gebhard, P. Incidence of overt homosexuality in the United States and Western Europe. In J. M. Livingwood (Ed.), *National Institute of Mental Health Task Force on Homosexuality: Final report and background papers.* Rockville, Md.: National Institute of Mental Health, 1972.

Gelles, R. J. *The violent home: A study of physical aggression between husbands and wives.* Beverly Hills, Calif.: Sage, 1972.

Gelles, R. J. Violence in the American family. In J. P. Martin (Ed.), *Violence and the family.* New York: John Wiley, 1978. (a)

Gelles, R. J. Violence toward children in the United States. *American Journal of Orthopsychiatry*, 1978, *48*, 580–592. (b)

Gelles, R. J. *Family violence.* Beverly Hills, Calif.: Sage, 1979.

Gelles, R. J., & Straus, M. A. Violence in the American family. *Journal of Social Issues*, 1979, *35*, 15–38.

Gelman, E. J. Conservation acquisition: A problem of learning to attend to relevant attributes. *Journal of Experimental Child Psychology*, 1969, *7*, 167–187.

Gelman, R. Cognitive development. In M. R. Rosenzweig & L. W. Porter (Eds.), *Annual review of psychology* (Vol. 29). Palo Alto, Calif.: Annual Reviews, 1978.

Gelman, R., & Gallistel, C. R. *The young child's understanding of number.* Cambridge, Mass.: Harvard University Press, 1978.

Gerber, M. The psycho-motor development of African children in the first year and the influence of maternal behavior. *Journal of Social Psychology*, 1958, *47*, 185–195.

Gerbner, G. Violence in television drama: Trends and symbolic functions. In G. A. Comstock & E. A. Rubenstein (Eds.), *Television and social behavior* (Vol. 1). Washington, D.C.: U.S. Government Printing Office, 1972.

Gesell, A. *The mental growth of the pre-school child.* New York: Macmillan, 1925.

Gesell, A. *Infancy and human growth.* New York: Macmillan, 1937.

Gesell, A. *Wolf-child and human child.* New York: Harper & Row, 1940.

Gesell, A., & Amatruda, C. S. *Developmental diagnosis: Normal and abnormal child development.* New York: Hoeber, 1941.

Getzels, J. W. On the transformation of values: A decade after Port Huron. *School Review*, 1972, *80*, 505–519.

Getzels, J. W., & Jackson, P. W. *Creativity and intelligence.* New York: John Wiley, 1962.

Gewirtz, J. L. The course of infant smiling in four child-rearing environments in Israel. In B. M. Foss (Ed.), *Determinants of infant behavior III.* London: Methuen, 1965.

Gewirtz, J. L., & Boyd, E. F. Mother-infant interaction and its study. In H. W. Reese (Ed.), *Advances in child development and behavior*, 1976, *11*, 142–160.

Gibson, E. J., & Walk, R. D. The "visual cliff." *Scientific American*, 1960, *202*, 64–71.

Gil, D. G. *Violence against children: Physical child abuse in the United States.* Cambridge, Mass.: Harvard University Press, 1970.

Ginsberg, H., & Opper, S. *Piaget's theory of intellectual development* (2nd ed.). Englewood Cliffs, N.J.: Prentice-Hall, 1978.

Ginzberg, E. Toward a theory of occupational choice: A restatement. *Vocational Guidance Quarterly,* 1972, *20,* 169–176.

Ginzberg, E., et al. *Occupational choice.* New York: Columbia University Press, 1951.

Glick, P. G., & Norton, A. J. Marrying, divorcing and living together in the U.S. today. *Population Bulletin,* 1978, *32,* 328–399.

Goddard, H. H. *Feeble-mindedness: Its causes and consequences.* New York: Macmillan, 1914.

Goldfarb, W. Childhood psychosis. In P. H. Mussen (Ed.), *Carmichael's manual of child psychology* (Vol. 2). New York: John Wiley, 1970.

Golding, W. *Lord of the flies.* New York: Coward, McCann & Geoghegan, 1962.

Goode, E. (Ed.). *Marijuana.* New York: Atherton Press, 1969.

Goodwin, R. Two decades of research into early language. In J. Sants (Ed.), *Developmental psychology and society.* London: Macmillan, 1980.

Gorn, G. J., Goldberg, M. E., & Kanungo, R. N. The role of educational television in changing the intergroup attitudes of children. *Child Development,* 1976, *47,* 277–280.

Gottesman, I. I. Schizophrenia and genetics: Toward understanding uncertainty. *Psychiatric Annuals,* 1979, *9,* 54–78.

Gottesman, I. I., & Shields, J. *The schizophrenic puzzle.* New York: Cambridge University Press, 1982.

Gottman, J. M. Toward a definition of social isolation in children. *Child Development,* 1977, *48,* 513–517.

Gould, R. L. The phases of adult life: A study in developmental psychology. *American Journal of Psychiatry,* 1972, *129,* 521–531.

Gould, R. L. *Transformations: Growth and change in adult life.* New York: Simon & Schuster, 1978.

Gould, S. J. *The mismeasure of man.* New York: W. W. Norton, 1981.

Graham, F. K., Ernhart, C. B., Thurston, D. L., & Craft, M. Development three years after perinatal anoxia and other potentially damaging experiences. *Psychological Monographs,* 1962, *76* (No. 522).

Grambs, J. D., & Waetjen, W. B. *Sex: Does it make a difference?* North Scituate, Mass.: Duxbury Press, 1975.

Greenacre, P. Play in relation to creative imagination. *Psychoanalytic Studies of the Child,* 1959, *14,* 61–80.

Greene, J. *Thinking and language.* London: Methuen, 1975.

Gronlund, N. E., & Holmlund, W. S. The value of elementary school sociometric status scores for predicting a pupil's adjustment in high school. *Educational Administration and Supervision,* 1958, *44,* 255–260.

Grossman, J. J. (Ed.). *Manual on terminology and classification in mental retardation, 1973 revision.* Washington, D.C.: American Association on Mental Deficiency, 1973.

Grotevant, M. D., Scarr, S., & Weinberg, R. A. *Intellectual development in family constellations with adopted and natural children: A test of the Zajonc and Markus model.* Paper presented at a meeting of the Society for Research in Child Development, New Orleans, 1977.

Gruman, G. J. Cultural origins of present-day age-ism: The modernization of the life cycle. In S. F. Spicker, K. M. Woodward, & D. D. Van Tassel (Eds.), *Aging and the elderly: Humanistic perspectives in gerontology.* Atlantic Highlands, N. J.: Humanities Press, 1978.

Guilford, J. P. Creativity. *American Psychologist,* 1950, *5,* 444–454.

Guilford, J. P. Three faces of intellect. *American Psychologist,* 1959, *14,* 469–479.

Gurland, B., Bennett, R., & Wilder, D. Reevaluating the place of evaluation in planning for alternatives to institutional care for the elderly. *Journal of Social Issues,* 1981, *37,* 51–70.

Gurney, R. *Language, brain and interactive processes.* London: Edward Arnold, 1973.

Gutmann, D. The cross-cultural perspective. In J. E. Birren & K. W. Schaie (Eds.), *Handbook of the psychology of aging.* New York: Van Nostrand, 1977.

Haan, N., Smith, N. B., & Block, J. Moral reasoning of young adults: Political-social behavior, family background, and personality correlates. *Journal of Personality and Social Psychology,* 1968, *10,* 183–201.

Haith, M. M., & Campos, J. J. Human infancy. In M. R. Rosenzweig & L. W. Porter (Eds.), *Annual review of psychology* (Vol. 28). Palo Alto, Calif.: Annual Reviews, 1977.

Hall, G. S. The contents of children's minds on entering school. *Paediatric Seminars,* 1891, *1,* 139–173.

Hall, G. S. *Senescence: The last half of life.* New York: Appleton-Century-Crofts, 1922.

Hallahan, D. P., & Heins, E. D. Issues in learning disabilities. In J. M. Kauffman & D. P. Hallahan (Eds.), *Teaching children with learning disabilities: Personal perspectives.* Columbus, Ohio: Charles E. Merrill, 1976.

Hallahan, D. P., & Kauffman, J. M. *Introduction to learning disabilities: A psychobehavioral approach.* Englewood Cliffs, N.J.: Prentice-Hall, 1976.

Hallahan, D. P., & Kauffman, J. M. *Exceptional children: Introduction to special education.* Englewood Cliffs, N.J.: Prentice-Hall, 1978.

Halonen, J. S., & Passman, R. H. Pacifiers' effects upon play and separations from the mother for the one-year-old in a novel environment. *Infant Behavior and Development,* 1978, *1,* 70–78.

Halverson, H. M. An experimental study of prehension in

infants by means of systematic cinema records. *Genetic Psychology Monographs*, 1931, *10*, 107–286.

Hanson, J. W., Streissguth, A. P., & Smith, D. W. The effects of moderate alcohol consumption during pregnancy on fetal growth and morphogenesia. *Journal of Pediatrics*, 1978, *92*, 457–460.

Harger, R. N. The sojourn of alcohol in the body. In R. G. McCarthy (Ed.), *Alcohol education for classroom and community*. New York: McGraw-Hill, 1964.

Harlow, H. F. The nature of love. *American Psychologist*, 1958, *12*, 673–685.

Harlow, H. F. Love in infant monkeys. *Scientific American*, 1959, *200*, 68–74.

Harlow, H. F., Harlow, M. K., & Suomi, S. J. From thought to therapy: Lessons from a primate laboratory. *American Scientist*, 1971, *59*, 538–549.

Harlow, H. F., McGaugh, J. L., & Thompson, R. F. *Psychology*. San Francisco: Albion, 1971.

Harlow, H. F., & Zimmerman, R. R. Affectional responses in the infant monkey. *Science*, 1959, *130*, 421–432.

Harper, L. V. The young as a source of stimuli controlling caretaker behavior. *Developmental Psychology*, 1971, *4*, 73–88.

Harrell, R. F., Woodyard, E., & Gates, A. *The effect of mothers' diets on the intelligence of the offspring*. New York: Bureau of Publications, Teachers College, 1955.

Hartshorne, H., & May, M. A. *Studies in the nature of character* (3 vols.). New York: Macmillan, 1928–1930.

Hartup, W. W. The origins of friendship. In M. Lewis & L. A. Rosenblum (Eds.), *Friendship and peer relations*. New York: John Wiley, 1975.

Hartup, W. W. Children and their friends. In H. McGurk (Ed.), *Issues in childhood social development*. London: Methuen, 1978.

Hartup, W. W., Glazer, J. A., & Charlesworth, R. Peer reinforcement and sociometric status. *Child Development*, 1967, *38*, 1017–1024.

Hartup, W. W., & Lempers, J. A problem in life span development: The interactional analysis of family attachments. In P. B. Baltes & K. W. Schaie (Eds.), *Life span developmental psychology: Personality and socialization*. New York: Academic Press, 1973.

Hatfield, J. S., Ferguson, L. R., & Alpert, R. Mother-child interaction and the socialization process. *Child Development*, 1967, *38*, 365–414.

Havighurst, R. J., & Gottlieb, D. Youth and the meaning of work. In R. J. Havighurst & P. H. Dreyer (Eds.), *Youth: The seventy-fourth yearbook of the National Society for the Study of Education*. Chicago: University of Chicago Press, 1975.

Havighurst, R. J., Neugarten, B. L., & Tobin, S. S. Disengagement and patterns of aging. In B. L. Neugarten (Ed.), *Middle age and aging*. Chicago: University of Chicago Press, 1968.

Hayden, T. L. *One child*. New York: G. P. Putnam's, 1980.

Hayes, K. J., & Hayes, C. Intellectual development of a home-raised chimpanzee. *Proceedings of the American Philosophical Society*, 1951, *95*, 105–109.

Hayflick, L. Why grow old? *Stanford Magazine*, September 1975, pp. 36–43.

Haywood, H. C., Meyers, C. E., & Switzky, H. N. Mental retardation. In M. R. Rosenzweig & L. W. Porter (Eds.), *Annual review of psychology* (Vol. 33). Palo Alto, Calif.: Annual Reviews, 1982.

Hebb, D. O. *The organization of behavior*. New York: John Wiley, 1949.

Hebb, D. O. *A textbook of psychology* (2nd ed.). Philadelphia: W. B. Saunders, 1966.

Heinonen, O. P., Slone, D., & Shapiro, S. *Birth defects and drugs in pregnancy*. Littleton, Mass.: Publishing Sciences Group, 1977.

Henderson, N. D. Human behavior genetics. In M. R. Rosenzweig & L. W. Porter (Eds.), *Annual review of psychology* (Vol. 33). Palo Alto, Calif.: Annual Reviews, 1982.

Hendry, L. S. *Cognitive processes in a moral conflict situation*. Unpublished doctoral dissertation, Yale University, 1960.

Hepner, R. Maternal nutrition and the fetus. *Journal of the American Medical Association*, 1958, *168*, 1774–1777.

Herman, J. Father-daughter incest. *Professional Psychology*, 1981, *12*, 76–80.

Herman, J., & Hirschman, L. Families at risk for father-daughter incest. *American Journal of Psychiatry*, 1981, *138*, 967–970.

Herrnstein, R. J. *IQ in the meritocracy*. Boston: Little, Brown, 1973.

Herold, E. S., & Goodwin, M. R. The adoption of oral contraceptives among adolescent females: Reference group influence. In K. Ishwaran (Ed.), *Childhood and adolescence in Canada*. Scarborough, Ont.: McGraw-Hill Ryerson, 1979.

Herr, E. L., & Cramer, S. H. *Career guidance through the life span: Systematic approaches*. Boston: Little, Brown, 1979.

Herzog, E., & Sudia, C. *Boys in fatherless homes*. Washington, D.C.: U.S. Department of Health & Human Services, 1970.

Heston, L. L. Psychiatric disorders in foster home children of schizophrenic mothers. *British Journal of Psychiatry*, 1966, *112*, 819–825.

Hetherington, E. M. Effects of paternal absence on sex-typed behaviors in Negro and white preadolescent males. *Journal of Personality and Social Psychology*, 1966, *4*, 87–91.

Hetherington, E. M. Effects of paternal absence on personality development in adolescent daughters. *Developmental Psychology*, 1972, *7*, 313–326.

Hetherington, E. M. Divorce: A child's perspective. *American Psychologist*, 1979, *34*, 851–858.

Hetherington, E. M., Cox, M., & Cox, R. Play and social interaction in children following divorce. *Journal of Social Issues*, 1979, *35*, 26–49.

Hetherington, E. M., & McIntyre, C. W. Developmental psychology. In M. R. Rosenzweig & L. W. Porter (Eds.), *Annual review of psychology* (Vol. 26). Palo Alto, Calif.: Annual Reviews, 1975.

Himmelweit, H. T., Oppenheim, A. N., & Vince, P. *Television and the child*. New York: Oxford University Press, 1958.

Hindley, C. B., Filliozat, A. M., Klackenberg, G., Nicolet-Meister, D., & Sand, E. A. Differences in age of walking in five European longitudinal samples. *Human Biology*, 1966, *38*, 364–379.

Hite, S. *The Hite report*. New York: Dell, 1976.

Hoffman, L. W. Early childhood experiences and women's achievement motives. *Journal of Social Issues*, 1972, *28*, 129–155.

Hoffman, L. W. Maternal employment: 1979. *American Psychologist*, 1979, *34*, 859–865.

Hoffman, M. L. Developmental synthesis of affect and cognition and its implications for altruistic motivation. *Developmental Psychology*, 1975, *11*, 607–622.

Hoffman, M. L. Empathy, role-taking, guilt, and development of altruistic motives. In T. Likona (Ed.), *Moral development: Current theory and research*. New York: Holt, Rinehart & Winston, 1976.

Hoffman, M. L. Personality and social development. In M. R. Rosenzweig & L. W. Porter (Eds.), *Annual review of psychology* (Vol. 28). Palo Alto, Calif.: Annual Reviews, 1977.

Holbrook, S. H. *Dreamers of the American dream*. New York: Doubleday, 1957.

Holland, J. L. Major programs of research on vocation behavior. In H. Borow (Ed.), *Man in a world at work*. Boston: Houghton Mifflin, 1964.

Holland, J. L. *The psychology of vocational choice*. Waltham, Mass.: Blaisdell, 1966.

Holland, J. L. *Vocational preference inventory (VPI)*. Palo Alto, Calif.: Consulting Psychologists Press, 1975.

Holland, J. L., Magoon, T. M., & Spokane, A. R. Counseling psychology: Career interventions, research, and theory. In M. R. Rosenzweig & L. W. Porter (Eds.), *Annual review of psychology* (Vol. 32). Palo Alto, Calif.: Annual Reviews, 1981.

Hollander, M. J., & Macurdy, E. A. *Alcohol and drug use among Vancouver secondary school students: 1970, 1974, 1978. Summary of findings*. Vancouver, B.C.: Alcohol and Drug Commission of British Columbia, 1978.

Holstein, C. B. Irreversible, stepwise sequence in the development of moral judgment: A longitudinal study of males and females. *Child Development*, 1976, *47*, 51–61.

Honzik, M. P. Verbalization as a factor in learning. *Child Development*, 1932, *3*, 108–113.

Horn, J. L. Psychometric studies of aging and intelligence. In S. Gerscon & A. Raskin (Eds.), *Aging: Genesis and treatment of psychological disorders in the elderly* (Vol. 2). New York: Raven, 1975.

Horn, J. L. Human abilities: A review of research and theory in the early 1970's. In M. R. Rosenzweig & L. W. Porter (Eds.), *Annual review of psychology* (Vol. 27). Palo Alto, Calif.: Annual Reviews, 1976.

Horn, J. L., & Donaldson, G. Cognitive development in adulthood. In O. G. Brim, Jr., & J. Kagan (Eds.), *Constancy and change in human development*. Cambridge, Mass.: Harvard University Press, 1980.

Horner, M. Woman's will to fail. *Psychology Today*, 1969, *3*, 36–38.

Horowitz, F. D. The relationship of anxiety, self-concept, and sociometric status among fourth, fifth, and sixth grade children. *Journal of Abnormal and Social Psychology*, 1962, *65*, 212–214.

Hunt, J. M. *Intelligence and experience*. New York: Ronald Press, 1961.

Hunt, J. M. The psychological basis for using pre-school enrichment as an antidote for cultural deprivation. *Merrill-Palmer Quarterly*, 1964, *10*, 209–248.

Hunt, M. *Sexual behavior in the 1970's*. Chicago: Playboy Press, 1974.

Hurlock, E. B. *Child development* (4th ed.). New York: McGraw-Hill, 1964.

Huston-Stein, A., & Higgins-Trenk, A. Development of females from childhood through adulthood: Career and feminine role orientations. In P. B. Baltes (Ed.), *Life-span development and behavior* (Vol. 1). New York: Academic Press, 1978.

Hutt, S. J., Lenard, H. G., & Prechtl, H. F. R. Psychophysiology of the newborn. In L. P. Lipsitt & H. W. Reese (Eds.), *Advances in child development and behavior*. New York: Academic Press, 1969.

Huyck, M. H., & Hoyer, W. H. *Adult development and aging*. Belmont, Calif.: Wadsworth, 1982.

Ilg, F. L., & Ames, L. B. *School readiness*. New York: Harper & Row, 1965.

Inhelder, B., & Piaget, J. *The growth of logical thinking from childhood to adolescence*. New York: Basic Books, 1958.

Involvement in developmental psychology today. Del Mar, Calif.: C.R.M. Books, 1971.

Irwin, D. M., & Bushnell, M. M. *Observational strategies for child study*. New York: Holt, Rinehart & Winston, 1980.

Isabell, B. J., & McKee, L. Society's cradle: An anthropological perspective on the socialization of cognition. In J. Sants (Ed.), *Developmental psychology and society*. London: Macmillan, 1980.

Jackson, C. N. Some aspects of form and growth. In W. J. Robbins, S. Brody, A. G. Hogan, C. N. Jackson, & C. W. Green (Eds.), *Growth*. New Haven, Conn.: Yale University Press, 1928.

Jacobs, R. H. *Life after youth*. Boston: Beacon Press, 1979.

Jacobson, S. W., & Kagan, J. Interpreting "imitative" responses in early infancy. *Science*, 1979, *205*, 215–217.

Jaffe, B. F., & Luterman, D. M. The child with a hearing loss. In A. P. Scheiner & I. F. Abroms (Eds.), *The practical management of the developmentally disabled child*. St. Louis: C. V. Mosby, 1980.

Jarvik, L. F., Klodin, V., & Matsuyama, S. S. Human aggression and the extra Y chromosome: Fact or fantasy? *American Psychologist*, 1973, *28*, 674–682.

Jenkins, C. D., Zyzanski, S. J., & Rosenman, R. H. Progress toward validation of a computer-scored test of the type A coronary-prone behavior pattern. *Psychosomatic Medicine,* 1971, *33*, 192–202.

Jensen, A. R. Social class, race, and genetics: Implications for education. *American Educational Research Journal*, 1968, *5*, 1–42.

Jensen, A. R. Kinship correlations reported by Sir Cyril Burt. *Behavior Genetics*, 1974, *4*, 1–28.

Jersild, A. T. *The psychology of adolescence* (2nd ed.). New York: Macmillan, 1963.

Johnson, H. R., Myhre, S. A., Ruvalcaba, R. H. A., Thuline, H. C., & Kelley, V. C. Effects of testosterone on body image and behavior in Klinefelter's syndrome: A pilot study. *Developmental Medicine and Child Neurology*, 1970, *12*, 454–460.

Johnson, N. Through the video-screen darkly. *Christian Science Monitor*, February 1969.

Johnson, R. D. Measurements of achievement in fundamental skills of elementary school children. *Research Quarterly*, 1962, *33*, 94–103.

Johnson, S. W., & Morasky, R. L. *Learning disabilities* (2nd ed.). Boston: Allyn & Bacon, 1980.

Johnson, W., Brown, S. F., Curtis, J. F., Edney, C. W., & Keaster, J. *Speech handicapped school children*. New York: Harper & Row, 1948.

Jones, H. E. Adolescence in our society. In Community Service Society of New York, *The family in a democratic society*. New York: Columbia University Press, 1949.

Jones, M. C. The later careers of boys who are early- or late-maturing. *Child Development*, 1957, *28*, 113–128.

Jones, M. C. Psychological correlates of somatic development. *Child Development*, 1965, *36*, 899–911.

Jones-Witters, P., & Witters, W. *Drugs and society: A biological perspective*. Belmont, Calif.: Wadsworth, 1983.

Joy, L. A., Kimball, M., & Zabrack, M. L. *Television exposure and children's aggressive behavior*. Paper presented at the annual meeting of the Canadian Psychological Association, Vancouver, British Columbia, June 1977.

Jung, C. G. *Psychological types*. New York: Harcourt Brace Jovanovich, 1923.

Kagan, J. S. Biological aspects of inhibition systems. *American Journal of Diseases of Children*, 1967, *114*, 507–512.

Kagan, J. S. Inadequate evidence and illogical conclusions. *Harvard Educational Review* (Reprint Series No. 2), 1969, 126–129.

Kagan, J. S. The parental love trap. *Psychology Today*, August 1978, pp. 54–61; 91.

Kagan, J. S. The construct of difficult temperament: A reply to Thomas, Chess, and Korn. *Merrill-Palmer Quarterly*, 1982, *28*, 21–24.

Kagan, J. S., Kearsley, R. B., & Zelaza, P. R. The effects of infant day care on psychological development. *Educational Quarterly*, 1977, *1*, 109–142.

Kagan, S., & Madsen, M. C. Experimental analyses of cooperation and competition of Anglo-American and Mexican children. *Developmental Psychology*, 1972, *6*, 49–59.

Kahn, A., & Blum, D. Phenothiazines and sudden infant death syndrome. *Pediatrics*, 1982, *70*, 75–78.

Kalat, J. W. *Biological Psychology*. Belmont, Calif.: Wadsworth, 1981.

Kalish, R. A. *Death, grief, and caring relationships*. Monterey, Calif.: Brooks/Cole, 1981.

Kalish, R. A. *Late adulthood: Perspectives on human development* (2nd ed.). Monterey, Calif.: Brooks/Cole, 1982.

Kalish, R. A., & Reynolds, D. K. *Death and ethnicity: A psychocultural study*. Los Angeles: University of Southern California Press, 1976.

Kamin, L. J. *The science and politics of IQ*. Hillsdale, N.J.: Lawrence Erlbaum, 1974.

Kanter, R. M. *Men and women of the corporation*. New York: Basic Books, 1977.

Katchadourian, H. *The biology of adolescence*. New York: W. H. Freeman, 1977.

Kato, T. Chromosome studies in pregnant rhesus monkeys macaque given LSD-25. *Diseases of the Nervous System*, 1970, *31*, 245–250.

Kellogg, W. N. Communication and language in the home-raised chimpanzee. *Science,* 1968, *162*, 423–427.

Kellogg, W. N., & Kellogg, L. A. *The ape and the child: A study of environmental influence upon early behavior*. New York: McGraw-Hill, 1933.

Kelly, G. A. *The psychology of personal constructs*. New York: W. W. Norton, 1955.

Kelly, T. J., Bullock, L. M., & Dykes, M. K. Behavior disorders: Teachers' perceptions. *Exceptional Children*, 1977, *43*, 316–318.

Kempe, R. S., & Kempe, C. H. *Child abuse*. Cambridge, Mass.: Harvard University Press, 1978.

Keniston, K. Do Americans really like children? *Childhood Education*, 1975, *52*, 4–12.

Kennell, J. H., Trause, M. A., & Klaus, M. H. Evidence for a sensitive period in the human mother. *Parent-Infant Interaction* (Ciba Foundation Symposium, new series), 1975, *33*, 87–102.

Keogh, J. F. Motor performance in elementary school children. *Monographs*. Los Angeles: University of California, Department of Physical Education, 1965.

Keogh, J. F. *A rhythmical hopping task as an assessment of motor deficiency*. Paper reported at the 2nd International Congress of Sports Psychology, Washington, D.C., 1968.

Kessen, W. *The child*. New York: John Wiley, 1965.

Kett, J. F. *Rites of passage: Adolescence in America, 1790 to the present*. New York: Basic Books, 1977.

Kiff, R. D., & Lepard, C. Visual response of premature infants. *Archives of Ophthalmology*, 1966, *75*, 631–633.

King, K., Balswick, J. O., & Robinson, I. E. The continuing premarital sexual revolution among college females. *Journal of Marriage and the Family*, 1977, *39*, 455–459.

Kinsey, A. C., Pomeroy, W. B., & Martin, C. E. *Sexual behavior in the human male.* Philadelphia: W. B. Saunders, 1948.

Kinsey, A. C., Pomeroy, W. B., Martin, C. E., & Gebhard, P. H. *Sexual behavior in the human female.* Philadelphia: W. B. Saunders, 1953.

Kirk, S. Educating exceptional children (3rd ed.). Boston, Mass.: Houghton Mifflin, 1979.

Kirk, S. A., & McCarthy, J. J. *The Illinois test of psycholinguistic abilities: An approach to differential diagnoses.* Urbana: University of Illinois Press, 1961.

Klagsbrun, F. *Too young to die: Youth and suicide.* Boston: Houghton Mifflin, 1976.

Klaus, M., & Kennell, J. *Maternal-infant bonding.* St. Louis: C. V. Mosby, 1976.

Klaus, M., Kreger, N., McAlpine, W., Steffa, M., & Kennell, J. Maternal attachment: Importance of the first post-partum days. *New England Journal of Medicine*, 1972, *286*, 460–463.

Kleemeier, R. Intellectual changes in the senium. *Proceedings of the Social Statistics Section of the American Statistical Association*, 1962, *1*, 290–295.

Klein, D. M., Jorgensen, S. R., & Miller, B. C. Research methods and developmental reciprocity in families. In R. M. Lerner & G. B. Spanier (Eds.), *Child influences on marital and family interaction.* New York: Academic Press, 1978.

Klusman, L. E. Reduction of pain in childbirth by alleviation of anxiety during pregnancy. *Journal of Consulting and Clinical Psychology*, 1975, *43*, 162–165.

Knight, B. M. *Enjoying single parenthood.* Toronto: Van Nostrand, 1980.

Knight, G. P., & Kagan, S. Development of prosocial and competitive behaviors in Anglo-American and Mexican-American children. *Child Development*, 1977, *48*, 1385–1394.

Knutson, J. F. Child abuse as an area of aggression research. *Journal of Pediatric Psychology*, 1978, *3*, 20–27.

Koch, H. L. Some personality correlates of sex, sibling position, and sex of sibling among five- and six-year-old children. *Genetic Psychology Monographs*, 1955, *52*, 3–50.

Koch, K. *I never told anybody.* New York: Random House, 1977.

Kohlberg, L. A. Development of moral character and moral ideology. In M. L. Hoffman & L. W. Hoffman (Eds.), *Review of Child Development Research* (Vol. 1). New York: Russell Sage Foundation, 1964.

Kohlberg, L. A. Cognitive-development analysis of children's sex-role concepts and attitudes. In E. Maccoby (Ed.), *The development of sex differences.* Stanford, Calif.: Stanford University Press, 1966.

Kohlberg, L. A. Stage and sequence: The cognitive-developmental approach to socialization. In D. Gosslin (Ed.), *Handbook of socialization theory and research.* Chicago: Rand McNally, 1969.

Kohlberg, L. A. Moral stages and moralization. In T. Likona (Ed.), *Moral development: Current theory and research.* New York: Holt, Rinehart & Winston, 1976.

Kohlberg, L. A. Revisions in the theory and practice of moral development. *New Directions for Child Development*, 1978, *2*, 83–87.

Kohlberg, L. A., & Turiel, E. *Research in moral development: A cognitive developmental approach.* New York: Holt, Rinehart & Winston, 1971.

Kolata, G. B. Behavioral teratology: Birth defects of the mind. *Science*, 1978, *202*, 732–734.

Kopp, C. B., & Parmelee, A. H. Prenatal and perinatal influences on infant behavior. In J. D. Osofsky (Ed.), *Handbook of infant development.* New York: John Wiley, 1979.

Kopplin, D. A., & Greenfield, T. K. Changing patterns of substance use on campus: A four-year follow-up study. *International Journal of Addictions*, 1977, *12*, 73–94.

Kotelchuck, M. The infant's relationship to the father: Experimental evidence. In M. Lamb (Ed.), *The role of the father in child development.* New York: John Wiley, 1976.

Krauss, R. M., & Glucksberg, S. Social and nonsocial speech. *Scientific American*, 1977, *236*, 100–105.

Krech, D., Crutchfield, R. S., & Livson, N. *Elements of psychology* (2nd ed.). New York: Alfred A. Knopf, 1969.

Krech, D., Rosenzweig, M., & Bennett, E. Effects of environmental complexity and training on brain chemistry. *Journal of Comparative and Physiological Psychology*, 1960, *53*, 509–519.

Krech, D., Rosenzweig, M., & Bennett, E. Relations between brain chemistry and problem-solving among rats in enriched and impoverished environments. *Journal of Comparative and Physiological Psychology*, 1962, *55*, 801–807.

Krech, D., Rosenzweig, M., & Bennett, E. Environmental impoverishment, social isolation, and changes in brain chemistry and anatomy. *Physiology and Behavior*, 1966, *1*, 99–104.

Krech, D., Rosenzweig, M., Bennett, E., & Krueckel, B. Enzyme concentrations in the brain and adjustive behavior patterns. *Science*, 1954, *120*, 994–996.

Kreinberg, N., & Chow, S. H. L. (Eds.). *Configurations of change: The integration of mildly handicapped children into the regular classroom.* Sioux Falls, S.D.: Adapt Press, 1973.

Krishna Singh, B., Walton, B. L., & Williams, J. S. Extra-marital sexual permissiveness: Conditions and contingencies. *Journal of Marriage and the Family*, 1976, *38*, 701–713.

Kron, R. E., Kaplan, S. L., Phoenix, M. D., & Finnegan, L. P. Behavior of infants born to narcotic-dependent mothers: Effects of prenatal and postnatal drugs. In J. L. Rementaria (Ed.), *Drug abuse in pregnancy and neonatal effects*. St. Louis: C. V. Mosby, 1977.

Kron, R. E., Stein, M., & Goddard, K. E. Newborn sucking behavior affected by obstetric sedation. *Pediatrics*, 1966, *37*, 1012–1016.

Kübler-Ross, E. *On death and dying*. New York: Macmillan, 1969.

Kübler-Ross, E. *Questions and answers on death and dying*. New York: Macmillan, 1974.

Kuder, F. *Activity, interests, and occupational choice*. Chicago: Science Research Associates, 1977.

Kuhn, D. Mechanisms of change in the development of cognitive structures. *Child Development*, 1972, *43*, 833–844.

Kurtines, W., & Grief, E. B. The development of moral thought: Review and evaluation of Kohlberg's approach. *Psychological Bulletin*, 1974, *81*, 453–470.

Lamaze, F. *Painless childbirth: The Lamaze method*. New York: Pocket Books, 1972.

Lamb, M. E. Interactions between eight-month-olds and their fathers and mothers. In M. E. Lamb (Ed.), *The role of the father in child development*. New York: John Wiley, 1976. (a)

Lamb, M. E. (Ed.). *The role of the father in child development*. New York: John Wiley, 1976. (b)

Lamb, M. E. Twelve-month-olds and their parents: Interaction in a laboratory playroom. *Developmental Psychology*, 1976, *12*, 237–244. (c)

Lamb, M. E. The development of parent-infant attachments in the first two years of life. In F. A. Pedersen (Ed.), *The father-infant relationship: Observational studies in the family setting*. New York: Praeger, 1980.

Lambert, W., Yackley, A., & Hine, R. N. Child training values of English Canadian and French Canadian parents. *Canadian Journal of Behavioral Science*, 1971, *3*, 217–236.

Landis, J. T., & Landis, M. G. *Building a successful marriage*. Englewood Cliffs, N.J.: Prentice-Hall, 1963.

Landreth, C. *Early childhood: Behavior and learning* (2nd ed.). New York: Alfred A. Knopf, 1967.

Lane, H. *The wild boy of Aveyron*. London: Allen & Unwin, 1977.

Langer, E. J., & Rodin, J. The effects of choice and enhanced personal responsibility for the aged. *Journal of Personality and Social Psychology*, 1976, *34*, 191–198.

Larsen, A. D., & Miller, J. B. The hearing impaired. In E. L. Meyen (Ed.), *Exceptional children and youth: An introduction*. Denver, Colo.: Love Publishing, 1978.

Lawton, M. P. The relative impact of congregate and traditional housing on elderly tenants. *Gerontologist*, 1976, *16*, 237–242.

Lawton, M. P. Community supports for the aged. *Journal of Social Issues*, 1981, *37*, 102–115.

Layzer, D. Heritability analyses of IQ scores: Science or numerology? *Science*, 1974, *183*, 1259–1266.

Leaf, A. Getting old. *Scientific American*, September 1973, *299*, pp. 44–53.

Leboyer, F. *Birth without violence*. New York: Random House, 1975.

Lee, E. S. Negro intelligence and selective migration: A Philadelphia test of the Klineberg hypothesis. *American Sociological Review*, 1951, *16*, 227–233.

Lefkowitz, M., Eron, L., Walder, L., & Huesmann, L. R. Television violence and child aggression: A follow-up study. In G. A. Comstock & E. A. Rubinstein (Eds.), *Television and social behavior* (Vol. 3). Washington, D.C.: U.S. Government Printing Office, 1972.

Lefrancois, G. R. *Developing creativity in high school students*. Unpublished M.Ed. thesis, University of Saskatchewan, Saskatoon, Saskatchewan, Canada, 1965.

Lefrancois, G. R. Jean Piaget's developmental model: Equilibration-through-adaptation. *Alberta Journal of Educational Research*, 1967, *13*, 161–171.

Lefrancois, G. R. A treatment hierarchy for the acceleration of conservation of substance. *Canadian Journal of Psychology*, 1968, *22*, 277–284.

Lefrancois, G. R. *Adolescents* (2nd ed.). Belmont, Calif.: Wadsworth, 1981.

Lefrancois, G. R. *Psychology for teaching: A bear rarely faces the front* (4th ed.). Belmont, Calif.: Wadsworth, 1982.

Lefrancois, G. R. *Psychology* (2nd ed.). Belmont, Calif.: Wadsworth, 1983.

Lehman, H. C. *Age and achievement*. Princeton, N.J.: Princeton University Press, 1953.

LeMasters, E. E. *Parents in modern America* (3rd ed.). Homewood, Ill.: Dorsey Press, 1977.

Lenneberg, E. H. *Biological foundations of language*. New York: John Wiley, 1967.

Lenneberg, E. H. On explaining language. *Science*, 1969, *164*, 635–643.

Lenneberg, E. H., Nichols, I. A., & Rosenberger, E. F. Primitive stages of language development in mongolism. In *Disorders of communication: Research publications, A.R.N.M.D.* (Vol. 42). Baltimore: Williams & Wilkins, 1964.

Lenz, W. Malformations caused by drugs in pregnancy. *American Journal of Diseases in Children*, 1966, *112*, 99–106.

Leon, J. Trends in drug use among young people in Oshawa: Prevalence and responses. *Canada's Mental Health*, 1977, *25*, 6–10.

Lepper, M. R. Intrinsic and extrinsic motivation in children: Detrimental effects of superfluous social controls. In W. A. Collins (Ed.), *Aspects of the development of competence: The Minnesota symposium on child psychology* (Vol. 14). Hillsdale, N.J.: Lawrence Erlbaum, 1981.

Lepper, M. R., & Greene, D. Turning play into work: Effects of adult surveillance and extrinsic rewards on children's intrinsic motivation. *Journal of Personality and Social Psychology*, 1975, *31*, 479–486.

Lepper, M. R., & Greene, D. Overjustification research and beyond: Towards a means-ends analysis of intrinsic and extrinsic motivation. In D. Greene & M. R. Lepper (Eds.), *The hidden costs of reward*. Hillsdale, N.J.: Lawrence Erlbaum, 1978.

Lepper, M. R., Greene, D., & Nisbett, R. E. Undermining children's intrinsic interest with extrinsic rewards: A test of the "overjustification" hypothesis. *Journal of Personality and Social Psychology,* 1973, *28,* 129–137.

Lerner, R. M. *Concepts and theories of human development*. Reading, Mass.: Addison-Wesley, 1976.

Lerner, R. M., & Korn, S. J. The development of body-build stereotypes in males. *Child Development*, 1972, *43,* 908–920.

Leslie, G. R. *The family in social context* (4th ed.). New York: Oxford University Press, 1979.

Levinson, D. J. Middle adulthood in modern society: A sociopsychological view. In G. Direnzo (Ed.), *Social character and social change*. Westport, Conn.: Greenwood Press, 1977.

Levinson, D. J. *The seasons of a man's life*. New York: Alfred A. Knopf, 1978.

Levinson, D. J. The midlife transition: A period in adult psychosocial development. In L. D. Steinberg (Ed.), *The life cycle: Readings in human development*. New York: Columbia University Press, 1981.

Levinson, D. J., Darrow, C. M., Klein, E. B., Levinson, M. H., & McKee, B. Periods in the adult development of men: Ages 18 to 45. *The Counseling Psychologist*, 1976, *6,* 21–25.

Lewin, R. Starved brains. *Psychology Today*, September 1975, pp. 29–33.

Lewis, M. Parents and children: Sex role development. *School Review*, 1972, *80,* 229–240.

Lewis, M. (Ed.). *Origins of intelligence: Infancy and early childhood*. New York: Plenum Press, 1976.

Lewis, M., & Lee-Painter, S. An interactional approach to the mother-infant dyad. In M. Lewis & L. A. Rosenblum (Eds.), *The effect of the infant on its caregiver*. New York: John Wiley, 1974.

Lewis, M., & Rosenblum, L. A. (Eds.). *Friendship and peer relations*. New York: John Wiley, 1975.

Lewis, T. L., & Maurer, D. *Newborns' central vision: Whole or hole?* Paper presented at the meeting of the Society for Research in Child Development, New Orleans, March 1977.

Liben, L. *Perspective-taking skills in young children: Seeing the world through rose-colored glasses*. Paper presented at the meeting of the Society for Research in Child Development, Denver, April 1975.

Liebert, R. M., & Baron, R. A. Short-term effects of televised aggression on children's aggressive behavior. In J. P. Murray, E. A. Rubinstein, & G. A. Comstock (Eds.), *Television and social behavior* (Vol. 2). Washington, D.C.: U.S. Government Printing Office, 1972.

Liebert, R. M., & Schwartzberg, N. S. Effects of mass media. In M. R. Rosenzweig & L. W. Porter (Eds.), *Annual review of psychology* (Vol. 28). Palo Alto, Calif.: Annual Reviews, 1977.

Lipsitt, L. P., Engen, T., & Kaye, H. Developmental changes in the olfactory threshold of the neonate. *Child Development*, 1963, *34,* 371–376.

Lipsitt, L. P., & Levy, N. Electrotactual threshold in the neonate. *Child Development*, 1959, *30,* 547–554.

Little, A. A longitudinal study of cognitive development in young children. *Child Development*, 1972, *43,* 1024–1034.

Little, L. J. The learning disabled. In E. L. Meyen (Ed.), *Exceptional children and youth: An introduction*. Denver, Colo.: Love Publishing, 1978.

Lloyd, R. E. Parent-youth conflicts of college students. *Sociology and Social Research*, 1954, *38,* 227–230.

Locke, J. Some thoughts concerning education (4th ed.). London: A. & J. Churchills, 1699.

Loehlin, J. C., & Nichols, R. C. *Heredity, environment, and personality: A study of 850 sets of twins*. Austin: University of Texas, 1976.

Looft, W. R. Egocentrism and social interaction in adolescence. *Adolescence*, 1971, *6,* 485–494.

Lopata, H. Z. The meaning of friendship in widowhood. In L. D. Steinberg (Ed.), *The life cycle: Readings in human development*. New York: Columbia University Press, 1981.

Louria, D. *Nightmare drugs*. New York: Pocket Books, 1966.

Loving parents given right to let boy die. *Edmonton Journal*, March 12, 1983, p. A-1.

Lowenthal, M. F., & Haven, C. Interaction and adaptation: Intimacy as a critical variable. In L. D. Steinberg (Ed.), *The life cycle: Readings in human development*. New York: Columbia University Press, 1981.

Luckey, E. B., & Nass, G. D. The comparison of sexual attitudes and behavior in an international sample. *Journal of Marriage and the Family*, 1969, *31,* 364–378.

Ludeman, K. The sexuality of the older person: Review of the literature. *Gerontologist*, 1981, *21,* 203–308.

Lunde, D. T., & Lunde, M. R. *The next generation: A book on parenting*. New York: Holt, Rinehart & Winston, 1980.

Lyle, J., & Hoffman, H. R. Children's use of television and other media. In E. A. Rubinstein, G. A. Comstock, & J. P. Murray (Eds.), *Television and social behavior* (Vol. 4). Washington, D.C.: U.S. Government Printing Office, 1972.

Lynn, D. B. *The father: His role in child development*. Monterey, Calif.: Brooks/Cole, 1974.

Lynn, D. B. *Daughters and parents: Past, present and future*. Monterey, Calif.: Brooks/Cole, 1979.

MacArthur, R. S. Some ability patterns: Central Eskimos and Nsenga Africans. *International Journal of Psychology*, 1973, *8,* 239–247.

MacArthur, R. S. *Differential ability patterns: Inuit, Nsenga, Canadian Whites*. Paper presented at 2nd meeting of International Association for Cross-Cultural Psychology, Kingston, Ontario, August 1974.

MacArthur, R. S. *Ecology, culture, and cognitive development: Canadian native youth*. Paper presented at meeting of Canadian Ethnic Studies Association, Winnipeg, Manitoba, October 1975.

Macaulay, R. K. S. The myth of female superiority in language. *Journal of Child Language*, 1977, *5*, 353–363.

Maccoby, E. E. Woman's intellect. In S. M. Farber & R. H. L. Wilson (Eds.), *Man and civilization: The potential of woman*. New York: McGraw-Hill, 1963.

Maccoby, E. E., & Jacklin, C. N. *The psychology of sex differences*. Stanford, Calif.: Stanford University Press, 1974.

Macklin, E. Heterosexual cohabitation among unmarried college students. *The Family Coordinator*, 1972, *21*, 463–472.

Magrab, P. For the sake of the children: A review of the psychological effects of divorce. *Journal of Divorce*, 1978, *1*, 233–245.

Malmquist, C. P. *Handbook of adolescence*. New York: Jason Aronson, 1978.

Mander, J. *Four arguments for the elimination of television*. New York: William Morrow, 1978.

Marcia, J. E. Development and validation of ego-identity status. *Journal of Personality and Social Psychology*, 1966, *3*, 551–558.

Marcia, J. E., & Friedman, M. L. Ego identity status in college women. *Journal of Personality*, 1970, *38*, 249–269.

Markides, K., & Martin, H. A causal model of life satisfaction among the elderly. *Journal of Gerontology*, 1979, *34*, 86–93.

Markman, E. M. Classes and collections: Conceptual organization and numerical abilities. *Cognitive Psychology*, 1979, *11*, 395–411.

Markman, E. M., Horton, M. S., & McLanahan, A. G. Classes and collections: Principles of organization in the learning of hierarchical relations. *Cognition*, 1980, *8*, 227–241.

Marks, P. A., & Haller, D. L. Now I lay me down for keeps. *Journal of Clinical Psychology*, 1977, *33*, 390–399.

Martin, H. *The abused child*. Cambridge, Mass.: Ballinger, 1976.

Martin, J., Martin, D. C., Lund, C. A., & Streissguth, A. P. Maternal alcohol ingestion and cigarette smoking and their effects on newborn conditioning. *Alcoholism: Clinical and Experimental Research*, 1977, *1*, 243–247.

Martin, J. P. Introduction. In J. P. Martin (Ed.), *Violence and the family*. New York: John Wiley, 1978.

Maslow, A. H. *Motivation and personality*. New York: Harper & Row, 1954.

Maslow, A. H. *Motivation and personality* (2nd ed.). New York: Harper & Row, 1970.

Masters, J. C. Interpreting "imitative" responses in early infancy. *Science*, 1979, *205*, 215.

Masters, W. H., & Johnson, V. E. *Human sexual inadequacy*. Boston: Little, Brown, 1970.

Maykovich, M. K. Attitudes versus behavior in extramarital sexual relations. *Journal of Marriage and the Family*, 1976, *38*, 693.

McCain, G., & Segal, E. M. *The game of science* (4th ed.). Monterey, Calif.: Brooks/Cole, 1982.

McCarthy, D. Language development. In L. Carmichael (Ed.), *Manual of child psychology* (2nd ed.). New York: John Wiley, 1954.

McClelland, D., Constantian, C. S., Regalado, D., & Stone, C. Making it to maturity. *Psychology Today*, June 1978, pp. 42–53; 114.

McCurdy, H. G. The childhood pattern of genius. *Journal of the Elisha Mitchell Scientific Society*, 1957, *73*, 448–462.

McDaniel, E., Guay, R., Ball, L., & Kolloff, M. *A spatial experience questionnaire and some preliminary findings*. Paper presented at the Annual Meeting of the American Psychological Association, Toronto, Ontario, 1978.

McGraw, M. B. *The neuromuscular maturation of the human infant*. New York: Columbia University Press, 1943.

McKee, J. P., & Leader, F. The relationship of socio-economic status and aggression to the competitive behavior of pre-school children. *Child Development*, 1955, *26*, 135–142.

McNeill, D. *The acquisition of language: The study of developmental psycholinguistics*. New York: Harper & Row, 1970.

McPhail, P., Ungoed-Thomas, J. R., & Chapman, H. *Moral education in the secondary school*. London: Longmans, 1972.

McTavish, D. G. Perceptions of old people: A review of research, methodologies and findings. *Gerontologist*, 1971, *11*, 90–101.

Mead, M. *Sex and temperament in three primitive societies*. New York: New American Library, 1935.

Mead, M. (Ed.). *Cooperation and competition among primitive peoples*. New York: McGraw-Hill, 1937.

Mead, M. Marriage in two steps. In H. A. Otto (Ed.), *The family in search of a future*. New York: Appleton-Century-Crofts, 1970.

Meadow, K. P. Development of deaf children. In E. M. Hetherington (Ed.), *Review of child development research* (Vol. 5). Chicago: University of Chicago Press, 1975.

Meier, G. W., Bunch, M. E., Nolan, C. Y., & Scheilder, C. H. Anoxia, behavioral development, and learning ability: A comparative experimental approach. *Psychological Monographs*, 1960, *74* (1, Whole No. 488).

Meiselman, K. *Incest*. San Francisco: Jossey-Bass, 1978.

Meissner, S. J. Parental interaction of the adolescent boy. *Journal of Genetic Psychology*, 1965, *107*, 225–233.

Melican, G. J., & Feldt, L. S. An empirical study of the Zajonc-Markus hypothesis for achievement test score declines. *American Educational Research Journal*, 1980, *17*, 5–19.

Meltzoff, A. N., & Moore, M. K. Imitation of facial and manual gestures by human neonates. *Science*, 1977, *198*, 75–78.

Meltzoff, A. N., & Moore, M. K. Interpreting "imitative" responses in early infancy. *Science*, 1979, *205*, 217–219.

Mercer, C. D., & Snell, M. E. *Learning theory research in mental retardation: Implications for teaching.* Columbus, Ohio: Charles E. Merrill, 1977.

Mercer, J. R. *Labeling the mentally retarded.* Berkeley: University of California Press, 1973.

Meredith, H. V. Somatic changes during prenatal life. *Child Development*, 1975, *46*, 603–610.

Meyen, E. L. (Ed.). *Exceptional children and youth: An introduction.* Denver, Colo.: Love Publishing, 1978.

Miller, J., & Taylor, G. The teaching force is aging. *The Canadian School Executive*, 1983, *2*, 12–14.

Miller, N. E. Behavioral medicine: Symbiosis between laboratory and clinic. *Annual review of psychology* (Vol. 34). Palo Alto, Calif.: Annual Reviews 1983.

Miller, S. A. *Certainty and necessity in the understanding of Piagetian concepts.* Paper presented at the Society for Research in Child Development Meetings, Boston, April 1981.

Miller, W. B. Lower class culture as a generating milieu of gang delinquency. *Journal of Social Issues*, 1958, *14*, 5–19.

Mindel, C. H., & Vaughan, C. E. A multidimensional approach to religiosity and disengagement. *Journal of Gerontology,* 1978, *33*, 103–108.

Minuchin, S., Rosman, B. L., & Baker, L *Psychosomatic families: Anorexia nervosa in context.* Cambridge, Mass.: Harvard University Press, 1978.

Mischel, W. *Personality and assessment.* New York: John Wiley, 1968.

Mischel, W. On the future of personality measurement. *American Psychologist*, 1977, *32*, 246–254.

Mischel, W. On the interface of cognition and personality: Beyond the person-situation debate. *American Psychologist*, 1979, *34*, 740–754.

Mitchell, G. D., Arling, G. L., & Moller, G. W. Long term effects of maternal punishment on the behavior of monkeys. *Psychonomic Science*, 1967, *8*, 209–210.

Moffitt, A. R. Consonant cue perception by 20–24 week old infants. *Child Development*, 1971, *42*, 717–731.

Money, J. Counselling in genetics and applied behavior genetics. In K. W. Schaie, V. F. Anderson, G. F. McClearn, & J. Money (Eds.), *Developmental human behavior genetics.* Lexington, Mass.: D. C. Heath, 1975.

Money, J., & Ehrhardt, A. A. Prenatal hormonal exposure: Possible effects on behavior in man. In R. P. Michael (Ed.), *Endocrinology and human behavior.* London: Oxford University Press, 1968.

Montemayor, R., & Eisen, M. The development of self-conceptions from childhood to adolescence. *Developmental Psychology*, 1977, *13*, 314–319.

Montemayor, R., & Van Komen, R. Age segregation of adolescents in and out of school. *Journal of Youth and Adolescence*, 1980, *9*, 371–381.

Monthly vital statistics, final mortality statistics, No. 79, 1120. Hyattsville, Md.: U.S. Department of Health & Human Services, 1979.

Morgan, C. L. *Introduction to comparative psychology.* London: Scott, 1894.

Morgan, C. L. *Habit and instinct.* London: Arnold, 1896.

Morris, D. *Intimate behavior.* New York: Random House, 1971.

Morris, D. *Manwatching: A field guide to human behaviour.* London: Jonathan Cape, 1977.

Morrison, J. R., & Stewart, M. A. The psychiatric status of the legal families of adopted hyperactive children. *Archives of General Psychiatry*, 1973, *28*, 888–891.

Morse, W. C. Serving the needs of children with behavior disorders. *Exceptional Children*, 1977, *44*, 158–164.

Moskowitz, B. A. The acquisition of language. *Scientific American*, 1978, *239*, 92–108.

Moss, H. A., & Susman, E. J. Longitudinal study of personality development. In O. G. Brim, Jr., & J. Kagan (Eds.), *Constancy and change in human development.* Cambridge Mass.: Harvard University Press, 1980.

Mowat, F. *People of the deer.* Boston: Little, Brown, 1952.

Moyer, K. E. *The psychobiology of aggression.* New York: Harper & Row, 1976.

Mulhern, R. K., & Passman, R. H. The child's behavioral pattern as a determinant of maternal punitiveness. *Child Development*, 1979, *15*, 417–423.

Murchison, C. (Ed.). *A history of psychology in autobiography* (Vol. 3). Worcester, Mass.: Clark University Press, 1936.

Murdock, G. P. World ethnographic sample. *American Anthropologist,* 1957, *59*, 676–688.

Murray, H. A. *Explorations in personality.* New York: Oxford University Press, 1938.

Murray, J. P. Television and violence: Implications of the Surgeon General's research program. *American Psychologist*, June 1973, pp. 472–478.

Mussen, P., & Eisenberg-Berg, N. *Roots of caring, sharing, and helping: The development of prosocial behavior in children.* New York: W. H. Freeman, 1977.

Muuss, R. E. *Theories of adolescence* (3rd ed.). New York: Random House, 1975.

Naeye, R. L. Sudden infant death. *Scientific American*, 1980, *242*, 56–62.

Nagy, M. H. The child's theories concerning death. *Journal of Genetic Psychology,* 1948, *73*, 3–27.

National Advisory Committee on Handicapped Children. Conference sponsored by the Bureau of Education of the Handicapped. U.S. Office of Education, Washington, D.C., September 28, 1968.

Nesselroade, J. R., & Baltes, P. B. Adolescent personality development and historical change: 1970–1972. *Monographs of the Society for Research in Child Development* 1974, *39* (1, Serial No. 154).

Neugarten, B. L. *Personality in middle and late life.* New York: Atherton Press, 1964.

Neugarten, B. L. (Ed.). *Middle age and aging: A reader in*

social psychology. Chicago: University of Chicago Press, 1968.

Neugarten, B. L. The wise of the young-old. In R. Gross, B. Gross, & S. Seidman (Eds.), *The new old: Struggling for decent aging.* New York.: Doubleday-Anchor, 1978.

Neugarten, B. L., & Datan, N. The subjective experience of middle age. In L. D. Steinberg (Ed.), *The life cycle: Readings in human development.* New York: Columbia University Press, 1981.

Newcomb, A. F., Brady, J. E., & Hartup, W. W. Friendship and incentive condition as determinants of children's task-oriented social behavior. *Child Development,* 1979, *50,* 878–881.

Newman, H. H., Freeman, F. N., & Holzinger, K. J. *Twins: A study of heredity and environment.* Chicago: University of Chicago Press, 1937.

Newsweek, January 6, 1969, p. 37.

Nichols, M. M. Acute alcohol withdrawal syndrome in a newborn. *American Journal of Diseases of Children,* 1967, *113,* 714–715.

Nock, S. L. The family life cycle: Empirical or conceptual tool? *Journal of Marriage and the Family,* 1979, *41,* 15–26.

Nolan, C. Y. The visually impaired. In E. L. Meyen (Ed.), *Exceptional children and youth: An introduction.* Denver, Colo.: Love Publishing, 1978.

Novak, L. Aging, total body potassium, fat-free mass, and cell mass in males and females between ages 18 and 85 years. *Journal of Gerontology,* 1972, *27,* 438–443.

Noyes, A. B. *My father's house: An Oneida boyhood.* New York: Farrar, Straus & Giroux, 1937.

Nucci, L. P., & Turiel, E. Social interactions and the development of social concepts in preschool children. *Child Development,* 1978, *49,* 400–407.

O'Donnell, P. A., & Bradfield, R. H. *Mainstreaming: Controversy and consensus.* San Rafael, Calif.: Academic Therapy Publications, 1976.

Oliver, J. E., & Taylor, A. Five generations of ill-treated children in one family pedigree. *British Journal of Psychiatry,* 1971, *119,* 473–480.

O'Neill, N., & O'Neill, G. *Open marriage: A new lifestyle for couples.* New York: M. Evans, 1972.

Opper, S. Concept development in Thai urban and rural children. In P. R. Dasen (Ed.), *Piagetian psychology: Cross-cultural contributions.* New York: Gardner Press, 1977.

Osborn, A. *Applied imagination.* New York: Charles Scribner's, 1957.

Osgood, C. E. A behavioristic analysis of perception and language as cognitive phenomena. In *Contemporary approaches to cognition.* Cambridge, Mass.: Harvard University Press, 1957.

Ottinger, D. R., & Simmons, J. E. Behavior of human neonates and prenatal maternal emotions. *Psychological Reports,* 1964, *14,* 391–394.

Ovcharchyn, C. A., Johnson, H. H., & Petzel, T. P. Type A behavior, academic aspirations, and academic success. *Journal of Personality,* 1981, *49,* 248–256.

Packard, V. *The sexual wilderness.* New York: Pocket Books, 1968.

Page, E. B., & Grandon, G. M. Family configuration and mental ability: Two theories contrasted with U.S. data. *American Educational Research Journal,* 1979, *16,* 257–272.

Palmore, E. Physical, mental, and social factors in predicting longevity. *Gerontologist,* 1969, *9,* 103–108.

Palmore, E., & Cleveland, W. Aging, terminal decline, and terminal drop. *Journal of Gerontology,* 1975, *31,* 76–81.

Papalia, D. F. The status of several conservative abilities across the life-span. *Human Development,* 1972, *15,* 229–243.

Parke, R. D. Perspectives on father-infant interaction. In J. D. Osofsky (Ed.), *Handbook of infant development.* New York: John Wiley, 1979.

Parke, R. D., & Collmer, C. W. Child abuse: An interdisciplinary analysis. In E. M. Hetherington (Ed.), *Review of child development research* (Vol. 5). Chicago: University of Chicago, 1975.

Parke, R. D., & O'Leary, S. Father-mother-infant interaction in the newborn period: Some findings, some observations, and some unresolved issues. In K. Riegal & J. Meacham (Eds.), *The developing individual in a changing world* (Vol. 2). The Hague: Mouton, 1975.

Parke, R. D., & Sawin, D. B. The family in early infancy: Social interactional and attitudinal analyses. In F. A. Pedersen (Ed.), *The father-infant relationship: Observational studies in the family setting.* New York: Praeger, 1980.

Parnes, S. J., Noller, R. B., & Biondi, A. M. *Guide to creative action* (Rev. ed. of *Creative behavior guidebook*). New York: Charles Scribner's, 1977.

Parten, M. B. Social participation among pre-school children. *Journal of Abnormal Social Psychology,* 1932, *27,* 243–270.

Passman, R. H. *The effects of mothers and security blankets upon learning in children (Should Linus bring his blanket to school?).* Paper presented at the annual meeting of the American Psychological Association, New Orleans, September 1974.

Passman, R. H. Arousal reducing properties of attachment objects: Testing the functional limits of the security blanket relative to the mother. *Dewvelopmental Psychology,* 1976, *12,* 468–469.

Passman, R. H. Providing attachment objects to facilitate learning and reduce distress: Effects of mothers and security blankets. *Developmental Psychology,* 1977, *12,* 25–28.

Passman, R. H., & Erck, T. W. Permitting maternal contact through vision alone: Films of mothers for promoting play and locomotion. *Developmental Psychology,* 1978, *14,* 512–516.

Passman, R. H., & Mulhern, R. K. Maternal punitiveness as affected by situational stress: An experimental analogue of child abuse. *Journal of Abnormal Psychology,* 1977, *86,* 565–569.

Passman, R. H., & Weisberg, P. Mothers and blankets as agents for promoting play and exploration by young children in a novel environment: The effects of social and nonsocial attachment objects. *Developmental Psychology*, 1975, *11*, 170–177.

Patterson, F. Conversations with a gorilla. *National Geographic*, 1978, *54*, 438–465.

Paulson, F. L. Teaching cooperation on television: An evaluation of "Sesame Street" social goals programs. *A.V. Communication Review*, 1974, *22*, 229–246.

Pavlov, I. P. *Conditioned reflexes*. London: Oxford University Press, 1927.

Pearce, J. C. *The crack in the cosmic egg*. New York: Fawcett Books, 1971.

Pearce, J. C. *Magical child: Rediscovering nature's plan for our children*. New York: Bantam Books, 1977.

Pearse, W. H. Trends in out-of-hospital births. *Obstetrics and Gynecology*, 1982, *60*, 267–270.

Peck, R. C. Psychological developments in the second half of life. In B. L. Neugarten (Ed.), *Middle age and aging*. Chicago: University of Chicago Press, 1968.

Pedersen, F. A. (Ed.). *The father-infant relationship: Observational studies in the family setting*. New York: Praeger, 1980.

Pember, D. R. *Mass media in America* (2nd ed.). Chicago: Science Research Associates, 1977.

Peskin, H. Influence of the developmental schedule of puberty on learning and ego functioning. *Journal of Youth and Adolescence*, 1973, *2*, 273–290.

Peters, R. *The place of Kohlberg's theory in moral education*. Paper presented at the 1st International Conference on Moral Development and Moral Education, Leicester, England, August 19–26, 1977.

Petretic, P. A., & Tweney, R. D. Does comprehension precede production? The development of children's responses to telegraphic sentences of varying grammatical complexity. *Journal of Child Language*, 1977, *4*, 201–209.

Phillips, J. L. *The origins of intellect*. San Francisco: W. H. Freeman, 1969.

Piaget, J. *The moral judgment of the child*. London: Kegan Paul, 1932.

Piaget, J. *Play, dreams and imitation in childhood*. New York: W. W. Norton, 1951.

Piaget, J. *The origins of intelligence in children*. New York: International Universities Press, 1952.

Piaget, J. *The construction of reality in the child*. New York: Basic Books, 1954.

Piaget, J. Intellectual development from adolescence to adulthood. *Human Development*, 1972, *15*, 1–12.

Pinard, A., & Laurendeau, M. A scale of mental development based on the theory of Piaget: Description of a project (A. B. Givens, Trans.). *Journal of Research and Science Teaching*, 1964, *2*, 253–260.

Pinard, A., & Sharp, E. I.Q. and point of view. *Psychology Today*, June 1972, pp. 65–90.

Pines, M. *Revolution in learning: The years from birth to six*. New York: Harper & Row, 1966.

Pines, M. Invisible playmates. *Psychology Today*, September 1978, pp. 38–42, 106.

Pines, M. Superkids. *Psychology Today*, January 1979, pp. 53–63.

Pines, M. Baby, you're incredible. *Psychology Today*, February 1982, pp. 48–53.

Pingree, S., & Hawkins, R. P. Children and media. In M. Butler & W. Paisley (Eds.), *Women and the mass media: Sourcebook for research and action*. New York: Human Sciences Press, 1980.

Plomin, R. The difficult concept of temperament: A response to Thomas, Chess, and Korn. *Merrill-Palmer Quarterly*, 1982, *28*, 25–33.

Plomin, R., DeFries, J. C., & McClearn, G. E. *Behavior genetics: A primer*. New York: W. H. Freeman, 1980.

Potter, E. L. Pregnancy. In M. Fishbein & R. J. R. Kennedy (Eds.), *Modern marriage and family living*. New York: Oxford University Press, 1957.

Prado, W. *Appraisal of performance as a function of the relative-ego-involvement of children and adolescents*. Unpublished doctoral dissertation, University of Oklahoma, 1958.

Pratt, K. C. The neonate. In L. Carmichael (Ed.), *Manual of child psychology* (2nd ed.). New York: John Wiley, 1954.

Premack, A. J., & Premack, D. Teaching language to an ape. *Scientific American*, 1972, *227*, 92–99.

Pritchard, J., & MacDonald, P. *Williams obstetrics* (16th ed.). New York: Appleton-Century-Crofts, 1980.

Provine, R. R., & Westerman, J. A. Crossing the midline: Limits of early eye-hand behavior. *Child Development*, 1979, *50*, 804–814.

Pulaski, M. A. Toys and imaginative play. In J. L. Singer (Ed.), *The child's world of make-believe*. New York: Academic Press, 1973.

Pyles Honzik, M. K. Verbalization as a factor in learning. *Child Development*, 1932, *3*, 108–113.

Quetelet, A. *Sur l'homme et le développement de ses facultés* (2 vols.). Paris: Badielier, 1835.

Quinlans have no regret—lawyer. *Edmonton Journal*, March 19, 1983, p. A2.

Quinn, R. P., Staines, G. L., & McCullough, M. *Job satisfaction: Is there a trend?* U.S. Department of Labor, Manpower Research Monograph No. 30. Washington, D.C.: U.S. Government Printing Office, 1974.

Ramey, J. W. Emerging patterns of innovative behavior in marriage. *The Family Coordinator,* 1972, *21*, 435–456.

Ramsay, D., & Campos, J. Memory by the infant in an object notion task. *Developmental Psychology*, 1975, *11*, 411–412.

Rank, O. *The trauma of birth*. New York: Harcourt Brace Jovanovich, 1929.

Rawlings, G., Reynolds, E. O. R., Steward, A., & Strang, L. B. Changing prognosis for infants of very low birth weight. *The Lancet*, 1971, *1*, 516–519.

Rawlings, S. Perspectives on American husbands and wives. In *Current Population Reports: Special Studies, Series P-23, No. 77*. Washington, D.C.: U.S. Bureau of the Census, 1978.

Rayburn, W., Wilson, G., Schreck, J., Louwsma, G., & Hamman, J. Prenatal counseling: A state-wide telephone service. *Obstetrics and Gynecology*, 1982, *60*, 243–246.

Reardon, R. C., & Burck, H. D. (Eds.). *Facilitating career development: Strategies for counselors.* Springfield, Ill.: Charles C. Thomas, 1975.

Rebelsky, F., & Hanks, C. Fathers' verbal interaction with infants in the first three months of life. *Child Development*, 1972, *121*, 49–57.

Reeder, S., et al. *Maternity nursing* (14th ed.). Philadelphia: J. B. Lippincott, 1980.

Reese, H. W., & Overton, W. F. Models and theories of development. In L. R. Goulet & P. B. Baltes (Eds.), *Life-span developmental psychology: Research and theory.* New York: Academic Press, 1970.

Reisman, J. M. *The development of clinical psychology.* New York: Appleton-Century-Crofts, 1966.

Reiss, I. L. *The social context of premarital sexual permissiveness.* New York: Holt, Rinehart & Winston, 1966.

Rheingold, H. L., & Cook, K. V. The contents of boys' and girls' rooms as an index of parents' behavior. *Child Development*, 1975, *46*, 459–463.

Rice, B. The Hawthorne defect: Persistence of a flawed theory. *Psychology Today*, February 1982, pp. 71–74.

Riegel, K. F. The language acquisition process: A reinterpretation of selected research findings. In L. R. Goulet & P. B. Baltes (Eds.), *Life-span developmental psychology: Research and theory.* New York: Academic Press, 1970.

Riegel, K. F. Influence of economic and political ideologies on the development of developmental psychology. *Psychological Bulletin*, 1972, *78*, 129–141.

Riegel, K. F. Dialectic operations: The final period of cognitive development. *Human Development*, 1973, *16*, 346–370. (a)

Riegel, K. F. Language and cognition: Some life-span developmental issues. *Gerontologist*, 1973, *13*, 478–482. (b)

Riegel, K. F. The dialectics of human development. *American Psychologist*, 1976, *31*, 689–700.

Riegel, K. F., & Riegel, R. M. Development, drop, and death. *Developmental Psychology*, 1972, *6*, 306–319.

Rincover, A., & Koegel, R. L. Research on the education of autistic children: Recent advances and future directions. In B. B. Lahey & A. E. Kazdin (Eds.), *Advances in child clinical psychology.* New York: Plenum, 1977.

Ringler, N. M., Kennell, J. H., Jarvella, R., Navojosky, B. J., & Klaus, M. H. Mother to child speech at two years: Effects of early post-natal contact. *Journal of Pediatrics*, 1975, *86*, 141–144.

Roazen, P. *Freud and his followers.* New York: Alfred A. Knopf, 1975.

Roberts, D. F., & Bachan, C. M. Mass communication effects. In M. R. Rosenzweig & L. W. Porter (Eds.), *Annual review of psychology* (Vol. 32). Palo Alto, Calif.: Annual Reviews, 1981.

Robinson, J. T., Chitham, R. G., Greenwood, R. M., & Taylor, J. W. Chromosome aberrations and LSD: A controlled study in 50 psychiatric patients. *British Journal of Psychiatry*, 1974, *125*, 238–244.

Robinson, N. M., & Robinson, H. B. *The mentally retarded child: A psychological approach* (2nd ed.). New York: McGraw-Hill, 1976.

Roethlisberger, S. J., & Dickson, W. J. *Management and the worker.* Cambridge, Mass.: Harvard University Press, 1939.

Rogers, C. R. *Client-centered therapy: Its current practice, its implications, and theory.* Boston: Houghton Mifflin, 1951.

Rogers, C. R. *Freedom to learn.* Columbus, Ohio: Charles E. Merrill, 1969.

Rollins, B. C., & Feldman, H. Marital satisfaction over the family life cycle. In L. D. Steinberg (Ed.), *The life cycle: Readings in human development.* New York: Columbia University Press, 1981.

Rosenbaum, A. L., Churchill, J. A., Shakhashiri, Z. A., & Moody, R. L. Neuropsychologic outcome of children whose mothers had proteinuria during pregnancy. A report from the collaborative study of cerebral palsy. *Obstetrics and Gynecology*, 1969, *33*, 118–123.

Rosenberg, M. *Society and the adolescent self-image.* Princeton, N.J. Princeton University Press, 1965.

Rosenkrantz, P. S., Vogel, S. R., Bee, H., Broverman, I., & Broverman, D. Sex-role stereotypes and self-concepts in college students. *Journal of Consulting and Clinical Psychology*, 1968, *32*, 287–295.

Rosenman, R. H., Brand, R. J., Jenkins, C. D., Friedman, M., Straus, R., & Wurm, M. Coronary heart disease in the western collaborative group study: Final follow-up experience of 8½ years. *Journal of the American Medical Association*, 1975, *233*, 872–877.

Rosenthal, R. Experimenter expectancy and the reassuring nature of the null hypothesis decision procedure. *Psychological Bulletin Monographs Supplement*, 1969–1970, pp. 30–47.

Rosenthal, R., & Fode, K. L. The effect of experimenter bias on the performance of the albino rat. *Behavioral Science*, 1963, *8*, 183–189.

Rosenthal, R., & Jacobson, L. *Pygmalion in the classroom: Teacher expectations and pupils' intellectual development.* New York: Holt, Rinehart & Winston, 1968. (a)

Rosenthal, R., & Jacobson, L. Teacher expectations for the disadvantaged. *Scientific American*, 1968, *218*, 19–23. (b)

Rosenthal, T. L., & Zimmerman, B. J. Modeling by exemplification and instruction in training conservation. *Developmental Psychology*, 1972, *6*, 392–401.

Rosenwaks, Z. Estrogen replacement therapy. *Proceedings of the Conference on Health Issues of Older Women: A*

Projection to the Year 2000. Stony Brook, N.Y.: School of Allied Health Professions, State University of New York, 1981.

Rosett, H. L., & Sander, L. W. Effects of maternal drinking on neonatal morphology and state regulation. In J. D. Osofsky (Ed.), *Handbook of infant development*. New York: John Wiley, 1979.

Ross, A. O. *Psychological aspects of learning disabilities and reading disorders*. New York: McGraw-Hill, 1976.

Ross, A. O. *Psychological disorders of children: A behavioral approach to theory, research, and therapy* (2nd ed.). New York: McGraw-Hill, 1980.

Ross, A. O., & Pelham, W. E. Child psychopathology. In M. R. Rosenzweig & L. W. Porter (Eds.), *Annual review of psychology* (Vol. 32). Palo Alto, Calif.: Annual Reviews, 1981.

Rossi, A. S. Aging and parenthood in the middle years. In P. B. Baltes & O. G. Brim, Jr. (Eds.), *Life-span development and behavior* (Vol. 3). New York: Academic Press, 1980.

Rossman, I. Anatomic and body composition changes with aging. In C. Finch & L. Hayflick (Eds.), *Handbook of the biology of aging*. New York: Van Nostrand Reinhold, 1977.

Rothbart, M. K. The concept of difficult temperament: A critical analysis of Thomas, Chess, and Korn. *Merrill-Palmer Quarterly,* 1982, *28*, 35–40.

Rothman, E. P. *Troubled teachers*. New York: David McKay, 1977.

Rothstein, E. The scar of Sigmund Freud. *New York Review of Books*, October 9, 1980, pp. 14–20.

Rousseau, J. J. *Emile, or on education* (B. Foxley, trans.). London: Dent, 1911. (Originally published, 1762.)

Rubin, I. The "sexless older years": A socially harmful stereotype. *Annals of the American Academy of Political and Social Science*, 1968, *376*, 86–95.

Rubin, K. H., Attewell, P. W., Tierney, M. C., & Tumolo, P. Development of spatial egocentrism and conservation across the life-span. *Developmental Psychology*, 1973, *9*, 432.

Rubinstein, E. A., Comstock, G. A., & Murray, J. P. (Eds.). *Television and social behavior* (5 vols.). Washington, D.C.: U.S. Government Printing Office, 1972.

Rubovits, P. C., & Maehr, M. L. Pygmalion analyzed: Toward an explanation of the Rosenthal-Jacobson findings. *Journal of Personality and Social Psychology*, 1971, *19*, 197–203.

Rubovits, P. C., & Maehr, M. L. Pygmalion black and white. *Journal of Personality and Social Psychology*, 1973, *25*, 210–218.

Rumbaugh, D. M. (Ed.). *Language learning by a chimpanzee: The Lana project*. New York: Academic Press, 1977.

Russell, J. A., & Ward, L. M. Environmental psychology. In M. R. Rosenzweig & L. W. Porter (Eds.), *Annual review of psychology* (Vol. 33). Palo Alto, Calif.: Annual Reviews, 1982.

Rutter, M., Birch, H. G., Thomas, A., & Chess, S. Temperamental characteristics in infancy and the later development of behavioral disorders. *British Journal of Psychiatry,* 1964, *110*, 651–661.

Rutter, M., & Lockyer, L. A five to fifteen year follow-up study of infantile psychosis. I. Description of sample. *British Journal of Psychiatry*, 1967, *113*, 1167–1182.

Sachs, J., & Truswell, L. Comprehension of two-word instructions by children in the one-word stage. *Journal of Child Language,* 1978, *5*, 17–24.

Sagan, C. *The dragons of Eden*. New York: Ballantine Books, 1977.

Sampson, E. E. Birth order, need achievement, and conformity. *Journal of Abnormal and Social Psychology*, 1962, *64*, 155–159.

Sato, S., Dreifuss, F. E., & Penry, J. K. Prognostic factors in absence seizures. *Neurology*, 1976, *26*, 788.

Scanzoni, L. D., & Scanzoni, J. *Men, women, and change: A sociology of marriage and family* (2nd ed.). New York: McGraw-Hill, 1981.

Scarr, S., & Salapatek, P. Patterns of fear development during infancy. *Merrill-Palmer Quarterly*, 1970, *16*, 56–90.

Scarr, S., & Weinberg, R. A. Intellectual similarities within families of both adopted and biological children. *Intelligence*, 1977, *1*, 170–191.

Scarr-Salapatek, S., & Williams, M. L. The effects of early stimulation on low-birth-weight infants. *Child Development*, 1973, *44*, 94–101.

Schaefer, C. E. Imaginary companions and creative adolescents. *Developmental Psychology*, 1969, *1*, 747–749.

Schaefer, E. S. Children's reports of parental behavior: An inventory. *Child Development*, 1965, *36*, 413–424.

Schaffer, H. R. The onset of fear of strangers and the incongruity hypothesis. *Journal of Child Psychology and Psychiatry*, 1966, 7, 95–106.

Schaffer, H. R. (Ed.). *Studies in mother-infant interaction*. London: Academic Press, 1977.

Schaffer, H. R., Collis, G. M., & Parsons, G. Vocal interchange and visual regard in verbal and pre-verbal children. In H. R. Schaffer (Ed.), *Studies in mother-infant interaction*. London: Academic Press, 1977.

Schaffer, H. R., & Emerson, P. E. The development of social attachment in infancy. *Monographs of the Society for Research in Child Development*, 1964 (Whole No. 94).

Schaie, K. W. A general model for the study of developmental problems. *Psychological Bulletin*, 1965, *64*, 92–107.

Schaie, K. W. Translations in gerontology—from lab to life: Intellectual functioning. *American Psychologist*, 1974, *29*, 802–807.

Schaie, K. W. The primary mental abilities in adulthood: An exploration in the development of psychometric intelligence. In P. B. Baltes & O. G. Brim, Jr. (Eds.), *Life-span development and behavior*. New York: Academic Press, 1979.

Schaie, K. W., & Gribbin, K. Adult development and aging. In M. R. Rosenzweig & L. W. Porter (Eds.), *Annual review of psychology* (Vol. 26). Palo Alto, Calif.: Annual Reviews, 1975.

Schaie, K. W., & Labouvie-Vief, G. Generational versus ontogenetic components of change in adult cognitive behavior: A fourteen year cross-sequential study. *Developmental Psychology*, 1974, *10*, 305–320.

Scheiner, A. P., & McNabb, N. A. The child with mental retardation. In A. P. Scheiner & I. F. Abroms (Eds.), *The practical management of the developmentally disabled child*. St. Louis: C. V. Mosby, 1980.

Scheinfeld, A. *Your heredity and environment*. Philadelphia: J. B. Lippincott, 1965.

Schmidt, G., & Sigusch, V. Women's sexual arousal. In J. Zubin & J. Money (Eds.), *Contemporary sexual behavior: Critical issues in the 1970s*. Baltimore: Johns Hopkins University Press, 1973.

Schramm, W., Lyle, J., & Parker, E. G. *Television in the lives of our children*. Stanford, Calif.: Stanford University Press, 1961.

Schulz, D. A. *The changing family: Its function and future*. Englewood Cliffs, N.J.: Prentice-Hall, 1982.

Schulz, D. A., & Rodgers, S. F. *Marriage, the family, and personal fulfillment* (2nd ed.). Englewood Cliffs, N.J.: Prentice-Hall, 1980.

Schweinhardt, L. J., & Weikart, D. P. Can preschool education make a long lasting difference? *Bulletin of the High/Scope Educational Research Foundation*, 1977, No. 4.

Searle, L. V. The organization of hereditary maze-brightness and maze-dullness. *Genetic Psychology Monographs*, 1949, *39*, 279–325.

Sears, R. R., Maccoby, E. P., & Lewin, H. *Patterns of Child Rearing*. New York: Harper & Row, 1957.

Sebeok, T. A., & Umiker-Sebeok, J. Performing animals: Secrets of the trade. *Psychology Today*, November 1979, pp. 78–91.

Sebeok, T. A., & Umiker-Sebeok, D. J. (Eds.). *Speaking of apes: A critical anthology of two-way communication with man*. New York: Plenum, 1980.

Seiden, R. H. Campus tragedy: A study of students' suicide. *Journal of Abnormal Psychology*, 1966, *71*, 389–399.

Seligman, M. E. P. *Helplessness: On depression, development, and death*. New York: W. H. Freeman, 1975.

Shaffer, D. R. *Social and personality development*. Monterey, Calif.: Brooks/Cole, 1979.

Shantz, C. U. The development of social cognition. In E. M. Hetherington (Ed.), *Review of child development research* (Vol. 5). Chicago: University of Chicago Press, 1975.

Shapira, A., & Madsen, M. C. Between and within group cooperation and competition among kibbutz and non-kibbutz children. *Developmental Psychology*, 1974, *10*, 140–145.

Shearer, L. Children bearing children. *Parade Magazine*, June 5, 1977, p. 16.

Sheehy, G. *Passages: Predictable crises of adult life*. New York: E. P. Dutton, 1976.

Sheppard, H. Work and retirement. In R. Binstock & E. Shanas (Eds.), *Handbook of aging and the social sciences*. New York: Van Nostrand Reinhold, 1976.

Sherman, M. *Hollow folk*. New York: Crowell, 1933.

Sherman, M., & Key, C. B. The intelligence of isolated mountain children. *Child Development*, 1932, *3*, 279–290.

Sherman, M., & Sherman, I. C. *The process of human behavior*. New York: W. W. Norton, 1929.

Shirley, M. M. *The first two years: A study of 25 babies* (Vol. 1). Institute of Child Welfare Series, No. 6. Minneapolis: University of Minnesota Press, 1933.

Shock, N. W. Biological theories of aging. In J. E. Birren and K. W. Schaie (Eds.), *Handbook of the psychology of aging*. New York: Van Nostrand Reinhold, 1977.

Short, J. F., Jr., & Nye, F. I. Reported behavior as a deviant behavior. *Social Problems*, 1957–1958, *5*, 207–213.

Shotland, R. L., & Straw, M. K. Bystander response to an assault: When a man attacks a woman. *Journal of Personality and Social Psychology*, 1976, *3*, 65–74.

Shuttleworth, F. K. The physical and mental growth of girls and boys age 6 to 19 in relation to age at maximum growth. *Monographs of the Society for Research in Child Development*, 1939, *4*(Serial No. 3).

Siegel, E., & Morris, N. M. Family planning: Its health rationale. *American Journal of Obstetrics and Gynecology*, 1974, *118*, 995.

Siegler, R. S., & Liebert, R. M. Effects of presenting relevant rules and complete feedback on the conservation of liquid quantity task. *Developmental Psychology*, 1972, 7, 133–138.

Signori, E. I., Butt, D. S., & Kozak, J. F. Dimensions in attitudes toward the aged. *Canadian Counsellor*, 1980, *14*, 88–92.

Silverman, S. R. The education of deaf children. In L. E. Davis (Ed.), *Handbook of speech pathology and audiology*. Englewood Cliffs, N.J.: Prentice-Hall, 1971.

Simmons, L. Aging in preindustrial societies. In C. Tibbitts (Ed.), *Handbook of social gerontology*. Chicago: University of Chicago Press, 1960.

Singer, D. G., & Revenson, T. A. *How a child thinks: A Piaget primer*. New York: New American Library, 1978.

Singer, J. L. (Ed.). *The child's world of make-believe: Experimental studies of imaginative play*. New York: Academic Press, 1973.

Singer, J. L., & Singer, D. B. Come back, Mister Rogers, come back. *Psychology Today*, March 1979, pp. 56–60.

Singer, R. S. Childhood, aggression and television. *Television and Children*, 1982, *5*, 57–63.

Singh, J. A., & Zingg, R. N. *Wolf-children and feral man*. New York: Harper & Row, 1942.

Skinner, B. F. *Science and human behavior*. New York: Macmillan, 1953.

Skinner, B. F. *Verbal behavior*. New York: Appleton-Century-Crofts, 1957.

Skinner, B. F. *Cumulative record* (rev. ed.). New York: Appleton-Century-Crofts, 1961.

Skolnick, A. The myth of the vulnerable child. *Psychology Today*, February 1978, pp. 56–60; 65.

Skolnick, A. Married lives: Longitudinal perspectives on marriage. In D. H. Eichorn, J. A. Clausen, N. Haan, M. P. Honzik, & P. H. Mussen (Eds.), *Present and past in middle life*. New York: Academic Press, 1981.

Slobin, D. I. Universals of grammatical development in children. In G. B. Flores D'Arcais & W. J. M. Levelt (Eds.), *Advances in Psycholinguistics*, Amsterdam: North Holland, 1970.

Slobin, D. I. They learn the same way all around the world. *Psychology Today*, July 1972, pp. 71–74; 82.

Smedslund, J. The acquisition of conservation of substance and weight in children: 1. Introduction. *Scandinavian Journal of Psychology*, 1961, *2*, 11–20. (a)

Smedslund, J. The acquisition of conservation of substance and weight in children: 2. External reinforcement of conservation of weight and of operations of addition and subtraction. *Scandinavian Journal of Psychology*, 1961, *2*, 71–84. (b)

Smedslund, J. The acquisition of conservation of substance and weight in children: 3. Extinction of conservation of weight acquired "normally" and by means of empirical controls on a balance scale. *Scandinavian Journal of Psychology*, 1961, *2*, 85–87. (c)

Smedslund, J. The acquisition of conservation of substance and weight in children: 4. An attempt at extinction of visual components of the weight concept. *Scandinavian Journal of Psychology*, 1961, *2*, 153–155. (d)

Smedslund, J. The acquisition of conservation of substance and weight in children: 5. Practice in conflict situations without external reinforcement. *Scandinavian Journal of Psychology*, 1961, *2*, 156–160. (e)

Smith, B. E., & Steinfield, J. The hippie communal movement: Effects on childbirth and development. *American Journal of Orthopsychiatry*, 1970, *40*, 527–530.

Smith, D. W., & Wilson, A. A. *The child with Down's syndrome (mongolism)*. Philadelphia: W. B. Saunders, 1973.

Smith, M. E. An investigation of the development of the sentence and the extent of vocabulary in young children. *University of Iowa Studies in Child Welfare*, 1926, *3*(5).

Smith, M. K. Measurement of the size of general English vocabulary through the elementary grades and high school. *Genetic Psychology Monographs*, 1941, *24*, 311–345.

Smoking imperils the unborn. *Science News*, January 27, 1979, p. 55.

Sobol, M. Commitment to work. In F. Nye & L. Hoffman (Eds.), *The employed mother in America*. Chicago: Rand McNally, 1963.

Sontag, L., & Wallace, R. I. Preliminary report of the Fels Fund: A study of fetal activity. *American Journal of Diseases of Children*, 1934, *48*, 1050–1057.

Sorensen, R. C. *Adolescent sexuality in contemporary America*. New York: World Publishing Co., 1973.

Spelt, D. K. The conditioning of the human fetus in utero. *Journal of Experimental Psychology*, 1948, *38*, 375–376.

Spitz, R. A. Hospitalism: An inquiry into the genesis of psychiatric conditions in early childhood. Part 1. *Psychoanalytic Studies of the Child*, 1945, *1*, 53–74.

Spitz, R. A. Unhappy and fatal outcomes of emotional deprivation and stress in infancy. In I. Galdston (Ed.), *Beyond the germ theory*. Washington, D.C.: Health Education Council, 1954.

Spring, C., & Sandoval, J. Food additives and hyperkinesis: A critical evaluation of the evidence. *Journal of Learning Disabilities*, 1976, *9*, 560–569.

Sroufe, L., & Waters, E. The ontogenesis of smiling and laughter: A perspective on the organization of development in infancy. *Psychological Review,* 1976, *83*, 173–189.

Sroufe, L., & Wunsch, J. The development of laughter in the first year of life. *Child Development*, 1972, *43*, 1326–1344.

Standing. L. Learning 10,000 pictures. *Quarterly Journal of Experimental Psychology,* 1973, *25*, 207–222.

Starr, R. H., Jr. Child abuse. *American Psychologist*, 1979, *34*, 872–878.

Starr, R. H., Jr. A research-based approach to the prediction of child abuse. In R. H. Starr, Jr. (Ed.), *Child abuse prediction: Policy implications*. Cambridge, Mass.: Ballinger, 1982.

Starr, R. H., Jr., Dietrich, K. N., & Fischhoff, J. *The contribution of children to their own abuse*. Paper presented at a meeting of the Society for Research in Child Development, Boston, April 1981.

Statistical Office of the United Nations, Department of Economic and Social Affairs. *Demographic Yearbook, 1978*. New York: United Nations, 1979.

Stayton, D., Ainsworth, M. D. S., & Main, M. Development of separation behavior in the first year of life: Protest, following and greeting. *Developmental Psychology*, 1973, *9*, 213–225.

Stein, S. B. *New parents' guide to early learning*. New York: New American Library, 1976.

Stein, Z., Susser, M., Saenger, G., & Marolla, F. *Famine and human development: The Dutch hunger winter of 1944–1945*. New York: Oxford University Press, 1975.

Stern, C. Hereditary factors affecting adoption. In *A Study of Adoption Practices* (Vol. 2). New York: Child Welfare League of America, 1956.

Stewart, R. B., Cluff, L. E., & Philp, R. *Drug monitoring: A requirement for responsible drug use*. Baltimore: Williams & Wilkins, 1977.

Stolk, M. V. Who owns the child? *Childhood Education*, 1974, *50*, 259–265.

Straus, M. A. Wife-beating: How common and why? In M. A.

Straus & G. T. Hotaling (Eds.), *The social causes of husband-wife violence*. Minneapolis: University of Minnesota Press, 1980. (a)

Straus, M. A. The marriage license as a hitting license: Evidence from popular culture, law, and social science. In M. A. Straus & G. T. Hotaling (Eds.), *The social causes of husband-wife violence*. Minneapolis: University of Minnesota Press, 1980. (b)

Strauss, A. *On social psychology: Selected papers.* Chicago: University of Chicago Press, 1964.

Strauss, B. V. The dynamics of ordinal position. *Quarterly Journal of Child Behavior*, 1959, *3*, 133–145.

Strean, H. S. *The extramarital affair.* New York: Free Press, 1980.

Streissguth, A. P., Herman, C. S., & Smith, D. W. Intelligence, behavior, and dysmorphogenesis in the fetal alcohol syndrome: A report on 20 patients. *Journal of Pediatrics*, 1978, *92*(3), 363–367.

Stuart, R. B. Critical reappraisal and reformulation of selected "mental health" programs. In L. A. Hamerlynck, P. O. Davidson, & L. E. Acker (Eds.), *Behavior modification and mental health services*. Calgary, Alberta: University of Calgary Press, 1969.

Sullivan, E. V. *A study of Kohlberg's structural theory of moral development: A critique of liberal social science ideology*. Unpublished manuscript, Ontario Institute for Studies in Education, Toronto, 1977.

Sullivan, E. V., & Quarter, J. Psychological correlates of certain postconventional moral types: A perspective on hybrid types. *Journal of Personality*, 1972, *40*(2), 149–161.

Sullivan, H. S. *The interpersonal theory of psychiatry.* New York: W. W. Norton, 1953.

Suls, J., & Kalle, R. J. Children's moral judgments as a function of intention, damage, and an actor's physical harm. *Developmental Psychology*, 1979, *15*, 93–94.

Super, D. E. *The psychology of careers.* New York: Harper & Row, 1957.

Super, D. E. Vocational maturity theory. In D. E. Super (Ed.), *Measuring vocational maturity for counseling and evaluation*. Washington, D.C.: National Vocational Guidance Association, 1974.

Super, D. E., & Hall, D. T. Career development: Exploration and planning. In M. R. Rosenzweig & L. W. Porter (Eds.), *Annual review of psychology* (Vol. 29). Palo Alto, Calif.: Annual Reviews, 1978.

Sutton-Smith, B., Roberts, J. W., & Rosenberg, B. G. Sibling associations and role involvement. *Merrill-Palmer Quarterly*, 1964, *10*, 25–38.

Swift, P. High school drunks. *Parade Magazine*, February 9, 1975, p. 13.

Talbert, G. B. Aging of the reproductive system. In C. Finch & L. Hayflick (Eds.), *Handbook of the biology of aging*. New York: Van Nostrand Reinhold, 1977.

Tallmer, M., Formanek, R., & Tallmer, J. Factors influencing children's concepts of death. *Journal of Clinical Child Psychology*, 1974, *3*, 17–19.

Tan, A. S. TV beauty ads and role expectations of adolescent female viewers. *Journal Questionnaire*, 1976, *53*, 271–279.

Tanner, J. M. *Growth at adolescence.* Springfield, Ill.: Charles C. Thomas, 1955.

Tanner, J. M. *Fetus into man: Physical growth from conception to maturity.* Cambridge, Mass.: Harvard University Press, 1978.

Teahan, J., & Kastenbaum, R. Subjective life expectancy and future time perspective as predictors of job success in the "hard core unemployed." *Omega*, 1970, *1*, 189–200.

Telfer, M. A., Baker, D., Clark, G. R., & Richardson, C. E. Incidence of gross chromosomal errors among tall, criminal American males. *Science*, 1968, *159*, 1249–1250.

Templin, M. C. *Certain language skills in children.* Minneapolis: University of Minnesota Press, 1957.

Terkel, S. *Working.* New York: Random House, 1972.

Terman, L. M., assisted by B. T. Baldwin and others. *Genetic studies of genius* (Vol. 1). Stanford, Calif.: Stanford University Press, 1925.

Terman, L. M., & Merrill, M. A. *Revised Stanford-Binet intelligence scale* (2nd ed.). Boston: Houghton Mifflin, 1973.

Terrace, H. S. Can an ape create a sentence? *Science*, November 23, 1979. (a)

Terrace, H. S. How Nim Chimpsky changed my mind. *Psychology Today*, November 1979, pp. 65–76. (b)

Terrace, H. S. *Nim: A chimpanzee who learned sign language.* New York: Alfred A. Knopf, 1980.

Tessman, L. H. *Children of parting parents.* New York: Aronson, 1978.

Thomas A., Chess, S., & Birch, H. G. *Temperament and behavior disorders in children.* New York: New York University Press, 1968.

Thomas, A., Chess, S., & Birch, H. G. The origin of personality. *Scientific American*, 1970, *223*, 102–109.

Thomas, A., Chess, S., & Korn, S. J. The reality of difficult temperament. *Merrill-Palmer Quarterly*, 1982, *28*, 1–20.

Thomas, J. W. Agency and achievement: Self-management and self-regard. *Review of Educational Research*, 1980, *50*, 213–240.

Thomas, R. M. *Comparing theories of child development.* Belmont, Calif.: Wadsworth, 1979.

Thompson, R. F. *Introduction to physiological psychology.* New York: Harper & Row, 1975.

Thorndike, R. L., & Hagen, E. *Measurement and evaluation in psychology and education* (4th ed.). New York: John Wiley, 1977.

Tibbetts, S. L. Sex role stereotyping in the lower grades: Part of the solution. *Journal of Vocational Behavior*, 1975, *6*, 255–261.

Timiras, P. S. *Developmental physiology and aging.* New York: Macmillan, 1972.

Tittle, C. K. Career counseling in contemporary U.S. high schools: An addendum to Rehberg and Hotchkiss. *Educational Researcher*, 1982, *11*, 12–18.

Tobin, S. S., & Kulys, R. The family in the institutionalization of the elderly. *Journal of Social Issues*, 1981, *37*, 145–157.

Toffler, A. *Future shock*. New York: Random House, 1970.

Torrance, E. P. *Guiding creative talent*. Englewood Cliffs, N.J.: Prentice-Hall, 1962.

Torrance, E. P. Torrance's tests of creative thinking. *Norms technical manual*. Princeton, N.J.: Personnel Press, 1966.

Torres, D. A. Youths and alcohol abuse: A continuing phenomenon. *Journal of Alcohol and Drug Education*, 1982, *27*, 74–82.

Travis, L. D. *Conservation acceleration through successive approximations*. Unpublished master's thesis, University of Alberta, Edmonton, 1969.

Trent, J. W., & Crais, J. L. Commitment and conformity in the American college. *Journal of Social Issues*, 1967, *22*, 34–51.

Trent, J. W., & Medsker, L. L. *Beyond high school: A study of 10,000 high school graduates*. Berkeley: Center for Research and Development in Higher Education, University of California, 1967.

Troll, L. E. *Continuations: Adult development and aging*. Monterey, Calif.: Brooks/Cole, 1982.

Troll, L. E., Miller, S., & Atchley, R. C. *Families of later life*. Belmont, Calif.: Wadsworth, 1979.

Troll, L. E., & Nowak, C. "How old are you?"—The question of age bias in the counseling of adults. *Counseling Psychologist*, 1976, *6*, 41–44.

Trost, J. Married and unmarried cohabitation: The case of Sweden, with some comparisons. *Journal of Marriage and the Family*, 1975, *37*, 677–682.

Tryon, R. C. Genetic differences in maze learning in rats. *Yearbook of the National Society for Studies in Education*, 1940, *39*, 111–119.

Tucker, B. Pregnancy and drugs. *Addictions*, 1975, *22*, 2–19.

Tuddenham, R. D. Studies in reputation: 3. Correlates of popularity among elementary school children. *Journal of Educational Psychology*, 1951, *42*, 257–276.

Turiel, E. Distinct conceptual and developmental domains: Social-convention and morality. In *Nebraska Symposium on Motivation*, 1977, *25*, 77–116.

Turner, B. F., & McCaffrey, J. H. Socialization and career orientation among black and white college women. *Journal of Vocational Behavior*, 1974, *5*, 307–319.

Uguroglu, M. E., & Walberg, H. J. Motivation and achievement: A quantitative synthesis. *American Educational Research Journal*, 1979, *16*, 375–389.

U.S. Department of Commerce, Bureau of the Census. *Social indicators III: Selected data on social conditions and trends in the United States*. Washington, D.C.: U.S. Government Printing Office, 1980.

U.S. Department of Health & Human Services. *Alcohol and health: New knowledge*. Second special report to the U.S. Congress. Washington, D.C.: U.S. Government Printing Office, June 1974.

U.S. Department of Labor. *The dictionary of occupational titles* (3rd ed.). Washington, D.C.: U.S. Government Printing Office, 1965.

U.S. Department of Labor. *The dictionary of occupational titles* (4th ed.). Washington, D.C.: U.S. Government Printing Office, 1978.

U.S. Office of Education. *Estimated number of handicapped children in the United States, 1974–1975*. Washington, D.C.: Bureau of Education for the Handicapped, 1975.

Uzgiris, I. C., & Hunt, J. *Assessment in infancy: Ordinal scales of psychological development*. Urbana: University of Illinois Press, 1975.

Vaillant, G. *Adaptation to life*. Boston: Little, Brown, 1977.

Van den Daele, L. D. Modification of infant state by treatment in a rockerbox. *Journal of Psychology*, 1970, *74*, 161–165.

Vaz, E., & Lodhi, A. *Crime and delinquency in Canada*. Scarborough, Ontario: Prentice-Hall, 1979.

Velandia, W., Grandon, G. M., & Page, E. B. Family size, birth order, and intelligence in a large South American sample. *American Educational Research Journal*, 1978, *15*, 399–416.

Vernon, P. E. *Intelligence, heredity and environment*. New York: W. H. Freeman, 1979.

Veroff, J. Social comparison and development of achievement motivation. In C. P. Smith (Ed.), *Achievement related motives in children*. New York: Russell Sage Foundation, 1969.

Vincent, C. E. Teenage unwed mothers in American society. *Journal of Social Issues*, 1966, *22*, 22–23.

von Hofsten, C., & Lindhagen, K. Observations on the development of reaching for moving objects. *Journal of Experimental Child Psychology*, 1979, *28*, 158–173.

Waddington, C. H. *The evolution of an evolutionist*. Edinburgh: Edinburgh University Press, 1975.

Wade, N. IQ and heredity: Suspicion of fraud beclouds classic experiment. *Science*, 1976, *194*, 916–919.

Walker, E. L. *Conditioning and instrumental learning*. Belmont, Calif.: Brooks/Cole, 1968.

Walker, J. J. The gifted and talented. In E. L. Meyen (Ed.), *Exceptional children and youth: An introduction*. Denver, Colo.: Love Publishing, 1978.

Wallerstein, J. S., & Kelly, J. B. The effects of parental divorce: The adolescent experience. In E. J. Anthony & C. Koupernik (Eds.), *The child in his family: Children at psychiatric risk* (Vol. 3). New York: John Wiley, 1974.

Wallerstein, J. S., & Kelly, J. B. The effects of parental divorce: Experiences of the preschool child. *Journal of the American Academy of Child Psychiatry*, 1975, *14*, 600–616.

Wallerstein, J. S., & Kelly, J. B. The effects of parental divorce: Experiences of the child in later latency. *American Journal of Orthopsychiatry*, 1976, *46*, 256–269.

Walsh, B. T. Endocrine disturbance in anorexia nervosa and depression. *Psychosomatic Medicine*, 1982, *44*, 85–91.

Ward, R. A *The aging experience: An introduction to social gerontology*. Philadelphia: J. B. Lippincott, 1979.

Wardhaugh, R. *The contents of language.* Rowley, Mass.: Newbury House, 1976.

Waring, J. *The middle years: A multidisciplinary view.* New York: Academy for Educational Development, 1978.

Wasserman, G. The nature and function of early mother-infant interaction. In B. L. Blum (Ed.), *Psychological aspects of pregnancy, birthing, and bonding.* New York: Human Sciences Press, 1980.

Watson, J. B. *Behavior: An introduction to comparative psychology.* New York: Holt, Rinehart & Winston, 1914.

Watson, J. B., & Rayner, R. Conditioned emotional reactions. *Journal of Experimental Psychology,* 1920, *3,* 1–14.

Watson, J. D. Involvement of RNA in the synthesis of proteins. *Science,* 1963, *140,* 17–26.

Wechsler, D. *The measurement and appraisal of adult intelligence* (4th ed.). Baltimore: Williams & Wilkins, 1958.

Weideger, P. *Menstruation and menopause: The physiology and psychology, the myth and the reality.* New York: Alfred A. Knopf, 1976.

Weikart, D. P., & Lambie, D. Z. Preschool intervention through a home teaching program. In J. Hellmuth (Ed.), *Disadvantaged child: Head Start and early intervention* (Vol. 2). Seattle, Wash.: Special Child Publications, 1968.

Weikart, D. P., Lambie, D. Z., Wozniak, R., Hull, W., Miller, N., & Jeffs, M. *Ypsilanti-Carnegie infant education project: Progress report.* Ypsilanti, Mich.: Department of Research and Development, Ypsilanti Public Schools, September 1969.

Weiner, B. A theory of motivation for some classroom experiences. *Journal of Educational Psychology,* 1979, *71,* 3–25.

Weiner, B. *Human motivation.* New York: Holt, Rinehart & Winston, 1980. (a)

Weiner, B. The role of affect in rational (attributional) approaches to human motivation. *Educational Researcher,* 1980, *9,* 4–11. (b)

Weininger, B., & Menkin, E. L. *Aging is a lifelong affair.* Los Angeles: Guild of Tutors Press, 1978.

Weisberg, P., & Russell, J. E. Proximity and interactional behavior of young children to their "security" blanket. *Child Development,* 1971, *42,* 1575–1579.

Weitz, R. The public, the primary physician, and genetic counselling. *Patient Counselling and Health Education,* 1981, first quarter, 13–16.

Wertham, F. *Seduction of the innocent.* New York: Holt, Rinehart & Winston, 1954.

Werts, C. E. Maternal influence on career choice. *Journal of Counseling Psychology,* 1968, *15,* 48–52.

Wesley, F., & Wesley, C. *Sex-role psychology.* New York: Human Sciences Press, 1977.

Whelan, R. J. The emotionally disturbed. In E. L. Meyen (Ed.), *Exceptional children and youth: An introduction.* Denver, Colo.: Love Publishing, 1978.

White, B. L. *The first three years of life.* Englewood Cliffs, N.J.: Prentice-Hall, 1975.

Whiting, H. T. A. *Acquiring ball skill, a psychological interpretation.* London: G. Bell, 1969.

Whorf, B. L. The relation of habitual thought and behavior to language. In L. Spier (Ed.), *Language, culture and personality.* Salt Lake City: University of Utah Press, 1941.

Whorf, B. L. *Language, thought and reality.* New York: John Wiley, 1956.

Wiener, G. The relationship of birth weight and length of gestation to intellectual development at ages 8 to 10 years. *Journal of Pediatrics,* 1970, *76,* 694.

Wiley, J. A psychology of auditory impairment. In W. M. Cruickshank (Ed.), *Psychology of exceptional children and youth* (3rd ed.). Englewood Cliffs, N.J.: Prentice-Hall, 1971.

Willemsen, E. *Understanding infancy.* New York: W. H. Freeman, 1979.

Willerman, L. Activity level and hyperactivity in twins. *Child Development,* 1973, *44,* 288–293.

Williams, R. L., & Long, J. D. *Toward a self-managed life style* (2nd ed.). Boston: Houghton Mifflin, 1978.

Wilson, R. S. Synchronies in mental development: An epigenetic perspective. *Science,* 1978, *202,* 939–948.

Winick, M. Nutrition and cell growth. *Nutrition Review,* 1968, *26,* 195–197.

Witkin, H. A., Mednick, S. A., Schulsinger, F., Bakkestrom, E., Christiansen, K. O., Goodenough, D. R., Hirschhorn, K., Lundesteen, C., Owen, D. R., Philip, J., Rubin, D. B., & Stocking, M. Criminality in XYY and XXY men. *Science,* 1976, *193,* 547–555.

Wohlwill, J. F. Methodology and research strategy in the study of developmental change. In L. R. Goulet & P. B. Baltes (Eds.), *Life-span developmental psychology: Research and theory.* New York: Academic Press, 1970.

Wohlwill, J. F. *The study of behavioral development.* New York: Academic Press, 1973.

Wolff, P. H. Observations on newborn infants. *Psychosomatic Medicine,* 1959, *21,* 110–118.

Wolff, P. H. Observations of the early development of smiling. In B. M. Foss (Ed.), *Determinants of infant behavior 2.* London: Methuen, 1963.

Wolff, P. H. The causes, controls, and organization of behavior in the neonate. *Psychological Issues,* 1966, *5*(1) (Whole No. 17), 1–105.

Wolff, P. H. The natural history of crying and other vocalizations in early infancy. In B. Foss (Ed.), *Determinants of infant behavior 4.* London: Methuen, 1969.

Wood, B. S. *Children and communication: Verbal and nonverbal language development.* Englewood Cliffs, N.J.: Prentice-Hall, 1976.

Wortis, H., Heimer, C. B., Braine, M., Redlo, M., & Rue, R. Growing up in Brooklyn: The early history of the premature child. *American Journal of Orthopsychiatry,* 1963, *33,* 535–539.

Wright, H. F. Observational child study. In P. H. Mussen (Ed.), *Handbook of research methods in child development.* New York: John Wiley, 1960.

Wurtman, R. J., & Wurtman, J. J. (Eds.). *Nutrition and the brain* (Vol. 1). New York: Raven Press, 1977.

Yager, J. Family issues in the pathogenesis of anorexia nervosa. *Psychosomatic Medicine*, 1982, *44*, 43–60.

Yankelovich, D. *The changing values on campus*. New York: Washington Square Press, 1972.

Yankelovich, D. The new psychological contracts at work. *Psychology Today*, May 1978, pp. 46–50.

Yarrow, L. J. Research in dimensions of early maternal care. *Merrill-Palmer Quarterly*, 1963, 9, 101–114.

Yarrow, L. J., & Goodwin, M. S. The immediate impact of separation: Reactions of infants to a change in mother figures. In L. J. Stone, H. T. Smith, & L. B. Murphy (Eds.), *The competent infant: Research and commentary*. New York: Basic Books, 1973.

Yarrow, M. R., Scott, P. L., & Zahn-Waxler, C. Learning concern for others. *Developmental Psychology*, 1973, *8*, 240–260.

Yarrow, M. R., & Zahn-Waxler, C. The emergence and functions of prosocial behaviors in young children. In R. Smart & M. Smart (Eds.), *Readings in child development and relationships* (2nd ed.). New York: Macmillan, 1977.

Yensen, R. On the measurement of happiness and its implications for welfare. In L. Levi (Ed.), *Emotions: Their parameters and measurement*. New York: Raven Press, 1975.

Zajonc, R. B. Family configuration and intelligence. *Science*, 1976, *192*, 227–236.

Zajonc, R. B., & Markus, G. B. Birth order and intellectual development. *Psychological Review*, 1975, *82*, 74–88.

Zamenhof, S., van Marthens, E., & Margolis, F. L. DNA (cell number) and protein in neonatal brain: Alteration by maternal dietary protein restriction. *Science*, 1968, *160*, 322–323.

Zeligs, R. *Children's experience with death*. Springfield Ill.: Charles C. Thomas, 1974.

Zingg, R. N. Reply to Professor Dennis. *American Journal of Psychology*, 1941, 54, 432–435.

PHOTO CREDITS

Freyberg, J. T., 210
Friedan, B., 222
Friedman, A. S., 345
Friedman, M. L., 342
Frisch, R. E., 302
Furniss, J., 345
Furry, C. A., 451
Furth, H. G., 243, 282, 309

Gallagher, J. J., 249
Gallistel, C. R., 243, 245
Galton, Francis, 69, 220
Garbarino, J., 226
Gardner, B. T., 186–187
Gardner, H., 209
Gardner, R. A., 186–187
Garmezy, N., 286
Garretson, M. D., 282
Gates, A., 103
Gayford, J. J., 429
Gebhard, D. H., 337, 417–418, 421, 448
Gelles, R. J., 225–227, 428
Gelman, R., 182, 243, 245
Gerber, M., 126
Gerbner, G., 259
Gesell, A., 60, 124, 174–175, 261
Getz, S. K., 261
Getzels, J. W., 216, 413
Gewirtz, J. L., 148, 159
Gibson, E. J., 129
Gil, D. G., 225–228
Ginzberg, E., 410
Giordani, B., 397
Glazer, J. A., 251
Glick, P. G., 214, 416
Glucksberg, S., 200
Goddard, H. H., 70
Goddard, K. E., 100
Goldberg, M. E., 261
Goldfarb, W., 284
Goode, E., 347
Goodwin, M. R., 338
Goodwin, M. S., 163, 165
Goodwin, R., 194
Gordon, M., 421
Gorn, G. J., 261
Gottesman, I. I., 80
Gottlieb, D., 408
Gottlieb, J., 292
Gottmans, J. M., 251
Gould, R. L., 372–373
Gould, S. J., 70, 77, 84–85, 267
Graham, F. K., 113
Grandon, G. M., 220–221
Greenacre, P., 210
Greenberg, R., 155
Greenberg, R. P., 33
Greene, D., 48
Greene, J., 275
Greenfield, T. K., 347
Greenwood, R. M., 348
Greif, E. B., 316

Gribbin, K., 393
Griffin, E. J., 131
Gronlund, N. E., 330
Grossman, J. J., 287
Grotevant, M. D., 221
Gruman, G. J., 438
Guay, R., 336
Guilford, J. P., 272–273
Gurland, B., 455
Gurney, R., 186
Gussow, J. D., 114
Gutmann, D., 396

Haan, N., 317
Hagen, E., 271
Haith, M. M., 134
Hall, D. T., 410, 413
Hall, G. Stanley, 11, 12
Hall, I. N., 300
Hallahan, D. P., 278, 285, 289, 291
Haller, D. L., 351
Halonen, J. S., 164
Halversen, H. M., 127
Hamman, J., 66
Hanks, C., 161
Hanson, J. W., 101
Harding, B., 307
Harger, R. N., 350
Harlow, H. F., 156, 247, 249
Harlow, M. K., 247
Harper, L. V., 145
Harrell, R. F., 103
Harrington, D. M., 272
Harroff, P. B., 422
Hartshorn, J., 307
Hartshorne, H., 314
Hartup, W. W., 152, 249, 251, 328
Haskell, W. L., 388
Hatfield, J. S., 216
Haven, C., 459
Harighurst, R. J., 408, 457
Harighurst, W. M., 345
Hawkins, R. P., 260
Hayes, C., 185
Hayes, K. J., 185
Hayflick, L., 442, 444
Haywood, H. C., 288
Hebb, D. O., 71, 151, 183, 267
Heimer, C. B., 114
Heinonen, O. P., 99
Heins, E. D., 285
Henderson, N. D., 80–82
Hendry, L. S., 313
Henry VIII, 62
Henry, W. H., 454
Hepner, R., 102
Herman, C. S., 101
Herman, J., 227
Herold, E. S., 338
Herr, E. L., 409
Herrnstein, R. J., 82
Herzog, E., 345

Heston, L. L., 80
Hetherington, E. M., 223–224, 335
Higgins-Trenk, A., 415
Himmelweit, H. T., 258
Hindley, C. B., 18
Hine, R. N., 335
Hippocrates, 105
Hirschman, L., 227
Hoffman, H. R., 257–258, 260
Hoffman, Lois Wladis, 316–317n, 336, 414
Hoffman, Martin L., 316, 317n, 318, 320, 335
Hogan, K. A., 213
Holbrook, S. H., 70
Holland, J. L., 335, 409
Hollander, M. J., 347
Holmes, O. W., 105
Holmlund, W. S., 330
Holstein, C. B., 316
Holzinger, K. J., 80
Honzik, M. P., 387
Horn, J. L., 393–394
Horner, M., 335
Horowitz, F. D., 252
Horton, M. S., 179
Howard, Margaret, 82
Hsu, L. K. G., 307
Huesmann, L. R., 260
Hunt, J., 272
Hunt, J. M., 79, 162
Hunt, M., 421
Hunter, M. A., 131
Hurlock, E. B., 210
Huston-Stein, A., 415
Hutt, S. J., 146

Ilg, F. L., 174–175
Inhelder, B., 307
Isbell, B. J., 148
Itard, lawyer, 60

Jacklin, C. N., 195, 335
Jackson, P. W., 216
Jacobs, R. H., 374
Jacobson, L., 253, 254
Jacobson, S. W., 139
Jaffe, B. F., 279
James, William, 133
Jarvella, R., 158
Jarvik, L. F., 67, 79, 81
Jenkins, C. D., 397
Jersild, A. T., 301, 329
Jensen, A. R., 81, 82, 132
Johnson, D., 212
Johnson, H. H., 397
Johnson, H. R., 67
Johnson, Nicholas, 257
Johnson, Robert D., 238–240
Johnson, S. W., 290
Johnson, Virginia, 448
Johnson, W., 195

SUBJECT INDEX AND GLOSSARY

This glossary defines the most important terms and expressions used in this text. In each case the meaning given corresponds to the usage in the text. For more complete definitions, consult a standard psychological dictionary. Page numbers in italic refer to illustrations.

Antisocial influences, 258–261
Anxiety, coping with, *164*
Ape language controversy, 187
Apnea, 124–125
Appearance:
  in adolescence, *303*
  in adulthood, *385–386*
  in old age, 445, *446*, 447
Approval:
  need for, 52
  peers and, 251
Area, conservation of, *242*
Arteriosclerosis, 447
Arthritis, 447
Artificial insemination A breeding
  procedure often employed in
  animal husbandry and sometimes
  with humans. This procedure
  obviates the necessity for a physical
  union between a pair of opposite-
  sexed individuals. 59
Assimilation The act of incorporating
  objects or aspects of objects to
  previously learned activities. To
  assimilate is, in a sense, to ingest or
  to employ for something that is
  previously learned; more simply, it
  is the exercising of previously
  learned responses. 39, 42–43
  in learning, 133
Association The common expression
  for **associationism**, a term
  employed almost synonymously
  with stimulus-response learning.
  Associationism refers to the
  formation of associations or links
  between stimuli, between
  responses, or between stimuli and
  responses. 44–46
Asthma, 281
Attachment:
  in infant development, 155–161
  social-emotional development and,
  143–167
Attribution theory, 254–255
Authoritarianism, in child care, 219
Autism, 283, 284
Autoimmunity A malfunction in the
  body's disease-fighting capabilities
  whereby the body's own benign
  cells are identified as harmful and
  attacked. Autoimmunity is thought
  to be involved in some age-related
  diseases. 443
Autonomy, 35, *36*, 37, 360, 362
Autosome Any chromosome in mature
  sperm and ova other than the sex
  chromosome. Each of these cells
  therefore contains twenty-two
  autosomes. 61–62

B, type of behavior, 397
Babbling The relatively meaningless
sounds that young infants repeat.
187–188
Babinski reflex A reflex present in the
  newborn child, but disappearing
  later in life. It involves fanning the
  toes as a result of being tickled in
  the center of the soles of the feet.
  Normal adults curl their toes
  inward rather than fanning them
  outward. 95, 113
Bar (Bat) Mitzvah, 300n, *301*
Barbiturates, in pregnancy, 99–100
Bargaining, about dying, 461
Basic need An unlearned physiological
  requirement of the human
  organism. Specifically, the need for
  food, drink, and sex. 52
Beauty, need for, 52
Behavior-disordered children, 283
Behavioral disorders, prevalence and
  causes, 283
Behavior modification A general
  term for the application of
  behavioristic principles (primarily
  principles of operant conditioning)
  in systematic and deliberate
  attempts to change behavior. 51
Behavior therapies, 284
Behavioristic theory A general term
  for those theories of learning
  concerned primarily with the
  observable components of
  behavior (stimuli and responses).
  Such theories are labeled S-R
  learning theories and are
  exemplified in classical and
  operant conditioning. 51, 53
Belongingness, need for, 52
Bidirectionality:
  of influence, 145
  in language learning, 192–194
  of parent-child influence, 152, 218
Bigamy, 419
Biographical histories, in passages
  concept, 369
Biographical interviews (Levinson's),
  364–365
Biological aging, theories of, 441–443
Birth control, 338
Birth order The position a child
  occupies in a family (for example,
  first-, second-, or thirdborn).
  220–221
Birthing rooms, 110
Blacks, intelligence, 81–83
Blank slate concept, 10–*11*
Blind infants, 152, 189
Blindness, 281
  legal and functional, 279
Body proportions, changes, *132*
Body transcendence vs. body
  preoccupation, crisis, 363
Bowing, 189

Boys:
  adolescent abilities, 335
  friendship patterns, 250–251
  maturation, 304–305
  in middle childhood, 237–239
Brain damage, in childbirth, 111–112
Brainstorming, 274
Breech birth An abnormal
  presentation of the fetus at birth:
  buttocks first rather than head first.
  108

Caesarian delivery, 108
Canalization Waddington's term to
  describe the extent to which
  genetically determined
  characteristics are resistant to
  environmental influences. A highly
  canalized trait (such as hair color)
  remains unchanged in the face of
  most environmental influences; less
  highly canalized characteristics
  (such as manifested intelligence)
  are highly influenced by the
  environment. 67–68
Cancer, 281
  in old age, 447
Cannabis sativa, 347
Catalense people, imitation in, 206–207
Capabilities, in job satisfaction, 414
Careers, 407–416
  choices, 409–410, *411*, 412
  defined, 413
  serial, 409
  sexual stereotypes, 411–412
Categorization stage, in language
  development, 190, 191
Catharsis, television effect, 261
Causality, false assumption of, 15
Cells:
  lifespan and, 442
  meiosis, 62
  mitosis divisions, 61
Cephalocaudal Referring to the
  direction of development,
  beginning with the head and
  proceeding outward toward the
  tail. Early infant development is
  cephalocaudal because children
  acquire control over their heads
  prior to acquiring control over
  their limbs. 96, 125
Cerebral palsy, 279–282
  degrees of, 279
Cervix The small circular opening to
  the womb (uterus) that dilates
  considerably during birth. 107
Change of life, 387–389
Cheating, 314
Child/Children:
  childbirth and, 111–114
  heredity-environment studies, 72–81
  institutionalized, 75–76

Height (continued)
  age and, 173
  in middle childhood, 237
Helplessness, 255–256
Heredity The transmission of physical and personality characteristics and predispositions from parent to offspring. 8, 59–68
  environment and, 57–87
  influence of, 68–83
  mechanics of, 59–65
Heredity-environment studies, 69–70, 72–83
Heritability, 83
Heritability coefficient An index of the extent to which variation in characteristics is related to genetic factors. A heritability coefficient of 70 for intelligence does not indicate that 70 percent of intelligence is due to heredity; it indicates that 70 percent of the variation in intelligence test scores appears to be accounted for by genetic factors. In other words, a heritability coefficient is an index of variation rather than of absolute amount. 82
Heterosexual, defined, 417
Heterozygous Refers to the presence of different genes with respect to a single trait. One of these genes is dominant and the other is recessive. 64
Hollow Children, 73–74
Holophrases, 188
Home care, day care vs., 214–215
Homosexuality:
  adolescent attitudes, 339
  life style, 417–418
Homozygous Refers to an individual's genetic makeup. Individuals are homozygous with respect to a particular trait if they possess identical genes for that trait. 64
Honesty, in research, 20
Hospitalism A medical name for the syndrome (configuration of symptoms) associated with the failure of infants to survive in children's homes or hospitals. Symptoms of hospitalism include listlessness, inability to gain weight, unresponsiveness, and eventual death. 10
Human development, theories of, 26–56
Humanism A philosophical and psychological orientation primarily concerned with humanity--the worth of humans as individuals and those processes that augment their human qualities. 53, 472–473

Humanistic approaches, to development, 51–53
Humanitarianism Concern with the welfare of humans. 10
Huntington's disease A neurological disorder characterized by uncontrollable physical movements, emotional changes, and mental deterioration. Onset is usually between the ages of twenty to forty. Death is usually due to complications arising from debilitation. 65
Hunzukuts, longevity, 444
Husband beating, 428
Hyperactivity, 285
Hyperkinesis, 283
Hypertension, 447
Hypocrisy, 310, 312

I-Thou relationship, 474
Id One of the three levels of the human personality, according to Freudian theory. The id is defined as all the instinctual urges to which humans are heir; it is the level of personality that contains human motives. A newborn child's personality, according to Freud, is all id. 31, *33*, 34
Idealism, in adolescence, 309
Identical twins Twins whose genetic origin is a single egg. Such twins are genetically identical. 77
Identification, Freudian, 31, *32*
Identity A logical rule specifying that certain activities leave objects or situations unchanged. 34, 240–241
  in adolescence, 339–342
  genetic predetermination in, 470
  identity diffusion vs., 37–38
  personal, 471, 473
Identity diffusion, 342, 360, *362*
  identity vs., 37–38
Identity status, 342
Idiot, 279
Illogical thinking, 176
Imaginary audience One manifestation of adolescent egocentrism. A reflection of the adolescent belief that a wide range of individuals are always aware of the adolescent's behavior and very concerned about it. 310–312
Imaginary playmate, 210–211, 212
Imagination, implications of, 210–211
Imaginative play Activities that include make-believe games; these are particularly prevalent during the preschool years. 209–210
Imbecile, 279

Imitation The complex process of learning through observation of a model. *49*, 206, *207*, 208
  in early childhood, 206, *207*, 208
  in infant development, 139–140
Immature birth A miscarriage occurring sometime between the twentieth and the twenty-eighth weeks of pregnancy and resulting in the birth of a fetus weighing between one and two pounds. 105, 106
Immigration policies, ageism in, 438
Impotence, in old age, 449
Imprinting, attachment and, 159
Income, in job satisfaction, 414
Incongruence, 151
Independent stage, in adolescence, 326–328
Indoctrination, for morality, 318
Inductive reasoning, 178
Industry, inferiority vs., 36–37, 362
Independent variable The variable in an experiment that can be manipulated to observe its effect on other variables. 13
Infancy A period of development that begins a few weeks after birth and lasts until approximately two years of age. 9, 89–167
Infant emotions, 146–152
Infant mortality, 9–10
Infant states, 145–146
Inferiority, industry vs., 36–37
Influence:
  bidirectionality of, 145, 152
  family model, 162
Inhalants, 349
Inhibitory-disinhibitory effect Imitative behavior that results in either the suppression (inhibition) or appearance (disinhibition) of previously acquired deviant behavior. 50–51
Initiative, guilt vs. 35–36, 37, 360, *362*
Institutionalized children, 75–76
  social-emotional development, 163
Institutions, for the elderly, 455
Instrumental learning, 46
Intact nuclear family, 424
Integrity, despair vs., 37, 36l, *362*
Intellectual development:
  in middle childhood, 239–245
  in pregnancy, 103
Intellectual exceptionality, 286
Intellectual giftedness, 290
Intellectualization, 35
Intelligence, 267–272
  age and, 391–*393*, *394*
  animal experiments on, 70–72
  of blacks, 81–83
  culture and, 269

Intelligence (continued)
  in old age, 450–451
  Piaget-based measures of, 272
  prematurity and, 115
  studies of, 69–85
Intelligence scores, 77, 79, 80
  changes in, 77
  correlation, 79
Intelligence tests, 267, 268, 269
Interaction, heredity-environment,
  83–85
Internal orientation, 255–256
Interview, example, 19
Intimacy and solidarity vs. isolation,
  stage of, 37, 38, 360, *362*
Introverts, 395
Intuitive thinking, 177–180
Invulnerables, 286
In utero A Latin expression meaning
  inside the uterus. 61, 95
  world in, 98–99
IQ, 267–268
IQ constancy, 271
  scores, *270*
Isolation, intimacy vs., 37, 38

Jensen hypothesis The argument
  advanced by Jensen, based on
  some evidence regarding heredity
  and environment, that the most
  influential environmental factors
  regarding intelligence are prenatal
  and that racial and social-class
  differences in intelligence test
  scores cannot be accounted for by
  differences in environment alone.
  Hence genetic factors are assumed
  to be responsible for some of the
  observed differences among
  different racial groups. 81–82
Job/Jobs:
  defined, 413
  sexual stereotypes, 411–412
Job satisfaction, 413–414
Jukes family, 70
Justice, need for, 52

Kallikak family, 70
Kidney problems, in old age, 447
Kissing, 189
Klinefelters syndrome, 67
Knowing, in learning theory, 51
Knowledge, need for, 52
Kwakiutl, 50

Labels, 292
Labor The process during which the
  fetus, the placenta, and other
  membranes are separated from the
  woman's body and expelled. The
  termination of labor is usually
  birth. 105–108

Labor (work) force, males and females
  in, *415*
LAD, 192, 194
Ladder concept, 365–*366*, 367–368
Lamaze childbirth, 110
Language:
  arbitrary sounds in, 183, *184*
  communication and, 183, 186–187
  elements of, 184–185
  nunhumans and, 185
  thinking and, 195–*198*, 199
Language Acquisition Device (LAD)
  A label employed by Chomsky to
  describe the neurological
  something that corresponds to
  grammar and that children are
  assumed to have in their brains as
  they are learning language. 192
  neurological mechanism, 192–194
Language codes, 198
Language development:
  in children, 185–191
  in early childhood, 170–202
  explanations of, 191–194
  learning theory of, 191–192
  milestones in, 196–197
  mother-infant interaction, 192–194
  sequential stages (Wood), 189, 190
  sex differences in, 195
  stuttering in, 195
  in twins, 195
Lanugo Downy, soft hair that covers
  the fetus. Lanugo grows over most
  of the child's body some time after
  the fifth month of pregnancy and is
  usually shed during the seventh
  month. However, some lanugo is
  often present at birth, especially on
  the infant's back. 95, 97
Late adult transition, *366*, 367–368
Late adulthood age, 367–368
Late childhood, 235
Latent stage (latency) The fourth of
  Freud's stages of psychosexual
  development, characterized by the
  development of the superego
  (conscience) and by loss of interest
  in sexual gratification. This stage is
  assumed to last from the age of six
  to eleven years. 32, 34, 247
Laughing, 149, 189
Leadership, age ranges for, 384
Learning:
  age and, 390–391
  development as, 14
  early, reflexes and, 135–139
  in old age, 450
Learning disabilities, 289–290
Learning theory:
  approaches to development, 43–51,
  53
  on attachment, 159

criticism of, 42–43
  of language development, 191–192
Leboyer childbirth, 110
Length, conservation of, *242*
Libido A general Freudian term
  denoting sexual urges. The libido
  is assumed to be the source of
  energy for sexual urges. Freud
  considers these urges the most
  important force in human
  motivation. 30
Life cycle:
  family, 425, 426–432
  theory of, 38
Life expectancy The expected
  duration of a human life. An
  average of the ages at which
  individuals die. 441–442
Life styles, 416–419
Lifespan The total length of an
  individual life, not an expectancy,
  but the maximum attainable in the
  absence of accident and disease.
  life expectancy and, 441–443
  study of, 10–19
  summary of, 373
Lifespan developmental psychology, 5–6
Liquids, conservation of, *242*
"Liver spots," 446
"Living together," life style, 416–417
Living will, 463
Lodge-Thorndike Tests, 270
Logic, in middle childhood, 240
Logic of propositions, 309
Longevity, 443–*444*, 445
**Longitudinal cross-sectional
  approach** See *short-term
  longitudinal approach.*
Longitudinal study A research
  technique in the study of child
  development that observes the
  same subjects over a long period of
  time. 16–18
Love:
  in child care, 219–220
  in the human condition, 474
**LSD-25 (d-lysergic acid
  diethylamide tartrate)** A
  particularly powerful hallucinogenic drug, this inexpensive, easily
  made, synthetic chemical can
  sometimes have profound
  influences on human perception.
  In everyday parlance it is often
  referred to as "acid." 348–349
  adolescent use, 347
  in pregnancy, 101

Mainstreaming, 282, 291–292
Malnutrition, in pregnancy, 102–104,
  114
Management skills, 381–382

Peer group (continued)
in adolescence, 328–331
delinquency and, 345
development, *329*
in middle childhood, 246–253
Peers, *246*
influence, *246*, 247–249
monkey, 247
Perception-dominated thinking, 176
Perceptual development, of the infant, 127–132
Performance, in old age, 451, 452
Permutation changes, 191
Person, whole vs. categorized, 165–166
Personal fable The belief that we are unique, special, and right. This belief is sometimes exaggerated in adolescence, as a function of adolescent egocentrism. 310
Personal interests, in job satisfaction, 414
Personalism, 473
Personality The set of characteristics that we typically manifest in our interactions with others. It includes all the abilities, predispositions, habits, and other qualities that make each of us different. 152, 339
in adolescence, 339–342
age and, 394–396
Personality changes, 395–396
Personality differences, 152
Personality disorders, 285–286
Personality levels, *14*
Phallic stage The third stage in Freud's theory of psychosexual development. It begins at the age of eighteen months and lasts to the age of approximately six years. During this stage children become concerned with their genitals and may show evidence of the much discussed complexes labeled *Oedipus* and *Electra*. 32, 34
Phenotypes, 67–*68*
Phoneme The simplest unit of language, consisting of a single sound such as a vowel. 184
Phrase structure rules A modern grammatical phrase referring to the implicit (or explicit) rules that govern the formation of correct phrases. For example, a phrase structure rule might specify that correct noun phrases may consist of an article and a noun; an article, an adjective, and a noun; an adjective and a pronoun; and so on. 191
Phylogenetic development The evolutionary development of the species from its origins to its

present state. Phylogeny is contrasted to ontogeny, in the sense that it refers to the development of a species rather than to the development of an individual. 58
Physical changes, pubescent, 302
Physical development, in adulthood, 384–389
in adolescence, 300–304
in middle childhood, 235–239
Physical exceptionality, 279–282
Physical handicaps, 279, *280*
Physical resemblance, *64*
Physiological needs, 52
Placenta A flat, thick membrane attached to the inside of the uterus during pregnancy and to the developing fetus. The placenta connects the mother and the fetus by the umbilical cord. 94
Play May be defined as activities that have no goal other than the enjoyment derived from them.
in early childhood, 208–213
sex differences in, 212–213
Poliomyelitis, 101
Polyandry, 419–420
Polygamy A form of marriage that permits a husband to have more than one wife (polygyny) or a wife to have more than one husband (polyandry). 419–420
Polygyny, 419–420
Positive reinforcement A stimulus that increases the probability of a response recurring as a result of being added to a situation after the response has occurred. It usually takes the form of a pleasant stimulus (*reward*) that results from a specific response. 46
Postmature birth, 106
Poverty, feminization of, 222
Preadolescence, 235
Preadulthood age, 365
Preconcept The label given to the preconceptual child's incomplete understanding of concept, resulting from an inability to classify. 177, 178
Preconceptual thinking, 177–178
Pregnancy, 92–*96*, 97–105, 471
detecting, 94
premarital, 338–339
Pregnant An adjective describing a woman who has had an ovum (egg cell) fertilized and who, nature willing, will eventually give birth to a human child. 93
Prehension The ability to grasp. 127
Premarital intercourse, 337, *420*
Premature birth, 106

Prematurity, 114–*115*, 116
causes, 114
effects, 114
Premoral level, 315
Prenatal development The period of development beginning at conception and ending at birth. That period lasts approximately nine calendar months in the human female (266 days). Chickens develop considerably faster. 93–96, *97–98*
factors affecting, 96–105
Preoperational stage, 182–183
Preoperational thought The second of Piaget's four major stages, lasting from about two to seven or eight years. It consists of two substages: intuitive thinking and preconceptual thinking. 39–40, 176–178, *180*
Preoperations, 240
Preschool education, 182
Prespeech stage, in language development, 186–188
Primary aging, 445
Primary circular reaction An expression employed by Piaget to describe a simple reflex activity such as thumb sucking. 136
Primary reinforcer A stimulus that is reinforcing in the absence of any learning. Such stimuli as food and drink are primary reinforcers because presumably an organism does not have to learn that they are pleasurable. 46
Prime of life, 384–394
Principles, morality of, 315
Problem solving:
age and, 390–391
creative, 275–276
Procreation, in Freudian theory, 30–33
Productiveness, in language, 183–184
Projection, 35
Prolapsed cord A condition that sometimes occurs during birth, when the infant's umbilical cord becomes lodged between his body and the birth canal, thereby cutting off his supply of oxygen. The effect may be brain damage of varying severity, depending on the length of time until delivery following prolapsing of the cord. 112–113
Proposition, logic of, 309
Prosocial behavior:
in adolescence, 318–319, 321
development of, 256
Prosocial effects, of television, 261
Prosody Modes of expression, intonations, accents, and pauses

Rosenthal effect (continued)
individual's behavior. Rosenthal ostensibly demonstrated that teacher expectations could affect the general academic performance of students and also their intelligence test scores. 254

Rubella, 101

Rules, of games, 313–315

Saccadic motion Extremely rapid, involuntary movements of the eyeballs without which vision would rapidly become faint and blurred (also called *optokinetic nystagmus*). 130

Safety needs, 52

Sampling, 19

Satisfaction, *398, 399*
in adulthood, 396
age and, 400
in marriage, 422–424, 431
in old age, 457–*458*, 459

Scale, of intelligence, 267

Scheme (also *schema* or *schemata*)
The label employed by Piaget to describe a unit in cognitive structure. A scheme is, in one sense, an activity together with its structural connotations. In another sense, scheme may be thought of as an idea or a concept. It usually labels a specific activity: the looking scheme, the grasping scheme, the sucking scheme. 39, 133

Schizophrenia, 284

School, in middle childhood, 253–256

Science, theory and, 29

Scooting A form of locomotion employed by young children. It is similar to creeping or crawling, except that children propel themselves in a sitting position by using their hands and arms. 76, 126

Seasons theory (Levinson's), 364–368, 373–374

Secondary aging, 445, 450

Secondary circular reaction Infant responses that are circular in the sense that the response serves as a stimulus for its own repetition and secondary because the responses do not center on the child's body, as do primary circular reactions. 136

Security blankets, *164*

Sedatives, 349

Self The concept that an individual has of himself or herself. Notions of the self are often closely allied with individuals' beliefs about how others perceive them.

in adolescence, 339–342
development of, 37–38
mystery of the, 471, 473

Self-absorption, generativity and, 37, 38

Self-actualization The process or act of becoming oneself, developing one's potential, achieving an awareness of one's identity, fulfilling oneself. The term *actualization* is central to humanistic psychology. *472–473*
need for, 52–53

Self-centered objectives, 380–381

Self-concept, 339
in adolescence, 303
age and, 396
peers and, 251–252

Self-consciousness, adolescent, 310

Self-esteem The individual's desire to be held in high esteem by others and to maintain a high opinion of one's own behavior and person.
in adolescence, 340–342

Self-expectations, in middle childhood, 254–256

Self-management skills, 381–382

Senescence The state of being old or the process of aging. 445

Senile dementia, 447

Senior citizens, 441

Sense perceptions, in adulthood, 386–387

Sensorimotor development:
of the infant, 134–140
substages, 136

Sensorimotor intelligence, 176, 178

Sensorimotor period The first stage of development in Piaget's classification. It lasts from birth to approximately age two and is so called because children understand their world primarily through their activities toward it and sensations of it. *39–41*

Sensorimotor play Activity involving the manipulation of objects or execution of activities simply for the sensations that are produced. (See *play*.) 208–*209*

Sensory changes, in old age, 448

Sentencelike word, 189, 190

Seriation The ordering of objects according to one or more empirical properties. To seriate is essentially to place in order. 244, *245*

Settling down, 366–367

Sex:
in adolescence, 336–339
double standard, 420
Freudian view of, 336–337

Sex chromosome A chromosome contained in sperm cells and ova

responsible for determining the sex of the offspring. Sex chromosomes produced by the female are of one variety (X); those produced by the male may be either X or Y. At fertilization (the union of sperm and ovum), an XX pairing will result in a girl; an XY pairing will result in a boy. The sperm cell is essentially responsible for determining the sex of the offspring. 61–63

Sex differences:
in adolescence, 334–336
cross-cultural, 335
in divorce response, 224
in happiness, 400
in language development, 195
in play, 212–*213*

Sex roles Attitudes, personality characteristics, behavior, and other qualities associated with being male or female in a specific culture. Sex roles are, in effect, the groupings of qualities that define masculine and feminine. Since they are largely culturally defined, sex roles may be quite different in different cultures.
in adolescence, 331–336
changing, 332, *333*
determinants of, 334
learning in play, 214

Sex typing Learning behavior appropriate to the sex of the individual. The term refers specifically to the acquisition of masculine behavior for a boy and feminine behavior for a girl.
in play, 213
sex roles and, 331–333

Sexual abuse, 227

Sexual behavior, 337–339

Sexual frustration, adolescent, 343

Sexual functioning, age and, 388–389

Sexuality:
in Freudian theory, 30
in old age, 448

Shame, autonomy vs., 35, 37

Shaping The term employed to describe a technique whereby animals and people are taught to perform complex behaviors not previously in their repertoire. The technique reinforces responses that become increasingly closer approximations to the desired behavior. Also called the method of successive approximations or the method of differential reinforcement of successive approximations. 47

Vegetative reflex A reflex pertaining to the intake of food (for example, swallowing and sucking). 123

Version Turning the fetus manually to assist delivery. 108

Vicarious reinforcement The type of reinforcement that results from observing someone else being reinforced. In imitative behavior, the observers frequently act as though they were being reinforced, when in fact they are not being reinforced, but are aware or simply assume that the model is. 50

Vilcabambans, longevity, 444

Villi, 94

Violence:
   in the family, 428, *429, 430*
   television and, 259

Virginity, 420

Vision, development, 127–130

Visual acuity, in the newborn, 130

Visual cliff studies, 129, *131*

Visual contact, 152

Visual impairment, 279, 281
   in old age, 447, 448

Vital marriage, 422

Vocabulary:
   growth in children, 188
   of primates, 186–187
   size, 185–186

Vocation, defined, 413

Vocational Preference Inventory (Holland), 409

Wariness, 150–151

Wechsler Adult Intelligence Scale (WAIS), 271

Wechsler Intelligence Scale for Children Revised (WISGR), 271

Wechsler Preschool and Primary Scale of Intelligence (WPPSI), 271

Wechsler tests, 270–271

Weight:
   in adolescence, 302
   height and, 173
   in middle childhood, 237

Whales, 185

Whole person, 165–166

Wife beating, 428, *429, 430*

Wife swapping, 421

Wild children (frequently referred to as *feral children*) Children allegedly abandoned by their parents and adopted and reared by such wild animals as wolves, bears, or tigers. 60

Wisdom, in old age, 452, *453–454*

Women:
   career disadvantages, 412
   life expectancy, 441, 442
   marriage-career problem, 415–416
   as workers, 408, 414–415

Word, progression from babble, 188

Work Activities engaged in for gain rather than primarily for the pleasure derived from them. 407–416
   in adulthood, 380, *381*
   play vs., 208
   reasons for, 407, 408
   satisfaction in, 413–414
   women in, 414–415

Work opportunities, changes in, 408–416

Work selection, 410–*411*, 412

Work skills, 381–382

World in utero, 61, 98–99

Wrinkles, in old age, 446

XYY syndrome, 67

Youth:
   adult development in, 380–384
   defined, 380, 382

Ypsilanti project, 14–15

Zuni, 50

Zygote A fertilized egg cell, formed from the union of a sperm cell and an egg cell. A zygote contains a full complement of 46 chromosomes. 100, 101